Helicobacter pylori
Basic Mechanisms to Clinical Cure 1996

Helicobacter pylori

Basic Mechanisms to Clinical Cure 1996

Edited by

Richard H. Hunt
Professor of Medicine
Director, Division of Gastroenterology
McMaster University Medical Centre
1200 Main Street West
Hamilton, Ontario L8N 3Z5
Canada

Guido N. J. Tytgat
Professor, Department of
Gastroenterology and Hepatology
Academic Medical Centre
9 Meibergdreef
1105 AZ Amsterdam
The Netherlands

The proceedings of a symposium organised by AXCAN PHARMA,
held in Ottawa, June 10 –12, 1996

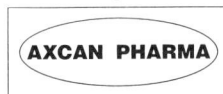

AXCAN PHARMA

KLUWER ACADEMIC PUBLISHERS
DORDRECHT / BOSTON / LONDON

Distributors

---

for the United States and Canada: Kluwer Academic Publishers, PO Box 358, Accord Station,
Hingham, MA 02018-0358, USA
for all other countries: Kluwer Academic Publishers Group, Distribution Center, PO Box 322,
3300 AH Dordrecht, The Netherlands

A catalogue record for this book is available from the British Library

ISBN 0-7923-8717-1

Contents

CONTENTS

WINNING POSTERS

List of Principal Contributors

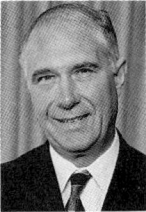

A. T. R. AXON
The Centre for Digestive Diseases
The General Infirmary at Leeds
Great George Street
Leeds LS1 3EX
UK

M. J. BLASER
Vanderbilt University School of Medicine
Division of Infectious Diseases
A-3310 Medical Centre
N 1161 21st Ave S
Nashville
TN 37232-2605
USA

T. J. BORODY
Centre for Digestive Diseases
144 Great North Road
Five Dock (Sydney)
NSW 2046
Australia

J. CALAM
Royal Postgraduate Medical School
Hammersmith Hospital
150 Du Cane Road
London W12 0NN
UK

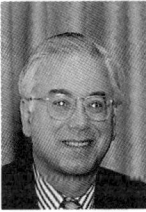

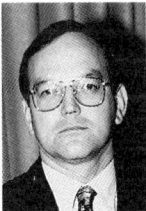

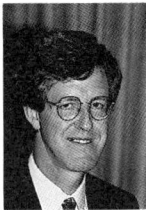

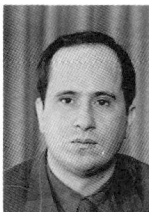

A. COVACCI
Immunobiological Research Institute
Department of Molecular Biology
Chiron-Biocine
Via Fiorentina 1
I-53100 Siena
Italy

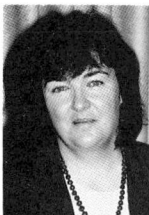

J. E. CRABTREE
Department of Clinical Medicine
St James's University Hospital
Clinical Sciences Building, Level 7
Leeds LS9 7TF
UK

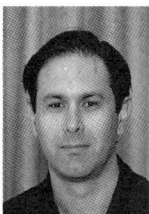

K. CROITORU
Department of Medicine
McMaster University
1200 Main Street W, Room 4W8
Hamilton
ON L8N 3Z5
Canada

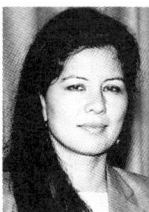

S. E. CROWE
Division of Gastroenterology
University of Texas Medical Branch
4.111 John Sealy Hospital
301 University Blvd.
Galveston
TX 77555-0564
USA

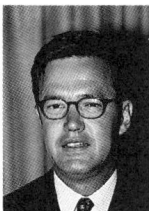

K. DEUSCH
Eberhard-Karls University
Department of General Surgery
Waldhörnlestr. 22
D-72072 Tübingen
Germany

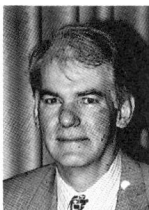

M. F. DIXON
Academic Unit of Pathology
University of Leeds
Centre for Digestive Diseases
The General Infirmary
Leeds LS2 9JT
UK

LIST OF PRINCIPAL CONTRIBUTORS

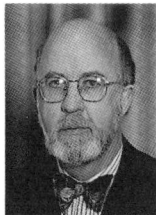

W. F. DOE
Division of Molecular Medicine
John Curtin School of Medical Research
Box 334
Canberra City
ACT 2601
Australia

B. DRUMM
Department of Pediatrics
University College of Dublin
Our Lady's Hospital for Sick Children
Crumlin (Dublin 12)
Eire

P. B. ERNST
Department of Pediatrics
University of Texas Medical Branch
Children's Hospital
Galveston
TX 77555-0366
USA

D. FORMAN
Centre for Cancer Research
University of Leeds
Arthington House
Cookridge Hospital
Leeds L310 0QD
UK

J. G. FOX
Division of Comparative Medicine
Massachusetts Institute of Technology
37 Vassar Street 45-106
Cambridge
MA 02139
USA

J. W. FRESTON
Department of Medicine
University of Connecticut
Health Center
Farmington
CT 06032
USA

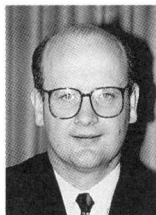

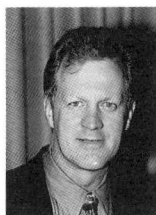

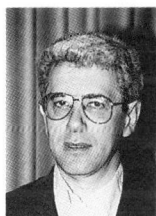

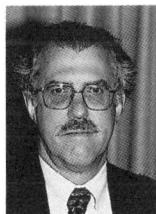

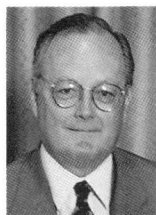

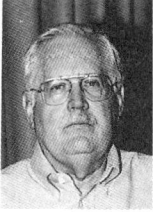

D. Y. GRAHAM
Baylor College of Medicine
VA Medical Center
2002 Holcombe Blvd.
Houston
TX 77030
USA

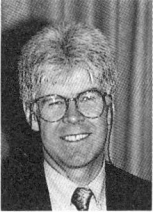

C. J. HAWKEY
Department of Medicine
Division of Gastroenterology
Queen's Medical Center
University Hospital
Nottingham NG7 2UH
UK

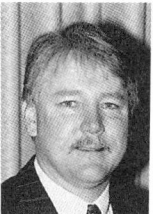

S. L. HAZELL
University of New South Wales
School of Microbiology and Immunology
PO Box 1
Kensington
Sydney
NSW 2033
Australia

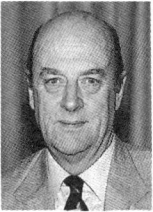

R. H. HUNT
Division of Gastroenterology
McMaster University Medical Centre
1200 Main Street W, Room 4W8
Hamilton
ON L8N 3Z5
Canada

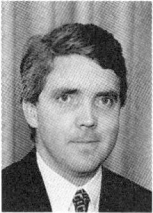

S. M. KELLY
York District Hospital
Wigginton Road
York YO3 7HE
UK

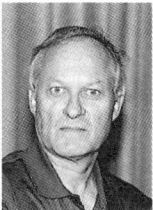

J.-P. KRAEHENBUHL
Biochemistry Institute
Swiss Institute for Experimental Cancer
Research
CH-1066 Epalinges
Switzerland

LIST OF PRINCIPAL CONTRIBUTORS

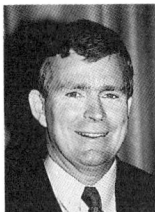

J. R. LAMBERT
Gastrointestinal Science Group
Mornington Peninsula Hospital
Frankston
Melbourne
VIC 3199
Australia

A. LEE
School of Microbiology and Immunology
University of New South Wales
PO Box 1
Kensington
Sydney
NSW 2033
Australia

L. M. LICHTENBERGER
The University of Texas Health Science Center
PO Box 20708
Houston
TX 77225
USA

P. MALFERTHEINER
Otto-von-Guericke-Universität
Medizinische Fakultät
Klinik Zentrum für Gastroenterologie, Hepatologie und Infektiologie
Liepziger Str. 44
D-39120 Maqdeburg
Germany

K. E. L. McCOLL
University of Glasgow
Department of Medicine and Therapeutics
Western Infirmary
Glasgow G11 6NT
UK

F. MÉGRAUD
CHU de Bordeaux
Laboratoire de Bactérologie – Enfants
Groupe Hospitalier Pellegrin
F-33076 Bordeaux Cedex
France

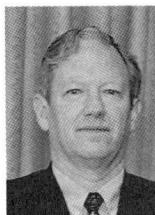

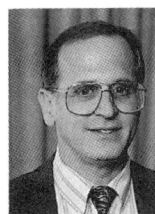

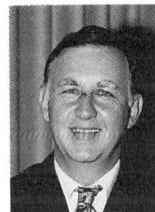

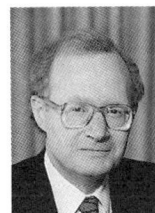

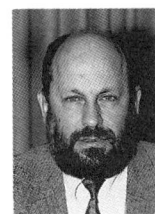

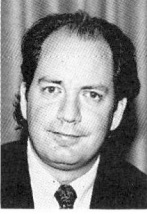

B. O'BRIEN
McMaster University
Centre for the Evaluation of Medicine
Father Sean O'Sullivan Research Centre
St Joseph's Hospital
50 Charlton Ave. E
Hamilton
ON L8N 4A6
Canada

C. A. O'MORAIN
Meath Hospital
Endoscopy Office
Heytesbury Street
Dublin 8
Eire

J. PARSONNET
Division of Infectious Diseases
Department of Medicine
Stanford University School of Medicine
Stanford
CA 94305-5092
USA

R. H. RIDDELL
McMaster University Medical Centre
1200 Main Street West
Hamilton
ON L8N 3Z5
Canada

G. SACHS
CURE VA Medical Center-Wadsworth
Bldg. 113, Room 324
Los Angeles
CA 90073
USA

K. P. SCHÄFER
Byk Gulden Pharmaceuticals
PO Box 10 013 10
D-78403 Konstanz
Germany

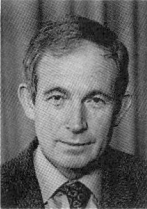

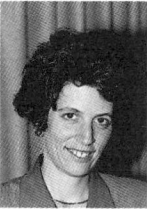

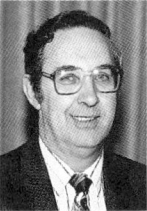

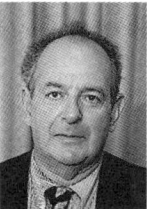

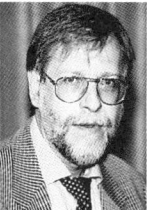

LIST OF PRINCIPAL CONTRIBUTORS

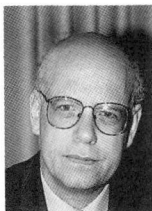

A. SONNENBERG
Gastroenterology Section
VA Medical Center 111-F
2100 Ridgecrest Drive SE
Alberquerque
NM 87108
USA

M. STOLTE
Institute of Pathology
Klinikum Bayreuth
Preuschwitzer Strasse 101
D-95455 Bayreuth
Germany

G. N. J. TYTGAT
Division of Gastroenterology and Hepatology
Academic Medical Center
9 Meibergdreef
1105 AZ Amsterdam
The Netherlands

J. L. WALLACE
The University of Calgary
Health Sciences Centre
3330 Hospital Drive NW
Calgary
AB T2N 1N1
Canada

N. A. WRIGHT
Department of Histopathology
Royal Postgraduate Medical School
Hammersmith Hospital
Du Cane Road
London W12 0NN
UK

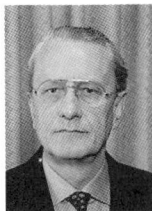

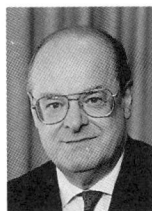

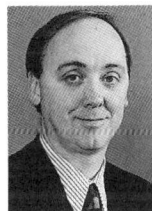

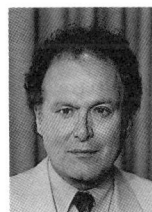

Preface

The impact of *Helicobacter pylori* on basic science and the clinical management of patients with the complications of this infection is bewildering. The explosion of new information both in the laboratory and at the bedside has progressed at an unprecedented rate.

Our main objective in furthering this progress has been to integrate this new information and organize a series of top-quality presentations and discussions between investigators and clinicians on all aspects of *H. pylori* research and to review the current position and future research directions. To that end, the second meeting '*Helicobacter pylori:* Basic Mechanisms to Clinical Cure' was organized in June 1996 in Ottawa, Canada, following the successful format of the first such meeting held in Amelia Island, Florida, in 1993. The meeting again focused on all timely aspects of *H. pylori* research. Internationally renowned basic and clinical scientists, all experts in their respective fields, explored in depth the spectrum of *H. pylori* infection and the related complications of gastritis, peptic ulcer, gastric cancer and lymphoma.

The presentations covered: the genetic heterogeneity of the organism, including the expression of virulence factors determined by the genetic pathogenicity island; the intricate cascade of chemokines and cytokines leading to mucosal inflammation; the complexities of the mucosal immune response, favoring a slight Th1 over Th2 lymphocyte imbalance; the fundamental issue of the apparent paradox of the induction of both apoptosis and epithelial hyperproliferation; the pathophysiological consequences of gastric mucosal inflammation with respect to the elevation of gastrin and the acid secretory response; the mechanisms leading to peptic ulcer disease, gastric carcinoma and gastric mucosa-associated lymphoid tissue (MALT) lymphoma; the established and novel therapeutic approaches to eradication and finally the prospects for successful therapeutic and preventative vaccination.

The comprehensive manuscripts in this book of the proceedings of the meeting reflect the most up-to-date information and state-of-the-art approaches to research and management of *H. pylori* infection and will provide an invaluable reference source. We thank all our colleagues for their excellent presentations and the timely delivery of their manuscripts which, with the help of Phil Johnstone and his colleagues at Kluwer Academic Publishers, has made rapid publication possible. We are confident that this book, like its predecessor, will be considered as 'The 1996 Reference on *Helicobacter pylori* Research'.

The Ottawa meeting was again generously supported by Léon and Diane Gosselin of Axcan Pharma, Mont-Saint-Hilaire, Canada. We all owe both of them and their staff at Axcan a great deal of gratitude for their superb organization and support.

Richard H. Hunt
McMaster University Medical Centre
Hamilton, Ontario, Canada

Guido N. J. Tytgat
Academic Medical Centre
Amsterdam, The Netherlands

Scientific Organizers and Co-Chairmen, Ottawa, June 1996

1
Mixed gastric infections and infection with other *Helicobacter* species

S. L. HAZELL

'The essence of science: ask an impertinent question and you are on the way to a pertinent answer' (Jacob Bronowski in *The Ascent of Man*)

INTRODUCTION

Helicobacter pylori is a spiral to helical, Gram-negative, microaerophilic bacterium that has been shown to be responsible for chronic active gastritis[1]. *H. pylori* infection is a necessary but not sufficient factor in gastric ulcer disease, duodenal ulcer disease and gastric adenocarcinoma[1,2]. *H. pylori* also provides the antigens that drive the development of gastric B cell MALT lymphomas[3].

Until recently most studies relating to *Helicobacter* infection and upper gastrointestinal disease in humans have focused on *H. pylori* as a single and unique entity. This perception is now being overturned with the developments in our understanding of gastric microbiology. In this review four interrelated topics will be discussed. These topics are: strain diversity of *H. pylori*, infection in an individual by multiple strains of *H. pylori*, infection with non-*H. pylori Helicobacter* spp. and finally, concomitant infection by *H. pylori* and other *Helicobacter* spp.

IS *HELICOBACTER PYLORI* A SINGLE SPECIES?

This may appear to be an impertinent question; however, as will become apparent below, the answer may be pertinent to our understanding of upper gastrointestinal disease.

As a result of the development of our understanding of the role of *H. pylori* in upper gastrointestinal pathology, numerous studies relating to the pathogenesis of this organism have appeared in the literature (please see Chapter 3). An important question arising from these studies relates to the strain diversity of *H. pylori*.

Molecular studies have shown a remarkable genetic diversity in this species. In addition, there have been reports of phenotypic differences between strains of *H. pylori* which have given rise to biotyping schemes for the organism[4,5]. However, such biotyping schemes do not appear to have become established in the study of disease related to these upper gastrointestinal pathogens. One scheme that has gained some acceptance is the use of the designation 'Type 1' and 'Type 2' strains; this designation being related to the phenotypic and genotypic characteristics of strains in terms of the cytotoxin gene (*vacA*) and the cytotoxin-associated gene (*cagA*)[6]. The question may be asked, does the designation of strains as either 'Type 1' or 'Type 2' relate to some taxonomic trait of *H. pylori*?

A variety of DNA-based methods have been used to identify and type *H. pylori*. Techniques such as ribotyping, random amplified polymorphic DNA-PCR (RAPD-PCR), restriction enzyme analysis (REA) and pulsed-field gel electrophoresis all attest to the considerable genomic variability between isolates of *H. pylori* from different individuals[7-12]. Further, in studies of the genetic arrangement of strains of *H. pylori* (physical–genetic maps) it has been noted that the gene order and rRNA gene copy number differ between strains[13,14]. Such data suggest that there exists a high level of genetic diversification between strains of *H. pylori*. Whether such diversification is of any taxonomic significance is a moot point, but one that is worthy of further examination.

Before we address further the question 'is *H. pylori* a single species?', we must come to some understanding of what makes a species. Chromosomal nucleotide similarity of >70% is considered to be the limit of speciation for many groups of bacteria[15]. Phylogenetic relationships are also determined by use of 'molecular chronometers'. The most widely used 'molecular chronometer' for the characterization of bacteria is the sequence of 16S rRNA[16]. Strains with >70% DNA relatedness usually have >97% sequence identity in their 16S rRNA[17].

To date, sequencing of the 16S rRNA gene has been used to place all of the known *Helicobacter* spp. into the genus. However, extensive evaluation of isolates of *H. pylori* to examine their relative taxonomic relationship has not yet been undertaken. Perhaps, given the evidence of genetic diversity within the species, this should now be undertaken. While the non-microbiologist may consider that a bacterium isolated from a human stomach, with the biochemical and morphological features of what we call now *H. pylori*, could be nothing else but *H. pylori*, such presumptions, while ostensibly satisfactory, belie current taxonomic experience.

To add further to the discussion of *H. pylori* taxonomy, we need to introduce an additional taxonomic tool. Multilocus (allozyme) enzyme electrophoresis (MEE) is a powerful tool that permits both intra-species and inter-species comparisons to be made, and has the power to reveal relationships available otherwise only through extensive sequencing of a large number of strains. Comparison of strains of bacteria by MEE, using a sufficiently large number of independent enzyme loci, provides a mechanism for estimating the chromosomal nucleotide similarity of strains and thus provides genetic data that are both statistically and biologically relevant[18]. This is because the net charge of a protein, and hence the rate of migration in a gel under non-denaturing conditions, is determined by the amino acid sequence. Variation in the mobility of alloenzymes can be equated directly with the alleles of specific gene loci[19].

2

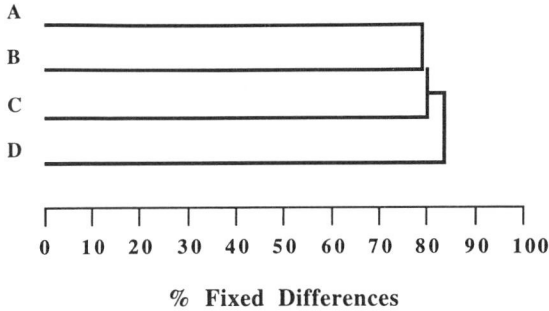

% **Fixed Differences**

Figure 1 Summary dendrogram based on 23 isolates showing the percentage fixed differences between clusters of four possible cryptic species within the *Helicobacter pylori* Complex. Dendrogram generated by the unweighted pair group method using arithmetic averages (UPGMA)[23]

To illustrate the power and utility of MEE we may use an example drawn from another infectious disease. Strains of *Haemophilus influenzae* biotype IV have been identified as important urogenital pathogens[20]. Genetic analysis of urogenital isolates of *Haemophilus influenzae* by MEE indicated that these bacteria may have belonged to a cryptic species (i.e. species not able to be differentiated on the basis of specific phenotypic characteristics) within the genus *Haemophilus*[21]. This observation was recently confirmed by 16S rRNA gene sequencing, where genital isolates were identified as being a cryptic species distinct from non-genital *Haemophilus influenzae* biotype IV and more closely related to *Haemophilus haemolyticus*[22]. Now that these species have been recognized, distinguishing traits may be identified and appropriate studies into their mechanisms of pathogenesis undertaken.

In a recent study we employed MEE to undertake a genetic analysis of selected isolates of *H. pylori*. We examined 23 isolates from patients suffering from peptic ulcer disease and non-ulcer dyspepsia. The data from our study indicated that the genetic diversity others have observed in *H. pylori* isolates may be sufficient to classify *H. pylori* strains into four or more (cryptic) species[23] (Figure 1). On the basis of this work we have proposed that strains currently identified as being *H. pylori* may belong to what may be more appropriately termed a '*Helicobacter pylori* Complex'. To determine the full scope of taxonomic diversity within this '*H. pylori* Complex', examination of a large sample of isolates will be required. Recently Xiang *et al.* proposed that isolates of *H. pylori* be designated as either 'Type 1' or 'Type 2' (based on *cagA* and *vacA* status)[6]. Given that our MEE data suggested that isolates associated with duodenal ulcer disease may not be monophyletic (i.e. disease may be induced by a number of cryptic species within the *H. pylori* Complex[23]), the designation of strains as either 'Type 1' or 'Type 2' may have no phylogenetic foundation. This is consistent with the results of biotyping studies by Owen and associates[5].

While the above data must be treated with appropriate caution until further studies are completed, we should bear in mind the recent study aimed at fixing the taxonomic position of '*Gastrospirillum hominis*' ('*Helicobacter heilmannii*') within the genus *Helicobacter*. Two morphologically identical isolates of

3

'*Helicobacter heilmannii*' were found to have distinct 16S rRNA gene sequences; indeed Solnick and associates commented that 'as we examine more clones, it becomes apparent that there are probably many species of these bacteria'[24]. Further comparative data come from studies of other *Helicobacter* spp. Morgan and Owen noted that while *H. pylori* was heterogeneous when assessed by DNA restriction endonuclear digestion, this was not the case for *Helicobacter mustelae*, the gastric helicobacter of ferrets[25]. The *Helicobacter pylori* Complex proposal may yet lead to new findings in relation to these important bacteria.

INFECTIONS WITH MULTIPLE STRAINS OF *HELICOBACTER PYLORI*

An area related to the issue of strain diversity is the issue of infection in a single individual by multiple strains of *H. pylori*. The occurrence of multiple strains in individuals has been the subject of a limited number of studies over the past 10 years. As our techniques for characterizing strains have improved, so has the evidence supporting multi-strain infections. Such multiple infections may have important implications with regard to pathology and pathogenic mechanisms.

As discussed earlier, *H. pylori* typing based on restriction fragment length polymorphism (RFLP), ribotyping and RAPD-PCR all indicate the hetero-geneous genetic nature of these bacteria[7-12]. Although it has been generally presumed that human disease occurs by infection with a single strain of *H. pylori*, over the past few years differences in DNA fingerprints of isolates from patients have been reported[7,8,10,26,27]. These data suggest that more than one strain of *H. pylori* may coexist within the human stomach at any one time.

One of the early studies in this area was conducted by Langenberg and associates, in the days when *H. pylori* was known as *Campylobacter pyloridis*, who initially reported that patients were only infected with one strain[28]. However, in a later study, this time when *H. pylori* was known as *Campylobacter pylori*, the same group noted differences between strains isolated from the same individual in one-third of their patients[26]. They concluded that these differences emanated from the coexistence in the stomach of subpopulations of bacteria with slightly different chromosomal DNAs, plasmids, or both.

Majewski and Goodwin showed profile differences with restriction enzyme analysis (REA) in pairs of isolates from 11 individuals, with the second isolate being markedly different in six subjects[10]. Taylor *et al.*, in a recent paper, reported 20% of patients to be infected with two or more strains of *H. pylori*[8]. Earlier, Owen and associates found, by ribotyping, a high degree of heterogeneity in isolates from three biopsies obtained from individual patients. This suggested different areas of the stomach may harbour distinct subpopulations of *H. pylori*. Only 2/13 patients had identical ribotypes of *H. pylori* at all three biopsy sites[27]. These data indicate that careful examination of gastric isolates does reveal distinct populations of *H. pylori* in the stomach.

In a recent study, aimed in part at addressing the question of strain diversity within infected individuals, we examined this issue by way of multiple biopsy specimens[29]. If different regions of the stomach do harbour distinct subpopu-lations of *H. pylori*, then multiple biopsy specimens should have provided a

Table 1 Strain diversity in multiple isolates from 17 patients infected with *Helicobacter pylori*

Number of strains	Number and percentage of patients colonized
One	4/17 (24%)
Two	5/17 (29%)
Three	3/17 (18%)
Four	3/17 (18%)
More than five	2/17 (11%)

further insight into the issue. In our study design we analysed two isolates per biopsy from up to 10 gastric biopsies per patient prior to, and following, therapy. Strains were fingerprinted by the use of RAPD-PCR, a technique which utilizes a single, randomly selected primer for DNA synthesis in a low-stringency PCR amplification cycle, generating a strain-specific fingerprint[9]. The observation of greater than one band difference in a RAPD fingerprint suggests there is sufficient polymorphic DNA diversity in an isolate to indicate that a new genomic variety is infecting a patient[30].

Our data[29] indicated, as others had observed, that patients may be colonized concurrently with a mixed population of *H. pylori* (Table 1). One isolate was found in 24% of cases (4/17). In the cases with multiple isolates the majority of patients were found to be infected by one predominant strain. In these patients the predominant strain was found to colonize the majority of biopsy sites, with other isolates being limited to one or two biopsy sites only. In some cases two strains were found to coexist at a single biopsy site. In one patient six strains were found to be colonizing the stomach.

Are these multiple isolates from the same individual all distinct strains of *H. pylori*, or are they subtypes of the predominant strain? It is possible that mutations or natural transformation may lead to changes in the RAPD-PCR profiles during the lifelong infection of a patient[12], although Nwokolo *et al.* noted a high degree of fingerprint stability in selected isolates from succeeding generations of the same family[31].

Thus the current evidence supports the hypothesis that individuals may be infected with multiple strains of *H. pylori*. Infection with multiple strains may occur during childhood, or be acquired over time during the life of an individual. This may have implications in regard to understanding the natural history of *H. pylori* infection and issues of pathogenesis. Also, given the possibility that persons may be infected with different species within the *H. pylori* Complex, we need to consider the impact of such infection and the interaction between such species.

GASTRIC INFECTIONS WITH *HELICOBACTER* SPECIES OTHER THAN *HELICOBACTER PYLORI*

Although, over the years, the majority of upper gastrointestinal infections have been attributed to *H. pylori*, there has been a steady stream of reports on the involvement of other *Helicobacter* spp., particularly '*Helicobacter heilmannii*'

('*Gastrospirillum hominis*'), in gastrointestinal pathology. While non-*H. pylori* infections have been documented, the prevalence of these infections is low. Notwithstanding, by a systematic examination of '*H. heilmannii*' we may be able to learn more about the host and bacterial factors in upper gastrointestinal disease.

Gastric tissues of cats are colonized by several large, morphologically distinct, spiral bacteria[32]. *Helicobacter felis* was isolated from cat gastric tissue in the late 1980s and later established as being a member of the *Helicobacter* genus[32,33]. Following these early animal studies, Dent and associates noted the occurrence of large spiral bacteria in the stomachs of a limited number of humans[34]. Serum collected from these patients was immunoreactive with *H. felis* antigens[35]; however, these bacteria were morphologically different from *H. felis* in that they lacked the periplasmic fibrils characteristic of *H. felis*[34,36]. The name '*Gastrospirillum hominis*' was proposed for these non-*H. felis* spiral bacteria[36].

Human infections involving '*Helicobacter heilmannii*' ('*Gastrospirillum hominis*')-like organisms are well documented; although the exact taxonomic status of these isolates remains to be determined[24]. Human infections with the related organism, *Helicobacter felis*, appear rare[37–43]. Over the years sporadic cases of gastritis associated with '*H. heilmannii*' have continued to appear in the literature[38–56]. One histopathologist, the late Konrad Heilmann, collected a large series of sections from infected patients and reported on clinical associations between infection with '*H. heilmannii*' and disease in humans[55,56]. The bacterium '*H. heilmannii*' has been named in his honour.

'Isolates' of '*H. heilmannii*' ('*Gastrospirillum hominis*') from human tissue have been available for some time by propagation of these organisms in the stomach of specific pathogen-free mice[57,58]. '*H. heilmannii*' has now been isolated by Hanninen *et al.* from gastric tissue of dogs[59], while a report of the isolation of a '*Helicobacter heilmannii*'-like organism ('*Gastrospirillum hominis*') from human gastric biopsy tissue has recently appeared[60].

Most cases of '*H. heilmannii*' infection are associated with mild chronic gastritis or active chronic gastritis; with some reports of acute presentations. Heilmann and associates noted in their study of 39 cases that 34/39 (87.2%) complained of upper abdominal discomfort. In relation to pathology, 5/39 patients (12.8%) had chronic gastritis while the majority, 34/39 (87.2%), had chronic gastritis with activity[56]. While inducing inflammation, these organisms were seen to be present deep in the gastric foveolae and intracellularly, and in parietal cells[55,56]. Bacteria were also seen to invade and damage gastric mucosal epithelial cells[55,56].

While the inflammation associated with '*H. heilmannii*' is usually mild, there have been at least three reports of gastric ulceration in association with infection by '*H. heilmannii*'; one of these reports being presented as an abstract to the European *Helicobacter* workshop in Brussels[49,61,62]. In one of these studies, Akin *et al.*[62] reported an '*H. heilmannii*' infection in a 16-year-old male subject who presented with abdominal pain, nausea and vomiting. The pertinent feature of this infection was the occurrence of four discrete gastric ulcers. These reports bring to the fore the issue of the relative importance of bacterial and host factors in the pathogenesis of peptic ulcer disease. Does '*H. heilmannii*' possess the unique virulence determinants now being identified in *H. pylori*? If not, we must be drawn back to a further examination of host factors as determinants of disease outcome. While these few cases of an association between ulcer disease and '*H.*

heilmannii' infection provide only limited anecdotal information, it will be very interesting to watch the developments in our understanding of disease in relation to both *H. pylori* and '*H. heilmannii*' over the next 5–10 years.

The prevalence of '*H. heilmannii*' infection in the general community is probably considerably less than 0.5% based on the reports of the prevalence of infection in symptomatic individuals presenting for endoscopic examination (prevalence range 0.07–1%)[39,43,47,56,63]. The spontaneous clearance of '*H. heilmannii*' appears to be another feature of this infection. This spontaneous resolution of infection may account for the low prevalence; however, it does suggest that the incidence of infection may be higher. Associations between contact with animals, particularly dogs and cats, and the occurrence of infection with '*H. heilmannii*' have been drawn from animal studies and anecdotal observations in the literature (i.e. '*H. heilmannii*' infection appears to be a zoonosis)[32–36,41,50–52,59]. Some sporadic symptomatic disease, particularly in pet owners, may therefore be associated with '*H. heilmannii*' infection; this is an issue worthy of further investigation.

MIXED INFECTIONS WITH *HELICOBACTER PYLORI* AND OTHER *HELICOBACTER* SPECIES

Reports in the literature of infections involving both *H. pylori* and other *Helicobacter* spp. are also rare[42,54,64,65]. Because of this, Stolte *et al.* suggested that infection with '*H. heilmannii*' may be protective in terms of *H. pylori* infection[54]. In a study of 912 patients, by Hilzenrat *et al.*, one of four cases found to be infected with '*H. heilmannii*' was shown also to have a concomitant infection with *H. pylori*[65]. The pathology in this case appeared unremarkable. Thus in this case, and in one reported by Queiroz *et al.*[42], infection with one species was not protective against infection with the other. Whether such co-infections would be stable over time remains a matter for conjecture.

In the prospective and retrospective studies of symptomatic individuals that have been reported, the prevalence of '*H. heilmannii*' infection has been only in the range of 0.07–1%[39,43,47,56,62]. This compares with a 30–60% infection with *H. pylori* in the same or similar patient populations. These figures probably overstate the prevalence of '*H. heilmannii*' infection in the general population, and we may therefore assume that the probability of coincident infection with '*H. heilmannii*' and *H. pylori* would be rare. The occurrence of one concomitant infection in four cases in the study by Hilzenrat *et al.* is consistent with the relative prevalence data for infections by *H. pylori* and '*H. heilmannii*'[65].

CONCLUSION

The subject of this review has been wide-ranging. The ideas put forward were in some cases provocative; however, the case has been made for the further systematic assessment of the taxonomy of *H. pylori*, and a review of the designation of these bacteria as part of a '*Helicobacter pylori* Complex'. Such an investigation offers the potential to reveal new data regarding epidemiology and pathogenesis associated with gastric infection. Review of the taxonomy of *H. pylori* would force a re-evaluation of the role, occurrence and significance of infections with multiple strains of *H. pylori*. Currently, data on mixed infection appear an interesting curiosity, yet these observations may force some significant re-evaluations of our understanding of the microecology of the human stomach.

As I have argued previously[66], data on human infection with '*H. heilmannii*' may provide new insights into the relative contribution of host and bacterial factors in human upper gastrointestinal disease. Tissue tropism, the role of toxins and host immune factors are some of the many areas that may be addressed using comparative data between '*H. heilmannii*' and *H. pylori*. A further review of this important area may be seen in a recent publication by Lee *et al.*[67].

References

1. Blaser MJ. *Helicobacter pylori* and the pathogenesis of gastroduodenal inflammation. J Infect Dis. 1989;161:626–33.
2. IARC Monographs on the evaluation of carcinogenic risks to humans, vol. 61. Lyon: World Health Organisation; 1994:177–240.
3. Parsonnet J, Hansen S, Rodriguez L *et al*. *Helicobacter pylori* infection and gastric lymphoma. N Engl J Med. 1994;330:1267–71.
4. Reina J, Alomar P. Biotypes of *Campylobacter pylori* isolated in gastroduodenal biopsies. Eur J Clin Microbiol Infect Dis. 1989;8:175–7.
5. Owen RJ, Bickley J, Moreno M, Costas M, Morgan DR. Biotype and macromolecular profiles of cytotoxin-producing strains of *Helicobacter pylori* from antral gastric mucosa, FEMS Microbiol Lett. 1991;63:199–204.
6. Xiang ZY, Censini S, Bayeli PF *et al*. Analysis of expression of CagA and VacA virulence factors in 43 strains of *Helicobacter pylori* reveals that clinical isolates can be divided into two major types and that CagA is not necessary for expression of the vacuolating cytotoxin. Infect Immun. 1995;63:94–8.
7. Hirschl AM, Richter M, Makristathis A *et al*. Single and multiple strain colonisation in patients with *Helicobacter pylori* associated gastritis: detection by macrorestriction DNA analysis. J Infect Dis. 1994;170:473–5.
8. Taylor NS, Fox JG, Akopyants NS *et al*. Long-term colonization with single and multiple strains of *Helicobacter pylori* assessed by DNA fingerprinting. J Clin Microbiol. 1995;33:918–23.
9. Akopyanz N, Bukanov NO, Westblom TU, Kresovich S, Berg DE. DNA diversity among clinical isolates of *Helicobacter pylori* detected by PCR-based RAPD fingerprinting. Nucl Acids Res. 1992;20:5137–40.
10. Majewski SIH, Goodwin CS. Restriction endonuclear analysis of the genome of *Campylobacter pylori* with a rapid extraction method: evidence for considerable genomic variation. J Infect Dis. 1988;157:465–71.
11. Rautelin H, Seppala K, Renkonen O, Vainio U, Kosunen TU. Role of metronidazole resistance in therapy of *Helicobacter pylori* infections. Antimicrob Agents Chemother. 1992;36:163–6.
12. Owen RJ, Bell GD, Desai M *et al*. Biotype and molecular fingerprints of metronidazole resistant strains of *Helicobacter pylori* from antral gastric mucosa. J Med Microbiol. 1993;38:6–12.
13. Taylor DE, Eaton M, Chang N, Salama SM. Construction of a *Helicobacter pylori* genome map and demonstration of diversity at the genome level. J Bacteriol. 1992;174:6800–6.
14. Bukanov NO, Berg DE. Ordered cosmid library and high-resolution physical–genetic map of *Helicobacter pylori* strain NCTC 11638. Mol Microbiol. 1994;11:509–23.
15. Wayne LG, Brenner DJ, Colwell RR *et al*. Report of the *ad hoc* committee on reconciliation of approaches to bacterial systematics. Int J Syst Bacteriol. 1987;37:463–4.
16. Woese CR. Bacterial evolution. Microbiol Rev. 1987;51:221–71.
17. Stackebrandt E, Goebel BM. A place for DNA–DNA reassociation and 16S rRNA sequence analysis in the present species definition in bacteriology. Int J Syst Bacteriol. 1994;44:846–9.
18. Richardson BJ, Baverstock PR, Adams, R. Allozyme electrophoresis: a handbook for animal systematics and population studies. Sydney: Academic Press; 1986.
19. Selander RK, Caugant DA, Ochman H, Musser JM, Gilmour MN, Whittam TS. Methods of

multilocus enzyme electrophoresis for bacterial population genetics and systematics. Appl Environ Microbiol. 1986;51:873–84.

20. Wallace RJ Jr, Baker CJ, Quinones FJ, Hollis DG, Weaver RE, Wiss K. Nontypable *Haemophilus influenzae* (biotype 4) as a neonatal, maternal, and genital pathogen. Rev Infect Dis. 1983;5: 123–36.

21. Musser JM, Barenkamp SJ, Granoff DM, Selander RK. Genetic relationships of serologically non-typable and serotype b strains of *Haemophilus influenzae*. Infect Immun. 1986;52:183–91.

22. Quentin R, Ruimy R, Rosenau A, Musser JM, Christen R. Genetic identification of cryptic geno-species of *Haemophilus* causing urogenital and neonatal infections by PCR using specific primers targeting genes coding for 16S rRNA. J Clin Microbiol. 1996;34:1380–5.

23. Hazell SL, Andrews RH, Mitchell HM, Daskalopoulous G. Genetic relationship among strains of *Helicobacter pylori*: identification of four cryptic species. J Infect Dis. (Submitted).

24. Solnick JV, O'Rourke J, Lee A, Paster BJ, Dewhirst FE, Tompkins LS. An uncultured gastric spiral organism is a newly identified *Helicobacter* in humans. J Infect Dis. 1993;168:379–85.

25. Morgan DD, Owen RJ. Use of DNA restriction endonuclease digest and ribosomal RNA gene probe patterns to fingerprint *Helicobacter pylori* and *Helicobacter mustelae* isolated from human and animal hosts. Mol Cell Probes. 1990;4:321–34.

26. Oudbier JH, Langenberg W, Rauws EA, Bruin Mosch C. Genotypical variation of *Campylobacter pylori* from gastric mucosa. J Clin Microbiol. 1990;28:559–65.

27. Owen RJ, Desai M, Figura N et al. Comparisons between degree of histological gastritis and DNA fingerprints, cytotoxicity and adhesivity of *Helicobacter pylori* from different gastric sites. Eur J Epidemiol. 1993;9:315–21.

28. Langenberg W, Rauws EA, Widjojokusumo A, Tytgat GN, Zanen HC. Identification of *Campylobacter pyloridis* isolates by restriction endonuclease DNA analysis. J Clin Microbiol. 1986;24:414–17.

29. Jorgensen M, Daskalopoulos G, Warburton V, Mitchell HM, Hazell SL. Multiple strain colonisation and metronidazole resistance in *Helicobacter pylori* infected patients; identification from sequential and multiple biopsy specimens. J Infect Dis. 1996 (In press).

30. Marshall DG, Chua A, Keeling PWN, Sullivan DJ, Coleman DC, Smyth CJ. Molecular analysis of *Helicobacter pylori* populations in antral biopsies from individual patients using randomly amplified polymorphic DNA (RAPD) fingerprinting. FEMS Immunol Med Microbiol. 1995;10: 317–24.

31. Nwokolo CU, Bickley J, Attard AR, Owen RJ, Costas M, Fraser IA. Evidence of clonal variants of *Helicobacter pylori* in three generations of a duodenal ulcer disease family. Gut. 1992;33: 1323–7.

32. Lee A, Hazell SL, O'Rourke J, Kouprach S. Isolation of a spiral-shaped bacterium from the cat stomach. Infect Immun. 1988;56:2843–50.

33. Paster BJ, Lee A, Fox JG et al. Phylogeny of *Helicobacter felis* sp. nov., *Helicobacter mustelae*, and related bacteria. Int J Syst Bacteriol. 1991;41:31–8.

34. Dent JC, McNulty CAM, Uff JC, Wilkinson SP, Gear MWL. Spiral organisms in the gastric antrum. Lancet. 1987;2:96.

35. Lee A, Dent J, Hazell S, McNulty C. Origin of spiral organisms in human gastric antrum. Lancet. 1988;1:300–1.

36. McNulty CAM, Dent JC, Curry A et al. New spiral bacterium in gastric mucosa. J Clin Pathol. 1989;42:585–91.

37. Lavelle J, Conklin F, Mitros S, Landas S. Transmission of a 'Gastrospirillum hominis' from cat to man. Gastroenterology. 1992;104:306.

38. Fischer R, Samisch W, Schwenke E. 'Gastrospirillum hominis', another four cases. Lancet. 1990;335:59.

39. Flejou JF, Diomande I, Molas G et al. Human chronic gastritis associated with non-*Helicobacter pylori* spiral organisms (*Gastrospirillum hominis*). Four cases and review of the literature. Gastroenterol Clin Biol. 1990;14:806–10.

40. Cayla R, Vialette G, Seurat PL et al. Role of non-*Helicobacter pylori* spiral organisms (*Gastrospirillum hominis*) in the human stomach. Ital J Gastroenterol. 1991;23(Suppl. 2):72.

41. Logan RP, Polson RJ, Baron JH, Walker MM. New spiral bacterium in the gastric mucosa: *Gastrospirillum hominis*. J Clin Pathol. 1990;43:262–3.

42. Queiroz DM, Cabral MM, Nogueira AM, Barbosa AJ, Rocha GA, Mendes EN. Mixed gastric infection by 'Gastrospirillum hominis' and *Helicobacter pylori*. Lancet. 1990;2:507–8.

43. Wegmann W, Aschwanden M, Schaub N, Aenishanslin W, Gyr K. Gastritis associated with *Gastrospirillum hominis* – assoziierte gastritis – einea zoonose? Schweiz Med Wochenschr. 1991;121:245–54.
44. Zhou DY, Yang Ht, Zhang WD. Gastritis due to *'Gastrospirillum hominis'*. Ital J Gastroenterol. 1991;23(Suppl. 2):83.
45. Kubonova K, Trupl J, Jancula L, Polak E, Viablik V. Presence of spiral bacteria (*'Gastrospirillum hominis'*) in the gastric mucosa. Eur J Clin Microbiol Infect Dis. 1991;10:459–60.
46. Ierardi E, Monno R, Mongelli A *et al. Gastrospirillum hominis* associated chronic active gastritis: the first report from Italy. Ital J Gastroenterol. 1991;23:86–7.
47. Oliva MM, Lazenby AJ, Perman LA. Gastritis associated with *Gastrospirillum hominis* in children – comparison with *Helicobacter pylori* and review of the literature. Mod Pathol. 1993;6:513–15.
48. Mazzuchelli L, Wildersmith CH, Ruchti C, Meyerwyss B, Berki HS. *Gastrospirillum hominis* in asymptomatic, healthy individuals. Dig Dis Sci. 1993;38:2087–9.
49. Debongnie JC, Donnay M, Mairesse J, Lamy V, Dekoninck X, Ramdani B. Acute gastric ulcerations and *Gastrospirillum hominis.* Another cause of gastric ulcer? Acta Gastro-Enterol Belg. 1993;56(Suppl.):56.
50. Lavelle J, Conklin F, Mitros S, Landas S. Transmission of *'Gastrospirillum hominis'* from cat to man. Gastroenterology. 1992;104:306.
51. Thomson MA, Storey P, Greer R. Cleghorn GJ. Canine–human transmission of *Gastrospirillum hominis.* Lancet. 1994;343:1605–7.
52. Curry A. Canine-to-human transmission of *Gastrospirillum hominis.* Lancet. 1994;344:190.
53. Debongnie JC. *Gastrospirillum hominis* prevalence. Dig Dis Sci. 1994;39:1618.
54. Stolte M, Wellens E, Bethke B, Ritter M, Eidt H. *Helicobacter heilmannii* (formerly *Gastrospirillum hominis*) gastritis: an infection transmitted by animals? Scand J Gastroenterol. 1994; 29:1061–4.
55. Heilmann KL, Borchard F. Further observations on human spirobacteria. In: Menge H, Gregor M, Tytgat GNJ, Marshall BJ, McNulty CAM, editors. *Helicobacter pylori* 1990. Berlin: Springer-Verlag; 1991:63–7.
56. Heilmann KL, Borchard F. Gastritis due to spiral shaped bacteria other than *Helicobacter pylori:* clinical, histological, and ultrastructural findings. Gut. 1991;32:137–40.
57. Lee A, Eckstein RP, Fevre DI, Dick E, Kellow JE. Non-*Campylobacter pylori* spiral organisms in the gastric antrum. Aust NZ J Med. 1989;19:156–8.
58. Dick E, Lee A, Watson G, O'Rourke J. Use of the mouse for the isolation and investigation of stomach-associated spiral shaped bacteria from man and other animals. J Med Microbiol. 1989; 29:55–62.
59. Hanninen ML, Jalava K, Saari S, Happonen J, Westermarck E. Culture of *'Gastrospirillum'* from gastric biopsies of dogs. Eur J Clin Microbiol Infect Dis. 1995;14:145–6.
60. Andersen LP, Nørgaard A, Holick S, Blom J, Elsborg L. Isolation of *'Helicobacter heilmannii'*-like organism from the human stomach. Eur J Clin Microbiol Infect Dis. 1996;15:95–6.
61. Chone L, Flejou JF, Gringnon Y, Bigard MA. *Helicobacter heilmannii:* new spiral shaped bacterium responsible for acute gastric ulcerations. Gastroenterol Clin Biol. 1995;19:447–8.
62. Akin OY, Tsou VM, Werner AL. *Gastrospirillum hominis*-associated chronic active gastritis. Pediatr Pathol Lab Med. 1995;15:429–35.
63. Monno R, Ierardi E, Valenza MA, Campanale A, Francavilla A, Fumarola L. *Gastrospirillum hominis* and human chronic gastritis. Microbiologica. 1995;18:441–4.
64. Hilzenrat N, Queiroz DM, Cabral MM *et al.* Mixed gastric infection by *'Gastrospirillum hominis'* and *Helicobacter pylori.* Lancet. 1990;2:507–8.
65. Hilzenrat N, Lamoureux E, Weintrub I, Lichter M, Alpert L. *Helicobacter heilmannii*-like spiral bacteria in gastric mucosal biopsies – prevalence and clinical significance. Arch Pathol Lab Med. 1995;119:1149–53.
66. Hazell SL. Isolation of *'Helicobacter heilmannii'* from human tissue. Eur J Clin Microbiol Infect Dis. 1996;15:4–9.
67. Lee A, O'Rourke J, Kellow JE. *Gastrospirillum hominis* (*Helicobacter pylori*) and other gastric infections of humans. In: Blaser MJ, Smith PD, Ravdin JI, Greenberg HB, Guerrant RL, editors. Infections of the gastrointestinal tract. New York: Raven Press; 1995:589–601.

2
In vivo studies of emergent issues in gastric *Helicobacter* pathogenesis and epidemiology

J. G. FOX

INTRODUCTION

Since the original description of the bacterium by Warren and Marshall in 1983, *Helicobacter pylori* is now causally linked to a variety of pathological conditions of the human stomach, such as chronic gastritis, peptic ulcer disease, gastric adenocarcinoma and, most recently, gastric mucosa-associated lymphoid tissue lymphoma[1-6]. The discovery of *H. pylori*, and its emerging importance in gastric disease, has generated an enormous interest in dissecting the pathogenesis and epidemiology of *H. pylori* infection[7,8]. Early studies failed to establish *H. pylori* in animal models and, surprisingly, Koch's postulates were initially fulfilled in two human volunteers[9 11]. These individuals suffered bouts of acute gastric symptomatology a few days after oral challenge with *H. pylori*, and in one of them a persistent gastritis was established[10,11].

Because investigators were unsuccessful in their attempts to establish *H. pylori* in the early 1980s in both conventional and germfree mice, as well as SPF guinea pigs, ferrets and rabbits[12-15], studies ensued to determine whether gastric disease occurred naturally in laboratory and domestic animals, and whether gastritis, if noted, was associated with an infectious aetiology. As a result of these efforts, six additional *Helicobacter* species have been isolated and identified from the stomachs of various mammals, including dogs, cats, ferrets, pigs, monkeys and cheetahs: these organisms, like *H. pylori*, are associated with various degrees of gastritis in their hosts[16-22].

Fortunately, experiments done in germfree piglets and dogs established that these animals would colonize with *H. pylori*, and that a gastritis was induced[12,23,24]. Also, certain macaque species are now known to be naturally infected with *H. pylori*, and these animals were also experimentally susceptible to the organism[25,26]. Thus these initial experiments were directed at convincing the research community that *H. pylori* was indeed a pathogen capable of eliciting a gastritis and immune response. The host range of naturally occurring *H. pylori* infections now includes a domestic animal, the cat[27,28]. Interestingly, as the ability to manipulate and grow *H. pylori in vitro* increased, so did the ability to colonize animal models. *H. pylori* has now experimentally produced gastritis in germfree athymic nude mice, and most recently in conventionally housed mice[29–31]. *H. pylori* has also been shown experimentally to produce gastritis in cats (Tables 1–3)[32].

  H. pylori, like all microbial pathogens, must engage in a number of general activities in order to establish long-term colonization in human hosts. These activities are: (a) entry and initial adherence; (b) localization to the preferred niche within the host; (c) avoidance of host defences; and (d) transmission to a new, susceptible individual[33]. Although most of the molecular factors involved in these activities with respect to *H. pylori* are still poorly defined in animal models, genetically manipulated *Helicobacter* spp. are now being constructed to address these properties. This chapter will therefore focus on several of these different animal models, both naturally occurring and experimentally produced, being used to help dissect the pathogenesis and epidemiology of *Helicobacter*-induced disease.

IN-VIVO MECHANISMS OF PATHOGENESIS

Germfree pigs

The germfree pig was the first animal model that was successfully colonized with *H. pylori*, and has proven to be very useful in studying pathogenic mechanisms[12,23]. Infected piglets developed a chronic antral gastritis with lymphoid follicles and a diffuse mononuclear infiltrate of the mucosa. Unfortunately, these germfree piglets can be used for only relatively short-term experiments (<30 days) because their rapid weight gain and size preclude their maintenance in germfree isolators for chronic studies. Nevertheless, they have proven to be very valuable in establishing the role of putative virulence factors in *H. pylori*.

The role of motility in colonization by *H. pylori*

Overlying the entire luminal surface of the stomach is a layer of mucus. While histological sections of gastric tissue from infected individuals reveal *H. pylori* in association with the epithelial cell surface, many bacteria colonize the mucus layer. Consequently, it has been suggested that motility in a viscous environment is important for colonization by *H. pylori*, and permits the bacteria to resist clearance by the host. The importance of motility was demonstrated in a gnotobiotic piglet study in which a highly motile *H. pylori* strain 26695 effectively colonized 100% of pigs, compared to the least motile strain (TX30) where only 17% of the piglets were colonized. Thus, these initial studies suggested that the ability of *H. pylori* to colonize and cause gastritis in gnotobiotic piglets correlated with motility[34].

  H. pylori is motile by means of multiple polar flagella. Two protein subunits which are components of the flagella have been identified, and the genes encoding these flagellins have been cloned[35,36]. Non-motile mutants, otherwise isogenic with

Table 1 *In-vivo* experimental infection with *H. pylori*

Animal	Age at dosing	Dose (cfu)	Frequency of dosing	Pre-dose treatment	Type of histological gastritis	Length of study	Immune response	Percentage infected and period of infection	Reference
Gnotobiotic pig	3 days	10^9	1×	Cimetidine	Acute (2 weeks) chronic thereafter	30 days	IgG ↑	100% 30 days	12
SPF pig	18 weeks	5×10^8	2×	Oral omeprazole 40 mg; 50 ml of fat per os	Chronic	6½ months	NR	75% 6 months	125
Barrier-maintained gnotobiotic pig, conventionalized at 24 days	3 days	10^9	1×	None	Chronic	40 days	IgG ↑ IgA ↑	75% 45 days 100% 60 days 100% 90 days	126
Gnotobiotic dogs	7 days	3×10^8	1×	None	Chronic	30 days	IgG ↑	30 days	24
Rhesus macaque	10 years	7 ml 10^9/ml	1×	None	Acute (2 weeks) chronic	64 weeks	IgG 1–5 months ↑	25% 10 weeks 0% 14 weeks	101
Japanese macaque	Adult	5 ml 10^9/ml	1×	Na bicarbonate famphotidine 20 mg/kg	Chronic	28 days 2 years	IgG ↑	58% 28 days 100% 2 years	100, 102
Domestic cat	Adult	3 ml 1.5×10^8 ml	3×EOD	Cimetidine	Chronic	7 months	IgG	100%	32

NR = not reported; EOD = every day; cfu = colony-forming units

13

Table 2 In-vivo experimental infection with other gastric Helicobacter species

Animal	Organism	Pre-dose treatment	Histological findings	Length of infection in study	Immune response	Chronic infection established	Reference
Ferret	H. mustelae 2×3 ml 1.5×10^8 c.f.u./ml	Cimetidine 10 mg/kg	Chronic, MAG	6 months – 3 years*	IgG ↑	100% 3 years	15, 86
Gnotobiotic mouse (Swiss Webster)	H. felis 3×2 day interval 0.5 ml $\sim 10^{10}$ c.f.u./ml	None	Active chronic	50 weeks	Early ↑ IgM IgG ↑	100% 50 weeks	113, 114
SPF mouse (Swiss Webster)	H. felis 3×2 day interval 0.5 ml $\sim 10^{10}$ c.f.u./ml	None	Active chronic	50 weeks	Early ↑ IgM IgG ↑	100% 50 weeks	113, 114
Gnotobiotic outbred rat	H. felis 0.5 ml $\sim 10^{10}$ c.f.u./ml	None	Chronic	10 weeks	↑ IgG Early ↑ IgM	100% 10 weeks	128
Gnotobiotic dog	H. felis 2 ml $\sim 10^9$ c.f.u./ml	None	Chronic	30 days	↑ IgG	100% 28 days	129
Balb/c	H. felis	None	MALT lymphoma	104 weeks	NR	100% 2 years	118
C57Bl/6	H. felis 3×2 day interval 0.5 ml $\sim 10^{10}$ c.f.u./ml		Chronic epithelial and mucus cell hyperplasia	12 months	IgG ↑	100% 1 year	117
Balb/c	GHLO from cheetah gastric homogenate (5.0 μm filtrate)		Chronic, gastric ulcers epithelial hyperplasia	12 months	NR	100% 1 year	127

MAG = Multifocal atrophic gastritis; NR = not reported; MALT = mucosa-associated lymphoid tissue
*Fox et al., unpublished observation, 1993

14

Table 3 Experimental infection in mice with *H. pylori*

Animal	Age at dosing	Dose	Type of histological gastritis	Immune response	Percentage infected and period of infection	Reference
Balb/c *nu/nu*	6 weeks	2 ml 10⁸/ml	Chronic	IgG ↑	100% 20 weeks	29
Balb/c Swiss Webster	NR	5×10^8	Chronic erosions *H. pylori* Cag-positive	IgG ↑	100% 8 weeks	57

NR = Not reported

15

wild-type *H. pylori*, have been constructed by allelic exchange[37,38]. A detailed *in-vitro* analysis of a *flaA*, a *flaB*, and a *flA flaB* double mutant, all isogenic with the N6 strain of *H. pylori*, revealed that both flagellin subunits are necessary for full motility[39]. While *flaA flaB* double mutants are completely non-motile, and are devoid of flagella, *flaA* mutants retain the residual motility of the parent strain and possess flagella which appear similar to those of the wild-type.

In gnotobiotic piglets both the *flaA* mutant and the *flaB* mutant were impaired in their ability to colonize with respect to the wild-type parental strain, but only the double mutant failed to colonize[40]. While these results are consistent with the motility patterns observed for these mutants *in vitro*, colonization was not assessed beyond 4 days post-inoculation (p.i.) in the piglets. Because the nature of the bacterial–mucosal surface interaction was not characterized – and the presence of low levels of mutant bacteria 4 days p.i. in a suckling piglet may represent residual luminal bacteria, rather than truly persistent colonization – studies of longer duration using these isogenic mutants in gnotobiotic piglets are needed.

The role of urease in colonization by *H. pylori*

It has been proposed that the abundant urease activity expressed by all *H. pylori* isolates is also important in gastric colonization, perhaps facilitating bacterial survival in an acidic environment[41,42]. In support of this hypothesis, an *H. pylori* mutant expressing very limited urease activity, which was isolated following MNNG mutagenesis, failed to colonize gnotobiotic piglets[43]. While providing tantalizing results, these studies were limited in that the bacterial strains used to infect the piglets were not genetically characterized, and the studies allowed only an analysis of acute colonization and infection.

Recently, however, isogenic urease-negative mutant strains of *H. pylori* have been constructed and administered to gnotobiotic piglets[44,45]. In this experiment a recombinant strain of *H. pylori* strain N6, one of the urease structural genes (*ureB*) was insertionally inactivated with the *Campylobacter* kanamycin resistance gene (*aph*)[44-46]. The isogenic N6 mutant expresses vacuolating cytotoxin activity and the cytotoxin-associated gene product, but it does not produce any detectable urease, nor is it impaired for growth *in vitro*. The identity of the chromosomal mutation in this strain was verified by Southern blot analysis and by polymerase chain reaction (PCR)[45]. These *in-vivo* studies clearly showed that urease activity in *H. pylori* was essential for colonization, but the mechanism by which urease allows colonization has not been determined[46]. Urease activity was considered important because the NH_3 generated by breakdown of urea could neutralize the gastric acid immediately surrounding the bacterium until it enters the protective barrier of the gastric mucus. A recent set of well-designed studies in achlorhydric gnotobiotic piglets, however, have partially discounted this hypothesis. Even in the presence of an achlorhydric stomach, urease-negative *H. pylori* organisms were found only in small numbers (10^2 c.f.u.), and were therefore considered incapable of colonizing the gastric mucosa[46]. This study also discounted the theory that urease plays a nutritional role by promoting nitrogen metabolism. The investigators demonstrated that only the wild-type *H. pylori* strain colonized the piglet stomach following administration of both wild-type and mutant strains in a co-colonization experiment[46]. In a separate experiment investigators also demonstrated that an *H. pylori* urease negative isogenic mutant was unable to colonize the stomach of nude mice[47].

THE ROLE OF VACUOLATING CYTOTOXIN AND THE CYTOTOXIN-ASSOCIATED GENE

Two bacterial determinants, which are not universally expressed by all *H. pylori* isolates, have been associated with peptic ulcer disease. These determinants are the vacuolating cytotoxin and the cytotoxin-associating gene. Approximately 50% of all *H. pylori* isolates produce a potent exotoxin which induces vacuole formation in cultured epithelial cells[48]. Of strains recovered from individuals suffering from duodenal ulceration or atrophic gastritis, >70% of the isolates elaborate this cytotoxic activity[49–51]. While individual strains exhibit a wide degree of variation in the amount of toxin produced, there is an association between the ability of an isolate to produce toxin and the severity of the inflammatory changes that the infected individual develops[52,53]. It is not clear if both toxin-producing strains and toxin-negative strains can infect susceptible individuals, or if the heterogeneous nature of toxin expression among strains is a consequence of an *in-vivo* adaptation by a subset of *H. pylori* isolates. While the precise mechanism of action has not been determined, the vacuolating cytotoxin has been shown to be sensitive to inhibition by bafilomycin A1[54]. This observation suggests a vacuolar-type proton ATPase, which results in acidification of an intracellular compartment within the epithelial cells. The gene encoding the vacuolating cytotoxin, designated *vacA*, has also been cloned[55]. The role of these gene products has not been directly tested in a chronic infection model. However, in the same gnotobiotic pig experiment which tested motility of *H. pylori*, the strains were also tested for *in-vitro* cytotoxin production[34]. Strain 26695 had high cytotoxin activity but TX30a did not; the 26695 strain also elicited more gastritis than did TX30a. The strain of *H. pylori* with the highest cytotoxin activity *in vivo*, but low motility, colonized only 40% of the germfree piglets. Although vacuolation of gastric epithelial cells was observed in infected as well as inoculated control pigs, the mean number of vacuoles per millimetre of mucosa was greater with *H. pylori* strain 26695[34]. More recently, in a well-controlled study, gnotobiotic piglets were given 10^9 c.f.u. of either strain 26695 or 26695 *vacA*:km (an isogenic toxin-negative mutant) by oral inoculation[56]. Piglets were euthanized 2 or 28 days post-inoculation (p.i.). All had *H. pylori* status and histological grading of inflammation and vacuolization scored semi-quantitatively. All piglets became colonized with *H. pylori* but, interestingly, there was no difference in colonization rate in piglets given tox+ or tox− *H. pylori*. Lymphocytic inflammation was observed in all piglets, and most had epithelial vacuolation with associated mild epithelial degeneration. Differences were not noted in colonization rate, inflammation, or epithelial vacuolization or degeneration in piglets given tox− *H. pylori* or tox+ *H. pylori*. In contrast to a pathogenic role proposed in mice, vacuolating cytotoxin in gnotobiotic piglets does not appear to play a role in colonization, vacuolization of epithelium or inflammation due to *H. pylori*[56].

EUTHYMIC AND ATHYMIC MICE

A preliminary report in 1991 indicated that fresh clinical isolates of *H. pylori*, but not isolates maintained in stock culture, colonized the stomach of athymic and euthymic mice for a short time interval[29]. Following this observation (a mouse model of acute tissue damage, using sonicates of isogenic strains), treatment with a sonicate of a vacuolating cytotoxin mutant failed to produce appreciable epithelial cell injury, whereas wild-type cytotoxin positive strains did[57]. The authors argued that this observation was consistent with the finding that culture supernatants from *H. pylori* strains which express the vacuolating cytotoxin cause a cytopathic effect on cultured epithelial cells, while supernatant from an isogenic mutant does not[58]. In addition the purified VacA cytotoxin caused gastric injury after oral administration to mice[59,60].

The mouse model was further developed to test the ability of *H. pylori* strains that expressed vacuolating cytotoxin (VacA) and the immunodominant cytotoxin-associated antigen (CagA) versus *H. pylori* strains that did not express the VacA and CagA antigens[31]. The ability of *H. pylori* to colonize was enhanced (over that of clinical isolates) by serial passage of *H. pylori* in mice. Thus *H. pylori* strains used in the experiments assessing gastric pathology were isolated from mice 2 weeks p.i., expanded *in vitro* and used in subsequent studies. The authors stated that the strains expressing the VacA and CagA experimentally produced gastritis, whereas the strain lacking these antigens did not produce gastric pathology[31]. The mice also had a systemic antibody response demonstrated by immunoblot to several dominant antigens, including a 55 kDa protein (probably representing a heat-shock protein, homologue to HSP60), a 26 kDa surface protein and the ureA subunit of urease[31]. However, the CagA antigen was not recognized, probably because of the early phase of infection in the mice. For example, the CagA immune response in humans was not noted in humans infected with CagA-positive *H. pylori* until 11 weeks after infection[61]. Immunological recognition of CagA (using NCTC 11637 as antigen), in twins infected with a CagA-positive strain of *H. pylori*, was noted 63 days after isolating *H. pylori* from one child, whereas the other twin did not respond to the antigen until day 857[62]. Interestingly using the CagA-positive *H. pylori* strain infecting the family as antigen, CagA antibody was not recognized throughout the study, for unknown reasons[62].

Another research group has recently described a mouse model of gastric *H. pylori* colonization in which the bacteria persist in some strains of mice for at least 5 months[63]. In general they noted the 'cleaner' the mouse (e.g. germfree animals or mice treated with antibiotics), the better the colonization rate. While all 17 strains of mice tested supported at least some colonization, and most clinical strains of *H. pylori* can colonize, successful gastric colonization was governed more by the growth medium and the frequency and size of dose and the host genotype. Although *H. pylori* could be isolated from all areas of the stomach, attaining levels up to 10^6 c.f.u./stomach, a marked predilection for the cardiac region was noted. Unfortunately, little or no meaningful gastritis was evident in these studies[63]. Several authors describing *H. pylori* in mice emphasize that fresh clinical specimens are required for colonization[29–31,63,64]. Thus to study pathogenesis the successful use of *H. pylori* isogenic mutants (which must be passaged numerous times *in vitro* to construct the mutant) a method must be developed to maintain the bacteria's virulence *in vitro* prior to inoculating these isogenic mutants into the mouse model. Despite these limitations the mouse model appears promising, and experiments to fully characterize the mouse model should be developed.

FERRETS

Natural infection

In 1985 a gastric campylobacter-like organism (GCLO) was isolated from a duodenal ulcer of a ferret (*Mustela putorius furo*)[65] and subsequently named *Helicobacter mustelae*[19]. Subsequently, in the United States, gastritis and peptic ulcers have been reported regularly in ferrets, colonized with *H. mustelae*[15,66]. Superficial gastritis was noted in the oxyntic gastric mucosa, whereas in the distal antrum the chronic inflammatory response occupied the full thickness of the mucosa. In the proximal antrum and tran-sitional mucosa, multifocal atrophic gastritis and regeneration were observed[67]. We have observed that virtually every ferret with chronic gastritis is also infected with *H. mustelae*, whereas SPF ferrets not infected with *H. mustelae* do not have gastritis, gastric ulcers, or detectable IgG antibody to the organism[15,67,68]. *H. mustelae* has also been isolated from the stomachs of ferrets living in England, Canada, and Australia, but not from ferrets in New Zealand[69,70]. The mild gastritis seen in ferret stomachs examined in England may indicate sparse colonization of *H. mustelae* strains in younger animals, or that the *H. mustelae* strains isolated from English ferrets are not as pathogenic as strains isolated from ferrets in the United States[69].

Adherence and adhesins

Ultrastructural examinations of ferret gastric tissue showed *H. mustelae* localized within the gastric pits with little evidence of bacteria on the external surface or in the overlying mucus layer[71], but very closely associated with the epithelial cells. Organisms were noted alongside microvilli and surfaces of the epithelium, perpendicular to the surface of the epithelial cells and, in some instances, penetrating these cells. Extensive loss of microvilli and the presence of adhesion pedestals were visible, and occasionally organisms were undergoing endocytosis and were localized intraepithelially within membrane-bound inclusions. A fibrous-like glyocalyx between epithelial cells and *H. mustelae* formed a very dense matrix when the two surfaces were very close together. Intercellular junctions also had *H. mustelae* present. However, this site did not have large numbers of bacteria, unlike that reported for *H. pylori*[41,72]. Thus close attachment of *H. mustelae*, like *H. pylori*, may play a role in peptic ulcer disease in the ferret.

In-vitro adhesin studies have shown that *H. mustelae*, like *H. pylori*, have specific ligand interactions with host lipid receptors[73,74]. Likewise, studies of cell surface properties of *H. mustelae* and *H. pylori* have indicated that these organisms have both hydrophobicity and hydrophilicity, depending on the specific assay being utilized[75]. Studies infer, however, that overall the cell surface of *H. mustelae* is relatively hydrophilic with distinct hydrophobic domains[75]. The ferret stomach is more hydrophobic than the large or small intestine of this species. Interestingly, the inflamed gastric mucosa infected with *H. mustelae* has an overall reduction in mucosal hydrophobicity which is consistent with findings observed in *H. pylori* infection[75,76]. This may be due to a reduction of hydrophobicity of the mucus layer overlying the gastric epithelia[76].

Electron microscopic analysis of *H. mustelae* demonstrates interesting differences when compared to *H. pylori*. While the flagella of *H. pylori* are restricted to the poles, *H. mustelae* has both polar and lateral flagella. Furthermore, the outer surface of the *H. mustelae* protoplasmic cylinder has an extensive array of ring-shaped structures that are not present on *H. pylori*. These have been characterized, and the major protein constituent of the rings has been identified[77]. Even though the surface rings do not align with a highly ordered symmetry, nor do they form a true crystalline array, or S layer, the relationship of the ring structures to the outer membrane, plus the structure of the rings themselves, have features indicating that the rings may be analogous to classical S layers. The rings appear to be primarily composed of a 150 kDa protein, designated Hsr (*Helicobacter* surface ring). Like most S layer proteins, Hsr is not covalently bound to the underlying membrane and treatment with EDTA releases the protein. The 8.5 nm diameter rings extend some 6 nm from the membrane, which is consistent with typical S layer subunits. These similarities suggest that the surface rings are also involved in functions that have been attributed to S layers, such as bacterial adherence and resistance to complement-mediated killing[78]. Affinity-purified antibody against the *H. mustelae* Hsr protein indicated that several strains of *H. pylori* and one strain of *H. felis* did not have crossreacting epitopes with *H. mustelae* Hsr. Although there are unanswered questions about the nature of the Hsr protein of *H. mustelae*, the abundance and surface location of the unusual ring structures make the protein a probable candidate for virulence. Although considerable research has focused on those factors that are common to all gastric *Helicobacter* species, determinants that are unique to one organism may provide a basis for comparison[79].

UREASE

Several virulence factors of *H. pylori* have also been identified in *H. mustelae*, including urease. An isogenic urease-negative mutant of *H. mustelae* was recently constructed to investigate the role of urease in the colonization of the gastric mucosa by *Helicobacter* organisms[80]. This isogenic urease-negative mutant strain of *H. mustelae* was used to infect specific pathogen-free ferrets. *Helicobacter mustelae* were orally dosed with either the wild-type parent strain of *H. mustelae*, the isogenic urease-negative mutant strain of *H. mustelae*, or sterile culture broth[81]. Infection status was monitored for 6 months by performing, sequentially, endoscopic gastric biopsy for urease activity, histopathology, and culture and serology. Negative control ferrets remained uninfected, as did ferrets receiving the isogenic negative mutant, whereas ferrets receiving the *H. mustelae* wild-type parent strain of *H. mustelae* remained infected throughout the study. The *H. mustelae*-infected ferrets exhibited diffuse mononuclear inflammation in the subglandular region and the lamina propria of the gastric mucosa, whereas uninfected ferrets showed no or minimal inflammation[81]. Thus the inability of urease-negative *Helicobacter mustelae* to colonize the gastric mucosa of ferrets confirms the studies in germfree piglets in which isogenic mutants at *H. pylori* lacking urease failed to colonize the stomach[46].

Flagella

H. mustelae, like *H. pylori*, possesses two flagellin molecules, FlaA and FlaB[37,39]. Isogenic mutant strains of *H. mustelae* were constructed by disruption of the *flaA* or *flaB* genes with a kanamycin resistance cassette or by introduction of both a kanamycin resistance cassette and a chloramphenicol resistance gene to produce a double mutant to determine whether one or both flagellin proteins were necessary for colonization and persistence of infection of *H. mustelae* in the ferret. Specific pathogen-free ferrets were given either the FlaA (moderately motile), FlaB (weakly motile) or FlaA/B (non-motile) mutant strain, the wild-type parent strain or sterile broth[82]. Gastric tissue samples were obtained during sequential gastric biopsies and during necropsy at 3 months post-infection. *H. mustelae* infection status was determined by culture and histology. The wild-type parent strain of *H. mustelae* infected all six ferrets at all time points (10^7 c.f.u./g). The FlaA mutant strain colonized at low levels (10^2–10^3 c.f.u./g) all three ferrets at 3 weeks, but at 7 and 11 weeks only one ferret in this group was culture-positive, whereas at 12 weeks two ferrets were positive for infection, but still with reduced numbers of organisms (10^4–10^5 c.f.u./g). The FlaB mutant strain infected all four ferrets at all time points. The number of *H. mustelae* was reduced at 3 weeks, while at 8 and 11 weeks the bacterial counts were comparable to the *H. mustelae*-infected control group (10^7 c.f.u./g). The FlaA/B double mutant strain was unable to colonize the ferret stomach at any time point.

Infection with the *H. mustelae* wild-type parent strains produced a mild lymphocytic and lymphofollicular gastritis. Infection with the FlaB mutant strain produced a similar gastritis while infection with the FlaA mutant strain produced only minimal to mild mononuclear cell gastritis. Thus the double mutant strain did not colonize, whereas the FlaA and FlaB single mutant strains initially colonized the ferret stomach at low levels, established a persistent infection, and the numbers of *H. mustelae* increased over time. The severity of gastritis produced by infection with these strains of *H. mustelae* also correlated with the number of gastric bacteria present. Therefore, flagellar-induced motility, like urease, is an important virulence factor for *H. mustelae*-induced pathogenesis in the ferret[82].

H. mustelae Cag homologue

Preliminary results indicate that strains of *H. mustelae* isolated from ferrets with severe gastritis in the United States have a Cag homologue, whereas strains of *H. mustelae* from British ferrets with a mild gastritis do not have the Cag homologue[83]. The *cag* gene has been more commonly linked to *H. pylori* strains isolated from duodenal ulcer patients; even though current data suggest this gene is only a biomarker of a pathogenesis island and not by itself a virulence determinant. Also, like humans infected with *H. pylori*, ferrets infected with *H. mustelae* have hypergastrinaemia, another feature which may be directly related to *H. mustelae*-induced ulcerogenesis in the ferret[84].

Epidemiology of natural infection

Faecal–oral transmission: isolation of H. mustelae in faeces

Weanling and adult ferret faeces have been screened for the presence of *H. mustelae* to determine whether faecal transmission could explain the 100% prevalence observed in weanling and adult ferrets[66,85]. *H. mustelae* was isolated from the faeces of eight of 74 9-week-old and three of eight 8-month-old ferrets. These results were based on biochemical and phenotypic criteria, as well as DNA probes and 16S RNA sequencing[85]. *H. mustelae* was not recovered from the faeces of 20-week-old ferrets which had been positive at weaning or from 1-year-old ferret faeces.

During experimental infection of ferrets with *H. mustelae*, a transient hypochlorhydria was observed approximately 4 weeks after the infection[86]. According to the urease tissue assay this period coincided with heavy *H. mustelae* colonization of the fundus. In the experimentally infected ferrets over time (>8 weeks), the organism, as in most naturally infected ferrets, colonizes the antrum in greater numbers[86]. To test whether hypochlorhydria enhanced faecal recovery of *H. mustelae*, oral omperazole was administered to adult ferrets in two separate experiments to pharmacologically induce gastric hypochlorhydria[86,87]. *H. mustelae* were isolated on sequential faecal sampling in 23 of 55 (41.8%) of the ferrets during omeprazole therapy, and their identification was confirmed by using standard biochemical tests and reactivity to specific *H. mustelae* DNA probes[87]. Faeces from the same ferrets, when not on omeprazole treatment and with acidic gastric pH, were positive for *H. mustelae* faeces in only six of 62 (9.3%) of the ferrets. Gastric biopsy samples from all ferrets were positive for *H. mustelae* and, in four of five ferrets, restriction enzyme patterns (using three restriction enzymes) of the gastric *H. mustelae* were identical to those of the faecal *H. mustelae* strains. These findings favour the hypothesis that hypochlorhydria promotes faecal–oral spread of *H. mustelae*. The successful isolation of *H. mustelae* from faeces intensified attempts to culture *H. pylori* from faeces. Indeed, although many laboratories have failed in their attempts to isolate the bacteria from faeces, *H. pylori* has now been successfully recovered from the faeces of both adults and children[88,89].

NON-HUMAN PRIMATES

Natural infection

Gastric *H. pylori*-like organisms (GHLO) were first noted in rhesus macaques in 1939[90]. Since then others have observed *H. pylori* in monkeys[25,90–92]. Additionally many old-world species are colonized with the large spiral gastric organisms '*H. heilmannii*'[93–95]. In the pigtail macaque, DNA–DNA homology studies from one gastric isolate indicated that this species showed less than 10% homology with *H. pylori*, and was given a novel designation, *H. nemistrinae*[16]. This new species was confirmed by further characterization by 16S rRNA of the type strain of *H. nemistrinae*[96].

In England and the United States, using SDS-PAGE analysis, antigenic and biochemical criteria, GHLO from rhesus monkeys were classified as *H. pylori*[26,92,94]. By using partial 16S rRNA sequencing and percentage similarity (99.2–100% with three human strains), a GHLO from a rhesus was identified conclusively as *H. pylori*[97]. Using restriction fragment length polymorphism (RFLP), each of 14 rhesus monkeys studied had from one to four strains identified. None of the 17 RFLP types corresponded to seven other RFLP types found among 16 other isolates cultured from 16 rhesus monkeys housed in a different colony. This indicated that, as in humans, *H. pylori* in rhesus monkeys are highly hetero-geneous[97].

H. pylori-associated gastritis in rhesus monkeys is often accompanied by a lymphocytic, plasmacytic gastritis, that apparently persists[25,26], but in one report only two of 14 rhesus monkeys with '*H. heilmannii*'-like organisms had gastric inflammation[95]. *H. pylori*-infected monkeys also have elevated specific *H. pylori* IgG serum levels, which decrease 1 month after antimicrobial therapy, as does the severity of gastritis in monkeys in which *H. pylori* has been eradicated; in animals in which *H. pylori* reinfection occurred, the gastritis returned, and *H. pylori* IgG levels remained elevated[26].

Rhesus monkeys successfully colonized with *H. pylori* produced gastritis, after the animals were orally challenged with an *H. pylori* strain isolated from a rhesus monkey. However, in four of five rhesus monkeys, and in none of four cynomolgus monkeys inoculated with a human *H. pylori* strain, colonization was unsuccessful[94]. The failure to colonize the monkeys with *H. pylori* may have been a host–parasite adaptive phenomenon. For example, human strains of *H. pylori*, when initially dosed into germfree piglets, did not colonize; however, on subsequent serial passage in piglets the strains adapted, successfully colonized and produced gastritis in the piglet[98]. Similar observations have been made in mice infected with *H. pylori*[31,64]. Thus, if subsequent oral challenge with the human *H. pylori* strain that initially colonized and was re-isolated from the one rhesus monkey was used, a higher percentage of human-strain *H. pylori* colonization may have occurred[94]. Nevertheless several studies indicate that successful experimental colonization occurred in chimpanzees and different macaque species orally dosed with human strains of *H. pylori*. The infection also reproduced the type of gastritis observed in naturally infected monkeys[99–102]. Importantly, in Japanese macaques, long-term colonization and persistence of gastritis induced by human strains of *H. pylori* has been established[103]. In Japanese macaques chronically infected with *H. pylori* the ammonia concentration in the gastric juice of infected monkeys versus controls is statistically higher, as is the gastritis score in the antrum and corpus[103]. Surprisingly, unlike what is observed in *H. pylori*-infected humans, the serum gastrin level between the two groups of monkeys was not significantly different (Table 4)[103].

Unfortunately the use of the primate to study pathogenesis has been limited because many non-human primates are colonized with the non-*H. pylori* helicobacters, which makes interpretation of experiments difficult. Cost of these animals also limits their widespread use.

Table 4 Effects of *H. pylori* infection on ammonia concentration in gastric juice, serum gastric levels, and gastritis score in Japanese monkeys

	Infected group (n = 6)	*Control group* (n = 7)
Ammonia concentration in gastric juice (μg/dl)	19 833 ± 3245*	6302 ± 3986
Gastritis score		
Antrum	5.8 ± 1.3*	2.1 ± 1.0
Corpus	4.0 ± 1.2**	2.3 ± 0.9
Serum gastrin levels (pg/ml)	108.8 ± 13.6	103.2 ± 18.2

Modified from ref. 103

CATS

H. pylori was recently identified in 100% of the stomachs examined from a group of specific pathogen-free cats, obtained from a commercial vendor[27]. The organism's identity was confirmed using phenotypic, biochemical, and 16S rRNA sequencing techniques[27]. By 16S rRNA sequence data the cat strain DO1 was 99.7% similar to that of the type strain of *H. pylori*. RFLP analysis of the *ureA* and *ureB* gene fragments of the cat *H. pylori* strain confirmed the presence of conserved regions when compared to human strains[28].

The presence of large numbers of *H. pylori* in the gastric mucosa of these cats was associated with a lymphofollicular gastritis, characterized by lymphoid aggregates and diffuse inflammation in the deep mucosa and lamina propria. The inflammatory cells consisted of lymphocytes, plasma cells and occasional neutrophils and eosinophils[27]. The inflammation was primarily located in the antrum, which corresponded to the heaviest concentration of *H. pylori* as judged by the presence of *H. pylori* histologically and by urease mapping. Ultrastructurally the organisms were numerous in the gastric mucus, and less frequently adhered tightly to gastric epithelia and formed pedestals between bacterial membranes and the epithelial microvilli[27]. This also highlights the value of these cats with a reduced natural gastric flora as *H. pylori* models.

The *H. pylori*-infected cats did not have large gastric spiral organisms colonizing the gastric mucosa. Competitive exclusion of *H. pylori* by the large gastric spiral organisms is a possibility; this phenomenon has also been suggested to account for the rare occurrence of dual infection in humans and non-human primates with large gastric spiral organisms and *H. pylori*[26,104,105].

Analyses of serum and mucosal secretions by ELISA in *H. pylori* naturally infected cats revealed an *H. pylori*-specific IgG response, and elevated IgA anti-*H. pylori* antibody levels in salivary and local gastric secretions[106].

Experimental inoculation of the feline *H. pylori* strain into naive cats without GHLO gastric infection, confirmed that *H. pylori* caused a gastritis identical to that noted in cats naturally infected with *H. pylori*[32]. In addition, persistent infection was demonstrated by the re-isolation of *H. pylori* on serial biopsies and at necropsy 7 months post-inoculation from all experimentally infected cats[32]. Studies have recently been completed which indicate that a Cag-positive human strain of *H. pylori* also infects and induces a persistent gastritis in cats (J. G. Fox, unpublished observations). These cats appear to be an ideal model to study pathogenesis and the effects of long-term colonization on gastric mucosa. It is important, however, to realize that many if not most cats, like dogs, are colonized with either *H. heilmannii*-like organisms or *H. felis*. Animals infected with the large gastric spirals, therefore, may not be suitable for experimental *H. pylori* studies[20,21,107,108].

EPIDEMIOLOGY OF NATURAL INFECTION

In a recent study, *H. pylori*-infected cats were screened by culture and PCR for the presence of *H. pylori* in salivary secretions, gastric juice, gastric tissue and faeces[106]. *H. pylori* was cultured from salivary secretions in six of 12 (50%) cats, and from gastric fluid samples in 11 of 12 (91%) cats. A 298 base-pair PCR product specific for an *H. pylori* 26 kDa surface protein was amplified from dental plaque samples from five of 12 (42%) cats, and from the faeces of four of five (80%) cats studied. Isolation of *H. pylori* from feline mucosal secretions suggests a zoonotic risk from exposure to personnel handling *H. pylori*-infected cats *in vivaria*[106]. Detailed studies using molecular, cultural and histological techniques are therefore needed to ascertain whether *H. pylori* does indeed naturally colonize the pet dog and cat.

INFLUENCE OF HOST GENOTYPE

Lee *et al.* isolated a spiral organism from the gastric mucosa of cats in 1988[20]. The bacterium was tightly coiled, with tufts of bipolar sheathed flagella and periplasmic fibres around the body, usually occurring in pairs[20]. The bacteria were urease-, catalase-, and oxidase-positive, typical biochemical features of other gastric helicobacters. In subsequent studies using 16S rRNA sequencing analysis and further biochemical characterization, the organism was named *Helicobacter felis*[21]. Gastric spiral bacteria with similar morphology (based on electron microscopy) have also been identified in the stomachs of dogs and cheetahs, and occasionally in the gastric tissue of humans[109-111]. The gastritis observed in infected dogs and cats is similar to that observed with *H. heilmannii*. Co-infection with *H. felis* and *H. heilmannii* in dogs and cats is often observed; indeed, it is impossible to distinguish the two organisms histologically by light microscopy.

Following the observations made by Solomon in 1896 that 'spirochaetes' from the stomachs of dogs, cats and rats could be transmitted to the mouse, where these organisms colonized the rodents' gastric mucosa, studies were undertaken to establish whether *H. felis* could colonize the mouse stomach and induce a gastritis[112]. In outbred Swiss germfree mice, *H. felis* selectively colonized the stomach and produced an active chronic gastritis that persisted in the mice for the 8-week duration of the study[113]. In subsequent studies using the same strain of *H. felis* and outbred mice (both germfree and barrier-maintained), it was shown that *H. felis* persistently colonized the stomach of mice for 1 year, and the infection elicited a chronic active gastritis as well as a sustained serum antibody response[114].

Previous investigators have pointed out that the gastric phenotype, as well as susceptibility to a variety of infectious agents, are strongly influenced by the genetic background of the mouse. For example, overexpression of transforming growth

Table 5   *H. felis* infection and inflammation in inbred mice

Mouse strain	Time p.i. (weeks)	H. felis positive glands/cm	H. felis max. organisms/ gland	Inflammation score*
Balb/c	2	4.0±3.7	2.6±3.5	1.1±0.5
C3H	2	4.4±4.3	4.6±4.2	4.5±2.7
C57BL/6	2	35.0±27.7	22.7±17.4	4.3±2.2
Balb/c	11	10.2±6.8	8.7±6.6	0.9±0.7
C3H	11	6.0±5.3	8.1±6.0	2.8±2.3
C57BL/6	11	16.0±19.6	12.4±10.3	6.2±0.9

Table modified from ref. 115
*Inflammation score (maximum=9) equals the sum of the grade of intensity of inflammation in the most inflamed area (0–3) and the longitudinal extent (0–3) and depth (0–3) of inflammation. Longitudinal extent and depth of inflammation were scored for the entire section

factor α in inbred FVB/N mice leads to much more severe gastric cystic hyperplasia compared with that observed in the outbred strain CD1[130]. Thus, studying the role of genetic factors in the pathogenesis of *Helicobacter*-associated gastritis by taking advantage of the wide range of inbred and other types of genetically defined mice was a logical next step in further exploration of *Helicobacter* pathogenesis using this model. Two different laboratories inoculated three inbred strains of mice with *H. felis* and tabulated the intensity of inflammation; in BALB/C mice inflammation was minimal, in C3H/He moderate and most severe in C57Bl/6 when examined 2–11 weeks p.i.[115,116] (Table 5). The authors also stated that C57Bl/6 mice had mucous cell hyperplasia in gastric fundic glands[115]. Furthermore, the study demonstrated that, by using congenic strains on the Balb/c and C57/Bl background, both MHC and non-MHC genes contributed to *H. felis*-associated gastritis[115].

Coincident with these studies, another report cited results of analysing the effect of chronic *H. felis* infection on p53 hemizygous C57Bl/6 and their wild-type counterpart C57Bl[117]. One year after infection with *H. felis*, the wild-type and p53 hemizygous mice showed severe adenomatous and cystic hyperplasia of the gastric surface foveolar epithelium. Infected mice also had a profound loss of parietal cells. BrdU uptake and PCNA staining were markedly increased in both sets of infected mice compared with controls, and infected p53 hemizygous mice had a higher proliferative index than the infected wild-type mice[117]. However, the mechanism for this proliferative effect (as well as that observed in *H. pylori* infection in humans) is unclear. One possible explanation, among others, is that an ongoing cycle of inflammation-mediated epithelial destruction is followed by activation of growth factors with subsequent epithelial regeneration leading to increased cell turnover. Regardless of the precise mechanisms involved, an increased proportion of gastric cells undergoing cell division could result in increased mitotic error, an increased mutation rate, and an increased risk of cancer formation.

Because loss of heterozygosity at the p53 locus has been found frequently in human gastric cancer specimens, and is thought to play a crucial role in cancer development, the results showing that mice lacking one copy of the *p53* gene had an increased (but not statistically significant) proliferative index, compared with wild-type controls, are of considerable interest. Reduction in the gene dosage, and consequently in the amount of p53 produced by the normal cell, did not seem to confer a significant growth advantage in the gastric epithelium in this mouse model. The development of frank neoplasia in this mouse model may require either additional mutations, genetic events, or a longer time period of infection. Homozygous p53 knockout mice in this study were not infected with *H. felis* because of their known diminished survival (3–6 months)[117].

In contrast, *H. felis* infection in BALB/c mice in another study caused a low-grade gastric lymphoma in mice. The presence of this lymphoid tumour was not evident until the mice had been infected for a 2-year period[118]. These studies, suggesting that particular inbred strains of mice have differing phenotypes of *H. felis*-induced gastritis, point to the importance of genetic make-up in determining the response to chronic infection with *H. felis*.

IMMUNIZATION STRATEGIES

Because of the high prevalence of *H. pylori* in developing countries, and the unacceptable relapse rate of *H. pylori* in patients treated with antimicrobials, an alternative strategy to control this gastric infection has been undertaken. The use of prophylactic oral vaccine was deemed a reasonable and achievable goal. In the past 5 years several laboratories have utilized the *H. felis* mouse model for immunization trials. Successful oral immunization with either whole-cell *H. felis* or *H. pylori* sonicate, plus a mucosal adjuvant (cholera toxin or LT) was achieved in early studies in mice challenged with *H. felis*[119,120]. Investigators have also employed recombinant urease or heat-shock proteins as antigens combined with mucosal adjuvants[121–123]. Using these immunization strategies, mice are protected experimentally after challenge with *H. felis*. This has also been used with success in the *H. pylori* mouse model. Therapeutic vaccination in experimental studies has also shown promise in preliminary results[124].

References

1. Marshall BJ, Warren JR. Unidentified curved bacillus on gastric epithelium in active chronic gastritis. Lancet. 1983;1:1273–5.
2. Correa P, Fox JG, Fontham E. *Helicobacter pylori* and gastric carcinoma: serum antibody prevalence in populations with contrasting cancer risks. Cancer. 1990;66:2569–74.
3. Graham DY. *Campylobacter pylori* and peptic ulcer disease. Gastroenterology. 1989;96:615–23.
4. Graham DY, Lew GM, Klein PD et al. Effect of treatment of *Helicobacter pylori* infection on the long-term recurrence of gastric or duodenal ulcer: a randomized controlled study. Ann Intern Med. 1992;116:705–8.
5. Parsonnet J, Friedman GD, Vandersteen DP. *Helicobacter pylori* infection and the risk of gastric carcinoma. N Engl J Med. 1991;325:1127–31.
6. Parsonnet J, Hanson S, Rodriguez L. *Helicobacter pylori* infection and gastric MALT lymphoma. N Engl J Med. 1994;330:1267–71.
7. Blaser MJ. *Helicobacter pylori*: its role in disease. J Clin Infect. 1992;15:386–93.
8. Lee A, Fox JG, Hazell S. Pathogenicity of *Helicobacter pylori*: a perspective. Infect Immun. 1993; 61:1601–10.
9. Fox JG. In vivo models of gastric *Helicobacter* infections. In: Hunt RH, Tytgat G, editors. *Helicobacter pylori*: Basic mechanisms to clinical cure. Dordrecht: Kluwer; 1994:3–27.

10. Marshall BJ, Armstrong JA, McGechie B, Glancy RJ. Attempt to fulfill Koch's postulates for pyloric *Campylobacter*. Med J Aust. 1985;142:436–9.
11. Morris A, Nicholson G. Ingestion of *Campylopyloridis* causes gastritis and raised fasting gastric pH. Am J Gastroenterol. 1987;82:192–9.
12. Krakowka S, Morgan DR, Kraft WG *et al*. Establishment of gastric *Campylobacter pylori* infection in the neonatal gnotobiotic piglet. Infect Immun. 1987;55:2789–96.
13. Yoshihiro F, Yamamoto I, Tonokatsu Y, Tamura K, Shimoyama T. Inoculation of animals with human *Helicobacter pylori* and long-term investigation of *Helicobacter pylori*-associated gastritis. Eur J Gastroenterol Hepatol. 1992;4:S39–44.
14. Cantorna MT, Balish E. Inability of human clinical isolates of *Helicobacter pylori* to colonize the alimentary tract of germ-free rodents. Can J Microbiol. 1990;36:237–41.
15. Fox JG, Otto G, Murphy JC *et al*. Gastric colonization of the ferret with *Helicobacter* species: natural and experimental infections. Rev Infect Dis. 1991;13(Suppl. 8):S671–80.
16. Bronsdon MA, Goodwin CS, Sly LI. *Helicobacter nemestrinae* sp. nov., a spiral bacterium found in the stomach of a pigtailed macaque (*Macaca nemestrina*). Int J Syst Bacteriol. 1991;41: 148–53.
17. Eaton KA, Dewhirst FE, Radin MJ. *Helicobacter acinonyx* sp. nov., isolated from cheetahs with gastritis. Int J Syst Bacteriol. 1993;43:99–106.
18. Fox JG, Taylor NS, Edmonds P. *Campylobacter pylori* subspecies *mustelae* subsp. nov. isolated from the gastric mucosa of ferrets (*Mustela putorius furo*), and an emended description of *Campylobacter pylori*. Int J Syst Bacteriol. 1988;38:367–70.
19. Fox JG, Chilvers T, Goodwin CS. *Campylobacter mustelae*, a new species resulting from the elevation of *Campylobacter pylori* subsp. *mustelae* to species status. Int J Syst Bacteriol. 1989;39: 301–3.
20. Lee A, Hazell SL, O'Rourke J. Isolation of a spiral-shaped bacterium from the cat stomach. Infect Immun. 1988;56:2843–50.
21. Paster BJ, Lee A, Fox JG. Phylogeny of *Helicobacter felis* sp. nov., *Helicobacter mustelae*, and related bacteria. Int J Syst Bacteriol. 1991;41:31–8.
22. Hanninen ML, Happonen I, Saari S. Culture and characteristics of *Helicobacter bizzozeronii*, a new canine gastric *Helicobacter* sp. Int J Syst Bacteriol. 1996;46:160–6.
23. Lambert JR, Borromes M, Pinkard KJ *et al*. Colonization of gnotobiotic piglets with *Campylobacter pyloridis* – an animal model? [letter]. J Infect Dis. 1987;155:1344.
24. Radin JM, Eaton KA, Krakowka S *et al*. *Helicobacter pylori* infection in gnotobiotic beagle dogs. Infect Immun. 1990;58:2606–12.
25. Baskerville A, Newell DG. Naturally occurring chronic gastritis and *C. pylori* infection in the rhesus monkey: a potential model for gastritis in man. Gut. 1988;29:465–72.
26. Dubois A, Fiala N, Heman-Ackah LM. Natural gastric infection with *Helicobacter pylori* in monkeys: a model for spiral bacteria infection in humans. Gastroenterology. 1994;106:1405–17.
27. Handt LK, Fox JG, Dewhirst FE *et al*. *Helicobacter pylori* isolated from the domestic cat: public health implications. Infect Immun. 1994;62:2367–74.
28. Handt LK, Fox JG, Stalis IH *et al*. Characterization of feline *Helicobacter pylori* strains and associated gastritis in a colony of domestic cats. J Clin Microbiol. 1995;33:2280–9.
29. Karita M, Kouchiyama T, Okita K, Nakazawa T. New small animal model for human gastric *Helicobacter pylori* infection: success in both nude and euthymic mice. Am J Gastroenterol. 1991; 86:1596–603.
30. Karita M, Li Q, Cantero D, Okita K. Establishment of a small animal model for human *H. pylori* infection using germ-free mouse. Am J Gastroenterol. 1994;89:208–13.
31. Marchetti M, Arico B, Burroni D, Figura N, Rappuoli R, Ghiara P. Development of a mouse model of *Helicobacter pylori* infection that mimics human disease. Science. 1995;267:1655–8.
32. Fox JG, Batchelder M, Marini RP *et al*. *Helicobacter pylori* induced gastritis in the domestic cat. Infect Immun. 1995;63:2674–81.
33. Finlay BB, Falkow S. Common themes in microbial pathogenicity. Microbiol Rev. 1989;53: 210–30.
34. Eaton KA, Morgan DR, Krakowka S. *Campylobacter pylori* virulence factors in gnotobiotic piglets. Infect Immun. 1989;57:1119–25.
35. Leying H, Suerbaum S, Geis G, Haas R. Cloning and genetic characterization of a *Helicobacter pylori* flagellin gene. Mol Microbiol. 1992;6:2863–74.
36. Kostrzynska M, Betts JD, Austin JW, Trust TJ. Identification, characterization, and spatial localization of two flagellin species in *Helicobacter pylori* flagella. J Bacteriol. 1991;173:937–46.

37. Suerbaum S, Josenhans D, Labigne A. Cloning and genetic characterization of the *Helicobacter pylori* and *Helicobacter mustelae* flaB flagellin genes and construction of *H. pylori* flaA- and flaB-negative mutants by electroporation-mediated allelic exchange. J Bacteriol. 1993;175: 3278–88.

38. Haas R, Meyer JF, Putten JPMV. A flagellated mutants of *Helicobacter pylori* generated by genetic transformation of naturally competent strains using transposon shuttle mutagenesis. Mol Microbiol. 1993;8:753–60.

39. Josenhans C, Labigne A, Suerbaum S. Comparative ultrastructural and functional studies of *Helicobacter pylori* and *Helicobacter mustelae* flagellin mutants: both flagellin subunits, FlaA and FlaB, are necessary for full motility in *Helicobacter* species. J Bacteriol. 1995;177:3010–20.

40. Eaton K, Suerbaum S, Josenhans C, Krakowka S. Colonization of gnotobiotic piglets by *H. pylori* deficient in two flagellin genes. Infect Immun. 1996;64:2445–8.

41. Hazell SL, Lee A, Brady L *et al*. *Campylobacter pyloridis* and gastritis: association with intercellular spaces and adaption to an environment of mucus as important factors in colonization of the gastric epithelium. J Infect Dis. 1986;153:658–63.

42. Hazell SL, Lee A. *Campylobacter pyloridis*, urease, hydrogen ion back diffusion and gastric ulcers. Lancet. 1986;2:15–17.

43. Eaton KA, Brooks CL, Morgan DR, Krakowka S. Essential role of urease in pathogenesis of gastritis induced by *Helicobacter pylori* in gnotobiotic piglets. Infect Immun. 1991;59:2470–5.

44. Labigne A, Cussac V, Courcoux P. Shuttle cloning and nucleotide sequences of *Helicobacter pylori* genes responsible for urease activity. J Bacteriol. 1992;173:1920–31.

45. Ferrero RL, Cussav C, Courcoux P, Labigne A. Construction of isogenic urease-negative mutants of *Helicobacter pylori* by allelic exchange. J Bacteriol. 1992;174:4212–17.

46. Eaton KA, Krakowka S. Effect of gastric pH on urease-dependent colonization of gnotobiotic piglets by *Helicobacter pylori*. Infect Immun. 1994;62:3604–7.

47. Tsuda M, Karita M, Morshed MG, Okira K, Nakazawa T. A urease-negative mutant of *Helicobacter pylori* constructed by allelic exchange mutagenesis lacks the ability to colonize the nude mouse stomach. Infect Immun. 1994;62:3586–9.

48. Leunk RD, Johnson PT, David BC, Kraft WG, Morgan DR. Cytotoxic activity in broth-culture filtrates of *Campylobacter pylori*. J Med Microbiol. 1988;26:93–9.

49. Figura N, Guglielmetti P, Rossolini A *et al*. Cytotoxin production by *Campylobacter pylori* strains isolated from patients with peptic ulcers and from patients with chronic gastritis only. J Clin Microbiol. 1989;27:225–6.

50. Fox JG, Correa P, Taylor NS *et al*. High prevalence and persistence of cytotoxin-positive *Helicobacter pylori* strains in a population at increased risk of gastric cancer. Am J Gastroenterol. 1992,87.1554–60.

51. Cover TJ, Vaughn SG, Cao P, Blaser MJ. Potentiation of *Helicobacter pylori* vacuolating toxin activity by nicotine and other weak bases. J Infect Dis. 1992;166:1073–8.

52. Covacci A, Censini S, Bugnoli M *et al*. Molecular characterization of the 128-kDa immunodominant antigen of *Helicobacter pylori* associated with cytotoxicity and duodenal ulcer. Proc Natl Acad Sci USA. 1993;90:5791–5.

53. Tummuru MK, Cover TL, Blaser MJ. Cloning and expression of a high molecular-mass major antigen of *Helicobacter pylori*: evidence of linkage to cytotoxicity. Infect Immun. 1993;61: 1799–809.

54. Papini E, Bugnoli M, Bernard MD, Figura N, Rappuoli R, Montecucco C. Bafilomycin-A1 inhibits *Helicobacter pylori*-induced vacuolization of HeLa cells. Mol Microbiol. 1993;7:323–7.

55. Schmitt W, Haas R. Genetic analysis of the *Helicobacter pylori* vacuolating cytotoxin: structural similarities with the IgA protease type of exported protein. Mol Microbiol. 1994;12:307–19.

56. Eaton KA, Cover T, Tummuru MKR, Blaser MJ, Krakowka S. The role of vacuolating cytotoxin in gastritis due to *H. pylori* in gnotobiotic piglets, abstr 2434. In: Abstracts of the Meeting of the American Gastroenterological Association 1996. American Gastroenterological Association, San Francisco, CA.

57. Ghiara P, Marchetti M, Blaser MJ, et al. Role of the *Helicobacter pylori* virulence factor vacuolating cytotoxin, CagA, and urease in a mouse model of disease. Infect Immun. 1995;63: 4154–60.

58. Phadnis SH, Ilver D, Janzon L, Normark S, Westblom TU. Pathological significance and molecular characterization of the vacuolating toxin gene of *Helicobacter pylori*. Infect Immun. 1994;62: 1557–65.

59. Telford JL, Dell'Orco M, Burroni D *et al.* Molecular analysis of the *Helicobacter pylori* cytotoxin gene. Eur J Gastroenterol Hepatol. 1993;5:S22–4.
60. Telford JL, Ghiara P, Dell'Orco M *et al.* Gene structure of the *Helicobacter pylori* cytotoxin and evidence of its key role in gastric disease. J Exp Med. 1994;179:1653–8.
61. Sobola GM, Crabtree JE, Dixon MF *et al.* Acute *Helicobacter pylori* infection: clinical features, local and systemic immune response, gastric mucosal histology, and gastric juice ascorbic acid concentration. Gut. 1991;32:1415–18.
62. Mitchell HM, Hazell SL, Kolesnikow R, Mitchell J, Frommer D. Antigen recognition during progression from acute to chronic infection with a *cagA*-positive strain of *Helicobacter pylori.* Infect Immun. 1996;64:1166–72.
63. McColm AA, Bagshaw J, O'Malley C, McLaren A. Development of a mouse model of gastric colonisation with *Helicobacter pylori.* Gut. 1995;37(Suppl. 1);A50.
64. Kleanthous H, Tibbitts T, Bakios TJ *et al. In vivo* selection of a highly adapted *H. pylori* isolate and the development of an *H. pylori* mouse model for studying vaccine efficacy and attenuating lesions. Gut. 1995;37(Suppl. 1);A94.
65. Fox JG, Edrise BM, Cabot E *et al. Campylobacter*-like organisms isolated from gastric mucosa of ferrets. Am J Vet Res. 1986;47:236–9.
66. Fox JG, Cabot EB, Taylor NS *et al.* Gastric colonization of *Campylobacter pylori* subsp. *mustelae* in ferrets. Infect Immun. 1988;56:2994–6.
67. Fox JG, Correa P, Taylor NS *et al. Helicobacter mustelae* associated gastritis in ferrets: an animal model of *Helicobacter pylori* gastritis in humans. Gastroenterology. 1990;99:352–61.
68. Gottfried MR, Washington K, Harrell LJ. *Helicobacter pylori*-like microorganisms and chronic active gastritis in ferrets. Am J Gastroenterol. 1990;85:813–18.
69. Tompkins DS, Wyatt JI, Rathbone BJ *et al.* The characterization and pathological significance of gastric *Campylobacter*-like organisms in the ferret: a model for chronic gastritis? Epidemiol Infect. 1988;101:269–78.
70. Morris A, Thomasen L, Tasman-Jones C *et al.* Failure to detect gastric *Campylobacter*-like organisms in a group of ferrets in New Zealand. NZ Med J. 1988;101:275.
71. O'Rourke J, Lee A, Fox JG. An ultrastructural study of *Helicobacter mustelae*: evidence of a specific association with gastric mucosa. J Med Microbiol. 1992;36:420–7.
72. Chen XG, Correa P, Offerhaus J *et al.* Ultrastructure of the gastric mucosa harboring *Campylobacter*-like organisms. Am J Clin Pathol. 1986;86:575–82.
73. Gold BD, Huesca M, Sherman PM *et al. Helicobacter mustelae* and *Helicobacter pylori* bind to common lipid receptors *in vitro.* Infect Immun. 1993;61:2632–8.
74. Gold B, Dytoc M, Huesca M *et al.* Comparison of *Helicobacter mustelae* and *Helicobacter pylori* adhesion to eukaryotic cells *in vitro.* Gastroenterology. 1995;109:692–700.
75. Gold BD, Islur P, Policova Z, Czinn S, Neumann AW, Sherman PM. Surface properties of *H. mustelae* and ferret gastrointestinal mucosa. Clin Invest Med. 1996;19:92–100.
76. Northfield TC. Decreased hydrophobicity of gastroduodenal mucosa due to *H. pylori* infection in humans. In: Hunt RH, Tytgat G, editors. *Helicobacter pylori*: basic mechanisms to clinical cure. Dordrecht: Kluwer; 1994:139–47.
77. O'Toole PW, Austin JW, Trust TJ. Identification and molecular characterization of a major ring-forming surface protein from the gastric pathogen *Helicobacter mustelae.* Mol Microbiol. 1994; 11:349–61.
78. Kay WW, Trust TJ. Form and function of the regular surface array of *Aeromonas salmonicida.* Experientia. 1991;47:412–14.
79. Schauer DB, Fox JG. Examining the surface of a gastric pathogen. Trends Microbiol. 1994;2: 219–20.
80. Solnick J, Josenhans C, Suerbaum S, Tompkins L, Labigne A. Construction and characterization of an isogenic urease-negative mutant of *Helicobacter mustelae.* Infect Immun. 1995;63: 3718–23.
81. Andrutis KA, Fox JG, Schauer DB *et al.* Identification of a *cagA* gene in *Helicobacter mustelae.* Gut. 1995;37(Suppl. 1):A30.
82. Andrutis KA, Fox JG, Josenhans C, Suerbaum S. Infection of the ferret stomach by isogenic flagellar mutant strains of *Helicobacter mustelae,* abstr 1203. In: Abstracts of the Meeting of the American Gastroenterological Association 1996. American Gastroenterological Association, San Francisco, CA.
83. Andrutis KA, Fox JG, Schauer DB *et al.* Inability of an isogenic urease-negative mutant strain of *Helicobacter mustelae* to colonize the ferret stomach. Infect Immun. 1995;63:3722–5.

84. Perkins SE, Fox JG, Walsh JH. *Helicobacter mustelae* associated hypergastrinemia in ferrets (*Mustelae putorius furo*). Am J Vet Res. 1996;57:147–50.

85. Fox JG, Paster BJ, Dewhirst FE *et al*. *Helicobacter mustelae* isolation from feces of ferrets: evidence to support fecal–oral transmission of a gastric *Helicobacter*. Infect Immun. 1992; 60:606–11.

86. Fox JG, Otto G, Taylor NS *et al*. *Helicobacter mustelae*-induced gastritis and elevated gastric pH in the ferret (*Mustela putorius furo*). Infect Immun. 1991;59:1875–80.

87. Fox JG, Blanco M, Yan L *et al*. Role of gastric pH in isolation of *Helicobacter mustelae* from the feces of ferrets. Gastroenterology. 1993;104:86–92.

88. Thomas JE, Gibson GR, Darboe MK *et al*. Isolation of *Helicobacter pylori* from human feces. Lancet. 1992;340:1194–5.

89. Kelly SM, Pitcher MCL, Farmery SM *et al*. Isolation of *Helicobacter pylori* from feces of patients with dyspepsia in the United Kingdom. Gastroenterology. 1994;107:1671–4.

90. Doenges JL. Spirochetes in the gastric glands of macacas rhesus and of man without related disease. Arch Pathol. 1939;27:469–77.

91. Bronsdon MA, Schoenknecht FD. *Campylobacter pylori* isolated from the stomach of the monkey, *Macaca nemistrina*. J Clin Microbiol. 1988;26:1725 –8.

92. Newell DG, Hudson MJ, Baskerville A. Isolation of a gastric *Campylobacter*-like organism from the stomach of four rhesus monkeys, and identification as *Campylobacter pylori*. J Med Microbiol. 1988;27:41–4.

93. Curry A, Jones DM, Eldridge J. Spiral organism in the baboon stomach. Lancet. 1987;2:634–5.

94. Euler AR, Zurenko GE, Moe JB *et al*. Evaluation of two monkey species (*Macaca mulatta* and *Macaca fascicularis*) as possible models for human *Helicobacter pylori* disease. J Clin Microbiol. 1990;28:2285–90.

95. Dubois A, Tarnawski A, Newell DG *et al*. Gastric injury and invasion of parietal cells by spiral bacteria in rhesus monkeys: are gastritis and hyperchlorhydria infectious diseases? Gastroenterology. 1991;100:884–91.

96. Sly LI, Bronsdon MA, Bowman JP *et al*. The phylogenetic position of *Helicobacter nemestrinae*. Int J Syst Bacteriol. 1993;43:386–7.

97. Drazek ES, Dubois A, Holmes RK. Characterization and presumptive identification of *Helicobacter pylori* isolates from rhesus monkeys. J Clin Microbiol. 1994;32:1799–804.

98. Akopyants NS, Eaton KA, Berg DE. Adaptive mutation and cocolonization during *Helicobacter pylori* infection of gnotobiotic piglets. Infect Immun. 1995;63:116–21.

99. Hazell SL, Eichberg JW, Lee RD *et al*. Selection of the chimpanzee over the baboon as a model for *Helicobacter pylori* infection. Gastroenterology. 1992;103:848–54.

100. Fujioka T, Shuto R, Kodama R *et al*. Experimental model for chronic gastritis with *Helicobacter pylori*: long term follow up study in *H. pylori*-infected Japanese macaques. Eur J Gastroenterol Hepatol. 1993;S1:S73–7.

101. Fukuda Y, Yamamoto I, Tonokatsu Y *et al*. Inoculation of rhesus monkeys with human *Helicobacter pylori*: a long-term investigation on gastric mucosa by endoscopy. Dig Endosc. 1992;4:19–30.

102. Shuto R, Fujioka T, Kubota I *et al*. Experimental gastritis induced by *Helicobacter pylori* in Japanese monkeys. Infect Immun. 1993;61:933–9.

103. Fujiyama K, Fujioka T, Murakami K *et al*. Effects of *Helicobacter pylori* on gastric mucosal defense factors in Japanese monkeys. J Gastroenterol. 1995;30:441–6.

104. Heilmann KL, Borchard F. Gastritis due to spiral shaped bacteria other than *Helicobacter pylori*: clinical, histological, and ultrastructural findings. Gut. 1991;32:137–40.

105. Stolte M, Wellens E, Bethke B. *Helicobacter heilmannii* (formerly *Gastrospirillum hominis*) gastritis: an infection transmitted by animals? Scand J Gastroenterol. 1994;29:1061–4.

106. Fox JG, Perkins S, Shen Z *et al*. Local immune response in *Helicobacter pylori* infected cats and identification of *H. pylori* in saliva, gastric fluid and feces. Immunology. 1996;88: 400–6.

107. Otto G, Hazell SH, Fox JG *et al*. Animal and public health implications of gastric colonization of cats by *Helicobacter*-like organisms. J Clin Microbiol. 1994;32:1043–9.

108. Henry GA, Long PH, Burns JL *et al*. Gastric spirillosis in beagles. Am J Vet Res. 1987;48: 831–6.

109. Eaton KA, Radin MJ, Kramer L *et al*. Epizoonotic gastritis associated with gastric spiral bacilli in cheetahs (*Acinonyx jubatus*). Vet Pathol. 1993;30:55–63.

110. Lockard VG, Boler RK. Ultrastructure of a spiraled microorganism in the gastric mucosa of dogs. Am J Vet Res. 1970;31:1453–62.
111. Lavelle JP, Landas S, Mitros FA *et al.* Acute gastritis associated with spiral organisms from cats. Dig Dis Sci. 1994;39:744–50.
112. Salomon H. Über das Spirillum des Säugetiermagens und sein Verhalten zu den Belegzellen. Zentralbl Baketeriol Parasitenkd Infektionskr Hyg Abt. 1898;119:422–41.
113. Lee A, Fox JG, Otto G *et al.* A small animal model of human *Helicobacter pylori* active chronic gastritis. Gastroenterology. 1990;99:1315–23.
114. Fox JG, Blanco M, Murphy JC *et al.* Local and systemic immune response in murine *Helicobacter felis* active chronic gastritis. Infect Immun. 1993;61:2309–15.
115. Mohammadi M, Redline R, Nedrud J *et al.* Role of the host in pathogenesis of *Helicobacter*-associated gastritis: *H. felis* infection of inbred and congenic mouse strains. Infect Immun. 1996;64:238–45.
116. Sakagami T, Shimoyama T, O'Rourke J *et al.* Back to the host: severity of inflammation induced by *Helicobacter felis* in different strains of mice. Am J Gastroenterol. 1994;89:1345 (abstract 241).
117. Fox JG, Li X, Cahill RJ *et al.* Hypertrophic gastropathy in *Helicobacter felis* infected wild type C57Bl/6 mice and p53 hemizygous transgenic mice. Gastroenterology. 1996;110:155–66.
118. Enno A, O'Rourke JL, Howlett CR, Jack A, Dixon MF, Lee A. MALToma-like lesions in the murine gastric mucosa after long-term infection with *Helicobacter felis*. Am J Pathol. 1995; 147:217–23.
119. Chen M-H, Lee A, Hazell S *et al.* Immunisation against gastric *Helicobacter* infection in a mouse/*Helicobacter felis* model [letter]. Lancet. 1992;339:1120–1.
120. Czinn SJ, Cai A, Nedrud JG. Protection of germ-free mice from infection by *Helicobacter felis* after active oral or passive IgA immunization. Vaccine. 1993;11:637–42.
121. Ferrero RL, Thieberge JM, Huerre M, Labigne A. Recombinant antigens prepared from the urease subunits of *Helicobacter* spp.: evidence of protection in a mouse model of gastric infection. Infect Immun. 1994;62:4981–9.
122. Michetti P, Corthesy-Theulaz I, Davin C *et al.* Immunization of BALB/c mice against *Helicobacter felis* infection with *Helicobacter pylori* urease. Gastroenterology. 1994;107: 1002–11.
123. Pappo J, Thomas W, Kabok Z, Taylor NS, Murphy JC, Fox JG. Effect of oral immunization with recombinant urease on murine *Helicobacter felis* gastritis. Infect Immun. 1995;63:1246–53.
124. Doidge C, Gust I, Lee A. Therapeutic immunization against *Helicobacter* infection (letter). Lancet. 1994;343:914–5.
125. Engstrand L, Rosberg K, Hubinette R, Berglindh T, Rolfsen W, Gustavsson S. Topographic mapping of *Helicobacter pylori* colonization in long-term infected pigs. Infect Immun. 1992; 60:653–6.
126. Eaton KA, Morgan DR, Krakowka S. Persistence of *Helicobacter pylori* in conventionalized piglets. J Infect Dis. 1990;161:1299–301.
127. Eaton KA, Radin MJ, Krakowka S. Animal model of gastric ulcer due to bacterial gastritis in mice. Vet Pathol. 1995;32:489–97.
128. Fox JG, Otto G, Lee A, Taylor NS, Murphy JC. *Helicobacter felis* gastritis in gnotobiotic rats: an animal model of *H. pylori* gastritis. Infect Immun. 1991;59:785–91.
129. Lee A, Krakowka S, Fox JG, Otto G, Murphy JC. *Helicobacter felis* as a cause of lympho-reticular hyperplasia in the dog stomach. Vet Pathol. 1992;29:487–94.
130. Takagi H, Jhappan C, Sharp R, Merlino G. Hypertrophic gastropathy resembling Menetrier's disease in transgenic mice overexpressing transforming growth factor α in the stomach. J Clin Invest. 1992;90:1161–7.

3
Genetic bases for heterogeneity of *Helicobacter pylori*

M. J. BLASER

INTRODUCTION

Diversity, a characteristic of all living things, has long been recognized among microorganisms and has been well appreciated among bacteria[1]. For pathogenic microbes, those whose lifestyle results in injury to their larger hosts, a central notion is that these often represent clonal populations. In this context clonality represents a common ancestry, and a very close if not identical genetic relationship among the members of a group.

It has been proposed that pathogens often began their existence as organisms of low virulence which then acquired a new genotype, conferring on them a selective advantage over their cousins that did not so change. For example, the first in a population of obligate parasites that acquires a new mechanism to efficiently extract iron from its larger host gains an important advantage over the other organisms in its ecological niche, allowing the favoured propagation of its genome. Over time, the organism with the favoured genome replaces the others in the niche because of its selective advantage. Examination of the population at this point would show a highly clonal distribution, unless there were on-going genetic exchange among members of the population[1].

Successful pathogens of humans that are highly clonal include *Mycobacterium tuberculosis* and *Shigella dysenteriae*[2,3]. Examination of strains of these organisms obtained from around the world shows only minute differences in their genome[2,3]. For *M. tuberculosis*, strains cannot be readily differentiated by examination of bacterial genes that encode a variety of housekeeping or virulence functions. Rather, they can be differentiated by examination of the location of a more-recently acquired genetic element, an insertion sequence (IS*610*), that has itself parasitized the *M. tuberculosis* chromosome[2]. For *Shigella dysenteriae* there are few genomic differences among strains distributed widely geographically and in time[3,4], and most of the variation observed involves plasmids, extra-chromosomal elements that replicate autonomously, and have vastly different phylogenetic origins. With these noted exceptions, these two human pathogens are highly clonal.

Table 1 Types of genomic diversity observed in *H. pylori* strains

Type	Example
Point mutations	RFLP and sequence variation (e.g. ureB)
Mosaicism	*vacA*
Non-conserved genes	*cag* island
Size polymorphism of particular genes	*cagA*
Insertion sequences	IS*605*
Chromosomal rearrangements	IS*605*-mediated
Plasmids	pHPM180

In contrast, the human pathogen *Helicobacter pylori* is highly diverse at a genetic level. Many different mechanisms contribute to its diversity (Table 1). In this chapter I will review the characteristics of this seeming paradox, and then explore reasons for the observations that have been made.

DIVERSITY DUE TO SINGLE BASE-PAIR VARIATION

Examination of the genome of *H. pylori* for restriction fragment length polymorphism (RFLP) shows that virtually every strain has its own profile. So strong and consistent is this observation that this phenomenon can be used for typing of *H. pylori* strains, whether by restriction endonuclease analysis (REA), or RFLP of polymerase chain reaction (PCR) products, or using random arbitrarily primed (RAP)-PCR[5-12]. Examination of the heterogeneity indicates that much of this phenomenon results from variation of single base-pairs. For example, in a study of the sequence of *ureC*, a highly conserved gene among all *H. pylori* strains, for a 210 bp region, each of 29 strains showed a different primary sequence[13]. Examination of these sequences indicates that much of the variation is synonymous (or silent), in which alternative codons will permit translation of the same amino acid in the expressed protein[12,13]. However, non-synonymous substitutions also exist. The ratio of synonymous to non-synonymous substitutions at a given locus provides a measure of the degree of conservation that is required at that locus. For *ureC*, part of the urease operon that is highly conserved not only among *H. pylori* strains, but also among other organisms, there clearly is much selective pressure to maintain particular protein sequence conservation. Nevertheless, the highly diverse nucleotide sequences, described by Kansau *et al.*[13], are indicative of the considerable variation among *H. pylori* strains. Whether these differences represent an ancient origin, a high mutation rate, and/or relatively inefficient DNA error-recognition or repair is presently unknown.

MOSAICISM OF *H. PYLORI* GENES

The structure of *vacA*, the gene encoding the vacuolating cytotoxin of *H. pylori*, represents a mosaic[14]. Although only about 50% of the *H. pylori* strains express this toxin *in vitro*, essentially all strains possess *vacA*; however, there is considerable heterogeneity in the structure of *vacA*. Two regions, one encoding the carboxyl-terminus of the pro-toxin and the other encoding a region near the amino terminus, appear relatively conserved from strain to strain. However, in two other regions considerable diversity exists. In the middle region there is sufficient diversity to define two allelic types, termed m1 and m2. In the region encoding the signal sequence there are three allelic types, termed s1a, s1b, and s2; the two former types are closely related to one another, yet distinct. With three s-types and two m-types, a total of six possibilities exist, and from examination of 62 isolates from US patients we have observed five of the combinations; however, we have not yet observed a strain of the s2m1 genotype[14]. The otherwise relatively random combinations of s- and m-types amid the relatively conserved regions of *vacA* observed among strains indicate that *vacA* is a mosaic gene. The origin of this mosaicism is not known; however, the most likely explanation is recombination among *H. pylori* strains with the recombinants possessing novel genotypes. One observation that supports this hypothesis is that *H. pylori* strains are naturally competent; that is, able to take up and incorporate foreign DNA from other strains into the genome through recombination[15,16].

NON-CONSERVED GENES

Certain *H. pylori* strains possess high (120–140kDa) molecular weight proteins that are highly antigenic[17,18]. These proteins have been called the CagA proteins, and they are encoded by *cagA*[19,20]. We now know that strains which do not express these proteins lack *cagA*; thus *cagA* was the first *H. pylori* gene to be described that is not conserved in all strains. The function of CagA is unknown. After *cagA* was identified, it became clear that it was part of a group of genes now called the *cag* pathogenicity island[21,22]. This region of about 40kb encodes approximately 20 genes including *cagA* and the adjacent *picA* and *picB*[23], and apparently has a different guanosine plus cytosine (G+C) content and third-codon preference than does the remainder of the *H. pylori* chromosome (Covacci A., personal communication, see Chapter 4 and Thompson S., personal communication), suggesting a different phylogenetic origin. For other pathogens the presence of a pathogenicity island represents a group of genes that enhance virulence, which may, in fact, be the reason for the clonality of those strains. Interestingly, strains possessing *cagA* and its adjacent genes are more virulent than *cagA⁻* strains. That the cag island is not present in all strains, and that its DNA content differs from the remainder of the genome, suggests that it was acquired after the ancestral chromosome.

VARIATION IN NUMBER OF INTRAGENIC CASSETTES

Examination of the structure of *cagA* indicates that a number of DNA repeats are present[19,20]. These elements, which range up to 102bp, have been found to be present in up to five copies, and account for the observed heterogeneity in the size of the *cagA* product. We have observed that, rather than being a fixed characteristic of each strain, size variation can occur, at least *in vitro*.

INSERTION SEQUENCES

Recognition of the *cag* island led to the identification of a novel insertion sequence, which has been named IS*605*. IS*605* includes two open reading frames, in opposite orientations that bear strong homology to the transposases of IS*200* and IS*1341*[24]. In studies of 85 strains from persons from seven countries we have found that IS*605* is present in 31%[25]. Interestingly, it is present at nearly equal frequency in strains that hybridize with a probe to *cagA*, indicating that it may be present independent of the *cag* island. A single strain may have multiple copies of IS*605*[24,25]. Whether IS*605* has retained the ability to transpose, or represents the remnant of a mobile genetic element, is not yet known.

CHROMOSOMAL REARRANGEMENTS

Comparison of physical maps of a variety of *E. coli* strains shows that each has a similar organization, in that position of various genes in relation to one another is highly conserved. In contrast, for *H. pylori*, genome maps of two different strains show completely different patterns[26,27]. This observation suggests that there has been extensive rearrangement of the chromosome of these two strains in relation to each other. That such rearrangement can occur has been documented by studies of the *cag* island. In strain NCTC 11367 the *cag* island exists in two parts, each bordered by IS*605*, but about 400 kb apart in the genome. In contrast, in the strains examined by Covacci *et al.* the island is intact. These findings suggest that rearrangement of *H. pylori* chromosomal DNA can occur through homologous recombination involving these repetitive IS*605* elements. Whether other mechanisms exist for chromosomal rearrangement has not been established.

PLASMIDS

Surveys of *H. pylori* strains have indicated that 35–75% possess plasmids[28–31]. In part, this range may reflect differences in techniques used by various investigators to isolate plasmid DNA. The nucleotide sequence of several plasmids is known, and there appears to be sequence conservation among a fraction of the plasmids[31,32]. Heterogeneity of plasmids may be useful for epidemiological analysis of *H. pylori* strains, as well as providing information on the evolution and virulence of these organisms.

CONCLUSIONS

The central question to consider is why a pathogenic organism such as *H. pylori* is so diverse. One possibility is that its diversity is an indication of the long duration of its interaction with humans and our ancestors. Observations consistent with an ancient origin of *H. pylori* are summarized in Table 2.

If the hypothesis that *H. pylori* infection of humans is ancient is correct, then it becomes easier to understand the profound diversity of these organisms.

Table 2 Evidence that *H. pylori* infection of humans is of ancient origin

1. Extensive genetic heterogeneity of *H. pylori*.
2. Digestive organs with acid-secreting epithelium (stomachs) arose early (300 million years) in vertebrate evolution.
3. Bacteria of *Helicobacter* genus are highly prevalent in the stomach of many vertebrates.
4. Organisms indistinguishable from *H. pylori* are widely present in the stomach of non-human primates.
5. Among human populations in developing countries *H. pylori* infection is nearly universally present.
6. *H. pylori* is adapted for persistence in humans, essentially for the lifetime of the host.
7. There appears to be little, if any, selection by *H. pylori* for human genes (unlike *P. falciparum*).

Explanations for lack of clonality may include colonization of exclusive niches by different subgroups of organisms. Another possibility is that polymorphism has allowed for the development of cooperativity between groups of organisms. Finally, since humans, their ancestors, their environments, and their diets are diverse, the diversity of *H. pylori* may reflect selection for a variety of phenotypic characteristics, so that, for the population of *H. pylori* at large, a balanced polymorphism exists. The natural competence of *H. pylori* provides a mechanism for transmission of variant genomic sequences to a variety of strains.

We are just at the beginning of understanding the microbiology of *H. pylori*. Further studies will both help us understand this important human pathogen, and permit development of a model of the selective pressures on organisms whose lifestyle involves persistent colonization of mucosal surfaces of mammals.

Acknowledgements

This work was supported in part by RO1 DK 50837 from the National Institutes of Health and the Medical Research Service of the Department of Veterans Affairs.

References

1. Smith JM. Population genetics: an introduction. In: Smith JM, Neidhardt FC, editors. *Escherichia coli* and *Salmonella*. Cellular and molecular biology. Washington, DC: ASM Press; 1996:2685–90.
2. Hermans PMW, Van Soolingen D, Dale JW *et al*. Insertion element IS*906* from *Mycobacterium tuberculosis*: a useful tool for diagnosis and epidemiology of tuberculosis. J Clin Microbiol. 1990;28:2051–8.
3. Blaser MJ, Miotto K, Hopkins JA. Molecular probe analysis of *Shigella dysenteriae* type I isolates from 1940 to 1987. Int J Epidemiol. 1992;21:594–8.
4. Strockbine NA, Paronnet J, Greene K, Kiehlbauch JA, Wachsmuth IK. Molecular epidemiologic techniques in analysis of epidemic *Shigella dysenteriae* type 1 strains. J Infect Dis. 1991;163:406–9.
5. Salama SM, Jiang Q, Chang N, Sherbaniuk RW, Taylor DE. Characterization of chromosomal DNA profiles from *Helicobacter pylori* strains isolated from sequential gastric biopsies. J Clin Microbiol. 1995;33:2496–7.
6. Xia HX, Windle HJ, Marshall DG, Smyth CJ, Keane CT, Omorain CA. Recrudescence of *Helicobacter pylori* after apparently successful eradication: novel application of randomly amplified polymorphic DNA fingerprinting. Gut. 1995;37:30–4.
7. Fujimoto S, Marshall B, Blaser MJ. PCR-based restriction fragment length polymorphism typing of *Helicobacter pylori*. J Clin Microbiol. 1994;32:331–4.

8. Tee W, Lambert J, Smallwood R, Schembri M, Ross BC, Dwyer B. Ribotyping of *Helicobacter pylori* from clinical specimens. J Clin Microbiol. 1992;30:1562–7.

9. Clayton CL, Kleanthous H, Morgan DD, Puckey L, Tabaqchali S. Rapid fingerprinting of *Helicobacter pylori* by polymerase chain reaction and restriction fragment length polymorphism analysis. J Clin Microbiol. 1993;31:1420–5.

10. Lopez CR, Owen RJ, Desai M. Differentiation between isolates of *Helicobacter pylori* by PCR-RFLP analysis of urease A and B genes and comparison with ribosomal RNA gene patterns. FEMS Microbiol Lett. 1993;110:37–43.

11. Prewett EJ, Bickley J, Owen RJ, Pounder RE. DNA patterns of *Helicobacter pylori* isolated from gastric antrum, body, and duodenum. Gastroenterology. 1992;102:829–33.

12. Foxall PA, Hu LT, Mobley HL. Use of polymerase chain reaction-amplified *Helicobacter pylori* urease structural genes for differentiation of isolates. J Clin Microbiol. 1992;30:739–41.

13. Kansau I, Raymond J, Bingen E. Genotyping of *Helicobacter pylori* isolates by sequencing of PCR products and comparison with the RAPD technique. Res Microbiol. 1996 (In press).

14. Atherton JC, Cao P, Peek RM, Tummuru MKR, Blaser MJ, Cover TL. Mosaicism in vacuolating cytotoxin alleles of *Helicobacter pylori*; association of specific *vacA* types with cytotoxin production and peptic ulceration. J Biol Chem. 1995;270:17771–7.

15. Wang Y, Roos KP, Taylor DE. Transformation of *Helicobacter pylori* by chromosomal metronidazole resistance and by a plasmid with a selectable chloramphenicol resistance marker. J Gen Microbiol. 1993;139:2485–93.

16. Ferrero RL, Cussac V, Courcoux P, Labigne A. Construction of isogenic urease-negative mutants of *Helicobacter pylori* by allelic exchange. J Bacteriol. 1992;174:4212–17.

17. Cover TL, Dooley CP, Blaser MJ. Characterization of, and human serologic response to, proteins in *Helicobacter pylori* broth culture supernatants with vacuolizing cytotoxin activity. Infect Immun. 1990;58:603–10.

18. Crabtree JE, Taylor JD, Wyatt JI et al. Mucosal IgA recognition of *Helicobacter pylori* 120 kDa protein, peptic ulceration, and gastric pathology. Lancet. 1991;338:332–5.

19. Tummuru MKR, Cover TL, Blaser MJ. Cloning and expression of a high molecular weight major antigen of *Helicobacter pylori*: evidence of linkage to cytotoxin production. Infect Immun. 1993;61:1799–809.

20. Covacci A, Censini S, Bugnoli M et al. Molecular characterization of the 128-kDa immuno-dominant antigen of *Helicobacter pylori* associated with cytotoxicity and duodenal ulcer. Proc Natl Acad Sci USA. 1993;90:5791–5.·

21. Akopyants JS, Kersulyte D, Berg DE. *Cag*II, a new multigene locus associated with virulence in *Helicobacter pylori*. Gut. 1995;37(Suppl. 1):A1.

22. Lang N, Censini S, Xiang Z et al. The *cagI* chromosomal region of *Helicobacter pylori* is type-1 specific and encodes exporter molecules and invasion genes. 8th International Workshop on Campylobacters, Helicobacter and Related Organisms. Winchester, UK: 1995;E2/3 (abstract).

23. Tummuru MKR, Sharma SA, Blaser MJ. *Helicobacter pylori picB*, a homolog of the *Bordetella pertussis* toxin secretion protein, is required for induction of IL-8 in gastric epithelial cells. Mol Microbiol. 1995;18:867–76.

24. Kersulyte D, Akopyants NS, Clifton S, Roe BS, Berg DE. IS605, a novel chimaeric transposable element from *Helicobacter pylori*. Abstracts of the Annual Meeting of the American Society of Microbiology. Washington, DC: ASM Press; 1996;B–62 (abstract).

25. Höök-Nikanne J, Tummuru MKR, Kersulyte D et al. IS605, a novel transposable element, suitable for typing *Helicobacter pylori* infection *in vivo* as assessed by quantitative culture and histology. Gastroenterology. 1996;A135 (abstract).

26. Taylor DE, Eaton M, Chang N, Salama SM. Construction of a *Helicobacter pylori* genome map and demonstration of diversity at the genome level. J Bacteriol. 1992;174:6800–6.

27. Bukanov NO, Berg DE. Ordered cosmid library and high-resolution physical–genetic map of *Helicobacter pylori* strain NCTC11638. Mol Microbiol. 1994;11:509–23.

28. Penfold SS, Lastovica AJ, Elisha BG. Demonstration of plasmids in *Campylobacter pylori* (letter). J Infect Dis. 1988;157:850–1.

29. Simor AE, Shames B, Drumm B, Sherman P, Low DE, Penner JL. Typing of *Campylobacter pylori* by bacterial DNA restriction endonuclease analysis and determination of plasmid profile. J Clin Microbiol. 1990;28:83–6.

30. Tjia TN, Harper WES, Goodwin CS, Grubb WB. Plasmids in *Campylobacter pyloridi*. Microbiol Lett. 1987;36:7–11.

31. Minnis JA, Taylor TE, Knesek JE, Peterson WL, McIntire SA. Characterization of a 3.5-kbp plasmid from *Helicobacter pylori*. Plasmid. 1995;34:22–36.
32. Kleanthous H, Clayton CL, Tabaqchali S. Characterization of a plasmid from *Helicobacter pylori* encoding a replication protein common to plasmids in gram-positive bacteria. Mol Microbiol. 1991;5:2377–89.

4

Mobilis in mobile: unexpected flexibility and quantum leaps in the *Helicobacter pylori* genome

A. COVACCI

THE LOST LANGUAGE OF BACTERIA

Disparate theories have been put forward to explain the origin of the genomic complexity in the Gram-negative bacterium *Helicobacter pylori*[1-3]. We are tempted to assume that the rates for molecular evolution are constant and that the forces acting on a gene apparently are not specific. We easily realize that, in the case of organisms different from primates, the study of the distribution of several selected genes on a world scale, the tracing of a population's map, will, in the end, not be corroborated by converging disciplines such as anthropology and linguistics.

HUMAN VARIABILITY

In the human population genes are relatively less diverse, with the exception of the genes for immunoglobulins and T cell receptor, where geographic variability probably reflects the great variability of the epidemics. For example, no variations were found in a 729 bp intronic sequence of the ZFY gene from 38 human males sampled world-wide. In contrast the age of the human DBR1 lineage (a member of the human leucocyte antigen, HLA) yields a rate of 1.06×10^{-9} nucleotide substitutions per site per year (as calculated on the divergence of orangutan lineage, African apes and *Homo erectus*). Moreover, the V beta gene segments from a single donor exhibit only 75% identity at nucleotide level. The DNA of every organism embodies unlimited information about their evolutionary history. Further, pseudogenes and repetitive sequences contribute to a dynamic view of the evolutionary changes occurring on a complex locus[4].

NEUTRAL MUTATIONS

A close inspection of *H. pylori* genes (Gene Bank update 1-7-96 and refs 5–9), from clinical isolates sampled in different continents, reveals frequencies observed in human genes and in pathogens such as *Neisseria gonorrhoeae*. The gene for *hspb* has 2.56% of mutations accumulated as SNP (single nucleotide polymorphisms) (42 mutations/1638 residues) and 1.28% of mutated amino acid residues (single amino acid polymorphisms or SAP) (7/546). The *urea* gene has a SNP value of 2.81% (20/714) and a SAP value of 1.26% (3/238). The *ureb* shows a 2.51% SNP (42/1678) and a 1.79% SAP (10/559). The *vaca* gene has a SNP value of 5.45% (212/3888) and a SAP value of 3.36% (45/1340). The *caga* gene SNP is 4.31% (153/3549) and SAP is 7.39% (85/1150). In the last case the ratio between the combined first and second position and the third position of the codon is approximately 1.1:0.9. This is indirect evidence that the selective pressure on *H. pylori* genes is not uniform. The observation that most of the mutations are neutral is probably true for all the selected genes with the exception of *caga*. This gene has a high degree of polymorphism, is under continuous selection (expansion of duplicated motifs)[8] and breaks the rule of mutations accumulated in the neutral part of a codon (third position). If we only consider numerical values for identities, the genes of *H. pylori* have a behaviour that is shared with organisms ranging from the unicellular level to vertebrates, but if we calculate the accumulation of mutations in the third position our picture is increasingly complex and represents a phenomenon that is not ubiquitous in population genetics. It is worth mentioning that the exception is again focused on a gene that is a specific marker for more virulent strains which are always associated with more severe forms of gastroduodenal diseases.

A UNIFIED CLASSIFICATION

H. pylori strains isolated from chronic active gastritis and from more severe gastric and duodenal disease such as peptic ulcer and distal adenocarcinoma differ regarding the expression of the immunodominant antigen CagA (cytotoxin associated gene A)[8]. The large majority of bacteria associated with the severe diseases contain the *caga* gene and express the CagA antigen. In association with this antigen bacteria produce the vacuolating toxin VacA (vacuolating toxin gene A) that is responsible for cytopathic effects *in vitro* and *in vivo*[10]. The co-expression of both CagA and VacA is a very frequent phenomenon in strains that contain the *caga* gene, but is independent from the presence of this gene, since null *caga* mutants still express the VacA protein[11]. In most of the industrialized countries bacteria expressing CagA are close to 80% of the total isolates and more than 90% in China, Africa and India[12,13]. Since virulence factors such as urease, superoxide dismutase or flagellins are commonly produced by *H. pylori* associated with severe and non-severe disease we have concluded that CagA and VacA are a subset of virulence factors specific for strains associated with severe diseases, and need to be differentiated by the more general virulence factors that are regarded as absolute requirements for infection and long-term colonization[14], but that are not involved in the later stages of organ damage. Using as a marker the *caga* and *vaca* genes, the CagA and VacA proteins and the *in-vitro* assay for vacuolating activity we have grouped 43 different clinical isolates into two broad families, Type I and Type II with intermediate strains that belong to the Type I family[15]. This classification was proposed with the aim of separating one population of more virulent from one population of less virulent bacteria, and to indicate that the intermediate phenotype is the result of a process of attenuation of the virulence. Due to the incomplete distribution of the *caga* gene, that remarkably is present only in strains associated with severe diseases, we have shown that the major differences between Type I and Type II strains are a consequence of genes associated with the *caga* trait, and that the phenotype usually ascribed to *caga* is dependent on polygenes[16].

The cag locus

The region containing *caga* was identified as a 40 kb locus named cag[17]. On the basis of the G+C content, the cag region possibly originated from a plasmid or a phage, but not from a *Helicobacter pylori* operon. The G+C content was approximately 35%, a value similar to sequences originated from plasmids. Sequences located in the chromosome of *H. pylori* have shown a G+C content fluctuating around 38–45%. In the reference strain CCUG 17874, the cag region was found split into two parts, cagI and cagII (cagII: D. Berg et al., submitted), by an intervening sequence flanked on both sides by a copy of the IS*605*, a newly discovered insertion sequence (ref. 17 and D. Berg et al., submitted). From a comparative analysis of clinical isolates we have observed cag organized in the following ways: (i) cagI and cagII separated by an intervening sequence flanked by two IS*605*; (ii) cagI and cagII separated by an IS*605*; (iii) cag I and cag II fused without IS*605*; (iv) partial or total deletion of cag I but not cag II against a background of multiple copies of IS*605*; (v) total absence of cag I and cag II and no IS*605* sequences. While (i), (ii), (iv) and (v) included more than one strain for each group, the group classified (iii) was the most abundant, with at least 14 different strains. The presence of the two direct repeats of 31 bp at the ends of cag without apparent duplicated sequences in the cagI/cagII interface, suggested that the cagI and cagII were acquired originally as a single unit, inserted into the glutamate racemase gene and that the presence of IS*605* into cag occurred more recently. The IS*605* was flanked by two ends having dyadic symmetry. This new IS included two transposases resembling analogous genes in Gram-negative and thermophyllic bacteria. More than 52% of the bacteria contained one copy of IS*605*, with several strains harbouring at least seven copies per genome equivalent.

The cag pathogenicity island

From the data collected we reached the conclusion that cag was a pathogenicity island (PAI)[18], a piece of horizontally transferred 'alien DNA', integrated into a very specific region of the chromosome, the last 31 nucleotides of the glutamate racemase gene (*glr*) and which contained more than 40 genes involved in virulence. The presence of direct repeats and a certain degree of instability in the cagI moiety suggested that cag was a member of the family of PAI that can be lost and have a clear integration sequence, like PAI-I and PAI-II from the uropathogenic strain 536 of *E. coli*[19] or PAI-pgm from *Yersinia pestis*[20]. Most of the deduced proteins were new and showed homologies with secretion proteases and translocases, with proteins associated with pilus or flagellum assembly and with sensors or permeases: they form a new secretion apparatus with features similar to type II, type III and type IV secretion systems[17,21-24]. The proteins encoded by genes located in the cag PAI probably participate in the formation of membrane pore complexes, forming a transfer system for the export of macro-molecules that could be involved in contacting recipient cells. The proposed *H. pylori* classification was enhanced and more subtly structured by the cag discovery.

cag as an evolutionistic engine

The origin of modern *Helicobacter* types from an ancestral proto-Type II *Helicobacter* evolved after the acquisition of the cag PAI: the newer Type I, growing twice as fast as a Type II strain, was exerting an evolutionary pressure probably responsible for recruiting new functions from old molecules. One example that was already discussed[9,17] is the *vacA* gene. The sequence of *vacA* in *bona-fide* Type II strains is only 50% identical to the allele present in Type I strains. Similarity between *vacA* genes in Type II strains is almost 90% identical and the same degree of similarity is observed after direct comparison of alleles from Type I strains. The association between VacA and CagA suggested that the presence of cag was the driving force for extracting a new function from an old protein, selecting spontaneous mutations that resulted in a completely new viru-lence factor. Type I strains can be now defined as cag-positive and Type II strains as cag-negative[17]. The evolutionary tree was further complicated by the acci-dental acquisition of an IS605 movable element. Only Type I strains were exposed and a new branch from the Type I strain indicated the intermediate lineage. The preferential integration site for IS605 was found within the cag PAI, but additional copies were also found outside this region. The insertion followed by homologous recombination generated the great variability observed within the intermediate type lineage. A consistent fraction of intermediate strains are phenotypically indistinguishable from Type I strains, but the instability of the cag PAI generates strains that resemble Type II strains. Inter-mediate strains are a typical population bottleneck, since they are responsible for the attenuation of virulence. The final picture is composed by: Type I strains (cag-positive, IS605-negative), intermediate strains (cag-positive, IS605-positive, different level of cag splitting and deletions) and Type II (cag-negative, IS605-negative). At any moment we can deduce if we are dealing with an intermediate strain with attenu-ated virulence or a Type II strain simply by using the IS605 as a marker, not present in the naturally less virulent Type II strains.

A world of PAIs

Pathogenicity islands have emerged from a status of mere curiosity to a central phenomenon in pathogenesis[18]. We are currently including in the growing list of PAIs groups of genes from very popular pathogens that have been acquired from phages or plasmids, but that are now stable elements of the main chromosome and are encapsulated from other virulence factors. PAIs can be grouped as stable and unstable (lost at the frequency of 10^{-4} in *E. coli* and 10^{-5} in *Y. pestis*) with no observed reversion rate[19,20]. They can be either flanked by direct repeats (very common in the unstable PAIs) or they do not have recognizable duplicated motifs (very stable PAIs). The absence of repeats can be due to accumulated mutations, since they were acquired very early in the process of speciation or by a different mechanism, based on sequences located within the genes flanking the insertions, that are always conserved. PAIs are characterized by a $G+C$ content that is different from the one observed in the host. PAIs DNA is 'alien', coming from a donor organism that we have not yet discovered, or that is possibly extinct and was never isolated in the intermediate form (as free molecules within the cell, like conjugative transposons or as an infectious form, like a phage particle or naked DNA). Pathogenicity islands were identified in Gram-negative bacteria and are associated with IS sequences (*Yersinia pestis* and *Helicobacter pylori*)[17–20]. The sizes range from 10 to 190kb with a middle value of 40kb. The PAIs are composed by multiple, high-density, virulence cassettes (20–40 different genes) that encode for haemolysins, p-related fimbriae, regulator for S-fimbrial expression, attaching and effacing determinants (in *E. coli*)[19] or type III secretory apparatus (in *Salmonella typhimurium*)[21] (see also refs 22–24).

Type III secretion systems

Type III secretion systems have similarities with genes required for flagellum assembly and have related functions: whether they originated from common ancestors or they have been transferred laterally to several bacterial species, functional constraints are evident. In flagellum biogenesis the proteins forming the P and L ring have cleaved signal peptides and are exported through the *sec*-dependent pathway. The external flagellar components are exported through a specialized pathway that needs to be considered as true secretion machinery. Four proteins have a direct role in this apparatus and three of them have a counterpart in type III secretion systems. Since the flagellar proteins are secreted by an apparatus encoded by flagellar genes, the type III secretion system itself is positioning all the members of the engine in a flagellum-like structure, with a channel that routes secreted proteins through the outer membrane. Flagellum biogenesis and type III secretion systems have nine components in common but additional genes are species-specific proteins that seem to be unique to one organism. Sensor-like proteins and two-component regulatory systems are part of type III secretion systems and, more generally, of PAIs. It should be noted that proteins of type III secretion systems are similar only over part of their lengths, that the sizes of the synthesized proteins are very different from the flagellar cognate molecules, that are frequently more similar to each other than to related flagellar proteins.

Integration and instability

The integration site of PAIs has been the subject of detailed analyses, with the aim of discovering the rules that dictate the acquisition and level of cross-talk with the host genes. The regions of the *E. coli* genome located at minutes 82 and 87, downstream of the gene for *selc* (encoding the tRNA for selenocysteine) and *leux* (encoding the tRNA for leucine), were mapped for prophage integration: retronphage phiR73 integrated at 82 and phage P4 at 87. Surprisingly PAI-I (70 kb) and PAI-II (190 kb) were discovered inserted in the same locations, at minutes 82 and 87, in the uropathogenic strain 536 of *E. coli*, a strain associated with chronic infection of the urinary tract. PAI-I and II encode for a haemolysin, for P-related fimbriae, for regulators of S fimbrial adhesins, for serum resistance factors and for virulence in the mouse[19]. The uroepithelial binding activity of the strain is totally dependent on the virulence factors contained in the PAI. At minute 82, when the region is not invaded by a retronphage or by PAI-I, the PAI-LEE can be integrated in the exact same way as PAI-I, with the exception that directed repeats are not found and the structure is remarkably stable[25]. *E. coli* strains possessing the LEE pathogenicity island are entheropathogenic and induce characteristic lesions in the intestinal epithelium named AE, attaching and effacing. All the elements required for degrading the apical structure, clustering cytoskeletal proteins and forming pedestals that cup single bacteria are included in a region of 35 kb. Enteropathogenic *E. coli* is recognized as the causative agent of severe infantile diarrhoea.

PAIs also have been identified in *Salmonella typhimurium* and renamed SPI1 and SPI2[26,27]. SPI1 is located at minute 63, between *fhlA* and *muts*, is 40 kb long and encodes a type III secretion system. Mutants in SPI1 are unable to effect entry into non-phagocytic cells and are virulent when administered i.p. SPI2 is located at minute 30.7, between *ydhe* and *pykf*, is also 40 kb in length and encodes a type III secretion system but mutants are attenuated after p.o. and i.p. inoculation, indicating that SPI2-dependent virulence factors are required after epithelial cell invasion. SPI1 and SPI2 do not have direct repeats and are stable.

Yersinia pestis strain KIM6+ has a Pgm+ phenotype that is lost in the strain KIM6. The Pgm phenotype was defined as: pesticin sensitivity (in a strain lacking the pesticin immunity protein), expression of iron-repressible outer membrane proteins and growth at 37°C in iron-limited medium. The phenotype is dependent on a 102 kb PAI, absent in Pgm⁻ strains, that is flanked by two copies of the IS*100*. Integration of the 102 kb PAI into the chromosome depends upon the presence of the insertion sequence; deletions are due to recombination between the flanking IS*100*[20].

PAIs are growing in number and variety: in the list are elements described in *Listeria monocytogenes* and *Dichelobacter nodosus*[28,29]. Two points deserve particular attention: (1) the observed instability and (2) PAIs potentiation. The instability can be easily explained by the presence of IS elements, such is the case of *H. pylori* and *Y. pestis*, or by repeats located in the integration site, as in *H. pylori* and *E. coli*. Moreover, direct repeats are not absolutely required for integration, since we observed integration even in the absence of a consensus sequence. There is more than one indirect observation that, in bacteria chronically persisting at the site of infection, the deletions of PAIs are very frequent and in a dynamic equilibrium with strains retaining the PAIs. This suggests that the instability is part of the infectious process and that it may act as a regulatory mechanism to reduce the virulence of the bacterial population in compromised hosts.

The emergence of a new pathogen

At the extreme of this phenomenon, new virulence determinants may potentiate the effect of the pathogenicity island, generating a pathogen with an increased spectrum and entirely new properties. We have previously described the LEE element and its effect in the recipient *E. coli* strain that is enteropathogenic (EPEC) and causes diarrhoea in children. But what about adding new functions into an EPEC strain? Scientists had the chance to assist in an event of microevolution in 1982, during an outbreak of haemorrhagic colitis. The causative agent was named enterohaemorrhagic *E. coli* strain O157:H7 (EHEC), and produced complex lesions on the surface of the enterocytes and on the vascular endothelium, causing the classical haemolytic/uraemic syndrome. Since the enterocyte lesions were identical to EPEC the strain was genetically dissected. The results indicated that EHEC was an EPEC strain that expressed *Shiga*-like cytotoxins after prophage insertion. The extraordinary adhesive properties were mediated by the acquisition of a plasmid encoding adherence factors. An important observation was the identification of *E. coli* strains with a single prophage insertion and *Shiga*-like phenotype, and rare isolates with plasmid-based adhesins[30]. After multiple rounds of intraspecies transfer (conjugation) the EHEC strain was selected (a *de-facto* new strain) and was clonally expanded into an intermediate host before diffusing in the humans. From this *in-vivo* genetic engineering experiment we have learned to reconsider the role of intermediate hosts for clonal expansion of new variants of mammalian pathogens, and more subtly our complete ignorance about the transfer of the pathogenicity islands from the donor organism/s to the actual host.

Mercator, the cartography of *H. pylori* genomic maps and the missing island

Mutation rates, virulent and attenuated strains, and virulence determinants lead, inevitably, to the structure of the genome of *Helicobacter pylori*. From the experiments with RAPD (random amplification of polymorphic DNA)[1] to gene mapping[3,31] we have had the opportunity to verify the supernatural level of gene rearrangement in different clinical isolates. In an extremely important paper[3] Diane Taylor recently determined the chromosomal structure of five different strains using PFGE (pulsed-field gel electrophoresis) and concluded that most of the genes have a different location in the circular chromosome of *H. pylori*, that is 1.7 Mb long. She was able to resolve the *cagA* gene but not the cag PAI that is conserved (in terms of structure and organization) in all Type I and intermediate strains that we have collected[17]. In addition she excluded from the work any Type II strain, so that we do not yet have a clear picture of the amount of Type I-specific sequences. However, the general message is very clear: genes are scrambled along the chromosome, rearranged, and functionally active. In an incidental way, she mentioned the possibility that this phenomenon depends upon the presence of repetitive sequences (the IS*605*) but this is very unlikely. In the first instance most of the strains have one or two copies of IS*605* and the level of permutation is too low to generate the very beautiful map she presented. In some special cases we have mapped six or seven IS*605*, but even seven copies are largely insufficient[17]. Also, the IS*605* is present in the intermediate strains but not in Type I or Type II strains, that show great variability in RAPD patterns. From the data that we have collected, scrambling is type-independent and ubiquitous. It diffused to a large majority of genes and gene clusters but is not acting on cag PAI. We can postulate easily the existence of hinge sequences as a target for recombination, leaving regulatory and coding sequences untouched, but an alternative explanation is based on conjugation and homologous recombination. The reassortment is compatible with a classification scheme, since the bacterial cells are homogeneous in terms of protein expression and encoded functions, and maintain the chromosome structure over very long periods. The level of macro-diversity is so pronounced that we are tempted to consider the existing population as a quasi-species, non-clonal in origin and evolving faster than most of the bacterial species. *H. pylori* may have evolved very strictly with an infected individual[32], infecting other members of the social nucleus, and may have followed, generation after generation, the destiny of his progeny over countries, distributed as a human marker. In a time when race is no longer included in human genetics textbooks, population genetics offer one hand to molecular genetics to trace the origin of another complexity: not human, but bacterial[4,33].

Acknowledgements

I thank Rino Rappuoli for helpful discussions, encouragement and suggestions. I gratefully acknowledge the precious collaboration of scientists working in my laboratory: Christina Lange for the work on functions associated with the pathogenicity island; Silvia Guidotti for the work on a new plasmid; Marta Marchetti for the commitment to the biology of the animal model; Stefano Censini for starting with me the work on the cag PAI, and for building the complete map of this region, including the signals for integration and for the hybridization studies. Special thanks to Douglas Berg (Washington University, St Louis) for exchanging data on cagII and IS*605* prior to publication and to Derya Unutmaz (Skirball Institute) for comments on the manuscript.

References

1. Akopyanz N, Bukanov NO, Westblom TU, Kresovich S, Berg DE. DNA diversity among clinical isolates of *Helicobacter pylori* detected by PCR-based RAPD fingerprinting. Nucl Acids Res. 1992;20:5137–42.
2. Akopyanz N, Bukanov NO, Westblom TU, Berg DE. PCR-based RFLP analysis of DNA sequence diversity in the gastric pathogen *Helicobacter pylori*. Nucl Acids Res. 1992;20:6221–5.
3. Jiang Q, Hiratsuka K, Taylor D. Variability of gene order in different *Helicobacter pylori* strains contribute to genome diversity. Mol Microbiol. 1966;20:833–42.
4. Cavalli-Sforza LL, Menozzi P, Piazza A. The history and geography of human genes. Princeton: Princeton University Press; 1994.
5. Labigne A, Cussac V, Courcoux P. Shuttle cloning and nucleotide sequences of *Helicobacter pylori* genes responsible for urease activity. J Bacteriol. 1991;173:1920–31.
6. Leying H, Suerbaum S, Geis G, Haas R. Cloning and genetic characterization of a *Helicobacter pylori* flagellin gene. Mol Microbiol. 1992;6:2863–74.
7. Telford JL, Ghiara P, Dell'orco M *et al*. Gene structure of the *Helicobacter pylori* cytotoxin and evidence of its key role in gastric disease. J Exp Med. 1994;179:1653–8.
8. Covacci A, Censini S, Bugnoli M *et al*. Molecular characterization of the 128-kDa immuno-

dominant antigen of *Helicobacter pylori* associated with cytotoxicity and duodenal ulcer. Proc Natl Acad Sci USA. 1993;90:5791–5.

9. Cover TL, Tummuru MKR, Cao P, Thompson SA, Blaser MJ. Divergence of genetic sequences for the vacuolating cytotoxin among *Helicobacter pylori* strains. J Biol Chem. 1994;269:10566–73.

10. Marchetti M, Arico B, Burroni D, Figura N, Rappuoli R, Ghiara P. Development of a mouse model of *Helicobacter pylori* infection that mimics human disease. Science. 1995;267:1655–8.

11. Tummuru MKR, Cover TL, Blaser MJ. Mutation of the cytotoxin-associated *cagA* gene does not affect the vacuolating cytotoxin activity of *Helicobacter pylori*. Infect Immun. 1994;62:2609–13.

12. Solnick JV, Tompkins LS. *Helicobacter pylori* and gastroduodenal disease: pathogenesis and host–parasite interaction. Infect Agents Dis. 1993;1:294–309.

13. Telford JL, Covacci A, Ghiara P, Montecucco C, Rappuoli R. Unravelling the pathogenic role of *Helicobacter pylori* in peptic ulcer: potential for new therapies and vaccines. Trends Biotechnol. 1994;12:420–6.

14. Boren T, Falk P, Roth KA, Larson G, Normark S. Attachment of *Helicobacter pylori* to human gastric epithelium mediated by blood group antigens. Science. 1993;262:1892–5.

15. Xiang ZY, Censini S, Bayeli PF *et al*. Analysis of expression of CagA and VacA virulence factors in 43 strains of *Helicobacter pylori* reveals that clinical isolates can be divided into two major types and that CagA is not necessary for expression of the vacuolating cytotoxin. Infect Immun. 1995;63:94–8.

16. Crabtree JE, Covacci A, Farmery SM *et al*. *Helicobacter pylori* induced interleukin-8 expression in gastric epithelial cells is associated with CagA positive phenotype. J Clin Pathol. 1995;48:41–5.

17. Censini S, Lange C, Xiang ZY *et al. cag*, a pathogenicity island of *Helicobacter pylori*, encodes Type I-specific and disease-associated virulence factors. (Submitted)

18. Lee CA. Pathogenicity islands and the evolution of bacterial pathogens. Infect Agents Dis. 1996;5:1–7.

19. Blum G, Ott M, Lischewski A *et al*. Excision of large DNA regions termed pathogenicity islands from tRNA-specific loci in the chromosome of an *Escherichia coli* wild-type pathogen. Infect Immun. 1994;62:606–14.

20. Fetherston JD, Schuetze P, Perry RD. Loss of the pigmentation phenotype in *Yersinia pestis* is due to the spontaneous deletion of 102 kb of chromosomal DNA which is flanked by a repetitive element. Mol Microbiol. 1992;6:2693–704.

21. Galan JE. Molecular genetic bases of *Salmonella* entry into host cells. Mol Microbiol. 1966;20:263–71.

22. Covacci A, Rappuoli R. Pertussis toxin export requires accessory genes located downstream from the pertussis toxin operon. Mol Microbiol. 1993;8:429–34.

23. Winans SC, Burns D, Christie PJ. Adaptation of a conjugal transfer system for the export of pathogenic macromolecules. Trends Microbiol. 1996;4:64–8.

24. Salmond GPC. Secretion of extracellular virulence factors by plant pathogenic bacteria. Annu Rev Phytopathol. 1994;32:181–200.

25. McDaniel TK, Jarvis KG, Donnenberg MS, Kaper JB. A genetic locus of enterocyte effacement conserved among diverse enterobacterial pathogens. Proc Natl Acad Sci USA. 1995;92:1664–8.

26. Bajaj V, Hwang C, Lee CA. *hilA* is a novel *ompT/toxR* family member that activates the expression of *Salmonella typhimurium* invasion genes. Mol Microbiol. 1995;18:715–27.

27. Shea JE, Hensel M, Gleeson C, Holden D. Identification of a virulence locus encoding a second type III secretion system in *Salmonella typhimurium*. Proc Natl Acad Sci USA. 1996;93:2593–7.

28. Gouin E, Mengaud J, Cossart P. The virulence gene cluster of *Listeria monocytogenes* is also present in *Listeria ivanovii*, an animal pathogen, and *Listeria seeligeri*, a nonpathogenic species. Infect Immun. 1994;62:3550–3.

29. Haring V, Billington SJ, Wright CL, Huggins AS, Katz ME, Rodd JI. Delineation of the virulence-related locus (*vrl*) of *Dichelobacter nodosus*. Microbiology. 1995;141:2081–9.

30. Whittam TS, Wolfe ML, Wachsmuth IK, Orskov F, Orskov I, Wilson RA. Clonal relationships among *Escherichia coli* strains that cause hemorrhagic colitis and infantile diarrhoea. Infect Immun. 1993;61:1619–29.

31. Bukanov NO, Berg DE. Ordered cosmid library and high-resolution physical-genetic map of *Helicobacter pylori* strain NCTC11638. Mol Microbiol. 1994;11:509–23.

32. Akopyants NS, Eaton KA, Berg DE. Adaptive mutation and cocolonization during *Helicobacter pylori* infection of gnotobiotic piglets. Infect Immun. 1995;63:116–21.
33. Bliska JB, Galan J, Falkow S. Signal transduction in the mammalian cell during bacterial attachment and entry. Cell. 1993;73:903–20.

5
Effect of gastric acid on *Helicobacter pylori* ecology

A. LEE, B. MELLGÅRD and H. LARSSON

INTRODUCTION

> 'Whereas the Top People have a duodenal ulcer, gastric ulcer has been regarded in Western Europe for the past half-century as an affliction of the materially and mentally under-privileged (Lancet, 30 May 1959)[1].

The discovery of *Helicobacter pylori* has altered for ever our perceptions of gastro-duodenal disease, and has dramatically influenced patient management. However, we have much to learn. We still cannot explain the rather politically incorrect observation of nearly 40 years ago which was referring to differences in distribution of peptic ulcers between the rich and the poor. While all would now accept *H. pylori* as a cause of peptic ulcer, most gastric ulcers (GU), many gastric cancers (GC) and all mucosa-associated lymphoid tissue (MALT) lymphomas, we cannot explain what is illustrated in Figure 1, i.e., that there are different patterns of *H. pylori*-associated disease and these patterns vary in different populations. Indeed, some of the pathways of disease appear to be mutually exclusive. In the developed world the pattern tends towards duodenal ulcer (DU), while in the developing world gastric cancer may be more likely to develop. In this latter group, gastric ulcers will outnumber duodenal ulcers, as is implied in the opening quote. This chapter attempts to address this issue by suggesting that a major difference in these populations is variation in local acid output.

THE OTHER FACTORS

With such multifactorial diseases it is unlikely that different disease profiles result from one property of host or bacterium. Thus, it is appropriate briefly to mention other factors that have been proposed and in some cases actively investigated. First, it is claimed that such differences result from the possession by *H. pylori* of varying virulence factors, introducing the idea of the ulcerogenic strain and the suggestion that more virulent strains may be present in some populations. Certainly, there do appear to be two broad categories of *H. pylori*. The so-called

1. Hp ingested

Duodenal ulcer

Gastric cancer or lymphoma

2. Acute gastritis

3. Active-Chronic gastritis

Gastric Ulcer

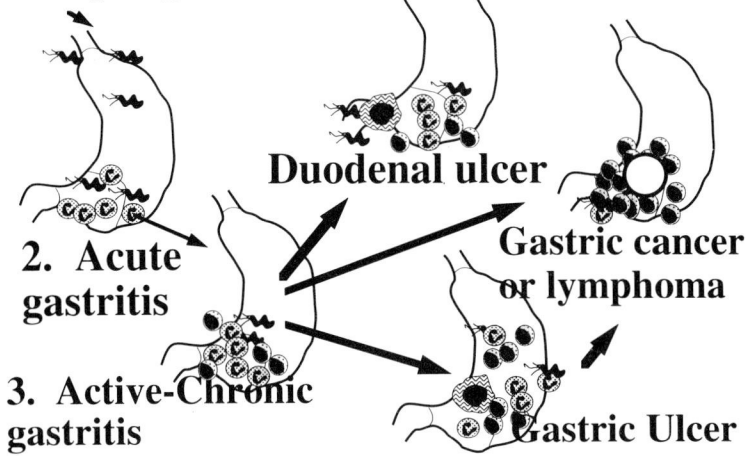

Figure 1 Patterns of *Helicobacter pylori*-associated disease

CagA[+] genotype is more frequently associated with DU disease and GC in some populations[2]. The explanation of increased virulence of cagA[+] strains appears to correlate with the co-expression with *cagA* of a gene named *picB*, which codes for a homologue of the *Bordetella pertussis* toxin secretion protein, and which induces the pro-inflammatory cytokine, IL-8 in gastric epithelium[3]. Certainly, if one assumes that the basis of any symptomatic disease caused by *H. pylori* is the underlying gastritis, then it is not surprising that a bacterium which induces a more severe inflammatory response will cause a greater proportion of DU and GC. However, distinction of CagA[+] and CagA[-] *H. pylori* strains cannot be the explanation for the different patterns of disease described above.

We have argued that host factors are important and have implied, based on animal studies, that different populations may respond differently with respect to their immunological reactivity to the presence of *H. pylori*[4]. The Japanese studies of Azuma and colleagues give support to this hypothesis, by showing differences in the allele frequency for genes of the major histocompatibility complex which control immune responses. Differences in HLA types should differ in their susceptibility to infection pathogens[5,6]. In this study genotypes for HLA-DQA1 were determined from allele-specific RFLP patterns. The allele frequency of HLA-DQA1 0102 was 62% in DU patients compared to 17% in *H. pylori*-negative controls. While these results are preliminary, and difficult to interpret, this will be a fruitful area for study in the future.

THE NEGLECTED HOST FACTOR IN *H. PYLORI* PATHOGENESIS: ACID OUTPUT

Based on a reading of the early literature, observation on *H. pylori*-infected populations and animal experimentation, we recently published an hypothesis which suggested acid output as most likely to be the dominant factor in determining the location of *H. pylori* pathology, and hence the pattern of symptomatic disease[7]. This chapter reviews the evidence for this hypothesis, adds to it, and puts down a challenge for experiments to be done to refute it.

THE ORIGINAL HYPOTHESES

1. The antrum is the preferred niche of the gastric helicobacters.
2. *H. pylori* can flourish only on non-acid-secreting gastric epithelium.
3. Bacteria in the antral-body border and the body of the stomach behave differently to bacteria in the antrum.

The concept is that *H. pylori* growth will be affected by the local acid conditions. In areas of high local acidity, while the organism may survive it will not multiply readily, and thus will produce different inflammatory products. Where acid levels are reduced, the bacterium may be more closely associated with the epithelium and/or will grow better, and so will produce more inflammatory products or deliver them more directly into the tissue. At intermediate areas of acid output, for example, as the antrum architecture changes to body architecture, a third state of bacterial growth will be encountered, once again with the possibility of different inflammatory potential. The assumption is one that is now becoming dominant in environmental microbiology and studies of bacterial pathogenesis[8,9]. Bacteria respond to environmental change by the switching-on of sets of genes best suited to survival in that local environment. So what is the evidence on which this hypothesis is based?

THE EVIDENCE

Pre-*H. pylori*

The literature in the first half of this century is full of meticulous observational studies on peptic ulcer disease that attempted to catalogue differences in order to try to understand these increasingly serious conditions. If we assume, which is now legitimate, that gastritis was caused by *H. pylori*, as were duodenal ulcer and gastric ulcer in those pre-NSAID days, then the differences seen must relate to differences in host response to *H. pylori*. Examples of these observations are:

1. DU and GU tend to be mutually exclusive. While 30% of patients with GU may have evidence of a previous DU, DU is hardly ever preceded by GU[10].
2. In the first half of the century, in Western countries, DU replaced GU, and ulcers became more common in males compared to females[11] (Figure 2).
3. Gastritis in DU patients is located in the antrum, whereas GU patients have a more widespread pangastritis[12].
4. In DU, acid tends to be increased, while in GU it is normal or reduced[13,14].
5. GU appear close to mucosal transitional zones, i.e. antrum/body cardia/body. Chronic ulceration occurs at sites nearest to the acid-secreting body mucosa, but rarely within it[15,16].

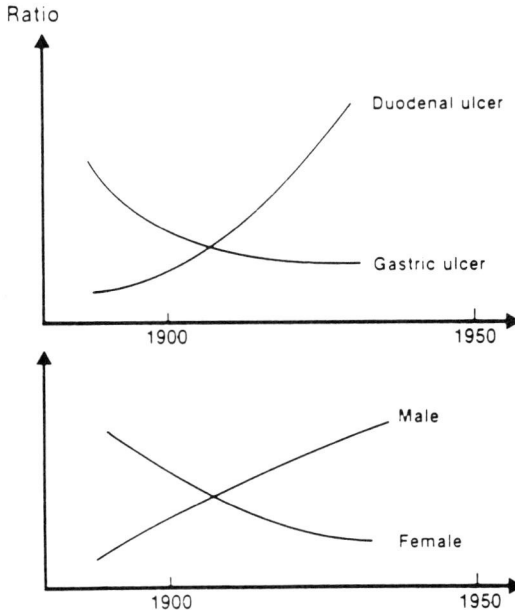

Figure 2 Changes in the ratios of duodenal ulcer/gastric ulcer in the Western world up until 1950 (taken from ref. 11)

6. Ulcers located in antral tissue which are further from the body mucosa are found in patients with elevated acid output[14].
7. The size of the transitional zone varies between GU and DU patients, being smaller in GU with possibly a more marked cut-off between body tissue parietal cells and antral tissue[17].

The excellent papers referred to in this section give many more relevant observations, but space restricts those selected to the above seven points. If the hypotheses are true how do they explain the above observations? Firstly we have to make a few assumptions: (a) Ulcers occur at transitional zones because at this area the mucosal defences are weakened due to structural differences such as local blood flow. (b) There is a threshold of inflammatory intensity that, once it is overcome at these sites, causes a small focus of weakness in the mucosa that allows acid damage and becomes the focus of the ulcer. Thus, in DU patients *H. pylori* can multiply only well enough to deliver inflammatory products close to the mucosa in the antrum. Acid output in the transitional zones restricts the *H. pylori*, such that damage is not caused at the weak spots, i.e. the area of most damaging inflammation is further down in the antrum away from the transitional zone and so no ulcers occur. However, down in the duodenal bulb, at the transitional zone between gastric metaplasia and duodenal tissue, the duodenitis may be so severe that a lesion occurs and the high acid levels from the stomach cause the damage which becomes the DU. With GU patients there is less local acid close to the transitional zone between antrum and body, so that *H. pylori* can thrive in this area. If the inflammation is intense enough, ulceration can occur in this weakened zone. Another consequence of this reduced acid is that the *H. pylori* is better able to multiply, grow or flourish in the body, so pangastritis results. This is the inflammation that can, over decades, result in destruction of parietal cells and chief cells, and so atrophy will occur.

The changes in DU/GU ratios in the Western world up until 1950 (Figure 2) are very unlikely to be due to infection with different strains of *H. pylori*[11,18]. However, if one hypothesized that increased standards of living, less disease and better nutrition results in an increased acid output on average, in a particular population, the shift from GU to DU can be explained. The female versus male change is less easy to explain, although one idea is worth reporting, for its novelty[19]. Up until 1910, ulcer was found more commonly in women than in men, and in 1857 the average age at which perforation was reported was 28 years compared to 43 in the male. The wearing of tight corsets by fashion-conscious women was suggested as being responsible, as in countries where tight lacing was not in vogue the incidence of perforated GU was often slightly higher in men!

The above explanation of the observations in terms of the hypothesis is not proof. What is lacking are experimental studies that showed that acid manipulation did indeed influence the behaviour and inflammatory potential of *H. pylori*. This evidence was forthcoming in the post-*H. pylori* era.

Post-*H. pylori*: human data

Once *H. pylori* had been discovered, and pathologists could now look for it, the correlations with the above observations were confirmed. With respect to the distribution of the bacteria in the different patient groups there is some confusion, possibly due to the quantitative measures used[20-24]. On balance most studies suggest that populations of *H. pylori* are greater in the antrum than in the body, although some would dispute this. All agree that the greater the number of *H. pylori* in the antrum, the greater the intensity of inflammation, and some suggest there are more bacteria in the antrum in DU patients compared to non-ulcer dyspepsia. All would also agree that there are large numbers of *H. pylori* in the body, so a clear statement with respect to the hypothesis cannot be made. The observations on the distribution of gastric inflammation are consistent. In the antrum, presence of *H. pylori* is always accompanied with inflammation, and in DU more bacteria seem to be associated with more severe gastritis. In DU patients the bacteria in the body are often associated with a normal epithelium. According to the hypothesis, deliberate interventions resulting in changes in acid output should result in changes in the distribution of gastritis and/or *H. pylori*. An elegant study of 20 DU patients pre- and post-vagotomy showed that acid suppression resulted in gastritis appearing in the body of the stomach[25]. A more recent study followed vagotomy patients 8 years post-surgery[26]. Major differences were seen between surgical patients and control patients with active ulcer; significant numbers of the acid-suppressed patients showed body gastritis and even atrophy, while the ulcer patients showed virtually no body gastritis.

Four studies have looked at the distribution of *H. pylori* and gastritis in patients on omeprazole, a proton pump inhibitor known to switch off local acid secretion very effectively. The first was by Vigneri *et al.*, who made the important observation that not only did *H. pylori* colonization increase in the body, but it decreased in the antrum[27]. Others confirmed this observation, and found correlation with the degree of inflammation. Thus, Kuipers *et al.* studied 50 patients with reflux oesophagitis on maintenance omeprazole therapy[28–30]. Seventeen *H. pylori*-negative patients had no gastritis before or after therapy. *H. pylori*-positive patients had predominant colonization and associated inflammation in the antrum before therapy. After therapy the infection mainly affected the body. The bacterial number and inflammation decreased in the antrum, and gastritis was seen in the body. Significantly, this body gastritis in a number of cases progressed to atrophy, thus mimicking the pattern of disease seen in the developed world simply by reducing local acid output. Importantly, and relevant to later discussion, the numbers of *H. pylori* in the body did not appear to go up; rather they remained stable. Logan and colleagues added a new dimension to the omeprazole studies when they also observed the fall in antral *H. pylori*, but claimed the increase in other areas of the stomach was a rise in both *H. pylori* numbers and severity of gastritis in the fundus[29]. They saw not much change in the corpus. These differences in the locations of colonization in different publications may indeed be due to the authors' use of different definitions with respect to body, corpus and fundus. Marzio *et al.*, who undertook a long-term study, showed that at the end of 4 weeks treatment with omeprazole 20 mg or 40 mg, almost all patients who initially had *H. pylori* in the antrum were found free of bacteria in the antrum, but had them in the body[30]. These changes remained constant for 1 year on ome-prazole 20 mg daily maintenance therapy, but if the maintenance dose was omeprazole 20 mg daily on alternate days, distribution returned to normal, slowly stabilizing at 8 months. After only 4 weeks of daily omeprazole therapy it still took 4 months to get back to the pre-omeprazole distribution.

The studies described above were the reason we used the word 'flourish' in the original hypothesis, as changes in acid secretion, while clearly causing changes in distribution of the gastritis, did not always correlate with apparent changes in the presence of the bacteria. We emphasized that the effect of acid is likely to be on bacterial behaviour, not simply on rate of multiplication. For example, the increase in body gastritis in the omeprazole-treated patients could be due to two possible variations in growth behaviour. First, the lack of an acid-suppressive effect on the bacteria in the body, resulting from proton pump inhibition, could result in the organism now being able to synthesize different metabolic products which could be more inflammatory. Alternatively, there could be a subtle change in niche brought about by changes in the pH of the local environment, with the bulk of the bacteria moving deeper into the mucus and so being closer to the tissue and thus more able to deliver inflammatory products. Certainly two colleagues have reported the anecdotal observation of *H. pylori* deep down in the gastric pits of body mucosa close to the parietal cells in patients on proton pump inhibitors. This is not normally observed (Wyatt and Stolte, personal communication).

Post-*H. pylori*: animal data

The authors have all had significant experience in the development of small animal models of *Helicobacter* infection. These models allow experimental manipulation of local pH, and an opportunity to closely monitor colonization of the whole stomach in a way which cannot be done in the human. It is these studies, more than any other, that convinced us of the major features of our thesis on acid effects on *H. pylori* ecology.

H. felis is a close relative of *H. pylori* and normally inhabits the canine and feline gastric mucosa[31]. The organism will colonize the stomach of rats and mice, thus providing us with convenient small animal models[32–36]. Presumably *H. felis* has adopted similar strategies to survival in the hostile gastric environment as *H. pylori*. Thus, the urease enzymes have a high degree of similarity, with 73% and 88% homology for the A and B subunits respectively[37]. However, when the gastric colonization of both rodents is mapped, differences compared with *H. pylori* in the human are seen, which are to our benefit when looking at acid-related effects[38]. *H. felis* colonization is antral predominant, with large numbers of bacteria which tend to go deeper into the tissue than *H. pylori*, being seen at the base of the pyloric glands. This deeper penetration is probably due to the inability of *H. felis* to adhere to the mucus neck region of the gland as does *H. pylori*. The only other area in the normal rodent stomach to be colonized by *H. felis* is the cardia, a small region of tissue close to the non-glandular region of the animals. Virtually no bacteria are seen in the body of the mouse stomach. An explanation for this distribution is that colonization is proportional to the number of parietal cells present in the gland. Cardia colonization is due to the lack of parietal cells in this tissue. This inverse relationship with acid-secreting capacity is best seen at the antral/body and cardia/body borders or transitional zones, where the bacteria are seen to taper off in numbers until none are seen once there are five parietal cells per gland. While the bacteria cause no gastritis in the mice used in this study due to host factors it is worth commenting that the pattern of colonization of *H. felis* in the mouse mimics exactly the pattern of gastritis seen in the *H. pylori*-infected human in the developed world; i.e. little body gastritis but significant inflammation in both the antrum and cardia.

To test the acid hypothesis, mice infected with *H. felis* were treated with either ranitidine or omeprazole[38]. Given the more complete acid-suppressive capacity of the proton pump inhibitor, it was expected there would be different effects of the two compounds on *H. felis* distribution (Figure 3). On omeprazole the bacterium was able to colonize the body in large numbers. Although all crypts in the antrum remained colonized there was a definite decline in bacterial numbers. Experiments in *H. felis*-infected rats show similar results[39]. With ranitidine similar effects were seen, but the decrease in bacterial numbers in the antrum did not occur. If one examined the sections closely it was clear that, in the body, *H. felis* was able to penetrate much more deeply into the gastric glands in the omeprazole-treated mice. On ranitidine the bacteria were seen more in the surface mucus and did not penetrate down to the parietal cells.

Thus the effects of acid suppression on the distribution of *H. felis* in the rodent stomach are equivalent to the effects of omeprazole on the distribution of the *H. pylori*-associated gastritis in the stomach of humans taking omeprazole. This is another reason why the term 'flourish' has been selected in the wording of our hypothesis, rather than 'grow'. We would argue that *H. felis* is more acid-labile than *H. pylori*, and so cannot grow in the body of the mouse stomach. While *H. pylori* can grow in the gastric body of the human, it is acid-restricted. Removal

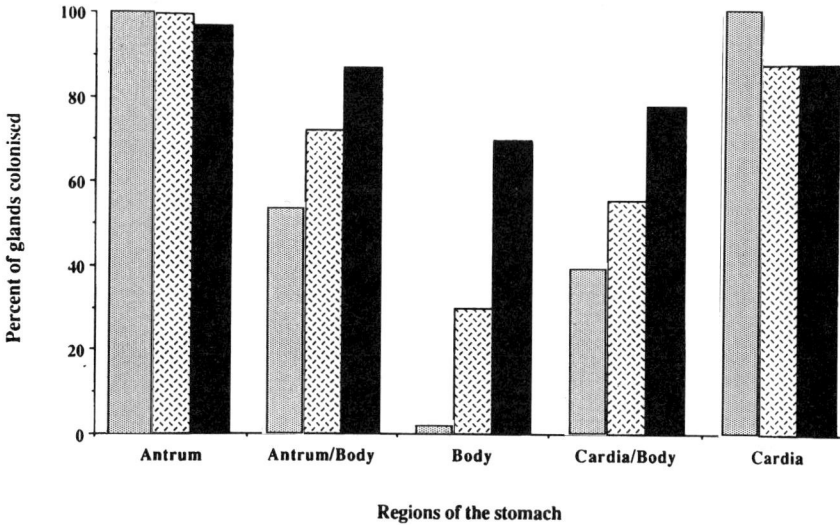

Figure 3 Effect of acid suppression on colonization of the mouse stomach with *Helicobacter felis*. Mice were infected with *H. felis* and treated with omeprazole or ranitidine. Stained sections of mouse stomach were coded and assessed 'blind' for colonization by measuring the percentage of glands infected. Areas assessed were antrum, body and the cardia equivalent (taken from ref. 38). ▨, *H. felis*; ▩, HF + ranitidine; ■, HF + omeprazole

of acid allows it to flourish and grow closer to the tissue. With both the *H. pylori* mouse models of the authors, *H. pylori* is seen more in the body of normal animals than is *H. felis* (O'Rourke and Mellgard, personal communication). When describing the effects of omeprazole on *H. pylori* it is not correct to say that the bacterium moves from antrum to body; rather growth is suppressed in the antrum and encouraged in the body.

H. pylori: controlling its own niche

H. pylori infection may have a direct effect on acid output and therefore an impact on its own habitat at different stages of the disease. Whether these mechanisms are a consequence of evolution, and so of benefit to the bacterium, or are simply secondary effects is unknown. On first infection, as well documented in cases of deliberate ingestion or accidental infection, a period of hypochlorhydria is observed, possibly due to the manufacture by the bacterium of specific anti-secretory products[40]. Significantly, where the histology has been reported in these individuals, the period of hypochlorhydria coincides with a pangastritis[41–44]. When the acid levels became normal the inflammation was restricted to the antrum. In the later stages of *H. pylori* infection, major disturbances in acid secretion can occur, probably due to impairment of inhibitory control as a consequence of inflammatory damage[45]. Thus DU patients have a six-fold increase in the acid response to gastrin-releasing peptide[46]. The resulting acid contributes to limitation of gastritis to the antrum.

57

The evidence: *in vitro* data

Whereas interpretation of *in-vitro* data is notoriously difficult with respect to understanding ecological data, as the conditions in a test tube rarely mimic the ecological niche, there are a number of important studies that highlight the complexity of acid sensitivity of *H. pylori*. The early studies identified the production of a modified urease enzyme as an important feature of adaptation to the acidic gastric environment. Three *Helicobacter* species, two which have been adapted to a gastric environment (*H. pylori* and *H. felis*) and one that is not normally seen in the stomach but which is primarily a lower bowel bacterium (*Helicobacter muridarum*), were all exposed to pH 2.0[47]. All three species died in 30 min. In contrast, in the presence of a concentration of urea (3 mmol/l) known to be found in the stomach, the gastric helicobacters were protected, while *H. muridarum* rapidly succumbed. The protective effect of urease in acid conditions has been confirmed recently using a wild-type strain of *H. pylori* and an isogenic urease negative mutant[48]. In the absence of urea, both strains survived well in pH from 4.5 to 7.2, but died at pH values below 4.5. Following addition of 10 mmol/l urea, the wild-type could now survive at pH 2.2, whereas the urease-negative mutant was killed. It has been shown that the higher the urea concentration the lower the pH at which *H. pylori* survives. At physiological urea concentrations the lowest pH at which the bacterium can survive long term is 4.5, or even slightly lower[49].

However, *in-vitro* studies have also revealed another facet of *H. pylori* and pH that demands a modification of our original hypothesis. While the bacterium can survive well in acid conditions in the presence of physiological urea concentrations, it is more vulnerable at more alkaline pH values. Thus, in a comprehensive set of papers from Glasgow, it was reported that rapid cell death on exposure to urea and citrate at pH 6.0 occurs in organisms with high urease activity such as *H. pylori* and *H. mustelae*. It was suggested that the cause of bacterial death was the failure of the citric acid cycle due to depletion of α-ketoglutarate caused by the incorporation of ammonia into glutamate[50-52]. In the studies with an isogenic mutant, Clyne and colleagues describe a similar phenomenon, but draw a different conclusion. They demonstrate that alkaline pH values are toxic to *H. pylori*, conclude that an acidic environment promotes the survival of *H. pylori* in the presence of urea, and say that the reason why *H. pylori* does not survive *in vitro* at pH above 4.0 in the presence of urea is the generation of alkaline pH conditions, and not ammonia toxicity[48]. The most recent study on acid effects *in vitro* also shows the vulnerability of *H. pylori* at alkaline pH values, and suggests that the presence of urea may set a limit to pH at the neutral/alkaline end at which the bacterium can survive. That these limitations, both at the low and high pH ends, were urease-dependent was demonstrated by the fact that urease inhibition decreased survival at low pH values, whereas it increased survival at high pH values in the presence of urea. A similar pattern for survival was observed with a urease-deficient mutant[49].

Out of these data appears an understanding of the complexity of *H. pylori* and pH which gives us a new appreciation of the human and animal *in-vivo* observations described above. Over the period of evolution *H. pylori* has evolved a strategy for survival in an acid environment that takes advantage of the continued presence of urea in the gastric mucosa and contents. As long as the stomach is functioning normally the bacterium survives. However, if there are major changes in the ecosystem such that the normally acid environment is no more, then possession of the urease enzyme becomes a liability and the organism self-destructs. Thus, in totally achlorhydric stomachs, such as seen in pernicious anaemia, the organism cannot survive. In reality *H. pylori* has a remarkably narrow pH range at which it will flourish. This then explains the different distribution in our animal models and the different patterns of gastritis in human populations. It is only in areas of gastric mucosa, where appropriate oxygen tension and the narrow pH range is present, that *H. pylori* will thrive and produce its inflammatory products close enough to the epithelial surface to cause gastritis. In different populations the local environmental conditions will vary, as will the disease manifestation.

The subtlety of these changes in the local niche, and the importance of the urease enzyme, is shown in one final, as yet unpublished, animal experiment. Here, *H. felis*-infected mice were treated with omeprazole and the colonization was mapped (Figure 4a). As expected, the bacterium appeared in the body and antral colonization was reduced. Given the comments above, we would conclude that in the antrum the local environment has become too alkaline to the detriment of the *H. felis*. In the body the pH is now very acceptable, with the urease enzyme maintaining the local pH within the optimum threshold. Co-administration of the omeprazole with a potent urease inhibitor, flurofamide, completely abolishes this effect, and colonization patterns resemble control-infected animals despite the reduced acid (Figure 4b).

All explanations with respect to acid resistance have to date concentrated on urease activity. However, a recent study looked at the capacity of *H. pylori* to maintain an appropriate trans-membrane ionic gradient at a low pH, and demonstrated a membrane gradient much more similar to acidophilic bacteria which grow at an acid pH, i.e. *Acidiphilium facilis* compared to acid-labile organisms such as *Escherichia coli*. This is an intriguing finding as it appears in conflict with the acquisition of urease as an alternative strategy, especially as *H. pylori* is not acid-resistant like *Acidiphilium* in the absence of urea[53].

THE HYPOTHESIS: AN ADDENDUM

To date our arguments have been based on the effects of an acid environment on *H. pylori* ecology. In reality the hypothesis should be amended to acknowledge the potential damaging effect of an alkaline milieu. Thus we add:

4. *H. pylori* has a narrow threshold of pH tolerance *in vivo*. Shifts to an increased pH in a local environment may have a significant impact on failure to flourish, as will a too-low pH.

An observation made by an astute researcher in our laboratory is worthy of repetition in the context of this point. 'What is the role of bicarbonate production in the ecology?' What indeed! (L. Aristoteli, personal communication).

THE CHALLENGES AHEAD

We and others have argued strongly that local acid conditions play a major role in the expression of *H. pylori*-associated gastroduodenal disease[7,21,54]. Yet this

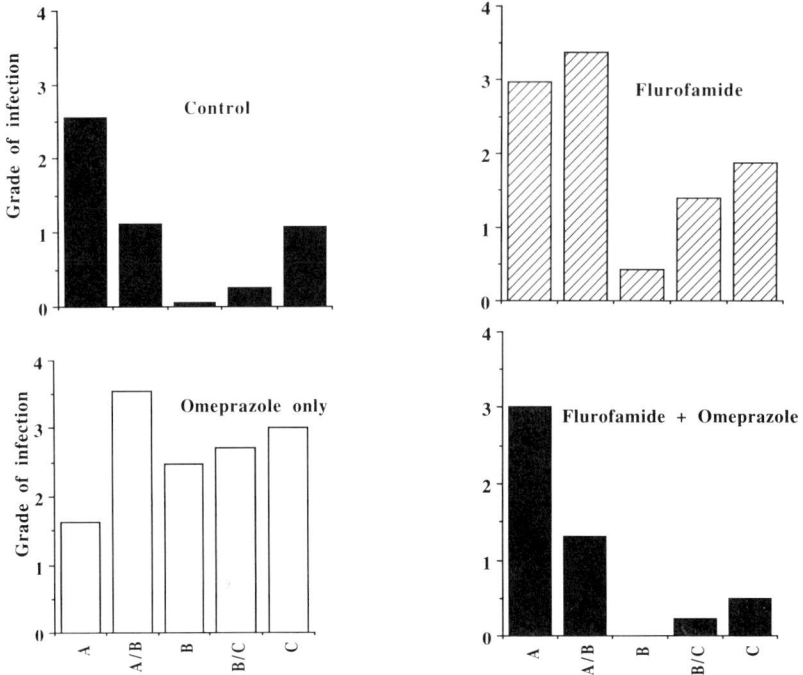

Figure 4 Effect of omeprazole and the urease inhibitor flurofamide on the colonization of the mouse stomach with *Helicobacter felis*. Stained sections of mouse stomach were coded and assessed 'blind' for colonization using a 1–4 grade of infection where 4=heavy colonization of all crypts and 1=occasional bacteria seen in a few crypts. Data shown represent the average for 20 mice per treatment group. The following areas of the stomach were graded: A=antrum, A/B=antral/body transitional zone, B=body, B/C=body/cardia border, C=cardia

topic has been largely ignored in most treatises of *H. pylori* pathogenesis. The worth of a good hypothesis is that it can be tested, confirmed, refuted and, if need be, discarded. Below we list the investigations that need to be done with respect to the hypotheses as formulated. We challenge the sceptics to prove us wrong!

If we are correct:

1. Different populations with different patterns of disease should have different local acid output. A surprising problem with respect to this investigation is that we have no precise non-invasive predictor of gastric acid output to use in large populations.
2. Genes expressed and inflammatory products produced by *H. pylori* should vary in different parts of the stomach in different populations.
3. *H. pylori* in the antrum, on average, will be more closely associated with the epithelium in DU patients than in the body. In GU patients this distinction will not be so obvious.

CONCLUSION

Better understanding of the influence of local pH on *H. pylori* colonization will not only explain the different patterns of gastroduodenal disease but, if exploited imaginatively, might open up novel therapies and more effective use of existing treatment regimens.

References

1. Anon. Gastric ulcer and the ulcer equation. Lancet. 1959;1:1131–3.
2. Crabtree JE. Gastric mucosal inflammatory responses to *Helicobacter pylori*. Aliment Pharmacol Ther. 1996;10(Suppl. 1):29–37.
3. Tummuru M, Sharma SA, Blaser MJ. *Helicobacter pylori* picb, a homologue of the *Bordetella pertussis* toxin secretion protein, is required for induction of IL-8 in gastric epithelial cells. Mol Microbiol. 1995;18:867–76.
4. Lee A. Peptic ulceration – *H. pylori*-initiated ulcerogenesis – look to the host. Lancet. 1993;341:280–1.
5. Azuma T, Konishi J, Ito Y *et al*. Genetic differences between duodenal ulcer patients who were positive or negative for *Helicobacter pylori*. J Clin Gastroenterol. 1995;21(Suppl. 1):S151–4.
6. Azuma T, Konishi J, Tanaka Y *et al*. Contribution of HLA-dqa gene to hosts response against *Helicobacter pylori*. Lancet. 1994;343:542–3.
7. Lee A, Dixon MF, Danon SJ *et al*. Local acid production and *Helicobacter pylori*: a unifying hypothesis of gastroduodenal disease. Eur J Gastroenterol Hepatol. 1995;7:461–5.
8. Miller JF, Mekalanos JJ, Falkow S. Coordinate regulation and sensory transduction in the control of bacterial virulence. Science. 1989;243:916–22.
9. Kroll JK. Bacterial virulence: an environmental response. Arch Dis Child. 1990;65:361–3.
10. Aagaard P, Andreassen M, Kurz L. Duodenal and gastric ulcer in the same patient. Lancet. 1959;1:1111–12.
11. Bonnevie O. Changing demographics of peptic ulcer disease. Dig Dis Sci. 1985;30:8–14S.
12. Schrager J, Spink R, Mitra S. The antrum in patients with duodenal and gastric ulcers. Gut. 1967;8:497–508.
13. Marks IN, Shay H. Observations on the pathogenesis of gastric ulcer. Lancet. 1959;1:107–11.
14. Ball PAJ. The secretory background to gastric ulcer. Lancet. 1961;1:1363–5.
15. Magnus HA. The pathology of simple gastritis. J Pathol Bacteriol. 1946;58.431–9.
16. Oi M, Oshida K, Sugimura S. The location of gastric ulcer. Gastroenterology. 1959;36:45–56.
17. Stave R, Brandtzaeg P, Nygaard K, Fausa O. The transitional body–antrum zone in resected human stomachs. Scand J Gastroenterol. 1978;13:685–91.
18. Sonnenberg A. Temporal trends and geographical variations of peptic ulcer disease. Aliment Pharmacol Ther. 1995;9(Suppl. 2):3–12.
19. Anon. Treatment of acid-related diseases. A century of change. Oxford: Oxford Clinical Communications; 1995.
20. Bayerdorffer E, Lehn N, Hatz R *et al*. Differences in expression of *Helicobacter pylori* gastritis in antrum and body. Gastroenterology. 1992;102:1575–82.
21. Stolte M, Eidt S, Ohnsmann A. Differences in *Helicobacter pylori* associated gastritis in the antrum and body of the stomach. Z. Gastroenterol. 1990;28:229–33.
22. Khulusi S, Mendall MA, Patel P, Levy J, Badve S, Northfield TC. *Helicobacter pylori* infection density and gastric inflammation in duodenal ulcer and non-ulcer subjects. Gut. 1995;37:319–24.
23. Thomas E, Farnum JB, Rohrbach M. *Helicobacter pylori* infection and inflammation of the gastric corpus. Gastroenterology. 1991;101:1454–5.
24. Genta RM, Robason GO, Graham DY. Inflammatory responses and intensity of *Helicobacter pylori* infection in patients with duodenal and gastric ulcer – histopathologic analysis with a new stain. Acta Histochem Cytochem. 1995;28:67–72.
25. Meikle DD, Taylor KB, Truelove SC, Whithead R. Gastritis duodenitis, and circulating levels of gastrin in duodenal ulcer before and after vagotomy. Gut. 1976;17:719–28.
26. Peetsalu A, Maaroos HI, Sipponen P, Peetsula M. Long-term effect of vagotomy on gastric mucosa and *Helicobacter pylori* in duodenal ulcer patients. Scand J Gastroenterol. 1991;26:77–83.

27. Vigneri S, Termini R, Scialabba A, Pisciotta G, di Mario F. Omeprazole therapy modifies the gastric localization of *Helicobacter pylori*. Am J Gastroenterol. 1991;86:1276.
28. Kuipers EJ, Uyterlinde AM, Pena AS *et al*. Increase of *Helicobacter pylori*-associated corpus gastritis during acid suppressive therapy – implications for long-term safety. Am J Gastroenterol. 1995;90:1401–6.
29. Logan RPH, Walker MM, Misiewicz JJ, Gummett PA, Karim QN, Baron JH. Changes in the intragastric distribution of *Helicobacter pylori* during treatment with omeprazole. Gut. 1995;36:12–16.
30. Marzio L, Biasco G, Cifani F *et al*. Short- and long-term omeprazole for the treatment and prevention of duodenal ulcer, and effect on *Helicobacter pylori*. Am J Gastroenterol. 1995;90:2172–6.
31. Paster BJ, Lee A, Fox JG *et al*. Phylogeny of *Helicobacter felis* sp. nov., *Helicobacter mustelae*, and related bacteria. Int J Syst Bacteriol. 1991;41:31–8.
32. Dick-Hegedus E, Lee A. Use of a mouse model to examine anti-*Helicobacter pylori* agents. Scand J Gastroenterol. 1991;26:909–15.
33. Lee A, Fox JG, Otto G, Murphy J. A small animal model of human *Helicobacter pylori* active chronic gastritis. Gastroenterology. 1990;99:1315–23.
34. Lee A. The use of a mouse model in the study of *Helicobacter* sp.-associated gastric cancer. Eur J Gastroenterol Hepatol. 1994;6(Suppl. 1):S67–71.
35. Michetti P, Corthesy-Theulaz I, Davin C *et al*. Immunisation of BALB/c mice against *Helicobacter felis* infection with *H. pylori* urease. Gastroenterology. 1994;107:1002–11.
36. Enno A, O'Rourke J, Lee A, Jack A, Dixon MF. Maltoma-like lesions in the stomach resulting from long-standing *Helicobacter* infection in the mouse. Am J Gastroenterol. 1994;1994:1357.
37. Ferrero RL, Labigne A. Cloning, expression and sequencing of *Helicobacter felis* urease genes. Mol Microbiol. 1993;9:323–33.
38. Danon SJ, O'Rourke JL, Moss ND, Lee A. The importance of local acid production in the distribution of *Helicobacter felis* in the mouse stomach. Gastroenterology. 1995;108:1386–95.
39. Mellgard B, Arvidsson S, Lee A, Sundell G, Larsson H. The *H. felis*-infected rat as a model for human *H. pylori* infection – colonisation pattern and inflammatory response. Am J Gastroenterol. 1994;89:1320.
40. Cave DR, King WW, Hoffman JS. Production of two chemically distinct and inhibitory factors produced by *H. pylori*. Eur J Gastroenterol Hepatol. 1993;5(Suppl.):23–7.
41. Morris A, Nicholson G. Ingestion of *Campylobacter pyloridis* causes gastritis and raised fasting gastric pH. Am J Gastroenterol. 1987;82:192–9.
42. Ramsey EJ, Carey KV, Peterson WL, Jackson JJ, Murphy FK, Read NWT. Epidemic gastritis with hypochlorhydria. Gastroenterology. 1979;76:1449–57.
43. Graham DY, Alpert LC, Smith JL, Yoshimura HH. Iatrogenic *Campylobacter pylori* infection is a cause of epidemic achlorhydria. Am J Gastroenterol. 1988;83:974–80.
44. Sobala GM, Crabtree JE, Dixon MF *et al*. Acute *Helicobacter pylori* infection: clinical features, local and systemic immune response, gastric mucosal histology, and gastric juice ascorbic acid concentrations. Gut. 1991;32:1415–18.
45. Graham DY, Lew GM, Lechago J. Antral G-cell and D-cell numbers in *Helicobacter pylori* infection – effect of *H. pylori* eradication. Gastroenterology. 1993;104:1655–60.
46. El-Omar E, Penman I, Ardill JES, Chittajallu RS, Howie C, McColl KEL. *Helicobacter pylori* infection and abnormalities of acid secretion in patients with duodenal ulcer disease. Gastroenterology. 1995;109:681–91.
47. Ferrero RL, Lee A. The importance of urease in acid protection for the gastric-colonising bacteria *Helicobacter pylori* and *Helicobacter felis* sp. nov. Microbiol Ecol Health Dis. 1991;4:121–34.
48. Clyne M, Labigne A, Drumm B. *Helicobacter pylori* requires an acidic environment to survive in the presence of urea. Infect Immun. 1995;63:1669–73.
49. Sjostrom JE, Larsson H. Factors affecting growth and antibiotic susceptibility of *Helicobacter pylori*: effect of pH and urea on the survival of a wild-type strain and a urease deficient mutant. J Med Microbiol. 1996;44:1–9.
50. Williams C, Neithercut WD, Hossack M, Hair J, McColl KEL. Urease-mediated destruction of bacteria is specific for *Helicobacter* urease and results in total cellular disruption. FEMS Immunol Med Microbiol. 1994;9:273–80.
51. Greig MA, Neithercut WD, Hossack M, McColl KE. Harnessing of urease activity of

Helicobacter pylori to induce self-destruction of the bacterium. J Clin Pathol. 1991;44:157–9.

52. Neithercut WD, Williams C, Hossack MS, McColl KEL. Ammonium metabolism and protection from urease mediated destruction in *Helicobacter pylori* infection. J Clin Pathol. 1993;46:75–8.

53. Matin A, Zychlinsky E, Keyhan M, Sachs G. Capacity of *Helicobacter pylori* to generate ionic gradients at low pH is similar to that of bacteria which grow under strongly acidic conditions. Infect Immun. 1996;64:1434–6.

54. Dixon M. Acid, ulcers, and *H. pylori*. Lancet. 1993;342:384–5.

6
Helicobacter pylori and the gastric environment

G. SACHS, K. MEYER-ROSBERG, D. R. SCOTT and K. MELCHERS

INTRODUCTION

The presence of acid secretion in the stomach was thought for many years not only to aid digestion but also to act as a barrier to bacterial infection. The isolation of *Helicobacter pylori* in the stomach has refuted this idea, at least in part[1,2]. The now-proven association of infection with this organism and the presence of duodenal and gastric ulcer disease has made eradication of *H. pylori* a central issue in the treatment of acid-related diseases[3,4]. The induction of gastritis by the organism, and the tendency towards atrophic gastritis with inflammation, points to an association of *H. pylori* infection and gastric cancer. Furthermore, the treatment of reflux disease with proton pump inhibitor drugs appears to accelerate atrophic gastritis in the body of the stomach of *H. pylori*-positive individuals[4,5].

It is not clear why the organism colonizes the stomach, and what special properties it must possess in order to be successful in the hostile acidic environment. These properties are likely to be many, but central to its survival must be the ability to resist at least a certain degree of acidity more efficiently than an aerobic bacterium such as *E. coli*.

Microorganisms can be classified as neutrophiles (those surviving at neutral pH), acidophiles (those surviving in highly acidic media) and alkalophiles (those surviving at highly alkaline pH). In turn there are obligate and facultative acidophiles or alkalophiles. The first question to resolve is whether *H. pylori* is possibly an acidophile.

Its optimal growth *in vitro* is between pH 6.0 and 7.0, and it does not grow at all at pH levels below 4.5–5.0 or at a pH above 8.0 *in vitro*[6]. These data alone show that this organism shows neutrophile characteristics and is not an acidophile. Yet it is present in the stomach of much of the adult population of the Western world, and in even more in the developing countries. It survives *in vitro* only between a medium pH of 4.0 and 8.2, in the absence of urea[7] (see below).

One explanation that has been entertained is that the actual gastric surface pH is surprisingly high. It has been suggested that gastric surface pH, irrespective of the rate of acid secretion, is close to 6.0 based on surface pH measurements using microelectrodes[8]. If this were correct, one might suppose that even *E. coli* would routinely colonize the stomach. Others have suggested that the ability of the gastric epithelium to elevate its pH to a value greater than that of the lumen is limited to when the pH of gastric contents is 3.0 or greater, i.e. not more than 1 mmol/L acid[9]. The ability of the gastric surface to neutralize luminal acidity is not only a function of the pH, but also of the volume of gastric contents. The mean diurnal pH in humans is about 1.4[10]. However, it must be remembered that this mean value is heavily skewed because of the relatively acidic pH at night, at which time there is a very low volume of a highly acidic secretion. There is also a need to separate the gastric fundus and gastric antrum in terms of the surface pH. Since the fundus secretes acid, its surface pH is likely to be more acidic as compared to the antrum, which does not secrete acid. In particular, in the base of the antral glands where there is not only a restricted diffusion path for the luminal acid, but also an ability to secrete HCO_3^-, it is likely that the pH is significantly higher than in the gastric lumen, particularly under conditions of low acid load. This would argue for a higher incidence of the organism in the antrum than in the fundus, and a higher incidence of the organism in the base of the antral gland than at the surface, which indeed appears to be the case[11]. Nevertheless, the organism must be able to resist considerable acidity for varying periods of time.

Another explanation for the gastric survival of the bacterium is its production of urease. The urease hydrolyses urea in the gastric contents to $2NH_3 + CO_2$, with resulting potential alkalinization of the environment to a pH as high as 9.0 in the absence of acid secretion or buffering. The enzyme itself is Ni^{2+}-dependent and consists of two subunits which also require Ni^{2+} for assembly. There does not appear to be a cleavable signal sequence to allow direct export of this protein. However, in addition the urease operon contains several other genes, two of which are clearly integral membrane proteins[12], but whose function is unknown. Urease is found on the exterior of *H. pylori* and, given the apparent absence of secretory mechanisms, the means whereby urease reaches the exterior of the organism is not known. One suggestion is that there is altruistic death of bacteria, with release and then binding of the urease from dead organisms to the surface of live organisms[13], but no direct experimental evidence has been obtained. The importance of the urease for *H. pylori* is emphasized by the finding that urease-negative mutants are not able to colonize the stomach. On the other hand, urease inhibitors are not successful in eradicating the organism once established (H. Larsson, personal communication). Measurement of urease activity is simple, either detecting alkalinization in the presence of urea or measuring CO_2 released from ^{14}C or ^{13}C urea. Further, since this is a constitutive enzyme for all infective strains of the organism, polymerase chain reaction amplification or ELISA tests are convenient means of detecting the presence of *H. pylori* in gastric biopsies.

Eradication of *H. pylori* is not a simple task and several drugs are required to be co-administered. The first triple therapy introduced includes bismuth and two antibiotics. The possible toxicity of bismuth, and the fact that no antisecretory medication is included, restricts the advisability for this medication to non-ulcer patients[14]. A newer formulation for bismuth is ranitidine–bismuth subcitrate, which increases the solubility of the bismuth but, again, two antibiotics are required to achieve reasonable rates of eradication[15]. However, this therapy does

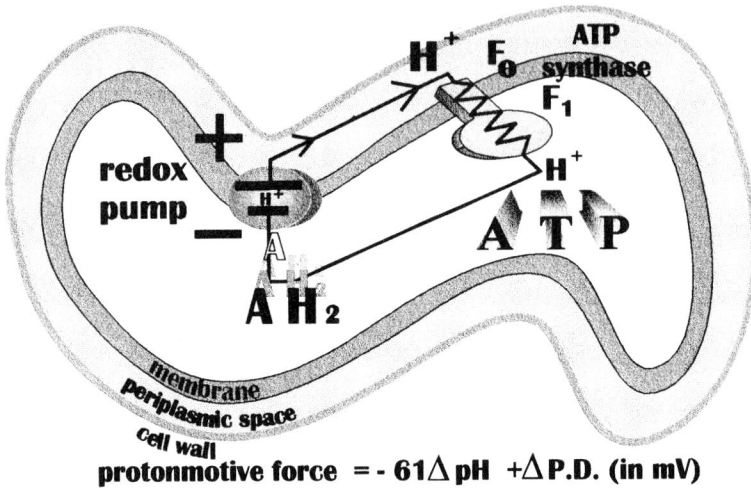

$$\text{protonmotive force} = -61\Delta\,\text{pH} + \Delta\,\text{P.D. (in mV)}$$

Figure 1 Model illustrating the concept of a proton-motive force. The redox pumps are represented as a battery generating a flow of H^+ to the exterior by substrate oxidation; the return circuit is by H^+ flux across the F_0F_1 ATP synthase generating ATP from ADP and Pi

include ranitidine for healing. The mechanism of action of Bi^{2+} is not known. It is retained for some considerable time in the stomach and it is cytotoxic if absorbed. However, it is relatively membrane-impermeable and presumably enters the organism during cell division.

Alternative triple therapies use a proton pump inhibitor with two antibiotics such as amoxycillin with either metronidazole or clarithromycin[16,17]. A proton pump inhibitor alone suppresses the organism in the antrum, but increases the incidence of the organism in the fundic or acid-secreting portion of the stomach[18]. This effect of proton pump inhibitors and their synergism with antibiotics is the topic of this short review, which focuses on the relationship between the membrane energetics of the bacterium and its environmental pH.

EXPERIMENTAL DESIGN

The adjustment of the bioenergetics of *H. pylori* to an acidic or alkaline environment is postulated to play an important role in its ability to survive in the stomach. Since it is neither an acidophile nor an alkalophile, it is most likely a neutrophile that has adapted to the acidic environment of the stomach. It would then be classified as an acid-tolerant neutrophile.

Aerobic bacteria generate an electrochemical gradient for protons, the proton-motive force, across their inner membrane. This is formed by oxidoreductases oriented across the bacterial membrane such that protons are driven outwards and electrons inwards, generating both a proton and electrical gradient (Figure 1). This electrochemical gradient for protons, the sum of the pH gradient and the electric gradient, is used to generate ATP by proton flux across the F_0F_1 ATP synthase in the membrane, and is also used to energize uptake of nutrients[19]. Neutrophiles such as *E. coli* maintain a relatively constant proton-motive force by adjusting the potential difference across the plasma membrane to compensate for the changes of pH gradient.

The proton-motive force, expressed in millivolts is:

$$\Delta \bar{\mu}_H{}^+ = -RT/nF \ln H_{out}/H_{in} + \Delta\psi = -61 \, \Delta pH + \Delta PD$$

The potential difference in neutrophiles is interior negative and the proton-motive force is usually about $-200 \, mV$.

Measurement of the proton-motive force requires evaluation of both the pH gradient and the potential difference. In bacteria and other small particles this measurement must be by indirect means. The distribution of a radioactive weak acid such as salicylate or a weak base such as benzylamine is measured, along with bacterial volume to provide an estimate of the internal pH. The distribution of a radioactive lipid-permeable cation such as Tl^+, ^3H-tetraphenylphosphonium or ^{86}Rb in the presence of the selective ionophore, valinomycin can be used to measure transmembrane potential[20]. This distribution is measured by either centrifugation or by flow dialysis[21]. Application of flow dialysis to measurement of the membrane potential of *H. pylori* gave a value of $-132 \, mV$ at pH 7.0 and the potential declined with the decrease of medium pH[22]. Flow dialysis is a slow response method and instead, in the work to be described, fluorescent probes of membrane potential and internal pH, as developed for mammalian cells, were used[23–25].

For pH measurements the fluorescent dye, BCECF, is added to a bacterial suspension in the form of BCECF-AM, a membrane-permeant, non-fluorescent form of the dye. Once inside a cell, or exposed to an esterase, the acetomethoxy group is removed and the free carboxylic acid groups generated. The dye is now fluorescent and trapped inside the cell or in the vicinity of the esterase. The dye is able to report on pH changes between about 5.8 and 7.8 by an increase in emission at 530 nm as the pH rises and the carboxylic group deprotonates.

$DiSC_3(5)$ is a positively charged lipophilic cation. It accumulates within negatively charged membrane-bounded spaces with an ensuing quench of fluorescence due to stacking of the dye at the solution–membrane interface. Hence this dye is able to measure internal negative, but not internal positive, potentials in isolated cells, bacteria and mitochondria.

These two dyes were applied to measuring internal pH and transmembrane potential in *H. pylori*. In particular the carbocyanine dye was used to measure transmembrane potential as a function of external pH. In all cases bacteria grown on blood agar plates were used.

Bacterial survival as a function of external pH was correlated with these measurements. Bacteria grown on blood agar plates were suspended in buffer and an aliquot suspended in strong buffer between pH 3.0 and 9.0 for 90 min, then diluted, and colony-forming units determined on blood agar plates in the absence of urea.

The pH-dependence of growth was determined by varying external pH again with strong buffers in the absence of urea. These methods are detailed elsewhere[26].

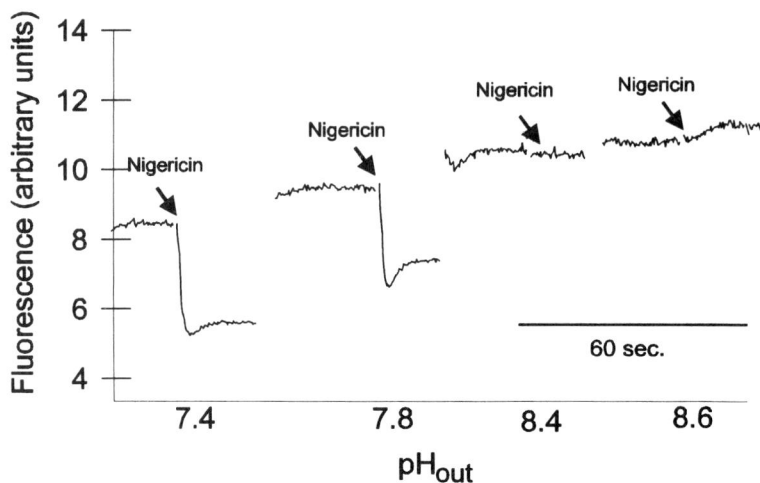

Figure 2 Use of a null-point method to calibrate the internal pH with BCECF. The bacteria are loaded with BCECF and placed in media at different pH with $[K] = 240$ mmol/L. After 1 min nigericin is added to equilibrate H_{in} and H_{out}. The external pH at which no change in fluorescence is seen is taken as the internal pH

RESULTS

Internal pH of *H. pylori*

The bacteria load well with BCECF-AM. They become visible as highly fluorescent spiral organisms. Much of the BCECF appears to be extracellular; thus changing medium pH results in a rapid change of fluorescence, and the addition of urea in weakly buffered medium also rapidly elevates fluorescence. If indeed the liberated dye is surface-bound, normal methods of calibration using the dual-excitation mode will report on medium and not intracellular pH.

In order to determine intracellular pH a null-point method was developed. Firstly, the internal [K] was determined in a batch of bacteria using the null-point method for $DiSC_3(5)$. Then the organism loaded with BCECF was added to media of different pH containing high K so that no K gradient should be present. After a short period of equilibration, the H for K exchanger, nigericin was added to equilibrate pH.

As shown in Figure 2 there was no change in fluorescence when the medium was at pH 8.4, but acidification of internal pH at 8.0 and lower, with alkalinization at pH 8.6 and above. From this, given that the internal and external [K] are exactly the same, the pH_{int} of *H. pylori* is 8.4. The same method used on *E. coli* spheroplasts gives a pH_{int} of 8.0, perhaps about $0.2 - 0.4$ pH units higher than those determined from weak base distribution. This would result if the $[K]_{in}$ was overestimated by the null-point method of calibration of potential difference.

Given that the BCECF is mainly extracellular, it is difficult to use this dye to estimate internal pH at lower pH values. However, as is discussed below, on the assumption that the proton-motive force is maintained constant, it is possible to

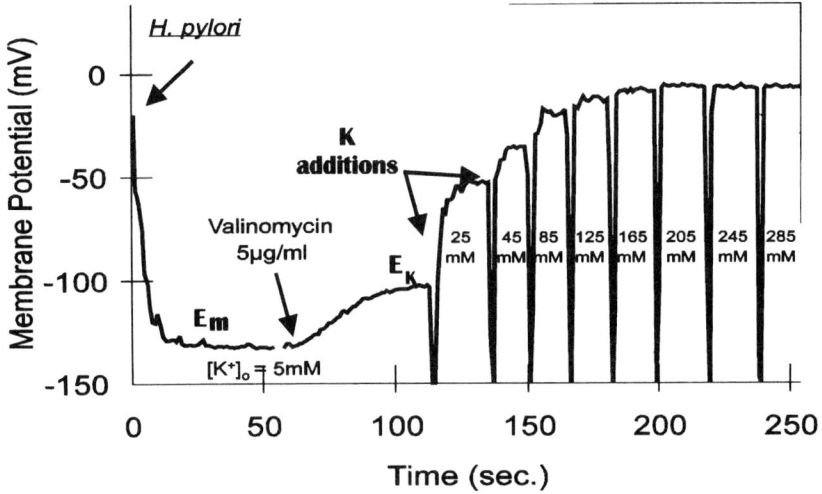

Figure 3 Null-point method to calibrate transmembrane potential using the fluorescent cationic dye, DiSC$_3$(5). The bacteria are added to a solution of DiSC$_3$(5), and uptake of the dye is indicated by a quench of fluorescence. Valinomycin is added to establish E_K and then external K is increased in a stepwise fashion until no further change in potential is seen. This then gives K$_{int}$ and, from that, the Nernst equation gives the transmembrane voltage in the presence of valinomycin as -101 mV, and the potential in the absence of valinomycin as -131 mV

calculate the change in internal pH as a function of external pH by the shortfall in change of membrane potential.

Transmembrane potential

Addition of *H. pylori* to medium containing the DiSC$_3$(5) dye results in a rapid uptake of the dye with a quench of fluorescence. Addition of the K$^+$ selective ionophore, valinomycin, results in an increase of fluorescence due to the establishment of the K$^+$ equilibrium potential, which is less than the membrane potential. Successive additions of K$^+$ to the medium result in increased fluorescence when the external [K$^+$] reaches between 200 and 240 mmol/L. At this point, therefore, the potential difference becomes zero when the internal and external K$^+$ concentrations are equal (Figure 3).

The concentration of internal K$^+$ allows calculation of the membrane potential with the external K$^+$ at 5 mmol/L when valinomycin is added and, by extrapolation, calculation of the resting membrane potential of *H. pylori* at pH 7.0. The value found is -131 mV, which is remarkably close to that (-132 mV) found using flow dialysis measurement of the distribution of the lipid-permeable cation, ^{3}H-TPMP[22].

The use of fluorimetry allows rapid measurement of the response of the organism to changes in medium pH, or to the addition of a variety of chemicals or drugs. If the organism is added to solutions containing DiSC$_3$(5) at different pH values, as shown in Figure 4, there is a progressive decrease in the potential difference

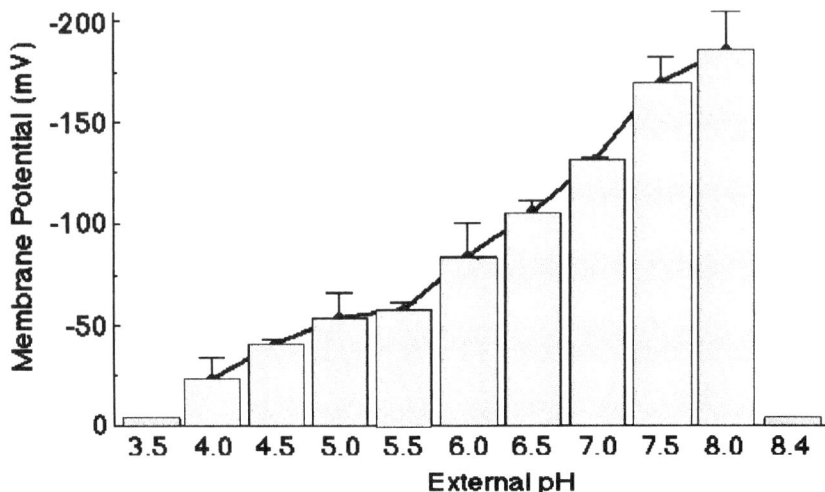

Figure 4 Variation of transmembrane potential as a function of external pH. The bacteria are placed in media of different pH and the potential difference measured using $DiSC_3(5)$. The zero potential in each experiment is obtained by adding 50 nmol/L tetrachlorsalicylanilide (TCS)

as the external pH decreases. This is best explained by the proton-motive force equation shown above, which predicts a reciprocal relationship between the potential difference and the pH gradient across the bacterial membrane.

From Figure 4 it can be seen that, between pH 8.0 and 5.0, there is a fall of transmembrane potential of about 120 mV. The theoretical fall would be 180 mV for the 3 pH unit shift if there were no change in the internal pH of the organism. If the carbocyanine dye is reporting linearly across this range of pH, the implication is that the internal pH has decreased by 1 unit as the pH changes from 8.0 to 5.0.

At pH 3.5 and 8.4, as emphasized in Figure 4, the potential difference is measured as zero. Whereas this measured value would be anticipated at the acidic pH, it is unexpected at the higher pH value. It is therefore important to define whether this loss of potential difference is readily reversed by restoring medium pH.

The method chosen to determine the reversibility was to place the organisms in the fluorimeter at either the acidic or the alkaline pH where no potential difference was seen. Then, after either 1 min or between 10 and 20 min, buffer was added to bring the organisms into a range at which a potential difference was present, to see whether this restoration of a viable pH was able to restore the potential difference.

Figure 5 shows that, when the organisms are placed in acidic pH at 3.5, the potential difference is close to zero. When the medium is brought up to a pH of 6.5, after 1 min there is a gradual restoration of the potential difference to the value expected at this pH. Hence it is possible to reverse the effect of short-term exposure to acid. However, after 5 min of exposure it is no longer possible to reverse the effect of acidification to pH 3.5. This result implies that the organism

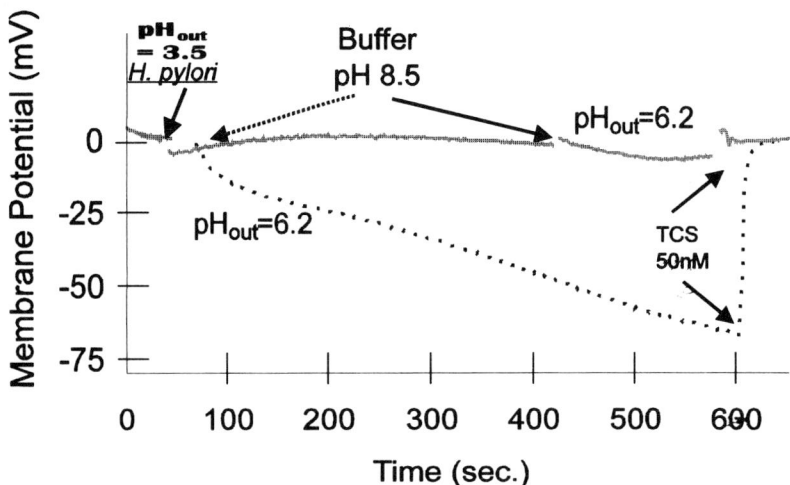

Figure 5 Effect of pH elevation on transmembrane potential after acid exposure for a short period of time (dashed line) and a longer period of time (solid line). At the end of each experiment TCS is added to set the potential to zero

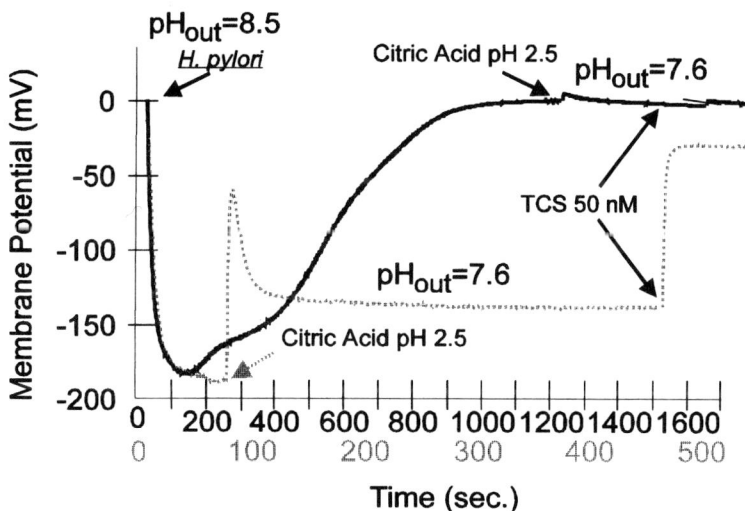

Figure 6 Effect of pH reduction on transmembrane potential after alkali exposure for a short period of time (dashed line) and a longer period of time (solid line). At the end of each experiment TCS is added to set the potential to zero

in the stomach is not routinely exposed to this pH at the surface of its plasma membrane for any length of time, presumably due to localized urease activity.

In turn, Figure 6 illustrates the effect of alkalinization to pH 8.5. If the organism is exposed to this pH for 1 min, and the medium reacidified, there is a rapid restoration of the potential difference down from the peak of about −180 mV. If, however, the alkalinity is allowed to collapse the potential difference to zero, reduction of the pH has no further effect. The proton-motive force in this organism can therefore resist transient alkalinization to a pH of 8.4, but not alkalinization of a long duration.

Survival of H. pylori

If the survival of H. pylori is measured at different pH values using strong buffer, so that the metabolism of the organism does not change the medium pH, the pH range over which the organism survives for 90 min is exactly the pH range over which it can maintain an effective proton-motive force or the capacity for oxidative synthesis of ATP. This is shown in Figure 7a. The inability of the organism to survive acidic pH may be ascribed to its inability to resist proton influx at a pH of 3.5 or below. Its inability to resist alkalinity may be due to the potential difference-dependent collapse of membrane integrity, as is found in artificial bilayers. Growth occurs over a more limited pH range, as shown in Figure 7b. Evidently maintenance of a proton-motive force alone is an insufficient condition for growth.

The effect of urea

The production of urease by H. pylori has long been recognized as a significant factor in enabling its gastric survival[27-29]. The hydrolysis of urea results in the formation of $(NH_4)_2CO_3$ with a pK_a of about 9, hence is able to elevate the pH in the immediate environment of the organism, to relatively neutral values in the presence of acid, and to alkaline values in neutral solutions. This is illustrated in Figure 8, which shows the effect of 5 mmol/L urea addition to acidic or neutral suspensions of H. pylori.

When 5 mmol/L urea is added to a suspension of H. pylori that have been maintained at a pH of 3.5, where there is no longer dye uptake, there is a rapid quenching of fluorescence and eventually the medium pH is about 6.0. The re-establishment of the normal transmembrane potential for a pH of 6.0 occurs more rapidly than the change of medium pH, and is also faster than when buffer is added to the medium (cf. Figure 5). This suggests that neutralization of the acid by urease activity is in a privileged compartment, such as the periplasmic space (Figure 8). Similar data were found for pH 3.0, but at pH 2.5 H. pylori was unable to reverse the potential difference. In the case of addition of 5 mmol/L urea to H. pylori suspended in weak buffer at pH 6 or 7, there is continuing alkalinization up to a pH of at least 8.4, with collapse of potential. These data show that, whereas urease is protective of the organism at mildly acidic pH, its activity is toxic at neutral pH in the absence of buffer.

The nature of H. pylori

Given that the organism survives over a pH range of 4–8, similar to that of E. coli, it must be considered as a neutrophile in terms of its bioenergetics. The

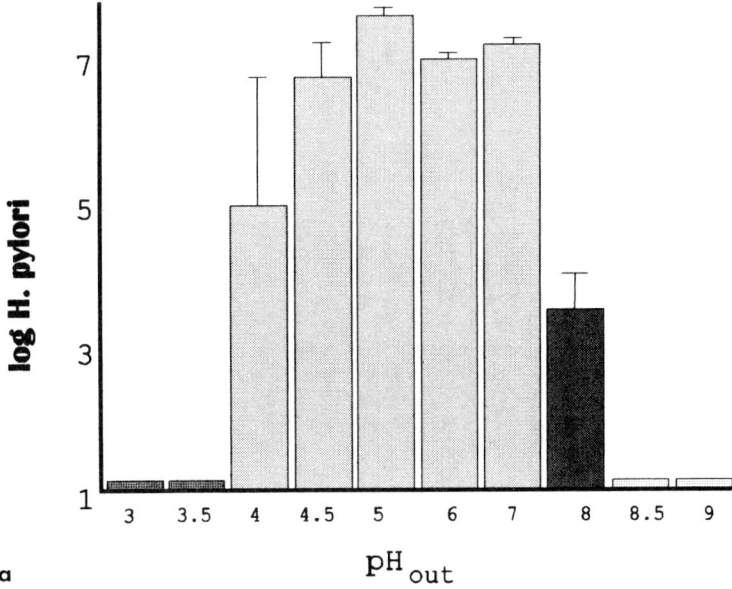

a

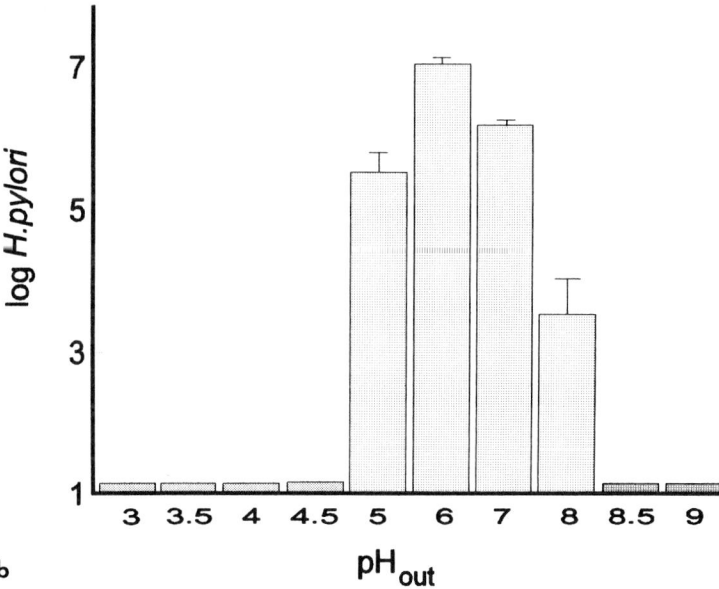

b

Figure 7 (a) Survival of *H. pylori* at different pH values in the absence of urea. (b) Growth of *H. pylori* at different pH values in the absence of urea

presence of urease allows survival down to a pH of 3.0, making it acid-tolerant. Urease activity also makes it relatively alkali-intolerant. The organism appears to survive in the stomach by adjusting its ability to generate its bioenergetic potential over a wider range of acidity than is usual for a neutrophile by the synthesis and

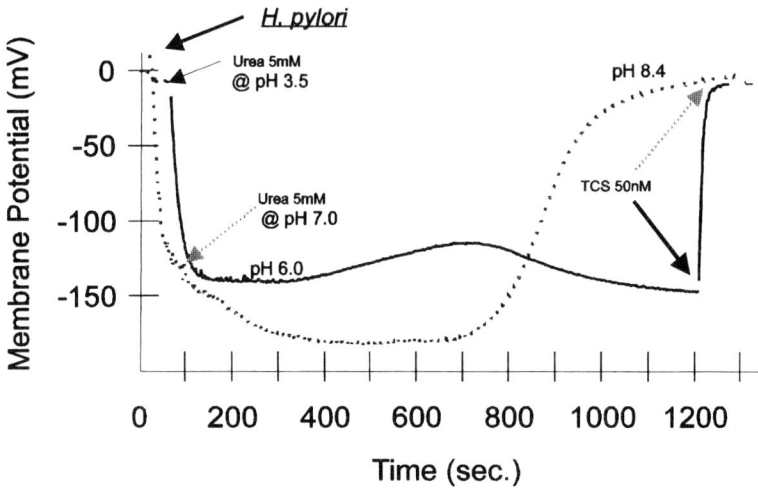

Figure 8 Effect of addition of urea under acidic (heavy line) and under neutral conditions of external pH (dashed line). At the end of each experiment TCS is added to set the potential to zero

activity of urease. The organism can therefore be classified as an *acid-tolerant* neutrophile.

DISCUSSION

The above findings explain, in part at least, the ability of *H. pylori* to survive in the acid environment of the stomach, as well as the effect of proton pump inhibitors (PPI) in suppressing the organism. Urease activity allows survival when the medium acidity is increased as due to acid secretion, to an environmental pH as low as 3.0, but not below. This defines the sites at which the organism can be found in the stomach, namely those regions where the pH is not lower than 3.0. The finding that survival occurs at pH 3.0 in the presence of urea, and that the organism is presently only in low numbers in the fundus, suggests that this region of the stomach has a surface pH of less than 3.0 for some considerable time, arguing against the pH electrode studies that have been interpreted as showing a surface pH of 6.0 or more. The prevalence of the organism in antral glands shows that there is not only survival in this region but also growth. Since growth is found *in vitro* only at a pH > 5.0, it would appear that, in the base of the antral glands, this pH is reached for some considerable fraction of the day.

The effect of proton pump inhibition on the organism in the stomach is readily explained by the findings discussed above. At standard therapy, on once-a-day treatment, after 3 days it may be anticipated that the pH at the base of antral glands, at least, may be elevated close to neutrality. At this pH urease activity could well result in elevation of pH into a toxic range. In fact there is significant suppression of *H. pylori* in the antrum with administration of omeprazole[3,18], consistent with the bioenergetic data. On the other hand the elevation of surface pH in the fundus by proton pump inhibition allows greater survival and even growth in this region, although not to the level found in the antrum. Overall, PPI administration would then result in suppression of the organism.

It is also possible to explain the synergism between PPI and either clarithromycin or amoxicillin based on the pH-dependent redistribution of the infective organism. The former is targeted to the ribosome and hence protein synthesis, the latter to cell wall biosynthesis. Both antibiotics are therefore most effective during the cell replication that occurs in log phase. Since PPI allow growth in the fundus, where previously there was none, the organisms in the fundus now become more sensitive to antibiotics, and both classes of drug inhibit the organism in the antrum.

At a pH of 4.0 to 5.0, at which the organism survives but does not grow, the organism is in stationary phase; at pH 5–7 the organism is able to grow, but has a long generation time of about 8 h. Since many antibiotics recommended for use in eradication of *H. pylori* require log phase for their bactericidal action, a pH-dependent alteration in the distribution of organisms between stationary and log phase will have significant effects on eradication results. However, PPI at current therapeutic levels will not fully inhibit acid secretion, and regions of acidity are likely to remain, where the organism is in stationary phase. For eradication, therefore, additional therapy will be required, such as a growth-independent antibiotic such as metronidazole, or even bismuth in addition. Clearly as more compounds are necessary, resistance, side-effects and compliance become increasingly important issues.

The measurement of the ability of *H. pylori* to maintain a proton-motive force has other implications. For example, adverse conditions of growth appear to result in coccoid formation. It is not known whether these coccoids are viable for a time, and whether they play any role in allowing survival of the bacteria. The ability of these ccccoids to maintain or re-establish a proton-motive force is therefore of importance in defining their viability.

On the other hand, there are many other factors that are probably of importance in determining gastric colonization of *H. pylori,* such as adherence to gastric epithelial cells. There appear to be specific receptors on these cells allowing tight adhesion, and once adhesion is established gastric cellular properties may aid survival of the organism. Bacterial motility also should play a role, in that random motion would allow the organism to escape from an inimical acidic or alkaline environment. H^+-dependent chemotaxis is unlikely but flagellar motors depend on the maintenance of a transmembrane electrochemical H^+ gradient and therefore motility is also linked to the ability to maintain a proton-motive force. Other enzymes also may be responsible for elevation of pH, especially inside the organism, such as deaminases.

Acknowledgements

This work was supported by USVA SMI funds and NIH grants DK40615, 41301 and 17294.

References

1. Warren JR, Marshall BJ. Unidentified curved bacilli on gastric epithelium in active chronic gastritis. Lancet. 1983;1:1273–5.

2. Graham DY. *Campylobacter pylori* and peptic ulcer disease. Gastroenterology. 1989;96:615–25.
3. Lee A, Dixon MF, Danon SJ *et al.* Local acid production and *Helicobacter pylori*: a unifying hypothesis of gastroduodenal disease. Eur J Gastroenterol Hepatol. 1995;7:461–5.
4. Walsh JH, Peterson WL. The treatment of *Helicobacter pylori* infection in the management of peptic ulcer disease. N Engl J Med. 1995;333:984–91.
5. Kuipers EJ, Lundell L, Klinkenberg-Knol EC *et al.* Atrophic gastritis and *Helicobacter pylori* infection in patients with reflux esophagitis treated with omeprazole or fundoplication. N Engl J Med. 1996;334:1018–22.
6. Morgan DR, Freedman F, Depew CE, Kraft WG. Growth of Campylobacter in liquid media. J Clin Microbiol. 1987;25:2123–5.
7. Clyne M, Labigne A, Drumm B. *Helicobacter pylori* requires an acidic environment to survive in the presence of urea. Infect Immun. 1995;63:1669–73.
8. Schade C, Flemstrom G, Holm I. Hydrogen ion concentration in the mucus layer on top of acid-stimulated and -inhibited rat gastric mucosa. Gastroenterology. 1994;107:180–8.
9. Engel E, Peskoff A, Kauffman GL Jr, Grossman MI. Analysis of hydrogen ion concentration in the gastric gel mucus layer. Am J Physiol. 1984;247:G321–38.
10. Burget DW, Chiverton SG, Hunt RH. Is there an optimal degree of acid suppression for healing of duodenal ulcers? A model of the relationship between ulcer healing and acid suppression. Gastroenterology. 1990;99:345–51.
11. Atherton JC, Cockayne A, Balsitis M, Kirk GE, Hawkey CJ, Spiller RC. Detection of the intra-gastric sites at which *Helicobacter pylori* evades treatment with amoxycillin and cimetidine. Gut. 1995;36:670–4.
12. Gerrero RL, Labigne A. Organization and expression of the *Helicobacter pylori* urease gene cluster. In: Goodwin CS, Wothey BW, editors. *Helicobacter pylori*: biology and clinical practice. Boca Raton, FLA: CRC Press; 1993:177–95.
13. Parma DH, Snyder M, Soboloevski S, Nawroz M, Gold L. The rex system of bacteriophage lambda and altruistic cell death. Genes Dev. 1992;6:497–510.
14. Thijs JC, van Zwet AA, Moolenaar W, Wolfhagen MJ, ten Bokkel Huinink J. Triple therapy vs amoxicillin plus omeprazole for treatment of *Helicobacter pylori* infection: a multicenter, prospective, randomized, controlled study of efficacy and side effects. Am J Gastroenterol. 1996;91:93–7.
15. Bardhan KD, Dekkers CP, Lam SK *et al.* GR122311X (ranitidine bismuth citrate), a new drug for the treatment of duodenal ulcer. Aliment Pharmacol Ther. 1995;9:497–506.
16. Yousfi MM, El-Zimaity HMT, Cole RA, Genta RM, Graham DY. Metronidazole, omeprazole and clarithromycin: an effective combination therapy for *Helicobacter pylori* infection. Aliment Pharmacol Ther. 1995;9:209–12.
17. Labenz J, Peitz U, Tillenburg B, Becker T, Boersch G, Stolte M. Short-term triple therapy with pantoprazole, clarithromycin and metronidazole for eradication of *Helicobacter pylori*. Leber Magen Darm. 1995;122:125–7.
18. Logan RPH, Walker MM, Misiewicz JJ, Kirk GE, Hawkey CJ, Spiller RC. Changes in the intra-gastric distribution of *Helicobacter pylori* during treatment with omeprazole. Gut. 1995;36:12–16.
19. Mitchell P. Chemiosmotic coupling in oxidative and photosynthetic phosphorylation. Biol Rev. 1966;41:445–502.
20. Ramos S, Schuldiner S, Kaback HR. The electrochemical gradient of protons and its relationship to active transport in *E. coli* membrane vesicles. Proc Natl Acad Sci USA. 1976;73:1892–6.
21. Kashket ER. The proton motive force in bacteria: a critical assessment of methods. Annu Rev Microbiol. 1985;39:219–42.
22. Matin A, Zychlinsky E, Keyahn M, Sachs G. The capacity of *Helicobacter pylori* to generate ionic gradients at low pH is similar to that of bacteria that grow under strongly acidic conditions. Infect Immun. 1996;64:1434–6.
23. Futsaether CM, Kjeldstad B, Johnsson A. Measurement of intracellular pH of *Propionumbacterium acne*: comparison between the fluorescent probe, BCECF and ^{31}P-NMR spectroscopy. Can J Microbiol. 1993;19:180–6.
24. Waggoner AS. Optical probes of membrane potential. J Membrane Biol. 1976;27:317–34.
25. Paradiso AM, Tsien RY, Machen TE. Digital image processing of intracellular pH in gastric oxyntic and chief cells. Nature. 1987;325:447–50.
26. Meyer-Rosberg K, Scott DR, Rex D, Melchers K, Sachs G. The effect of environmental pH on the proton motive force of *Helicobacter pylori*. Gastroenterology. 1996 (In press).

27. Eaton KA, Krakowka S. Effect of gastric pH on urease dependent colonisation of gnotobiotic piglets by *Helicobacter pylori*. Infect Immun. 1994;62:3604–7.
28. Eaton KA, Morgan DR, Brooks CL, Krakowka S. Essential role of urease in the pathogenesis of gastritis induced by *Helicobacter pylori* in gnotobiotic piglets. Infect Immun. 1991;59:2470–5.
29. Tsuda M, Karita M, Morshed MG, Okita K, Nakazawa T. A urease negative mutant of *Helicobacter pylori* constructed by allelic exchange mutagenesis lacks the ability to colonize the nude mouse stomach. Infect Immun. 1994;62:3586–9.

7
P-type ion motive ATPases of *Helicobacter pylori*

K. MELCHERS, W. STEINHILBER and K. P. SCHÄFER

INTRODUCTION

Helicobacter pylori is an acid-tolerant neutrophile isolated in 1983 by Warren and Marshall[1]. Today it is known as a human gastric pathogen associated with peptic ulcer as well as chronic gastritis which may predispose to gastric cancer[2,3]. The bacterium is unique in surviving in the human stomach which is dominated by the gastric proton pump, the H,K,ATPase. The stomach is notorious for providing a highly variable cationic environment. Thus, *H. pylori* must have developed specialized physiological strategies of both survival and pathogenicity. Rational strategies of *H. pylori* eradication need prior elucidation of these mechanisms to define possible molecular drug target sites.

The primary basis of *H. pylori* survival, as well as for other bacteria, is the proton motive force (p.m.f.) across the cytoplasmic membrane ensuring a continuous supply of energy by ATP synthesis[4]. Maintaining the p.m.f. requires that the proton concentration in the external medium stays within certain pH limits. Urease activity plays a central role in *H. pylori* acid tolerance by production of large amounts of ammonia due to cleavage of urea. Ammonia is a potent proton scavenger through formation of ammonium ions. The balance between acid secretion into the gastric lumen by the gastric H,K,ATPase, and urease activity is now thought to maintain the p.m.f. of *H. pylori* even under acidic conditions[5]. In conclusion, expression of urease is essential for survival and therefore is a prerequisite of *H. pylori* colonization as well as pathogenicity (Figure 1). Since urease is a nickel metalloenzyme expressed in large amounts[6,7] *H. pylori* needs an efficient management of nickel supplies. With respect to cellular homeostasis of ions the bacterium has to control the expression of selected ion transporters. **NixA**, a high-affinity Ni^{2+} uptake transport protein[8], and **hpn**, a cytoplasmic Ni^{2+} storage protein[9], are parts of the nickel management system of *H. pylori*. Moreover, as shown for other bacteria, expression of ion transporters is essential for turgor pressure, homeostasis of intracellular pH and ion composition as well as maintenance of transmembrane ion gradients as the basis of transport across the cytoplasmic membrane and generation of energy. Among these membrane

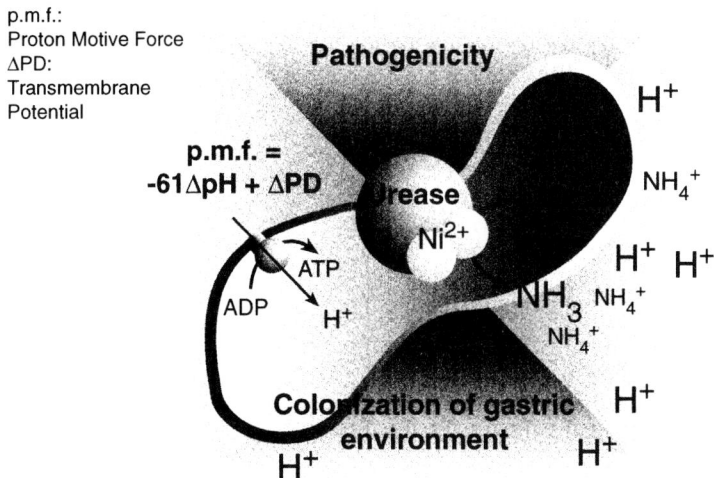

p.m.f.:
Proton Motive Force
ΔPD:
Transmembrane
Potential

p.m.f. =
-61ΔpH + ΔPD

Figure 1 Central role of urease for *H. pylori* survival. Urease is a nickel metalloenzyme constitutively expressed in large amounts in *H. pylori*. The enzyme plays a central role during colonization as well as pathogenicity. Urease neutralizes the gastric acid by production of ammonia which binds protons by forming ammonium ions. Urease activity therefore leads to elevated pH values in the microenvironment of the bacterium. This mechanism is thought to be essential during the initial step of colonization of the stomach by *H. pylori*. Enzymatic cleavage of urea stabilizes the pH difference (ΔpH) between the cytoplasm and the extracellular microenvironment of *H. pylori* under acidic conditions, allowing ATP synthesis driven by the p.m.f. even at low external pH values

transporters may be suitable targets for the development of drugs for *H. pylori* eradication.

ION PUMPS DETECTED IN *H. PYLORI*

Several ion transporters and ion pumps of *H. pylori* are now described in preliminary form, or have been cloned and analysed in more detail (Figure 2). Among these pumps are two transition metal ion pumps, ATPase-439 and ATPase-948 (the latter also referred to as Cop ATPase) cloned in our laboratory. These two pumps of 75 kDa (ATPase-439) or 81 kDa (ATPase-948) belong to the class of P-type ion motive ATPases. All known P-type ATPases contain an invariant aspartate residue, which forms the β-aspartyl phosphate intermediate during the catalytic cycle, embedded in a strictly conserved DKTGT consensus motif. We used this sequence motif to isolate the two genes from an *H. pylori* gene library by employing degenerate DNA oligonucleotides in a Southern blot screening method[10]. In other bacteria, members of this distinct family of ion transporters have been postulated to play important roles in a variety of environmental adaptation systems. Therefore, biochemical and functional analysis of the cloned ion pumps may give us further insights into *H. pylori* physiology and molecular biology.

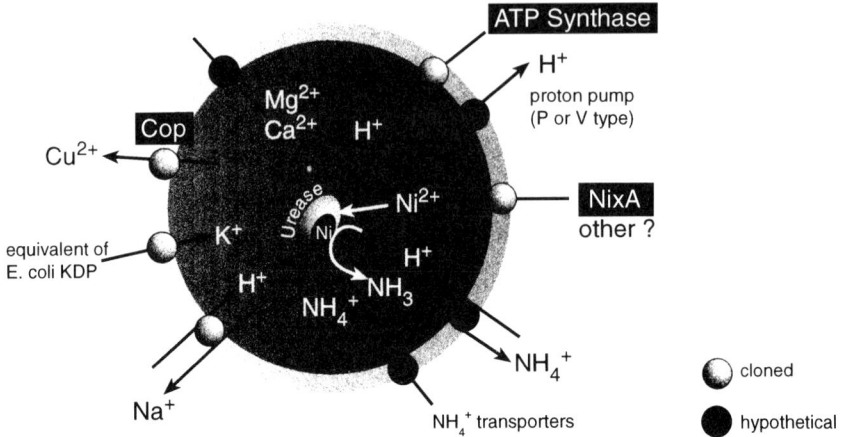

Figure 2 Central role of ion transport for *H. pylori* biology. Several ion-transport mechanisms are expected to be active in *H. pylori* maintaining intracellular ion composition, turgor pressure and intracellular pH. These mechanisms are essential for survival of the pathogen in the human stomach and include the action of transporter ATPases. Among those, some are expected to represent homologues of proteins also present in other bacteria (general ion-transport pathways), while others should be adapted to the special need of *H. pylori* in its unique environment. The latter, for example, comprise the expression of NixA, a high-affinity uptake transporter for Ni^{2+}. Shown in the figure are hypothetical transporters involved in the management of Mg^{2+}, Ca^{2+}, H^+ and NH_4^+. Others are described in preliminary reports, e.g. the homologue of the Kdp operon of *Escherichia coli*, the H^+,Na^+ antiporter and an F-type ATP synthetase (Clayton, C.L. *et al.*, abstract presented at Workshop of the European *H. pylori* Study Group, Edinburgh, 1995). Two P-type ion pumps, a Cu^{2+} ATPase and an ion pump involved in urease activity (ATPase-439) were cloned and analysed in more detail[11,16]

ATPase-439: a P-type ATPase involved in urease activity

This ion pump, which was the first full-length P-type ATPase cloned from *H. pylori,* consists of 686 amino acids including the conserved sites of phosphorylation and ATP binding[10]. From amino acid similarity and hydropathy analysis the enzyme was very similar to the bacterial Cu^{2+} and Cd^{2+} transition metal ion ATPases[11,12]. In collaboration with George Sachs from the University of California at Los Angeles (UCLA, USA) the topology of the pump was assayed by *in-vitro* translation of fusion vectors containing putative membrane-spanning sequences. This showed that the membrane domain of the pump is formed by at least eight transmembrane segments[10]. Transmembrane segment 6 (TM6) contained a Cys−Pro−Cys motif characteristic for transition metal ion pumps, also referred to as CPX-type ATPases[12]. The data from the topological analysis placed the large cytoplasmic ATP-binding and phosphorylation loop between TM6 and TM7. In this region the enzyme contained several cysteine and histidine residues, possibly indicative of ion binding. In the N-terminal region there is another putative ion-binding site present. The motif found here consists of a Cys−X−X−Cys motif preceded by a pair of histidine residues (HIHNLDCPDC). Cys/His sequences are assumed[13] to provide binding sites for cations such as Zn^{2+} or Ni^{2+}. These data are summarized in Figure 3.

In collaboration with Rainer Haas from the Max-Planck Institute of Biology at

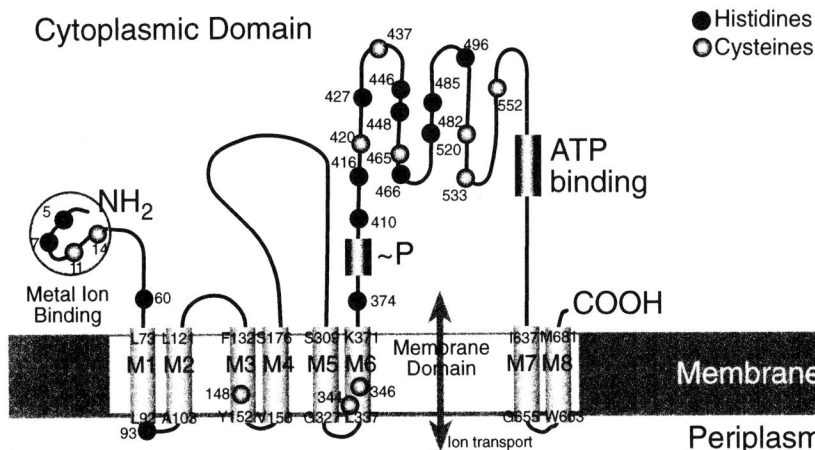

Figure 3 Model of ATPase-439. The ATPase consists of 686 amino acids. It carries a comparatively small membrane domain while most of the amino acid chain resides in the cytoplasm. The membrane domain is formed by four pairs of transmembrane segments, M1 through M8. M6 contains a conserved Cys^{344}–Pro–Cys^{346} motif characteristic for transition metal ion pumps. Also present is an N-terminal His/Cys ion-binding motif. The large cytoplasmic loop between transmembrane segment 6 (M6) and 7 (M7) carrying the conserved sequence elements of ATP binding and phosphorylation contains several cysteine and histidine residues while the membrane domain is relatively poor in Cys/His. ATPase-439 was isolated by Southern blot screening using degenerate DNA oligonucleotide probes targeted to the conserved phosphorylation region present in P type ATPases[11]

Tübingen (Germany) the ATPase-439 gene of an *H. pylori* strain was inactivated by transposon insertion. Preliminary data obtained by analysis of the *H. pylori* mutants containing inactivated ATPase-439 genes revealed that the mutants were strongly reduced in urease activity. Since this phenotype of the mutants could be reversed by growing the ATPase-439 deficient strains in medium supplemented with NiCl$_2$ it is likely that this ion pump is involved in the nickel transport mechanisms of *H. pylori*.

ATPase-948: a copper resistance pump

The first publication on the existence of a Cop ATPase in *H. pylori* was from Ge *et al.* in 1995[14]. They reported a Cop operon carrying two genes which encode a P-type ATPase of 611 amino acids, hpCopA, and a small divalent cation-binding protein referred to as hpCopP. Knockout mutation of the CopA gene rendered the *H. pylori* mutants more susceptible to Cu^{2+} ions, indicating a role in copper export of the CopA ion pump[14]. The *hpCopA* gene product, in contrast to the other Cu^{2+} ion pumps cloned so far[12], has been described to contain a membrane domain of only six transmembrane segments. Also missing is an N-terminal ion-binding motif characteristic for the transition metal ion pumps. Since a Cys–X–X–Cys ion-binding motif was found in the CopP gene associated with the hpCopA operon it was speculated that CopP provides the ion-binding site for the Cop ATPase. However, these irregularities, as reported previously[14], could be

81

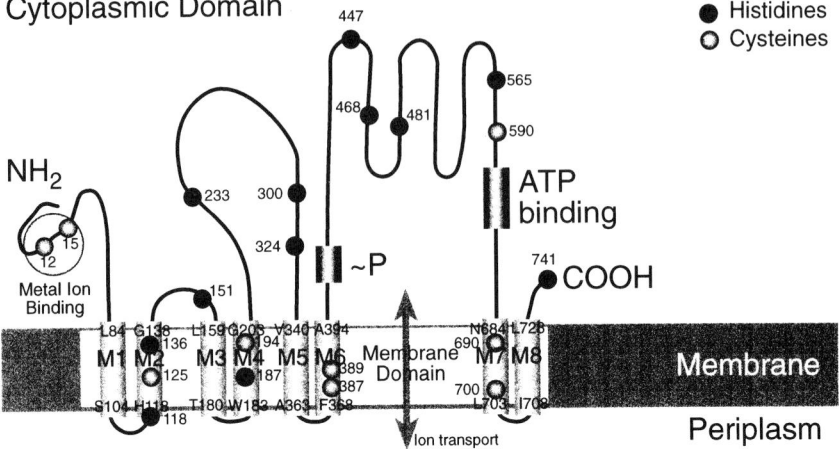

Figure 4 Model of ATPase-948 (Cop ATPase). This ion pump of *H. pylori*, also isolated by Southern blot screening[11], contains 741 amino acids. The transmembrane segments, M1–M8, were predicted by hydropathy analysis and homology to the other transition metal ion pumps. As found for ATPase-439, a Cys[387]–Pro–Cys[389] motif is present in M6 of Cop ATPase. An N-terminal ion binding motif of the Cys–X–X–Cys type was also found. The large loop of ATP binding and phosphorylation is located between transmembrane segments 6 and 7. This ATPase is most probably active as a copper export pump

due to cloning of an N-terminal truncated protein. Using the same strategy of P-type ion pump isolation we now have cloned the full-length Cop ATPase of *H. pylori* encoded by an open reading frame (ORF) of 2223 bp of plasmid pRH948 (ATPase-948). The gene predicts a membrane pump of 741 amino acids containing an N-terminal Cys–Ser–His–Cys ion-binding motif, as found in the other Cu^{2+}-transporting ATPases of bacteria and eukaryotic cells. The hydropathy profile predicts a membrane domain of eight hydrophobic segments. These data indicate that the Cop ATPase of *H. pylori* acts as a single subunit ATPase. Figure 4 summarizes the general structural features of Cop ATPase. The numbers of cysteine as well as histidine residues are similar when compared to ATPase-439, but their distribution along the amino acid sequence is different. Six out of nine cysteines are located in the membrane domain of ATPase-948 while most of the histidine residues reside in the cytoplasmic fraction of the enzyme.

CopP, also found to be associated with the Cop ATPase operon in pRH948, is homologous to another divalent cation binding protein, CopZ. The latter is contained in the *cop*YZAB operon of *Enterococcus hirae* encoding a Cu^{2+} import ATPase (CopA), a Cu^{2+} export pump (CopB) and two small regulators, CopY and CopZ, controlling Cop ATPase expression[15]. This finding suggests that, in *H. pylori*, CopP is involved in the regulation of Cop ATPase expression.

CONCLUSIONS

H. pylori contains a family of ion pumps adapted to the need of survival in the gastric environment. Among these pumps are the two single subunit P-type

82

Table 1 Properties of *H. pylori* P-type pumps

Enzyme properties	ATPase-439	ATPase-948
Amino acids in sequence	686	741
Predicted molecular weight	75 kDa	80 kDa
Transmembrane helices	8	8
Cys–Pro–Cys motif	+	+
N-terminal ion-binding motif	+	+
Single subunit ATPase	+	+
Putative function	Unknown, related to urease activity	Cu^{2+} transport

This table summarizes the major features of the two cloned ATPases, ATPase-439 and ATPase-948 (Cop ATPase). Both amino acid sequences are homologous to transition ion P-type ATPases (about 50% similarity). Transmembrane segments of ATPase-439 were identified by *in-vitro* translation. Transmembrane segments of Cop ATPase were determined by hydropathy and homology

ATPases described above. The features of the cloned ion pumps are summarized in Table 1.

Cop ATPase (ATPase-948) mediates the export of copper ions, and therefore represents a member of the bacterial metal ion-resistance pumps. In contrast to the enterococcal Cop operon the homologous operon of *H. pylori* does not contain the equivalent of CopA, the Cu^{2+} import ATPase of *E. hirae*. This finding may indicate that there are other genes encoding copper import proteins elsewhere in the genome of *H. pylori*. Another possibility may be that the efficient Ni^{2+} uptake system present in this pathogen is leaky for copper ions. In both cases *H. pylori* might need a Cu^{2+} ion export pump to avoid accumulation of toxic copper concentrations in the cytoplasm.

The other pump with homology to transition ion pumps cloned in our laboratory, ATPase-439, seems to be involved in expression of active urease. Since urease requires Ni^{2+} for catalysis and ATPase-439 carries putative Ni^{2+}-binding sites, the dependence of urease activity on ATPase expression may be due to the special nickel biology of *H. pylori*. In summary, both P-type ion motive ATPases contribute to specialized capacities of *H. pylori* physiology, namely efficient cation accumulation and expression of large amounts of urease.

Future experiments to test the ability of ATPase-deficient mutants for *in-vivo* infectivity will help to elucidate whether the cloned ion pumps are essential for survival of *H. pylori* in a gastric environment.

Acknowledgements

We thank Dr Rainer Haas for providing the *H. pylori* 69A gene library and for performing transposon shuttle mutagenesis of ATPase-439. We gratefully acknowledge invaluable support by Dr George Sachs in providing the M0/M1 insertion vectors in his unique laboratory environment during the experiments to determine ATPase membrane topology. Finally, we thank him for his untiring readiness for stimulating discussions.

References

1. Warren JR, Marshall B. Unidentified curved bacilli on gastric epithelium in active chronic gastritis. Lancet. 1983;4:1273–5.
2. Lee A, Fox J, Hazell SL. Pathogenicity of *Helicobacter pylori*: a perspective. Infect Immun. 1993;61:1601–10.
3. Blaser MJ, Perez-Perez GI, Kleanthous H *et al.* Infection with *Helicobacter pylori* strains possessing cagA is associated with an increased risk of developing adenocarcinoma of the stomach. Cancer Res. 1995;55:2111–15.
4. Mitchell P. Chemiosmotic coupling in oxidative and photosynthetic phosphorylation. Biol Rev. 1966;41:445–502.
5. Meyer-Rosberg K, Scott DR, Rex D, Melchers K, Sachs G. The bioenergetic profile of *Helicobacter pylori*. Gastroenterology. (In press).
6. Owen RJ, Martin SR, Borman P. Rapid urea hydrolysis by gastric Campylobacters (letter). Lancet. 1985;1:111.
7. Hawtin PR, Delves HT, Newell DG. The demonstration of nickel in the urease of *Helicobacter pylori* by atomic absorption spectroscopy. FEMS Microbiol Lett. 1991;77:51–4.
8. Mobley HLT, Garner RM, Bauernfeind P. *Helicobacter pylori* nickel-transport gene nixA: synthesis of catalytically active urease in *Escherichia coli* independent of growth conditions. Mol Microbiol. 1995;16:97–107.
9. Gilbert JV, Ramakrishna J, Sunderman FW, Wright A, Plaut AG. Protein Hpn: cloning and characterization of a histidine-rich metal-binding polypeptide in *Helicobacter pylori* and *Helicobacter mustelae*. Infect Immun. 1995;63:2682–8.
10. Melchers K, Weitzenegger T, Buhmann A, Steinhilber W, Sachs G, Schäfer KP. Cloning and membrane topology of a P type ATPase from *Helicobacter pylori*. J Biol Chem. 1996;271:446–57.
11. Silver S, Nucifora G, Phung LT. Human menkes X-chromosome disease and the straphylococcal cadmium-resistance ATPase: a remarkable similarity in protein sequences. Mol Microbiol. 1993;10:7–12.
12. Solioz M. In: Anderson JP, editor. Ion pumps. JAI Press; 1996:(in press).
13. Wu LF. Putative nickel-binding sites of microbial proteins. Res Microbiol. 1992;143:347–51.
14. Ge Z, Hiratsuka K, Taylor DE. Nucleotide sequence and mutational analysis indicate that two *Helicobacter pylori* genes encode a P-type ATPase and a cation-binding protein associated with copper transport. Mol Microbiol. 1995;15:97–106.
15. Odermatt A, Solioz M. Two *trans*-acting metalloregulatory proteins controlling expression of the copper-ATPases of *Enterococcus hirae*. J Biol Chem. 1995;270:4349–54.

8
Which is the most important factor in duodenal ulcer pathogenesis: the strain of *Helicobacter pylori* or the host?

D. Y. GRAHAM, R. M. GENTA, M. F. GO and H. MALATY

INTRODUCTION

Helicobacter pylori infection causes gastritis which is typically asymptomatic, but is a condition that underlies gastric ulcer, duodenal ulcer, gastric adenocarcinoma, and gastric mucosa-associated lymphoid tissue (MALT) lymphoma. These different diseases may be the result of differences in the host, the bacterial strain infecting the host, environmental factors interacting with the bacteria or the host, or a combination of these factors[1-3]. This review is concerned with the relationship between *H. pylori* infection and duodenal ulcer disease.

ROLE OF BACTERIA VIRULENCE FACTORS

Data obtained by using DNA/DNA hybridization in solution or repetitive extragenic palindromic–polymerase chain reaction (REP–PCR) suggest that strains from patients with duodenal ulcer disease differ from those with asymptomatic gastritis[4,5] These two techniques look at the entire bacterial genome and do not identify specific genes to evaluate for functional significance. Another approach has been to look for proteins that are expressed more commonly in strains from patients with duodenal ulcer than those without. This technique has led to the discovery of the *vacA* gene encoding the vacuolating cytotoxin and the *cagA* pathogenicity island[6,7]. Disease-specific bacterial factors are well known and include examples such as cholera toxin and cholera, shiga toxin and shigellosis, diphtheria toxin and diphtheria. All these factors show disease specificity (i.e. they are present in strains that cause the disease and absent from those that do not). Statistics are not needed to demonstrate the relationship, and the relationship is equally strong in different regions and populations. In contrast, none of the currently identified *H. pylori* putative virulence factors shows any disease

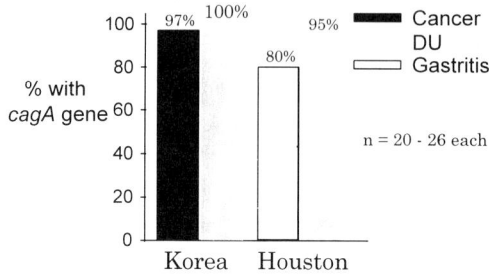

Figure 1 Frequency of the *cagA* gene detected by PCR based on detection of the gene by PCR amplification using a primer pair that amplifies a 297 bp region of the gene. The high prevalence of the *cagA* gene in both patients with asymptomatic gastritis and with symptomatic duodenal ulcer makes it unlikely that the gene has any disease specificity

specificity and, equally importantly, shows remarkable geographic variability in prevalence. Figure 1 shows the frequency of the *cagA* gene in Seoul, Korea, compared to that found in Houston, Texas[8,9]. Since duodenal ulcer protects against gastric cancer, one would not anticipate that if *cagA* were a disease-specific factor it would not be found in both diseases[10]. The prevalence of the *cagA* gene was also found in Houston to be similar in asymp-tomatic gastritis and patients with duodenal ulcer[8]. One is forced to conclude that, while the factors identified to date may have a role in modulating the degree of inflammation, or in other as yet undiscovered events, none of these effects is disease-specific. The determining factor for *H. pylori* duodenal ulcer disease may well relate to the host and not the strain of *H. pylori*.

ROLE OF THE HOST IN DUODENAL ULCER DISEASE

One approach to explore the role of the host versus the environment in the patho-genesis of a disease is to examine the presence of a particular disease in twins. An ideal study is one in which monozygotic and dizygotic twins, including twins separated at an early age and those reared together, are examined. In the pre-*H. pylori* era twin studies showed that duodenal ulcer disease had a genetic com-ponent[11,12]. Recent studies have confirmed a strong genetic component relating to susceptibility to *H. pylori* infection[13]. The twin studies have also been extended to duodenal ulcer disease in the *H. pylori* era, and have confirmed a strong genetic component[14]. Taken together, the data show that genetics of the host play a role, but not the only one, in the development of peptic ulcer disease.

ROLE OF ACID

The dictum 'no acid – no ulcer' has been proven to be literally true. The addition of 'no *H. pylori* – no ulcer'[15] has not invalidated this, and the large body of evidence relating to the importance of acid in ulcer disease cannot be ignored. Furthermore, it remains true that ulcers heal and tend not to recur if acid secretion is suppressed by drugs or selective vagotomy. Increasingly sophisticated studies of acid secretion

Table 1 Some factors previously related to acid secretion in patients with duodenal ulcer disease

Increased basal acid output
Increased maximum acid output (pentagastrin)
Increased ratio of basal to maximum acid output
Increased GRP-stimulated acid output
Increased ratio of GRP to pentagastrin-stimulated acid output
Decreased inhibition of acid secretion with antral distension or antral acidification
Exaggerated meal-stimulated gastrin secretion
Increased parietal cell mass
Increased serum pepsinogen I

have been performed over the last half-century in the search for a specific dysregulation of gastric acid secretion to explain duodenal ulcer disease. Table 1 lists some of the perturbations in gastric physiology that have been associated with duodenal ulcer. It has been consistently confirmed that patients with duodenal ulcer, on average, have a higher rate of acid secretion than do normal, healthy individuals. It has also been known for about a half-century that patients with duodenal ulcer have severe antral, but only minimal corpus, gastritis[15]. In the virtual absence of corpus gastritis, maximum acid output following pentagastrin stimulation provides an indirect measurement of the number of parietal cells, and patients with duodenal ulcer have more parietal cells than do normal subjects.

The concentration of acid in the stomach is the product of two components: the parietal cell component, which secretes acid at about 140 mmol/L, and a non-parietal cell component, which secretes an alkaline fluid rich in bicarbonate. Basal acid secretion reflects the number of parietal cells secreting, and can range from none to all, as in the case of a pathological secretory state such as Zollinger –Ellison syndrome. In 1971 it was suggested that exaggerated meal-stimulated gastrin was present in patients with duodenal ulcer disease[16]. It has recently been shown that this abnormality was related to *H. pylori* infection, not to duodenal ulcer, and that it was reversible following cure of the *H. pylori* infection[17].

Recently there has been renewed interest in the use of gastrin-releasing peptide (GRP), the mammalian equivalent of the frog skin peptide bombesin, as a stimulant of gastric acid secretion[17]. This peptide stimulates gastrin release as well as somatostatin release, and thus provided a new way of accessing the regulation of acid secretion. It was found that maximum GRP stimulation (approximately 40 picomoles per kilogram per hour) in normals resulted in secretion of about 30% of the maximum pentagastrin-stimulated acid output (MAO)[17]. In contrast, patients with *H. pylori* infection had a higher rate of stimulation, nearing 85–90% of the MAO. Cure of *H. pylori* infection resulted in the normalization of the gastric secretory response to GRP (Figure 2). These data initially interpreted were confusing, possibly because they were not directly compared to the previous elegant studies of bombesin-stimulated acid secretion[18]. Another potentially con-fusing factor was that, in these studies, the amount of acid secreted by normal subjects was compared to that of patients with duodenal ulcer disease, and dose–response curves were not presented. It would have been more appropriate to evaluate the effect of the stimuli in relation to the maximum amount of acid secretion possible in any individual (i.e. the percentage of pentagastrin-stimulated MAO). When the

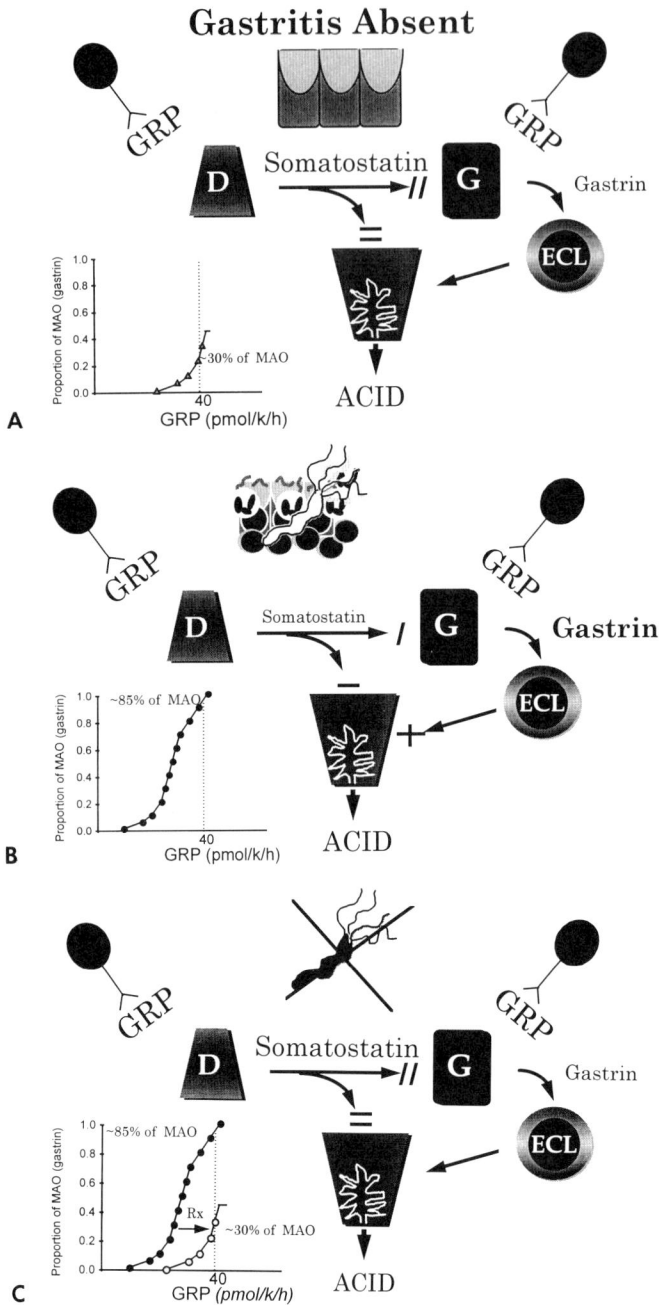

Figure 2 A: Summary of the current thinking about gastric acid secretion with the intravenous administration of gastrin-releasing peptide (GRP). Both somatostatin secreting D-cell and gastrin secreting G-cells are stimulated. Gastrin in turn stimulates the enterochromaffin-like cell to secrete histamine, which stimulates acid secretion from the parietal cells. Because somatostatin is inhibitory, the response to gastrin is blunted, resulting in only about 30% of pentagastrin-stimulated acid output. **B**: *H. pylori* infection, probably acting through cytokines, inhibits the D cell and stimulates the G cell, leading to enhanced acid secretion in response to GRP infusion. This is seen as an upward shift in the dose–response curve to GRP. **C**: Cure of the infection returns the response to GRP infusion back to normal

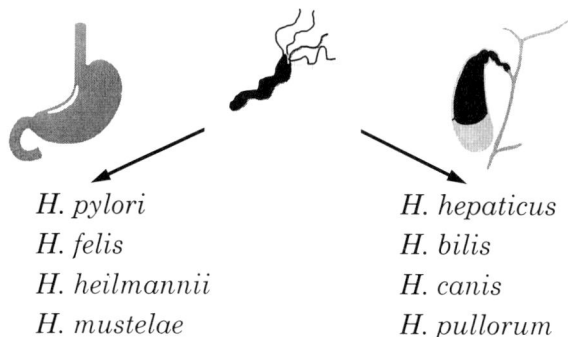

H. pylori	*H. hepaticus*
H. felis	*H. bilis*
H. heilmannii	*H. canis*
H. mustelae	*H. pullorum*

Figure 3 *Helicobacter* can be grouped into those whose growth is inhibited by bile and those that are resistant to bile. This figure shows some of the common species in each group

data were reinterpreted in this light, *H. pylori* infection, irrespective of the presence of duodenal ulcer, was found to increase the acid output in response to GRP from about 30% of MAO to 85–90% of MAO (i.e. there was an upward shift of the dose–response curve). Cure of the infection led to the return of the percentage of maximum acid secretion to the levels of normal uninfected individuals. With the exception of the exaggerated parietal cell mass in patients with duodenal ulcer, all other derangements of acid production have proved to be reversible epiphenomena related to *H. pylori* infection, rather than disease-specific abnormalities[17]. Thus, one must conclude that a greater-than-normal ability to secrete acid may be one of the genetic host factors that underlie duodenal ulcer disease. If acid secretion has a normal bell-shaped distribution, and the odds of infection are independent of the rate of acid secretion, one would then expect that about 15% of those who become infected will develop duodenal ulcer disease. Obviously, the actual situation is more complicated than this, but this crude calculation does approximate the actual situation in Western countries. These data suggest that the host is more important than the strain of *H. pylori*.

HOW MIGHT THE ABILITY TO MAKE LOTS OF ACID AND *H. PYLORI* INTERACT TO CAUSE DUODENAL ULCER?

Species of the genus *Helicobacter* can be divided into those that live in the stomach and those that live in the intestines. Recently, a group of *Helicobacter* that can also live in the liver or biliary ducts have been identified (Figure 3). We now recognize that *Helicobacter* can be divided into two major groups depending on the ability to grow in the presence of bile; those that grow in the liver and intestine and are resistant to bile. *H. pylori* growth is inhibited by bile; yet *H. pylori* can easily be demonstrated in areas of gastric metaplasia in or around the duodenal bulb in patients with duodenal ulcer, a site where bile is typically present[15]. One of the possible explanations for this conundrum is that the *H. pylori* that cause duodenal ulcer disease have acquired the ability to grow in the presence of bile. We tested that hypothesis by comparing the effect of bile on the growth of *H. pylori* isolates from patients with asymptomatic gastritis to those

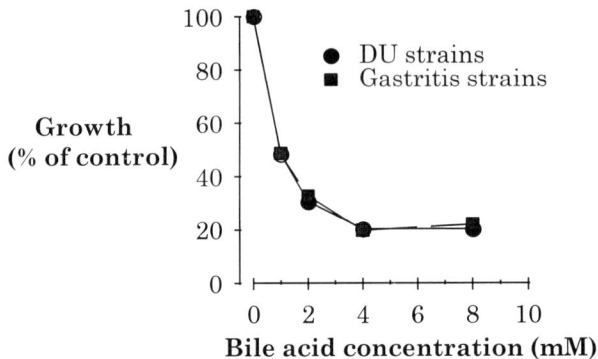

Figure 4 *H. pylori* obtained from patients with duodenal ulcer and isolates from patients with asymptomatic gastritis were compared for their ability to grow in the presence of bile salts. There was a dose-dependent inhibition of growth that was not different depending on from which disease the isolate was obtained

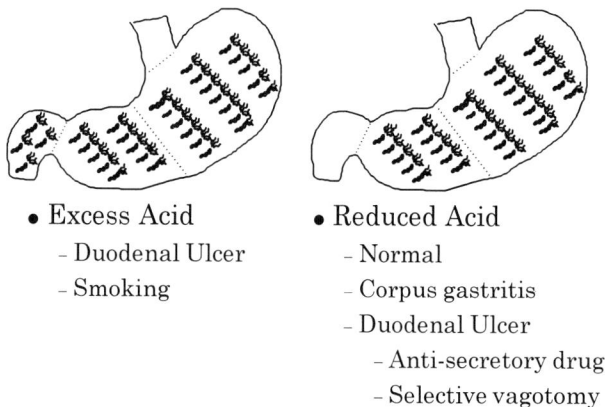

- Excess Acid
  - Duodenal Ulcer
  - Smoking

- Reduced Acid
  - Normal
  - Corpus gastritis
  - Duodenal Ulcer
    - Anti-secretory drug
    - Selective vagotomy

Figure 5 This figure summarizes the hypothesis that an excessive duodenal acid load would precipitate bile salts and allow *H. pylori* to thrive, whereas reducing acid output would allow bile in the duodenal bulb to inhibit *H. pylori* growth and promote ulcer healing

from patients with duodenal ulcer disease. Both sets of isolates showed identical dose-dependent inhibition of growth (Figure 4)[19]. Another possibility is that the duodenal bulb of patients with duodenal ulcer has less bile than that of normal subjects. Glycine-conjugated bile acids have a pK_a of between 4.3 and 5.2, and are thus insoluble (precipitated from solution) in acidic environments. Thus the combination of high prolonged acid secretion and rapid gastric emptying would promote development of gastric metaplasia in the bulb, as well as precipitating the deleterious bile acids allowing *H. pylori* to thrive. Any factor capable of increasing the duodenal acid load (e.g. smoking, which inhibits pancreatic bicarbonate secretion), could enhance the ability of *H. pylori* to grow in the duodenal bulb. Inhibition of acid by antisecretory therapy or highly selective vagotomy, stopping smoking, or any mechanism that results in an increase in duodenal bulb pH, would tend to inhibit the growth of *H. pylori* and result in healing of duodenal ulcer disease (Figure 5).

These data and speculations offer an explanation as to why duodenal ulcer occurs in only some people, those with high acid secretion, and suggest that the most important factor in the pathogenesis of duodenal ulcer 'is the host'.

Acknowledgements

This work was supported by a grant from NIH/NCI 5RO1CA67469, by the Department of Veterans Affairs, and by the generous support of Hilda Schwartz.

References

1. Go MF, Graham DY. Determinants of clinical outcome of *H. pylori* infection: duodenal ulcer. In: Hunt RH, Tytgat GNJ, editors. *Helicobacter pylori*: basic mechanisms to clinical cure. Dordrecht: Kluwer; 1994:421–8.
2. Go MF, Graham DY. How does *Helicobacter pylori* cause duodenal ulcer disease: the bug, the host, or both? J Gastroenterol Hepatol. 1994;9(Suppl. 1):S8–10.
3. Graham DY, Malaty HM, Go MF. Are there susceptible hosts to *Helicobacter pylori* infection? Scand J Gastroenterol Suppl. 1994;205:6–10.
4. Go MF, Chan KY, Versalovic J, Koeuth T, Graham DY, Lupski JR. Cluster analysis of *Helicobacter pylori* genomic DNA fingerprints suggests gastroduodenal disease-specific associations. Scand J Gastroenterol. 1995;30:640–6.
5. Yoshimura HH, Evans DG, Graham DY. DNA–DNA hybridization demonstrates apparent genetic differences between *Helicobacter pylori* from patients with duodenal ulcer and asymptomatic gastritis. Dig Dis Sci. 1993;38:1128–31.
6. Covacci A, Censini S, Bugnoli M *et al*. Molecular characterization of the 128-kDa immunodominant antigen of *Helicobacter pylori* associated with cytotoxicity and duodenal ulcer. Proc Natl Acad Sci USA. 1993;90:5791–5.
7. Tummuru MK, Cover TL, Blaser MJ. Cloning and expression of a high-molecular-mass major antigen of *Helicobacter pylori*: evidence of linkage to cytotoxin production. Infect Immun. 1993; 61:1799–809.
8. Go MF, Graham DY. The *cagA* gene is present in the majority of *H. pylori* strains independent of whether the individual has duodenal ulcer or asymptomatic gastritis. Helicobacter. 1996;1: 107–11.
9. Miehlke S, Kibler K, Kim JG *et al*. Allelic variation in the *cagA* gene of *Helicobacter pylori* obtained from Korea compared to the United States. Am J Gastroenterol. 1996 (In press).
10. Graham DY, Go MF, Genta RM. *Helicobacter pylori*, duodenal ulcer, gastric cancer: tunnel vision or blinders? Ann Med. 1995;27:589–94.
11. McConnell RB. Peptic ulcer: early genetic evidence – families, twins, and markers. In: Rotter JI, Samloff IM, Rimoin DL, editors. The genetics and heterogeneity of common gastrointestinal disorders. New York: Academic Press; 1980:31–41.
12. Gotlieb-Jensen K. Peptic ulcer: genetic and epidemiological aspects based on twin studies. Copenhagen: Munksgaard; 1972.
13. Malaty HM, Engstrand L, Pedersen NL, Graham DY. *Helicobacter pylori* infection: genetic and environmental influences. A study of twins [see comments]. Ann Intern Med. 1994;120:982–6.
14. Malaty H, Pedersen NL, Engstrand L, Isaksson I, Graham DY. Genetic and environmental influences of peptic ulcer disease. Gastroenterology. 1996;110:A184.
15. Graham DY. *Campylobacter pylori* and peptic ulcer disease. Gastroenterology. 1989;96:615–25.
16. McGuigan JE, Trudeau WL. Differences in rates of gastrin release in normal persons and patients with duodenal-ulcer disease. N Engl J Med. 1973;288:64–6.
17. Graham DY. *Helicobacter pylori* and perturbations in acid secretion: the end of the beginning. Gastroenterology. 1996;110:1647–50.
18. Hirschowitz BI, Tim LO, Helman CA, Molina E. Bombesin and G-17 dose responses in duodenal ulcer and controls. Dig Dis Sci. 1985;30:1092–103.
19. Han SW, Evans DG, El-Zaatari FAK, Go MF, Graham DY. The interaction of pH, bile and *Helicobacter pylori* may explain duodenal ulcer. Am J Gastroenterol. 1996;91:1135–7.

9
The effect of *Helicobacter pylori* on the surface hydrophobicity and phospholipid composition of the gastric mucosa

L. M. LICHTENBERGER

INTRODUCTION OF GASTRIC MUCOSAL HYDROPHOBICITY

In 1983 our laboratory reported that the canine gastric mucosa has clear hydrophobic properties as determined by contact angle analysis, which is routinely employed in industry to determine surface wettability[1]. This technique is schematically depicted in Figure 1, in which a microlitre droplet of water is applied to a test surface, and the contact angle at the air/liquid/solid interface is read through a telescopic eyepiece. A large contact angle reading is observed when the droplet beads up after it is applied to a hydrophobic surface, whereas minimal values are registered when the droplet is applied to, and attempts to coat, a wettable surface. Since this observation, reports from our laboratory and those of other investigators have indicated that the stomachs of all mammalian species tested to date, including humans, have non-wettable properties that appear to be attributable to the hydrophobic characteristics of the overlying mucus gel layer[1-7]. Biochemical and biophysical analyses indicate that this unique surface property appears to be attributable to the presence of surface-active phospholipids present within and coating the mucus gel layer, with phosphatidylcholine being the most prominent constituent, representing 40–60% of the total[8-10]. Ultrastructural studies employing special stains and fixatives to preserve and stain basic phospholipids indicate that surface-active phospholipids are synthesized and stored in specific organelles of gastric surface mucous cells, which are in turn secreted into the mucus gel layer upon stimulation[11-16]. Further these same phospholipidic structures are stored as lamellae or filamentous structures within the mucus gel layer where they are recruited to coat the luminal interface of the gel in a state of dynamic equilibrium. We have determined that the percentage of the mucus gel layer that is coated by these phospholipidic filamentous structures is statistically associated with the contact angle of the tissue[12].

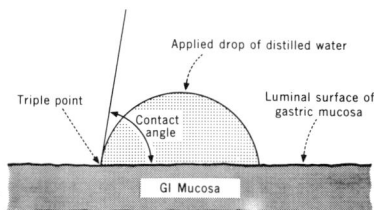

Figure 1   Schematic representation of contact angle analysis

Most of the evidence relating the hydrophobic/phospholipid properties of the gastric mucus gel layer to the barrier properties of the tissue are indirect and include:

1. the observation that tissues with the greatest acid resistivity (i.e. oxyntic mucosa) also possess the highest hydrophobicity[1];
2. the fact that all established damaging agents induce a rapid decrease in surface hydrophobicity of the canine and rodent gastric mucosa[7,17–19];
3. administration of gastroprotective prostaglandins maintains or enhances the non-wettable state of the tissue (even in the presence of a damaging agent) and stimulates the synthesis and secretion of surface-active phospho-lipids[7,12,17,18];
4. reports that the hydrophobic properties of the tissue and their barrier properties are highly significantly associated[7];
5. the fact that intragastric administration of phosphatidylcholine to rats both increases mucosal hydrophobicity and protects the animal from gastrointestinal ulceration and bleeding induced by a number of damaging agents and/or conditions such as stress[9,19,20].

EFFECT OF *H. PYLORI* ON THE SURFACE HYDROPHOBICITY AND PHOSPHOLIPID CONCENTRATION OF THE HUMAN GASTRIC MUCOSA

In 1990 Northfield and associates employed contact angle analysis of endoscopic biopsies to report that the hydrophobicity of the gastric antral mucosa of peptic ulcer patients was significantly lower by contact angle analysis than that recorded in healthy volunteers[5]. Subsequent studies, in which they stratified their subjects in accordance to *H. pylori* status, revealed that surface hydrophobicity was significantly lower in both asymptomatic and symptomatic individuals who were infected by the organism in comparison to age- and sex-matched uninfected controls[20,21]. Furthermore, treatment of infected patients with antibiotic/bismuth therapy resulted in a recovery of surface hydrophobicity to normal values, whereas treatment with H_2-receptor antagonists, although promoting ulcer healing in infected patients, had no discernible effects on increasing the patients' gastric surface hydrophobicity. This observation suggests that the decrease in surface hydrophobicity in peptic ulcer patients is directly related to infection with *H. pylori*, and not a secondary consequence due to inflammation or compromised

Table 1 Phospholipase enzyme activity of *H. pylori* lysates and growth medium (nmol/h per mg protein)

	PLA_2	PLC
H. pylori lysate	0.322	122
H. pylori growth medium	0.913	N.D.

gastric mucosal integrity. Go and associates, in collaboration with our laboratory, have confirmed these findings, and demonstrated a clear reduction in gastric mucosal hydrophobicity related to infection with *H. pylori* that rapidly responds to the eradication of the bacteria with medical therapy[22].

A number of laboratories have investigated the effects of *H. pylori* on the phospholipid composition of the gastric mucosa, with conflicting results. Two groups have reported preliminary data which suggest that *H. pylori* infection either decreases or has no effect on the phospholipid concentration of endoscopic gastric biopsy tissue[23,24]. The most comprehensive published study to date, however, has reported a clear decrease in mucosal phospholipid, phosphatidylcholine and phosphatidylethanolamine concentration of endoscopic gastric biopsies excised from *H. pylori*-infected subjects compared with values of age- and sex-matched uninfected controls[25].

Consistent with these biochemical and biophysical findings a number of laboratories have employed phospholipid-selective stains to demonstrate that the density of phospholipidic lamellae and filamentous structures within the mucus gel layer is decreased or absent in *H. pylori*-infected subjects[26,27]. Hills made the interesting observation, using special stains and techniques to preserve and identify phospholipids, that *H. pylori* present within the mucus gel layer are frequently coated by oligolamellae structures and contain dense phospholipid-reactive bodies intracellularly[28]. This led him to speculate that the *H. pylori* have the capacity to both engulf phospholipids secreted into the mucus gel layer and transfer these protective amphipathic molecules to their surface to increase the bacteria's resistance to luminal acid.

MOLECULAR MECHANISM BY WHICH *H. PYLORI* REDUCES GASTRIC MUCOSAL HYDROPHOBICITY

A number of investigators have reported that *H. pylori*, in addition to possessing urease and protease enzymes, have the capacity to catalyse the hydrolysis of both triglycerides and phospholipids[29,30]. Evidence from both our and other laboratories has documented the presence of phospholipase A_1, A_2 and C in *H. pylori* lysates and filtrates, with PLC being present primarily in bacterial membranes and PLA being detectable both in the membrane and filtrate fractions[29–31] (see Table 1). We also have evidence that *H. pylori* PLA_2 has a clear calcium-dependence, as in other membrane/bacterial systems, whereas PLC activity, although displaying some dependence on multivalent cations (zinc), is not affected by the calcium concentration of the incubation buffer[31]. We also have confirmed the findings of the Slomiany laboratory[29,30] that the phospholipase activity (both

PLC and PLA_2) are inhibited by the same bismuth salts that are routinely employed in classical bismuth-based triple therapies. Furthermore, our observation that the bismuth-induced inhibition in PLA_2 could be reversed by increasing the buffer's calcium concentration suggests that bismuth blocks enzymatic activity by competing with calcium for binding/activation sites on the enzyme molecule. We also demonstrated that *H. pylori* lysates have the capacity to remove a synthetic hydrophobic monolayer of phosphatidylcholine from a glass slide, and that this ability of the bacterial extract to transform an inert surface from a hydrophobic to a hydrophilic state could be blocked if the monolayer was generated in the presence of bismuth salts[31].

It is now well established that *H. pylori* possesses a very active urease enzyme that translocates to the bacteria's surface to convert urea to ammonia (NH_3) and bicarbonate[32]. Because of its high enzymatic activity and the presence of available substrate in the gastric lumen, NH_3 is present in millimolar concentrations (ranging from 2 to 40 mmol/L) in the gastric juice of *H. pylori*-infected individuals. Also, since gastric acidity is either normal or elevated during the chronic stages of infection prior to the onset of gastric atrophy, most if not all of the base will be converted to the positively charged NH_4^+ ion. Since the choline-based head group of the surface-active phospholipid, phosphatidylcholine, also possesses a positively charged (quaternary) ammonium group, we reasoned that the NH_4^+ generated by the bacteria may compete for and replace gastric phosphatidylcholine for negatively charged binding sites on the mucus gel layer. In a recent paper we presented both *in-vivo* and *in-vitro* evidence that this may occur, as we demonstrated that the addition of NH_4^+ salts, together with low doses of a mucolytic agent, rapidly decreased the hydrophobicity of the rat gastric mucosa and increased the stomach's sensitivity to luminal acid. In the same study we demonstrated that exposure of inert phospholipid-coated materials to a medium containing NH_4^+ salts (in millimolar concentrations) resulted in a decrease in surface hydrophobicity and an acceleration in the flux of HCl across those surfaces.

SUMMARY

The human gastric mucosa, like that of most mammalian species, is endowed with hydrophobic surface properties to protect the underlying tissue from luminal acid. This property appears to be, in part, attributable to the presence of surfactant-like phospholipids within and coating the mucus gel layer. The surface hydrophobic properties of gastric endoscopic biopsy tissues are clearly attenuated in individuals infected with *H. pylori*, and this increase in surface wettability may be responsible for an increase in acid-sensitivity of the affected tissue and a trigger to the development of gastritis. The mechanism by which *H. pylori* comprises the hydrophobic barrier properties of the stomach is still under study, and may relate to the hydrolysis of surface phospholipids by the bacteria's complement of phospholipase enzymes, and the urease-catalysed generation of ammonium salts, which displace phospholipids from the surface of the mucus gel layer, thereby inserting breaks (water channels) in the hydrophobic phospholipid lining of the stomach (see Figure 2 for a schematic depiction of the model).

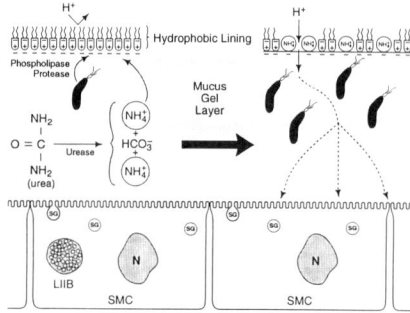

Figure 2 Schematic representation of molecular mechanisms by which *H. pylori* compromise gastric mucosal hydrophobicity. SMC = surface mucous cell; SG = secretory granule; LIIB = large infranuclear inclusion body. (From Annu Rev Physiol. 1995;57:565–83)

Acknowledgements

This work was supported by NIH grant DK 33239.

References

1. Hills BA, Butler BD, Lichtenberger LM. Gastric mucosal barrier: the hydrophobic lining to the lumen of the stomach. Am J Physiol: Gastrointest Liver Physiol. 1983;7:G561–8.
2. Dial EJ, Lichtenberger LM. Surface hydrophobicity of the gastric mucosa in the developing rat. Effects of corticosteroids, thyroxine and prostaglandin E_2. Gastroenterology. 1988;94:57–67.
3. Kao Y-CJ, Lichtenberger LM. Hydrophobic properties of the mucus cells of the stomach and submucosal glands. Gastroenterology. 1990;98:A67.
4. Mack DR, Neumann AW, Policova Z, Sherman PM. Surface hydrophobicity of the intestinal tract. Am J Physiol. 1992;262:G171–7.
5. Spychal RT, Goggin PM, Marrero JM *et al.* Surface hydrophobicity of gastric mucosa in peptic ulcer disease: relationship to gastritis and *Campylobacter pylori* infection. Gastroenterology. 1990; 98:1250–4.
6. Spychal RT, Marrero JM, Saverymuttu SH, Northfield TC. Measurement of the surface hydrophobicity of human gastrointestinal mucosa. Gastroenterology. 1989;97:104–11.
7. Goddard PJ, Kao Y-CJ, Lichtenberger LM. Luminal surface hydrophobicity of canine gastric mucosa is dependent on a surface mucous gel. Gastroenterology. 1990;98:361–70.
8. Wassef M, Lin Y, Horowitz M. Molecular species of phosphatidylcholine from rat gastric mucosa. Biochim Biophys Acta. 1973;573:222–6.
9. Lichtenberger LM, Graziani LA, Dial EJ, Butler BD, Hills BA. Role of surface-active phospholipids in gastric cytoprotection. Science. 1983;219:1327–9.
10. Butler BD, Lichtenberger LM, Hills BA. Distribution of surfactants in the canine GI tract and their ability to lubricate. Am J Physiol: Gastrointest Liver Physiol. 1983;7:G645–51.
11. Kao Y-CJ, Lichtenberger LM. Localization of phospholipid-rich zones in rat gastric mucosa: possible origin of a protective hydrophobic lining. J Histochem Cytochem. 1987;35:1285–98.
12. Kao Y-CJ, Goddard PJ, Lichtenberger LM. Morphological effects of aspirin and prostaglandin on the canine gastric mucosal surface: analysis with a phospholipid cytochemical stain. Gastroenterology. 1990;98:592–606.
13. Kao Y-CJ, Lichtenberger LM. A method to preserve extracellular surfacant-like phospholipids on the luminal surface of the rodent gastric mucosa. J Histochem Cytochem. 1990;38:427–31.
14. Kao Y-CJ, Lichtenberger LM. Phospholipid- and neutral-lipid-containing organelles of rat gastroduodenal mucous cells. Gastroenterology. 1991;101:7–21.
15. Lichtenberger LM, Ahmed TN, Barretto JC, Kao YC, Dial EJ. Use of fluorescent hydrophobic dyes in establishing the presence of lipids in the gastric mucus gel layer. J Clin Gastroenterol. 1992;14(Suppl. 1):S82–7.

16. Kao Y-CJ, Lichtenberger LM. Effect of 16,16 dimethyl prostaglandin E_2 on the lipidic organelles of rat gastric surface mucous cells. Gastroenterology. 1993;104:103–13.
17. Lichtenberger LM. Membranes and barriers: with a focus on the gastric mucosal barrier. Clin Invest Med. 1987;10:181–8.
18. Lichtenberger LM, Richards JE, Hills BA. Effect of 16,16 dimethyl prostaglandin E_2 on the surface hydrophobicity of aspirin-treated canine gastric mucosa. Gastroenterology. 1985;88: 308–14.
19. Lichtenberger LM, Romero JJ, Kao Y-CJ, Dial EJ. Gastric protective activity of mixtures of saturated polar and neutral lipids in rats. Gastroenterology. 1990;99:511–26.
20. Goggin PM, Marrero JM, Spychal RI, Jackson PA, Corbishley CM, Northfield TC. Surface hydrophobicity of gastric mucosa in *Helicobacter pylori* infection: effect of clearance and eradication. Gastroenterology. 1992;103:1486–90.
21. Goggin PM, Northfield TC, Spychal RI. Factors affecting gastric mucosal hydrophobicity in man. Scand J Gastroenterol. 1991;26(Suppl. 181):65–73.
22. Go MF, Lew GM, Lichtenberger LM, Genta RM, Graham DY. Gastric mucosal hydrophobicity and *Helicobacter pylori*: response to antimicrobial therapy. Am J Gastroenterol. 1993;88:1362–5.
23. Orchard JL, Smith W. Gastric mucosal phospholipid content in non-ulcer dyspepsia. Gastroenterology. 1992;102:A141.
24. Koyama T, Tadano J, Kawasaki S *et al*. Effect of *H. pylori* infection on phospholipids of gastric mucosa in patients with peptic ulcer. Gastroenterology. 1995;110:A162.
25. Nardone G, D'Armieto F, Corso G *et al*. Lipids of human gastric mucosa: effect of inflammatory infiltrates. *Helicobacter pylori* infection and non-alcoholic cirrhosis. Gastroenterology. 1994;107: 362–8.
26. Mauch F, Bode G, Ditschuneit H, Malfertheiner P. Demonstration of a phospholipid-rich zone in the human gastric epithelium damaged by *Helicobacter pylori*. Gastroenterology. 1993;105: 1698–704.
27. Sbarbati A, Deganello A, Tamassia G, Bertini M, Gaburro D, Osculati F. Surfactant-like material in the antral mucosa of children. J Pediatr Gastroenterol. 1994;13:279–84.
28. Hills BA. Gastric mucosal barrier: evidence for *Helicobacter pylori* ingesting gastric surfactant and deriving protection from it. Gut. 1993;34:588–93.
29. Slomiany BL, Kasinathan C, Slomiany A. Lipolytic activity of *Campylobacter pylori*: effect of colloidal bismuth subcitrate (De-Nol). Am J Gastroenterol. 1989;84:1273–7.
30. Langston SR, Cesareo SD. *Helicobacter pylori* associated phospholipase A_2 activity: a factor in peptic ulcer production? J Clin Pathol. 1982;45:221–4.
31. Ottlecz A, Romero JJ, Hazell SL, Graham DY, Lichtenberger LM. Phospholipase activity of *Helicobacter pylori* and its inhibition by bismuth salts: biochemical and biophysical studies. Dig Dis Sci. 1993;38:2071–80.
32. Hazell SL, Bordy T, Gal A, Lee A. *Campylobacter pylori* in gastritis. I: Detection of urease as a marker of bacterial colonization and gastritis. Am J Gastroenterol. 1987;82:292–6.
33. Lichtenberger LM, Romero JJ. Effect of ammonium ion on the hydrophobic and barrier properties of the gastric mucus gel layer. J Gastroenterol Hepatol. 1994;9:513–19.

10
Mediators of inflammation in *Helicobacter pylori* infection

K. BODGER and J. E. CRABTREE

INTRODUCTION

Helicobacter pylori infection is invariably associated with chronic gastric inflammation, representing the host immune response to the organism[1]. Mediators of inflammation, liberated by immune cells and by other host cells, play a pivotal role in determining the qualitative and quantitative aspects of any immune response. These cellular products include peptide messengers such as cytokines and growth factors, bioactive lipids such as leukotrienes and prostaglandins, and short-lived unstable molecules such as nitric oxide. An understanding of the various roles played by this multiplicity of cellular products in *H. pylori*-induced inflammation may provide important clues as to the mechanisms by which infection produces clinical disease.

H. PYLORI INTERACTIONS WITH THE HOST

When considering the mechanisms of *H. pylori*-induced inflammation, it is important to appreciate the potential routes by which the organism may interact with host cells to initiate an immune response. *H. pylori* colonizes the human gastric epithelium, living within the mucus layer in close proximity with the epithelial surface, to which it may adhere, but without invading the mucosa[2]. There are therefore two main mechanisms by which *H. pylori*, or its products, may induce the recruitment and activation of leucocytes to produce inflammation: direct stimulation of immune cells, and stimulation of epithelial chemokines.

Direct stimulation of immune cells

The diffusion of *H. pylori*-derived factors from the luminal surface into the underlying mucosa will allow direct contact of bacterial components with mucosal and circulating leucocytes, a process which may be facilitated by bacterial-induced damage to the protective epithelial cell lining. *In-vitro* experiments with peripheral

98

Table 1 Mucosal mediators associated with *H. pylori* infection *in vivo*

Mediator	References
Cytokines	
TNFα	27, 28, 29
IL-1 α/β	28, 30
IL-2	30
IL-6	27, 30, 29
IL-7	29, 31
IL-10	29, 32
IFNγ	33
Chemokines	
IL-8	24, 30, 31, 34, 35
GRO-α	36
RANTES	36
MIP-1α	36
Other molecules	
LT-B$_4$	37
LT-C$_4$	38
iNOS	39, 40

blood cells have shown that a variety of extracts of *H. pylori* strains are capable of inducing chemotaxis and activation of phagocytic cells[3–16] and proliferative responses in lymphocytes[17,18].

Epithelial cell chemokine response

The chemokine family of peptides are involved in the recruitment and activation of specific immune cells. Different chemokines show marked target cell specificity with members of the C-X-C subfamily (e.g. IL-8, GRO-α) having specific chemotactic activity for neutrophils and members of the C-C family (e.g. RANTES, MIP-1α) having effects on monocytes and lymphocytes[19]. The gastric epithelium is now known to be an important source of chemokines[20–25], which are released following direct interaction with *H. pylori* both in response to exogenous irritants such as *H. pylori*[20–25] and on exposure to endogenous proinflammatory mediators[26]. This chemokine response may be particularly important in the early stages of inflammation, with the epithelium acting as a crucial first line of defence against microbial infection.

MEDIATORS OF INFLAMMATION

The immune responses resulting from interactions between *H. pylori* and host cells will lead to the liberation of a range of inflammatory mediators. These immune cell products will have a major role in further amplifying and co-ordinating the immune response. In describing this multiplicity of immune mediators (Table 1)[27–40] it is useful to consider those products involved in natural immunity, which are largely concerned with the initial recruitment and subsequent

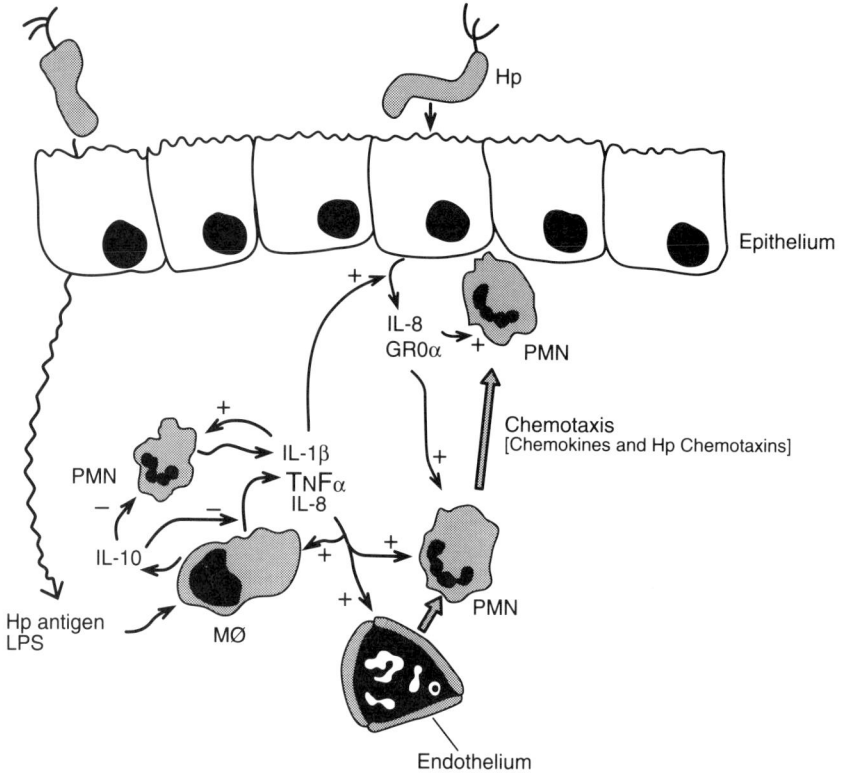

Figure 1 Cytokine mediators in non-specific (natural) immunity to *H. pylori*

activation of phagocytes (Figure 1), and those mediators which are released mainly during antigen-specific immune responses involving lymphocytes (Figure 2).

Mediators in natural immunity

Acquisition of *H. pylori* infection is thought usually to occur in early life where it passes unnoticed clinically[41]. Hence, the initial immunological events following gastric colonization are largely unknown. Phagocytic cells (neutrophils and macrophages) typically play a major role in acute responses to bacterial infections, constituting the immediate non-specific immune response (natural immunity). Isolated histological studies of acute *H. pylori* infection in adults suggest that there is indeed a marked neutrophilic component[42,43]. In some individuals this acute response may be effective in bacterial clearance[43]. The persistence of a neutrophil response in chronic *H. pylori* infection suggests that these cells play a major role in the inflammatory reactions to the organism.

H. pylori itself is a potent source of factors capable of directly inducing neutrophil chemotaxis and/or activation *in vitro*. An *H. pylori* water extract can

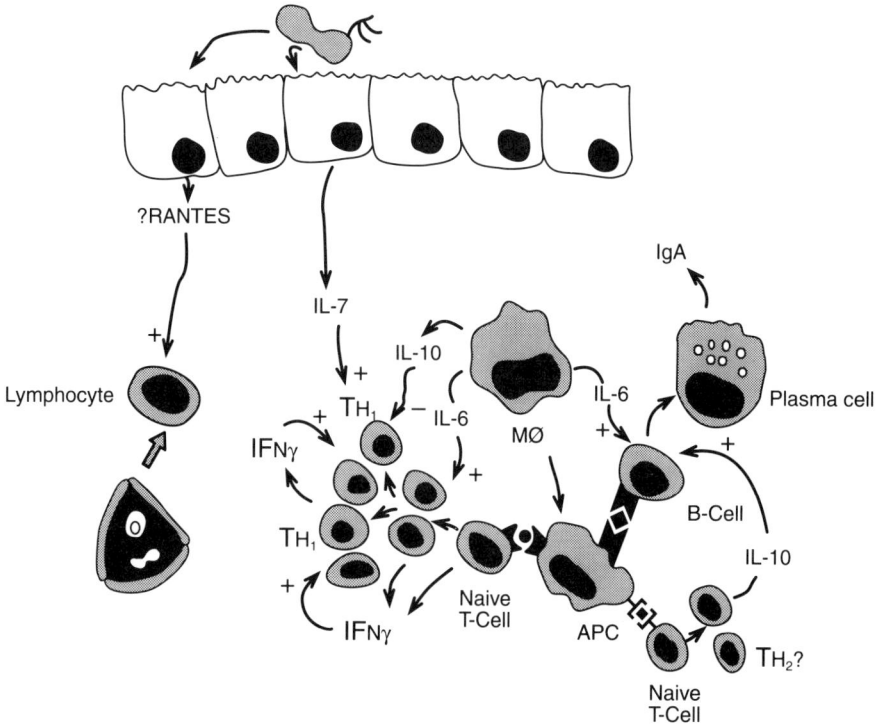

Figure 2 Cytokine mediators in antigen-specific immunity

induce adhesion and emigration of leucocytes from rat mesenteric venules[8], and *in-vitro* exposure of human neutrophils to components of *H. pylori* leads to changes in adhesion molecule expression, neutrophil degranulation and the generation of reactive oxygen metabolites[3–16]. All strains of *H. pylori* appear to possess a gene encoding for a 150 kDa neutrophil-activating protein (HP-NAP), which is present in water extracts of the organism[15]. In common with other Gram-negative bacteria, *H. pylori* possesses lipopolysaccharide (LPS) in its cell envelope which is capable of priming neutrophils for activation[9], although its biological activity is relatively weak[16]. Although *H. pylori* is usually regarded as non-invasive[2], diffusion of these various bacterial products into the mucosa is one putative mechanism for neutrophil recruitment and activation.

There is accumulating evidence that gastric epithelial cells play a key role in *H. pylori*-induced inflammation, particularly in relation to the neutrophilic response. The epithelial cell represents the first line of defence against microbial infection, and is likely to be particularly vulnerable to direct damage by *H. pylori* or its products. Gastric epithelium, in common with other mucosal epithelia[44,45], is a recognized source of chemokines such as interleukin-8[20–25] and GRO-α[25], which have target specificity for neutrophils.

In vitro, H. pylori induces gastric epithelial cell lines to increase IL-8 gene transcription and IL-8 secretion[20–23]. Bacterial induction of IL-8 is via a tyrosine kinase pathway[46], and involves NFkB activation[47]. Transcriptional regulation involves both NFkB and AP-1 binding regions in the promoting region of the IL-8 gene[46]. The *in-vitro* epithelial IL-8 response is observed specifically with strains of the CagA phenotype[20–23]. Studies with isogenic mutants show that CagA is not the direct inducer of epithelial chemokine responses[22,23]. *cagA*-positive strains of *H. pylori* co-express multiple other genes in a pathogenicity island which is absent from *cagA*-negative strains[48]. The products of multiple genes in this pathogenicity island are required for induction of IL-8[48], one of which includes the recently described *picB*[49] which is synonymous with *cagE*[48].

In vivo it is interesting to note that those patients infected with CagA-positive strains are most likely to have prominent neutrophil infiltration of the gastric mucosa reflecting 'active' gastritis[50], and consistent with an enhanced chemokine response. Furthermore, immunohistochemistry has revealed increased IL-8 immunoreactivity in the gastric epithelium of *H. pylori*-infected individuals[24,35], and recent biopsy studies have confirmed both increased gastric mucosal IL-8 mRNA expression and IL-8 protein content in CagA-positive compared to CagA-negative infection[29,30,51].

Mononuclear phagocytes play a pivotal role in early immune responses to bacteria, serving as a potent source of proinflammatory mediators and as important antigen-presenting cells involved in the initiation of specific immunity. *In-vitro* exposure of human peripheral blood monocytes to a variety of *H. pylori*-derived soluble antigens, including a lipopolysaccharide-free extract, results in monocyte activation, as measured by increased expression of HLA-DR and IL-2 receptors, production of the inflammatory cytokines IL-1 and tumour necrosis factor-alpha (peptide and mRNA), and secretion of superoxide anion[52]. Furthermore, short-term *in-vitro* culture of endoscopic antral biopsies has revealed enhanced secretion of three predominantly monocyte/macrophage-derived proinflammatory cytokines, namely tumour necrosis factor-α, IL-6[27] and IL-1β[28] in *H. pylori*-infected subjects. These macrophage-derived cytokines have a wide range of proinflammatory actions[53], with both TNF-α and IL-1 inducing the up-regulation of endothelial cell adhesion molecules, increasing neutrophil adhesiveness, and stimulating gastric epithelial chemokine release[26], all of which will contribute to the accumulation and activation of leucocytes.

In addition to cytokine production, the cells of natural immunity are involved in the secretion of bioactive lipids, which are also involved in the recruitment and activation of phagocytes. Some of these endogenous lipids, such as platelet-activating factor (PAF) and leukotrienes, have been specifically implicated in peptic ulcerogenesis[54]. Levels of leukotriene B_4 (LT-B_4), which induces neutrophil adhesion, chemotaxis, and degranulation *in vitro*, are elevated in the mucosa of *H. pylori*-infected subjects, particularly where there is active gastritis[37]. Levels of *in-vitro* LT-C_4 secretion from biopsies incubated with ionophore are increased in *H. pylori*-infected subjects, and fall following treatment with colloidal bismuth, suggesting that *H. pylori* infection is associated with an increased capacity to generate proinflammatory eicosanoids[38]. Prostaglandins, in contrast, are known to possess properties which may be protective to the gastrointestinal mucosa, such as the inhibition of acid secretion and cytoprotection against various experimental injuries. Data are conflicting as to whether mucosal prostaglandin levels are altered in *H. pylori* infection, with several studies reporting non-significant increases in prostaglandin in infected subjects[55,56], and one group suggesting that PGE_2 levels are depressed[57].

Hence, there is evidence to suggest *H. pylori* colonization of the mucosa leads to the stimulation and activation of innate defence mechanisms involving chemokines and other proinflammatory cytokines, as well as bioactive lipids, leading to phagocyte accumulation and activation within the gastric mucosa. As with the IL-8 response of the epithelium[20–23], the expression of some of these proinflammatory mediators may vary quantitatively, with different *H. pylori* strains, with *cagA*-positive strains evoking a more vigorous release of inflammatory mediators. For example, a recent report suggests that patients infected with *cagA*-positive organisms have enhanced IL-1β levels in antral mucosa compared to those with *cagA*-negative infection[51]. A number of clinical studies have now shown increased mucosal inflammatory cell infiltration to be associated with infection with *cagA*-positive strains[29,30,50,58,59].

Role of mediators in induction of specific immune responses

In addition to phagocytic cells, *H. pylori* chronic gastritis is characterized by infiltration of the mucosa by lymphocytes and plasma cells, suggesting the activation of antigen-specific cellular and humoral immunity. Analysis of lymphocyte surface markers in *H. pylori* gastritis supports the view that mucosal lymphocytes are involved in specific immune responses, with a significant elevation in CD45RO+ (antigen-committed) memory type T cells[60]. Furthermore, *H. pylori*-specific CD4+ (helper) lymphocyte clones have been obtained from peripheral blood and gastric biopsies[61]. Provisional work has suggested that mRNA expression for RANTES, a chemokine which selectively attracts CD4+, CD45RO+ T cells, is found more frequently in *H. pylori* gastritis than in controls[36].

The activation of CD4+ ('helper') T cells, which is a key event in antigen specific immune responses, leads to the liberation of a variety of cytokines. Originally based on experiments in mice, T-helper cells are classified into two main types depending on characteristic profiles of cytokine secretion: Th1 cells secrete IL-2 and interferon gamma (IFNγ), whereas Th2 cells produce IL-4, IL-5 and IL-10[62]. In some parasitic infections, Th1 responses appear protective, whereas Th2 cells appear to exacerbate disease[63]. Although this functional dichotomy of T cells is not so clear-cut in humans, work to date has suggested that Th1 responses may predominate in chronic gastritis. *H. pylori*-stimulated peripheral blood lymphocytes secrete IFNγ *in vitro*[64], and an increase in IFNγ-secreting cells but not IL-4-secreting cells has been described in both *H. pylori*-positive and -negative gastritis[65]. IFNγ has a wide range of proinflammatory effects, including the activation of vascular endothelial cells, macrophages, neutrophils, and cytotoxic NK cells, the up-regulation of MHC Class II molecule expression, and roles in T- and B-cell differentiation. *H. pylori* infection is also associated with increased mucosal expression of IL-7[29,31], one source of which is the human intestinal epithelial cell[66]. IL-7 is a potent regulatory factor for intestinal mucosal T lymphocytes[66] as well as B cells[67].

Mediators involved in down-regulation of immune responses

Despite initiating both natural and specific immune responses in the gastric mucosa, *H. pylori* infection persists long-term. Although this is likely to reflect, in part, the relatively inaccessible ecological niche occupied by the organism, which precludes direct attack by immune cells, there may also be an element of immune down-regulation. A number of studies have suggested that *H. pylori* may indeed possess some immunosuppressive actions. *H. pylori* extracts have been shown to inhibit mitogen-induced proliferation of peripheral blood mononuclear cells *in vitro*[68], and a whole cell inactivated *H. pylori* preparation has been shown to induce lower proliferative responses in blood mononuclear cells from *H. pylori*-infected subjects than from uninfected patients[18,64]. A possible mechanism for *H. pylori*-induced suppression of immunity is via the induction of counter-regulatory cytokine secretion. Increased levels of IL-10 (both secreted protein and mRNA) have been reported recently in *H. pylori*-infected human mucosa[29,32], with expression of IL-10 mRNA increasing with the severity of gastritis[29]. This potent inhibitor of both phagocyte and lymphocyte responses, which is produced by mononuclear phagocytes and Th2 cells, may represent one mechanism of immune down-regulation. While this may be protective, limiting tissue damage caused by inflammation, the induction of counter-regulatory cytokine release may also contribute towards failure of the immune response to eliminate infection[32].

Nitric oxide

Increased mucosal levels of inducible nitric oxide synthase (iNOS) have been reported in gut inflammation at various sites[40], including *H. pylori* gastritis[39,40]. Rachmilewitz *et al.* found elevated gastric mucosal iNOS activity in duodenal ulcer patients compared to controls, but levels were higher in *H. pylori*-infected ulcer patients than in infected subjects without ulcers, and did not fall after eradication of the organism[69]. The role of nitric oxide (NO) in gastrointestinal inflammation in general remains contentious. Some authors suggest NO has a protective role in the gut[70], while others regard it as a molecular aggressor, particularly in chronic inflammation[71].

CONCLUSION

A large array of immunologically active molecules have now been implicated in *H. pylori*-associated mucosal inflammation, which serve to augment, amplify and modulate immune cell function. Qualitative and/or quantitative differences in the production of these mediators, resulting from infection by *H. pylori* strains differing in pathogenicity, may explain the spectrum of clinical disease manifestations.

References

1. Crabtree JE. Gastric mucosal inflammatory responses to *Helicobacter pylori*. Aliment Pharmacol Ther. 1996;10(Suppl. 1):29–37.

2. Blaser M. Pathogenesis of infections due to persistent bacteria at mucosal surfaces. In: Northfield TC, Mendall M, Goggin PM, editors. *Helicobacter pylori* infection. London: Kluwer; 1993:33–9.

3. Yoshida N, Granger DN, Evans DJ *et al.* Mechanisms involved in *Helicobacter pylori*-induced inflammation. Gastroenterology. 1993;105:1431–40.

4. Norgaard A, Andersen LP, Nielsen H. Neutrophil degranulation by *Helicobacter pylori* proteins. Gut. 1995;36:354–7.

5. Mooney C, Keenan J, Munster D *et al.* Neutrophil activation by *H. pylori.* Gut. 1991;32:853–7.

6. Norgaard A, Nielsen H, Andersen LP. Activation of human phagocytes by *Helicobacter pylori.* A novel interaction with neutrophils and monocytes distinct from that of N-formylated oligopeptides. Int J Med Microbiol, Virol, Parasitol Infect Dis. 1993;280:86–92.

7. Neilsen H, Andersen LP. Chemotactic activity of *Helicobacter pylori* sonicate for human poly-morphonuclear leucocytes and monocytes. Gut. 1992;33:738–42.

8. Kurose I, Granger DN, Evans DJ *et al. Helicobacter pylori*-induced microvascular protein leakage in rats: role of neutrophils, mast cells and platelets. Gastroenterology. 1994;107:70–9.

9. Neilsen H, Birkholz S, Andersen LP, Moran AP. Neutrophil activation by *Helicobacter pylori* lipopolysaccharide. J Infect Dis. 1994;170:135–9.

10. Craig PM, Territo MC, Karnes WE, Walsh JH. *Helicobacter pylori* secretes a chemotactic factor for monocytes and neutrophils. Gut. 1992;33:1020–3.

11. Nielsen H, Andersen LP. Activation of human phagocytic oxidative metabolism by *Helicobacter pylori.* Gastroenterology. 1992;103:1747–53.

12. Enders G, Brooks W, Jan N von, Lehn N, Bayerdorffer E, Hatz R. Expression of adhesion molecules on human granulocytes after stimulation with *Helicobacter pylori* membrane proteins: comparison with membrane proteins of other bacteria. Infect Immun. 1995;63:2473–7.

13. Kozol R, McCurdy B, Czanko R. A neutrophil chemotactic factor present in *H. pylori* but absent in *H. mustelae.* Dig Dis Sci. 1993;38:137–41.

14. Rautelin H, Blomberg B, Fredlund H, Jarnerot G, Danielsson D. Incidence of *Helicobacter pylori* strains activating neutrophils in patients with peptic ulcer disease. Gut. 1993;34:599–603.

15. Evans DJ, Evans DG, Takemura T *et al.* Characterisation of a *Helicobacter pylori* neutrophil activating factor. Infect Immun. 1995;63:2213–20.

16. Moran AP. The role of lipopolysaccharide in *Helicobacter pylori* pathogenesis. Aliment Pharmacol Ther. 1996;10(Suppl. 1):39–50.

17. Birkholz S, Knipp U, Opferkuch W. Stimulatory effects of *Helicobacter pylori* on human peripheral blood mononuclear cells of *H. pylori* infected patients and healthy blood donors. Int J Med Microbiol, Virol, Parasitol Infect Dis. 1993;280:166–76.

18. Karttunen R, Andersson G, Poikonen K *et al. Helicobacter pylori* induces lymphocyte activation in peripheral blood cultures. Clin Exp Immunol. 1990;82:485–8.

19. Baggiolini M, Dewald B, Moser B. Interleukin-8 and related chemotactic cytokines – C-X-C and C-C chemokines. Adv Immunol. 1994;55:97–179.

20. Crabtree JE, Farmery SM, Lindley IJD, Figura N, Peichl P, Tompkins DS. CagA/cytotoxic strains of *Helicobacter pylori* and interleukin-8 in gastric epithelial cells. J Clin Pathol. 1994;47:945–50.

21. Crabtree JE, Covacci A, Farmery SM *et al. Helicobacter pylori* induced interleukin-8 expression in gastric epithelial cells is associated with CagA positive phenotype. J Clin Pathol. 1995;48:41–5.

22. Crabtree JE, Xiang Z, Lindley IJD, Tompkins DS, Rappuoli R, Covacci A. Induction of interleukin-8 secretion from gastric epithelial cells by cagA-negative isogenic mutant of *Helicobacter pylori.* J Clin Pathol. 1995;48:967–9.

23. Sharma SA, Tummuru MKR, Miller GG, Blaser MJ. Interleukin-8 response of gastric epithelial cell lines to *Helicobacter pylori* stimulation in vitro. Infect Immun. 1995;63:1681–7.

24. Crabtree JE, Wyatt JI, Trejdosiewicz LK *et al.* Interleukin-8 expression in *Helicobacter pylori,* normal and neoplastic gastroduodenal mucosa. J Clin Pathol. 1994;47:61–6.

25. Azuma A, Aihara M, Doi T, Funakoshi Y, Imagawa K, Kikuchi M. *Helicobacter pylori* induced chemokine production in human gastric carcinoma cell lines: effects of rebamipide. Gastro-enterology. 1996;110:A272.

26. Yashimoto K, Okamoto S, Mukaida N, Murakami S, Mai M, Matsushima K. Tumour necrosis factor-α and interferon-gamma induce interleukin-8 production in human gastric cancer cell line through acting concurrently on AP-1 and NF-kB-like binding sites of the IL-8 gene. J Biol Chem. 1992;267:22506–11.

27. Crabtree JE, Shallcross TM, Heatley RV, Wyatt JI. Mucosal tumour necrosis factor-alpha and interleukin-6 in patients with *Helicobacter pylori*-associated gastritis. Gut. 1991;44:768–71.

28. Noach LA, Bosma NB, Jansen J, Hoek FJ, van Deventer SJH, Tytgat GNJ. Mucosal tumour

necrosis factor-alpha, interleukin-1 beta, and interleukin-8 production in patients with *Helicobacter pylori* infection. Scand J Gastroenterol. 1994;29:425–9.

29. Yamaoka Y, Kita M, Kodama T, Sawai N, Imanishi J. *Helicobacter pylori cagA* gene and expression of cytokine messenger RNA in gastric mucosa. Gastroenterology. 1996;110:1744–52.

30. Peek RM Jr, Miller GG, Tham KT *et al.* Heightened inflammatory response and cytokine expression *in vivo* to CagA+ *Helicobacter pylori* strains. Lab Invest. 1995;73:760–70.

31. Yamaoka Y, Kita M, Kodama T, Sawai N, Kashima K, Imanishi J. Expression of cytokine mRNA in gastric mucosa with *Helicobacter pylori* infection. Scand J Gastroenterol. 1995;30:1153–9.

32. Bodger K, Heatley RV. Mucosal secretion of interleukin-10 in gastritis. Gut. 1996;38(Suppl. 1): A30.

33. Karttunen R, Karttunen T, Ekre H-PT, MacDonald TT. Interferon gamma and interleukin 4 secreting cells in the gastric antrum in *Helicobacter pylori* positive and negative gastritis. Gut. 1995;36:341–5.

34. Crabtree JE, Peichl P, Wyatt JI, Stachl U, Lindley IJD. Gastric IL-8 and IL-8 IgA autoantibodies in *Helicobacter pylori* infection. Scand J Immunol. 1993;37:65–70.

35. Crabtree JE, Lindley IJD. Mucosal interleukin-8 and gastroduodenal disease. Eur J Gastroenterol Hepatol. 1994;6(Suppl. 1):S33–8.

36. Yamaoka Y, Kita M, Kodama T, Sawai N, Imanishi J. Expression of chemokine mRNA in gastric mucosa with *Helicobacter pylori* infection. Gastroenterology. 1996;110:A1049.

37. Fukada T, Kimura S, Arakawa T, Kobayashi K. Possible role of leukotrienes in gastritis associated with *Campylobacter pylori*. J Clin Gastroenterol. 1990;12(Suppl. 1):S131–4.

38. Ahmed A, Holton J, Vaira D, Smith SK, Hoult JRS. Eicosanoid synthesis and *Helicobacter pylori* associated gastritis: increase in leukotriene C4 generation associated with *H. pylori* colonisation. Prostaglandins. 1992;44:75–86.

39. Rieder G, Hatz RA, Stolte M, Enders G. iNOS in *H. pylori*-associated gastritis: possible role in carcinogenesis. Gastroenterology. 1996;110;A1002.

40. Mannick E, Ribbons KA, Zhang XJ *et al.* Expression of inducible nitric oxide synthase is a general response to gut inflammation and is not disease or site specific. Gastroenterology. 1996;110: A955.

41. Neale KR, Logan RPH. The epidemiology and transmission of *Helicobacter pylori* infection in children. Aliment Pharmacol Ther. 1995;9(Suppl. 2):77–84.

42. Sobala GM, Crabtree JE, Dixon MF *et al.* Acute *Helicobacter pylori* infection. Clinical features, local and systemic immune responses, gastric mucosal histology and gastric juice ascorbic acid concentrations. Gut. 1991;32:1415–18.

43. Marshall B, Armstrong J, McGechie D, Glancy R. Attempt to fulfil Koch's postulate for pyloric *Campylobacter*. Med J Aust. 1985;152:436–9.

44. Eckmann L, Kagnoff MF, Fierer J. Epithelial cells secrete chemokine interleukin-8 in response to bacterial entry. Infect Immun. 1993;61:4569–74.

45. Massion PP, Inoue H, Richman-Eistenstat J *et al.* Novel *Pseudomonas* product stimulates interleukin-8 production in airway epithelial cells *in vitro*. J Clin Invest. 1994;93:26–32.

46. Aihara M, Tsuchimoto D, Imagawa K, Kikuchi M, Mukaida N, Matsushima K. Signal transduction pathway in the IL-8 production of gastric mucosal cell (MKN-45) induced by *H. pylori*. Gastroenterology. 1996;110:A48.

47. Keates S, Hitti Y, Bliss Jr CM, Kelly CP. NFkB, a transcriptional regulatory factor for IL-8 gene expression, is activated by *H. pylori* in AGS human gastric epithelial cells. Gastroenterology. 1996; 110:A936.

48. Censini S, Lange C, Xiang Z *et al. cag*, a pathogenicity island of *Helicobacter pylori*, encodes Type I-specific and disease-associated virulence factors. (Submitted.)

49. Tummuru MKR, Sharma SA, Blaser MJ. *Helicobacter pylori* picB, a homologue of the *Bordetella pertussis* toxin secretion protein, is required for induction of IL-8 in gastric epithelial cells. Mol Microbiol. 1995;18:867–76.

50. Crabtree JE, Taylor JD, Wyatt JI *et al.* Mucosal IgA recognition of *Helicobacter pylori* 120kDa protein, peptic ulceration, and gastric pathology. Lancet. 1991;338:332–5.

51. Yamaoka Y, Kita M, Kodama N, Sawai N, Kashima K, Imanishi J. *Helicobacter pylori cagA* gene and production of cytokine in gastric mucosa. Gastroenterology. 1996;110:A299.

52. Mai UEH, Perez-Perez GI, Wahl LM *et al.* Soluble surface proteins from *Helicobacter pylori* activate monocytes/macrophages by lipopolysaccharide-independent mechanism. J Clin Invest. 1991;87:894–900.

53. Nicola NA. Guidebook to cytokines and their receptors. Oxford: Oxford University Press; 1994.

54. Ackerman Z, Karmeli F, Ligumsky M, Rachmilewitz D. Enhanced gastric and duodenal platelet-activating factor and leukotriene generation in duodenal ulcer patients. Scand J Gastroenterol. 1990;25:925–34.

55. Taha AS, Boothman P, Holland P *et al.* Gastric mucosal prostaglandin synthesis in the presence of *Campylobacter pylori* in patients with gastric ulcers and non-ulcer dyspepsia. Am J Gastroenterol. 1990;85:47–50.

56. Hudson N, Balsitis M, Filipowicz F, Hawkey CJ. Effect of *Helicobacter pylori* colonisation on gastric mucosal eicosanoid synthesis in patients taking non-steroidal anti-inflammatory drugs. Gut. 1993;34:748–51.

57. Goren A, Fotherby KJ, Shorthouse M, Wright DGD, Hunter JO. *Campylobacter pyloridis* and acid secretion [Letter]. Lancet. 1989;2:212.

58. Crabtree JE, Wyatt JI, Perry S, Davies GR, Covacci A, Morgan AG. CagA seropositive *Helicobacter pylori* infected non-ulcer patients have increased frequency of intestinal metaplasia. Gastroenterology. 1996;110:A85.

59. Graham DY, Genta RM, Graham DP, Crabtree JE. Serum CagA antibodies in peptic ulcer and asymptomatic adults: lack of a correlation of presence of IgG antibody in patients with peptic ulcer disease or asymptomatic *H. pylori* gastritis. J Clin Pathol. 1996 (In press).

60. Hatz RA, Meimarakis G, Bayerdorffer E, Stolte M, Kirchner T, Enders G. Characterisation of lymphocytic infiltrates in *Helicobacter pylori* associated gastritis. Scand J Gastroenterol. 1996; 31:222–8.

61. Di Tommaso A, Xiang Z, Bugnoli M *et al.* *Helicobacter pylori* specific CD4+ T-cell clones from peripheral blood and gastric biopsies. Infect Immun. 1995;63:1102–12.

62. Mosmann CNL, Cherwinski H, Bond MW, Giedlin MA, Coffman RL. Two types of murine helper T cell clones. I. Definition according to profiles of lymphokine activities and secreted proteins. J Immunol. 1986;136:2348–57.

63. Sher A, Gazzinelli RT, Oswald IP *et al.* Role of T-cell derived cytokines in the down-regulation of immune responses in parasitic and retroviral infection. Immunol Rev. 1992;127:183–204.

64. Karttunen R. Blood lymphocyte proliferation, cytokine secretion and appearance of T-cells with activation markers in cultures with *Helicobacter pylori*. Clin Exp Immunol. 1991;83:396–400.

65. Karttunen R, Karttunen T, Ekre H-PT, MacDonald TT. Interferon gamma and interleukin 4 secreting cells in the gastric antrum in *Helicobacter pylori* positive and negative gastritis. Gut. 1995;36:341–5.

66. Watanabe M, Ueno Y, Yajima T *et al.* Interleukin-7 is produced by human intestinal epithelial cells and regulates the proliferation of intestinal mucosal lymphocytes. J Clin Invest. 1995;95: 2945–53.

67. Goodwin RG, Lupton S, Schmierer A *et al.* Human interleukin-7: molecular cloning and growth factor activity on human and murine B-lineage cells. Proc Natl Acad Sci USA. 1989;86:302–6.

68. Knipp U, Birkholz S, Kaup W, Opferkuch W. Immune suppressive effects of *Helicobacter pylori* on human peripheral blood mononuclear cells. Med Microbiol Immunol. 1993;182:63–7.

69. Rachmilewitz D, Karmeli F, Eliakim R *et al.* Enhanced gastric nitric oxide synthase activity in duodenal ulcer patients. Gut. 1994;35:1394–7.

70. Kubes P, Wallace JL. Nitric oxide as a mediator of gastrointestinal injury? – Say it ain't so. Mediat Inflam. 1995;4:397–405.

71. Miller JS, Grisham MB. Nitric oxide as a mediator of inflammation? - You had better believe it. Mediat Inflam. 1995;4:387–96.

11
Effects of abnormalities of gastrin and somatostatin in *Helicobacter pylori* infection on acid secretion

J. CALAM. I. L. P. BEALES, A. GIBBONS, M. GHATEI and
J. Del VALLE

INTRODUCTION

Before the discovery of *H. pylori* the aetiology of gastroduodenal diseases was largely viewed in terms of associated abnormalities of gastric secretion. Elevated acid secretion in patients with duodenal ulcers (DU) seemed likely to be damaging the duodenum, and diminished acid secretion in patients with gastric cancer allowed overgrowth of mitogen-producing bacteria. Consequently gastric cancer and DU rarely occurred in the same patient. Since it emerged that *H. pylori* plays a major role in these diseases, we and others have investigated the effect of this infection on gastric physiology. Initial work examined how *H. pylori* might elevate acid secretion in DU disease. As the link between *H. pylori* and gastric cancer emerged the acid-lowering effects of this infection became more interesting. One part of the work has explored patterns of acid secretion under specific conditions in the different patient groups. Other studies have used *in-vitro* systems to explore the cellular events which might underlie what is found in patients. We are learning how infection and inflammation affect endocrine and exocrine systems of the gastrointestinal tract. Knowledge remains rudimentary, and whilst we learn more about the effects of relevant factors on various cells it will become necessary to dissect which of these effects actually determine disease outcomes. Hopefully, knowledge of why *H. pylori* exerts opposite effects on acid in different individuals will help us to identify patients at particular risk of DU or cancer.

GASTRIC PATHOPHYSIOLOGY BEFORE THE DISCOVERY OF *H. PYLORI*

Before *H. pylori* was discovered, studies showed that acid secretion tended to be low in patients with gastric cancer[1] and high in DU disease. Two main abnormalities were found in DU patients. First, they were estimated to have, on average, about 2 billion parietal cells compared with 1 billion in controls, leading to a maximal acid-secretory capacity which is about twice normal[2,3]. Secondly, studies showed abnormalities of physiological control which appear to show a defect in inhibitory control. Basal acid secretion was increased even more than would be expected from the increased parietal cell mass[2]. A low intragastric pH inhibited peptone-stimulated acid secretion less than usual[4] and, perhaps because of this, acid secretion persisted for longer than usual after meals[5]. Also, acid secretion in response to bombesin, which is the amphibian equivalent of gastrin-releasing peptide (GRP), was found to be elevated in DU patients. More precisely, an inhibitory effect of high doses appeared lacking in DU patients[6,7]. This difference may be explained by a lack of bombesin-stimulated somatostatin release[8] in the DU group (see below). One finding suggested that such parameters may vary with time. Achord found that basal acid output was higher in DU patients whose ulcers were active as opposed to healed at the time of testing[9]. Acid secretion tended to fall as ulcers healed without treatment of *H. pylori*, but this trend was not statistically significant. Nevertheless, this finding raises the possibility that the pathophysiology of DU disease might be cyclical, and ulcers occur when the abnormality is maximal.

Hormonal abnormalities noted in DU disease before the discovery of *H. pylori*

Gastrin

Initial studies of hormonal control in DU disease examined the acid-stimulating antral hormone gastrin (see below). Elevated peak postprandial gastrin concentrations were found in DU patients in some centres[10,11], but not in others. In retrospect this probably depended on whether controls were infected with *H. pylori*. Other studies showed that a low intragastric pH inhibited peptone-stimulated gastrin release less in DU patients than in controls[4]. One stimulus that consistently produced higher plasma gastrin levels in DU patients than controls was bombesin[6,7].

Somatostatin

Decreased mucosal somatostatin was a more consistent finding in DU disease. Studies showed less immunoreactive somatostatin and fewer immunoreactive D cells in DU patients[12]. This was particularly interesting because it offered an explanation for the failure of acid-inhibitory reflexes in DU patients. However, the cause of the decreased mucosal expression of somatostatin in DU disease remained a mystery until the discovery of *H. pylori*.

Histamine

Mucosal histamine concentrations were found to be diminished in patients with DU[13]. This was thought to be due to an increased release of histamine, but this may be incorrect (see below).

109

EFFECTS OF *H. PYLORI* GASTRITIS ON THE ENDOCRINE AND EXOCRINE CELLS OF THE STOMACH

When it became clear that *H. pylori* is a major aetiological agent in DU disease we, and others, asked whether this infection causes some of the alterations in gastric physiology that had been reported in upper gastrointestinal diseases. This has proved to be the case, although the picture remains incomplete. The current knowledge will be examined cell by cell.

Gastrin and G cells

Gastrins[14] emanate from G cells which are located in the gastric antrum and to a lesser extent in the duodenum. The main forms are gastrin-34 (G34) and its C-terminal fragment gastrin-17 (G17). About 95% of antral gastrin is G17, whilst duodenal gastrin is about 60% G34[15]. G34 and G17 have similar agonist activity at the gastrin (alias CCK-B) receptor[16], but G34 is cleared more slowly from the circulation[16] and is therefore more potent, dose for dose. G cells release gastrin in response to luminal stimuli including products of protein digestion, and intramucosal stimuli including gastrin-releasing peptide[14]. Gastrin acts via the blood stream to increase acid secretion. It does this both directly by stimulating parietal cells[17], and indirectly by stimulating ECL cells to release histamine[18]. Gastrin also has a trophic effect on the gastric epithelium[19] and particularly on the ECL cells that it contains[20].

Gastrin in H. pylori *infection*

Elevation of gastrin release in association with *H. pylori* infection was first reported by Odera *et al.*[21], who found that plasma gastrin levels fall when this infection is treated in children. However, acid was not measured, and it seemed likely that the initial elevation of gastrin was related to low acid secretion following first infection. We reported elevations of postprandial gastrin levels and maximal acid output in infected versus uninfected DU patients, and proposed the 'gastrin link' between infection of the antrum and ulcers in the duodenum[22]. We, and others, then confirmed that gastric levels fall on eradication of *H. pylori*. Gastrin is elevated during fasting, and after stimulation with meals or gastrin-releasing peptide (GRP)[11,23,24]. Interestingly the excessive rise in gastrin after GRP[23] and after eating[25] is predominantly due to a rise in G17. This might be because the excessive gastrin emanates from the antrum where G17 predominates. Alternatively *H. pylori* might accelerate the cleavage of G34 to produce G17. Eradication of the infection restores the inhibitory effect of cholecystokinin on gastric release[26]. This reflex is believed to be mediated through release of somatostatin from antral D cells[27].

Possible mechanisms of increased gastrin release

A variety of mechanisms have been proposed to explain the increase in gastrin release.

1. Products of H. pylori *enzyme urease.* Urease might elevate gastrin release by generating alkali, or by producing ammonium ions. We originally proposed the role of alkali[22]. Acid inhibits gastrin release, probably by stimulating D cells to release somatostatin[28,29], so that local alkalinization might have the opposite effect. Direct measurements showed that the pH in the gastric mucus layer is more alkaline in *H. pylori* infection, but only by 0.3–0.8 of a pH unit[11]. Moreover, inhibition of urease by acetohydroxamic acid[30] did not decrease gastrin release in short-term experiments. These data are against the role of pH, but the possibility cannot be dismissed because some persisting production of ammonia during administration of acetohydroxamic acid[30] might have been sufficient to produce alkalinization. Also, if alkalinization is involved, the studies might have been too short. Plasma gastrin levels remain considerably elevated 3 h after acidification of the stomach of achlorhydric patients[31].

Ammonium ions might release gastrin independent of any effect on pH. Lichtenberger *et al.* found elevated plasma gastrin levels in rats whose diets had been supplemented with ammonium acetate for 2 weeks[32]. However, the amount of ammonium acetate given was sufficient to cause inflammation, which might have contributed. A study in Japan suggests that monochloramine may be a more potent stimulant of gastrin release than ammonia itself[33]. Ammonia released by *H. pylori* activates neutrophils to create oxidative bursts *in vitro*[34]. Oxidation of hydrochloric acid by neutrophils would be expected to produce hypochlorous acid, which then reacts with ammonia to produce monochloramine, NH_2Cl. This stimulated gastrin release and acid secretion more than ammonia in rats[33].

2. Inflammatory mediators. Inflammatory mediators released in *H. pylori* gastritis might also be responsible for an increased gastrin release. This infection increases the mucosal expression of many cytokines including: interleukins (IL) 1β, 6 and 8, tumour necrosis factor-α (TNFα), interferon-γ (IFNγ) and platelet-activating factor (PAF)[35]. Teichmann reported in a series of abstracts that several cytokines release gastrin from gastric antral preparations *in vitro*, including IL-1 and -2, TNFα, INFγ and leukotrienes C_4 and D_4[11]. We found that TNFα and IFNγ release gastrin from canine antral endocrine cells in primary culture[36]. Immuno-blockade of somatostatin, if anything, enhanced the effect, suggesting that the cytokines were not acting via D cells. Beales and Calam showed that TNFα increased gastrin release from slices of human antral biopsies in organ culture[37]. This effect was also resistant to immunoblockade of somatostatin. TNFα and *H. pylori* infection were both found to attenuate cholecystokinin (CCK)'s inhibitory effect on gastrin release in these preparations. This effect of CCK is believed to be mediated by release of somatostatin[27], so that these findings suggest that D-cell function was diminished. Schepp and colleagues found that TNFα releases gastrin from rabbit G cells, and found that IL-1β had a similar effect on this preparation[38]. Another study demonstrates the importance of synergism between stimuli; *H. pylori* sonicates do not release gastrin from canine antral cells when given alone, but strongly released gastrin to 230% above basal levels when given with IL-8. This chemokine, given alone, stimulated gastrin release to about 40% above basal level[39]. Interestingly the response to IL-8 plus *H. pylori* extract appeared to vary between strains of *H. pylori*.

Somatostatin and D cells

Somatostatin peptides[40] are released from D cells located throughout the gastro-intestinal tract and other organs. The two main forms, S28 and S14, both have high affinity for the various somatostatin receptors SSTR1–5[41]. Of these SSTR2 is most involved in the physiological inhibition of acid secretion[42]. D cells in the gastric antrum are 'open', with microvilli extending into the gastric lumen, while D cells of the gastric corpus are 'closed' and do not contact the lumen[40]. Somatostatin is released from the antrum by luminal factors, notably acid[28,43], but also by food[44]. Although antral D cells are in contact with the gastric lumen there is evidence that acid affects antral D cells indirectly, through a neural reflex which may involve CGRP[45].

Somatostatin is also released by neurotransmitters including epinephrine and a wide variety of peptides including gastrin-releasing peptide (GRP)/bombesin and CCK. Stimulation of somatostatin release by small intestinal hormones such as CCK is probably important in the inhibition of gastric secretion, which occurs in the late postprandial period. Somatostatin has widespread inhibitory effects on endocrine and exocrine cells, including G cells, ECL cells and parietal cells[40]. Expression of somatostatin is maximal when the intragastric pH is low and, during fasting, consistent with its inhibitory role[28,29,46].

Somatostatin in H. pylori infection

Several studies have shown that the decrease in the mucosal expression of somato-statin noted in DU patients is actually due to *H. pylori* infection. Kaneko *et al.*[47] showed diminished mucosal somatostatin peptide in association with this infection, and we showed that *H. pylori* infection also decreases mucosal somatostatin mRNA and the number of immunoreactive D cells[48]. Other groups have since confirmed the inhibitory effect of *H. pylori* on mucosal levels of somatostatin peptide[49–51], mRNA[50] and D-cell numbers[52]. Graham *et al.*[53] were unable to detect a difference in the number of D cells. Little is known of D-cell function in *H. pylori* infection. We compared the response of mucosal somatostatin mRNA to 3h infusions of GRP between infected and uninfected subjects[54]. The results showed a significant rise in somatostatin mRNA in the infected, but not in the uninfected, group. The reason for this difference awaits elucidation, but baseline somatostatin mRNA levels were considerably diminished in the infected group, so the difference might be due to diminished auto-inhibition of D cells by somatostatin itself[55]. Whatever the explanation the results do show that D cells are capable of responding to GRP in *H. pylori* infection. We found that eradication of *H. pylori* had no significant effect on somatostatin mRNA in the gastric corpus of DU patients, but that somatostatin mRNA was considerably diminished in the gastric corpus of non-ulcer subjects. This might be because corpus gastritis tends to be more severe in non-ulcer than in DU patients[56].

The finding that *H. pylori* infection diminishes mucosal somatostatin is interesting, firstly, because it explains diminished mucosal somatostatin in DU patients and secondly, since somatostatin is a potent inhibitor of G cells, ECL cells and parietal cells, it offers an explanation for other aspects of *H. pylori* pathophysiology. Diminished somatostatin expression in the gastric antrum may well cause the elevation in gastrin release. Similarly, diminished somatostatin in the corpus might increase acid secretion, but here the findings do not fit so well. Acid secretion is highest in DU patients who, on current evidence, have the least disturbance of corpus somatostatin levels.

Possible mechanisms of diminished mucosal somatostatin

It is unknown how *H. pylori* infection inhibits D cells, but we found that prolonged exposure of D cells to the cytokine TNFα has this effect. Exposure of elutriated canine corpus D cells in primary culture to TNFα for 2h weakly stimulated somatostatin release, but somatostatin release decreased by about 40% when these cells were exposed to TNFα for 24h. This was partly due to a fall in the cell content of somatostatin, which was too great to be explained by the initial increase in release. In addition, TNFα produced a selective inhibition in somato-statin release in response to CCK and gastrin. The percentage of cell content released by epinephrine was unaffected[57]. Therefore, TNFα released in infected mucosa might suppress D cells. Vuyyuru *et al.* studied the effect of histamine H_3-receptor stimulation and blockade on the release of somatostatin, gastrin and histamine from extracts of antral mucosa[58]. Stimulation of H_3 receptors decreased release of somatostatin and increased release of gastrin and histamine. H_3 blockade had the opposite effect. These studies used the specific H_3-receptor agonist R^α methylhistamine. The results raise the possibility that the less specific agonist N^α methylhistamine which *H. pylori* produces might cause the suppression of D cells seen in this infection.

Enterochromaffin-like (ECL) cells and histamine

Histamine is released from enterochromaffin-like (ECL) cells and stimulates acid secretion locally via histamine H_2 receptors on parietal cells. Histamine may also be released from mast cells. It is produced from histidine by histidine decarboxylase. ECL cells are stimulated to release histamine by factors including gastrin; thus ECL cells may contribute to gastrin-stimulated acid secretion even though gastrin receptors are present on the parietal cells themselves[17].

Histamine in H. pylori *infection*

Studies have shown that mucosal concentrations of histamine are diminished in *H. pylori* gastritis[59]. This has been interpreted as reflecting increased release of histamine. On the other hand mucosal levels of histidine decarboxylase are also diminished, suggesting that histamine synthesis may actually be diminished (see below)[60].

Possible mechanisms of altered ECL-cell function

1. Gastrin is known to stimulate ECL cells to proliferate and to release gastrin.
2. A recent abstract from Prinz *et al.* indicates that histamine release from ECL cells is decreased by IL-1β[61].
3. N^α methylhistamine.

Courillon-Mallet *et al.* recently showed that *H. pylori* produces the histamine metabolite N^α methylhistamine[60]. This is a potent histamine H_3 receptor agonist, but also stimulates H_1 and H_2 receptors. Infected mucosa contained much more N^α methylhistamine and the synthetic enzyme N^α histamine methyltransferase than did uninfected mucosa. Infected mucosa showed a lower capacity to bind [^{3}H]N^α methylhistamine and lower indices of ECL-cell function: histamine itself and the synthetic enzyme histidine decarboxylase. Mucosal somatostatin was also diminished[60]. Other work shows that a more selective H_3-receptor agonist inhibits acid secretion *in vivo*[62] and in isolated rabbit gastric glands *in vitro*[63]. The above is consistent with evidence that ECL cells possess inhibitory H_3 receptors[64]. Therefore N^α methylhistamine produced by *H. pylori* might cause diminished ECL-cell function in *H. pylori* gastritis, and thus tend to diminish acid secretion. On the other hand, infusions of N^α methylhistamine itself, into intact animals, stimulated acid secretion[65], consistent with its H_2-receptor agonist effect. Therefore, more work is required to determine the net effects of this interesting product.

Parietal cells

Parietal cells are located in the gastric glands and secrete acid into the lumen of the stomach in response to gastrin, acetylcholine and histamine. Parietal cells are inhibited by somatostatin. Factors which affect these cells will therefore have the most direct effect on acid secretion.

Potential modulators of parietal cell function in H. pylori infection

In-vitro studies have identified a variety of *H. pylori* products and inflammatory mediators which affect parietal cell function:

Inhibitors
1. Cave's group have identified two products which inhibit parietal cell function. One of these (AIF1) resembled nigericin; the other (AIF2) is a protein which has recently been purified and found to be a dimer with 46 kDa subunits. The gene encoding it has recently been cloned[66].
2. Beil *et al.* identified certain fatty acids which are produced by *H. pylori* and inhibit parietal cell function. These act partly as proton ionophores allowing protons to re-enter the cells, and partly by inhibiting the proton pump itself[67].
3. The cytokines $TNF\alpha$ and $IL-1\beta$ inhibit parietal cell function. Beales *et al.* have shown that they act through more than one pathway at the post-receptor level[68]. One feature of these results is that the cytokines are able to decrease the maximal response of parietal cell stimuli. This sort of result raises the possibility that 'maximal acid output' may actually be less fixed than was previously thought.

Stimulants
We examined the effect of N^α methylhistamine on elutriated rabbit parietal cells in primary culture because Courillon-Mallet *et al.* showed that *H. pylori* produces this, and other data suggested that parietal cells might possess inhibitory H_3 receptors. Our results showed that N^α methylhistamine acts on these cells purely

as an H_2 agonist to stimulate acid secretion[69]. This finding raises the possibility that *H. pylori* increases acid secretion through a direct effect of N^{α} methyl-histamine on parietal cells.

The effect of atrophic gastritis

The above relates to acute effects of various factors on parietal cell function. This is in the realm of physiology. However, it is also clear that histological changes can have a marked effect on the number of parietal cells present. *H. pylori* causes atrophic gastritis[70], which is characterized by a loss of parietal cells with the subsequent loss of acid secretory capacity.

EFFECTS OF *H. PYLORI* INFECTION ON GASTRIC ACID SECRETION

It has become clear that the effects of *H. pylori* on acid secretion depend on several variables:

1. The effect varies from patient to patient. For example, *H. pylori* infection elevates acid secretion in DU patients, but decreases it in patients who develop atrophic gastritis.
2. The effect varies from time to time within the same patient. For example, acid secretion is initially lost, but then returns[71].
3. The effect of *H. pylori* on acid secretion depends on the physiological conditions at the time of measurement. For example, *H. pylori* had no effect on meal-stimulated acid secretion when the intragastric pH was high, but elevated acid secretion when the intragastric pH was low[72].

One useful way to disentangle this subject is to divide acid secretion into:

A. Maximal acid output (MAO) which reflects the rate of acid secretion produced by maximal stimulation with agents such as pentagastrin or histamine.
B. The actual rate of acid secretion determined by physiological control mechanisms under the conditions of study, which will fall within the range from zero to the MAO.

Maximal acid output

Low acid secretion

MAO tends to be normal or slightly decreased in *H. pylori*-infected subjects without ulcers[73–76]. MAO is markedly abnormal in certain specific situations. It is decreased in patients who develop gastric cancer[77] and greatly diminished for weeks or months after first infection[71]. Gastric atrophy probably contributes to diminished acid secretion in the former. The latter is reversible, suggesting temporary suppression of parietal cells by *H. pylori* products or inflammatory mediators. Such factors might also contribute to the chronically low acid secretion seen in a minority of patients with chronic gastritis. This is supported by normalization of acid secretion in these subjects following successful eradication of *H. pylori*[78].

High acid secretion

Increased maximal acid output is seen in *H. pylori*-infected patients with DU disease. Until recently the increased MAO in these patients was regarded as being more or less fixed, because early studies showed no change 1 month after eradication of *H. pylori*[79,80]. However, two recent studies have shown that MAO eventually falls when *H. pylori* is eradicated from patients with DU disease[81,82]. The mechanism of this effect is currently unknown, but withdrawal of factors such as gastrin and N^α methylhistamine could be involved (see above). On the other hand, if it really does take 6 or 12 months for MAO to fall, a slower process might be involved. Withdrawal of a trophic effect of gastrin[19] (or some other growth factor or cytokine) on parietal cells also might be responsible.

Why do different patients react differently to the same infection?

It is unclear why the same infection produces different patterns of acid secretion in different individuals. There is no evidence to link any particular strain of bacteria to high or low acid secretion. More severe corpus gastritis might diminish parietal cell function, either acutely through cytokine release, or chronically by leading to gastric atrophy. Environmental factors associated with atrophy include lack of antioxidant vitamins[83], and a high-salt diet[84]. In addition we found HLA DQ5 to be over-represented in infected patients with atrophy[85]. Elevated MAO in DU disease might be due to a lack of such factors. It was recently reported that DU patients who were all infected with *H. pylori* had about 3 times as many ECL cells in their gastric mucosa as either infected non-ulcer patients, or uninfected controls[86]. This raises the possibility that elevated acid secretion in DU patients might be due to excessive histamine release from ECL cells in the gastric mucosa.

Disturbances of physiological control of gastrin release in *H. pylori* infection

H. pylori infection causes a defect in the reflex inhibition of acid secretion which was previously observed in patients with DU disease (see above). This is probably related to the paucity of mucosal somatostatin.

Basal acid secretion

We and others have seen a significant fall in basal acid secretion following successful eradication of *H. pylori* from DU patients[87,88] consistent with the fall in plasma gastrin, but have not seen the same change in non-ulcer patients[58,89], perhaps because an improvement in corpus gastritis led to an opposing increase in acid secretion.

Meal-stimulated acid secretion at a low intragastric pH

We found that *H. pylori* impairs the inhibition of peptone-stimulated acid secretion by a low intragastric pH. The low pH suppressed acid secretion by >80% in uninfected subjects but by <50% in *H. pylori*-infected volunteers[72]. Acid secretion stimulated by neutral peptone was similar in the infected and uninfected groups, indicating that the abnormality lies in the inhibitory pathway.

The inhibitory effect of antral distension

Antral distension normally inhibits pentagastrin-stimulated acid secretion, and this reflex is also attenuated by *H. pylori* infection[90].

Gastrin-releasing peptide-stimulated acid secretion

Infusions of gastrin-releasing peptide (GRP) normally exert a mixture of stimulatory and inhibitory effects on acid secretion. Stimulation is through gastrin release, while inhibition may be through somatostatin[8], which exogenous GRP probably releases indirectly via several routes, including locally released gastrin, mucosal nerves and small intestinal hormones, including CCK. Acid secretion stimulated by GRP is elevated about 3 times in *H. pylori* infection, and about 6 times in DU patients when compared with uninfected controls[91]. The more marked elevation of acid secretion in DU patients might be due to their greater parietal cell mass (see above). Elevated GRP-stimulated acid secretion disappears slowly during the first year after successful eradication. It was recently found that CCK infusions inhibit GRP-stimulated acid secretion less in *H. pylori*-infected persons[92]. This is consistent with a lack of CCK-stimulated somatostatin release.

Therefore, it is important to ask whether the changes are sufficient to affect the pH in the duodenum. Hamlet and Olbe[93] found that infected subjects did, indeed, have a lower intraduodenal pH during the second hour after neutral and acidic meals than did healthy controls. However, this was at least partly due to rapid gastric emptying, in addition to changes in acid secretion.

CONCLUSION

The work described above shows that products of *H. pylori* itself, and certain inflammatory mediators released in *H. pylori* gastritis, can modulate the behaviour of the endocrine and exocrine cells of the stomach. These effects presumably underlie the changes in acid secretion that *H. pylori* infection produces. It is likely that these changes in acid secretion contribute to the major clinical outcomes; ulcers, gastric atrophy and cancer. Therefore an understanding of the cellular events which determine acid output should help us to understand what leads to the various outcomes of this infection, and thus enable us to target therapy more accurately.

References

1. Carlborg L, Dahlgren S, Nordgren B. Gastric secretion of hydrochloric acid and sialic acid in patients with peptic ulcer and gastric cancer during intravenous infusion of histamine. Scand J Gastroenterol. 1970;5:427–31.
2. Blair AJ, Feldman M, Barnett C, Walsh JH, Richardson CT. Detailed comparison of basal and food-stimulated gastric acid secretion rates and serum gastrin concentrations in duodenal ulcer patients and normal subjects. J Clin Invest. 1987;79:582–7.
3. Cox AJJ. Stomach size and its relation to chronic peptic ulcer. Arch Pathol. 1952;54:407–12.

4. Walsh JH, Richardson CT, Fordtran JS. pH dependence of acid secretion and gastrin release in normal and ulcer subjects. J Clin Invest. 1975;55:462–8.
5. Malagelada JR, Longstreth GF, Deering TB, Summerskill WH, Go VL. Gastric secretion and emptying after ordinary meals in duodenal ulcer. Gastroenterology. 1977;73:989–94.
6. Hirschowitz BI, Tim LO, Helman CA, Molina E. Bombesin and G-17 dose responses in duodenal ulcer and controls. Dig Dis Sci. 1985;30:1092–103.
7. Helman CA, Hirschowitz BI. Divergent effects of bombesin and bethanechol on stimulated gastric secretion in duodenal ulcer and in normal men. Gastroenterology. 1987;92:1926–33.
8. Schubert ML, Jong MJ, Makhlouf GM. Bombesin/GRP-stimulated somatostatin secretion is mediated by gastrin in the antrum and intrinsic neurons in the fundus. Am J Physiol. 1991;261: G885–9.
9. Achord JL. Gastric pepsin and acid secretion in patients with acute and healed duodenal ulcer. Gastroenterology. 1981;81:15–18.
10. Taylor IL, Dockray GJ, Calam J, Walker RJ. Big and little gastrin responses to food in normal and ulcer subjects. Gut. 1979;20:957–62.
11. Moss S, Calam J. *Helicobacter pylori* and peptic ulcers: the present position. Gut. 1992;33: 289–92.
12. McHenry L Jr, Vuyyuru L, Schubert ML. *Helicobacter pylori* and duodenal ulcer disease: the somatostatin link? Gastroenterology. 1993;104:1573–5.
13. Man WK, Thompson JN, Baron JH, Spencer J. Histamine and duodenal ulcer: effect of omeprazole on gastric histamine in patients with duodenal ulcer. Gut. 1986;27:418–22.
14. Walsh JH. Gastrin. In: Walsh JH, Dockray GJ, editors. Gut peptides: biochemistry and physiology. New York: Raven Press; 1994:75–121.
15. Calam J, Dockray GJ, Walker RJ, Owens D. Molecular forms of gastrin in peptic ulcer: a comparison of serum and tissue concentrations of G17 and G34 in gastric and duodenal ulcer subjects. Eur J Clin Invest. 1980;10:241–7.
16. Eysselein VE, Maxwell V, Reedy T, Wunsch E, Walsh JH. Similar acid stimulatory potencies of synthetic human big and little gastrins in man. J Clin Invest. 1984;73:1284–90.
17. Kopin AS, Lee YM, McBride EW *et al*. Expression cloning and characterization of the canine parietal cell gastrin receptor. Proc Natl Acad Sci USA. 1992;89:3605–9.
18. Waldum HL, Sandvik AK, Brenna E, Petersen H. Gastrin–histamine sequence in the regulation of gastric acid secretion. Gut. 1991;32:698–701.
19. Ascencio F, Fransson LA, Wadstrom T. Affinity of the gastric pathogen *Helicobacter pylori* for the N-sulphated glycosaminoglycan heparan sulphate. J Med Microbiol. 1993;38:240–4.
20. Lehy T. Trophic effect of some regulatory peptides on gastric exocrine and endocrine cells of the rat. Scand J Gastroenterol. 1994;19(Suppl. 101):27–30.
21. Odera G, Holton J, Altare F, Vaira D, Ainley C, Ansaldi N. Amoxycillin plus tinidazole for *Campylobacter pylori* gastritis in children: assessment by serum IgG antibody, pepsinogen 1 and gastrin level. Lancet. 1989;1:690–2.
22. Levi S, Beardshall K, Haddad G, Playford R, Ghosh P, Calam J. *Campylobacter pylori* and duodenal ulcers: the gastrin link. Lancet. 1989;1:1167–8.
23. Beardshall K, Moss S, Gill J *et al*. Suppression of *Helicobacter pylori* reduces gastrin releasing peptide stimulated gastrin release in duodenal ulcer patients. Gut. 1992;33:601–3.
24. Graham DY, Opekun A, Lew GM, Klein PD, Walsh JH. *Helicobacter pylori*-associated exaggerated gastrin release in duodenal ulcer patients. The effect of bombesin infusion and urea ingestion. Gastroenterology. 1991;100:1571–5.
25. Mulholland G, Ardill JE, Fillmore D, Chittajallu RS, Fullarton GM, McColl KE. *Helicobacter pylori* related hypergastrinaemia is the result of a selective increase in gastrin 17. Gut. 1993;34: 757–61.
26. Konturek JW, Gillessen A, Konturek SJ, Domschke W. Eradication of *Helicobacter pylori* restores the inhibitory effect of cholecystokinin on postprandial gastrin release in duodenal ulcer patients. Gut. 1995;37:482–7.
27. Buchan AM, Meloche RM, Kwok YN, Kofod H. Effect of cholecystokinin and secretin on somatostatin release from cultured antral cells. Gastroenterology. 1993;104:1414–19.
28. Holst JJ, Jensen SL, Knuhtsen S, Nielsen OV, Rehfeld JF. Effect of vagus, gastric inhibitory polypeptide, and HCl on gastrin and somatostatin release from perfused pig antrum. Am J Physiol. 1983;244:G515–22.
29. Brand SJ, Stone D. Reciprocal regulation of antral gastrin and somatostatin gene expression by omeprazole-induced achlorhydria. J Clin Invest. 1988;82:1059–66.

30. el Nujumi AM, Dorrian CA, Chittajallu RS, Neithercut WD, McColl KE. Effect of inhibition of *Helicobacter pylori* urease activity by acetohydroxamic acid on serum gastrin in duodenal ulcer subjects. Gut. 1991;32:866–70.
31. Fahrenkrug J, Schaffalitzky de Muckadell OB, Hornum I, Rehfeld JF. The mechanism of hypergastrinemia in achlorhydria. Effect of food, acid, and calcitonin on serum gastrin concentrations and component pattern in pernicious anemia, with correlation to endogenous secretin concentrations in plasma. Gastroenterology. 1976;71:33–7.
32. Lichtenberger LM, Dial EJ, Romero JJ, Lechago J, Jarboe LA, Wolfe MM. Role of luminal ammonia in the development of gastropathy and hypergastrinemia in the rat. Gastroenterology. 1995;108:320–9.
33. Saita H, Murakami M, Dekigai H, Kita T. Effects of ammonia and monochloramine on gastrin release and acid secretion. Gastroenterology. 1993;104:A183.
34. Suzuki M, Miura S, Suematsu M et al. *Helicobacter pylori*-associated ammonia production enhances neutrophil-dependent gastric mucosal cell injury. Am J Physiol. 1992;263:G719–25.
35. Blaser MJ. Hypotheses on the pathogenesis and natural history of *Helicobacter pylori*-induced inflammation. Gastroenterology. 1992;102:720–7.
36. Lehmann FS, Golodner EH, Wang J et al. Mononuclear cells and cytokines stimulate gastrin release from canine antral cells in primary culture. Am J Physiol. 1996 (in press).
37. Beales ILP, Calam J. *Helicobacter pylori* infection and exogenous tumour necrosis factor alpha produce similar effects on gastrin release from human antral fragments. Gut. 1996;38(Suppl. 1): A12.
38. Weigert N, Schaffer K, Schusdziarra V, Classen M, Schepp W. Gastrin secretion from primary cultures of rabbit antral G cells: stimulation by inflammatory cytokines. Gastroenterology. 1996; 110:147–54.
39. Beales I, Srinivasan S, Blaser M et al. Effect of *Helicobacter pylori* constituents and inflammatory cytokines on gastrin release from isolated canine G-cells. Gastroenterology. 1995;108:A779.
40. Chiba T, Yamada T. Gut somatostatin. In: Walsh JH, Dockray GJ, editors. Gut peptides: biochemistry and physiology. New York: Raven Press; 1994:123–45.
41. Bruns C, Weckbecker G, Raulf F, Lubbert H, Hoyer D. Characterization of somatostatin receptor subtypes. Ciba Found Symp. 1995;190:89–101.
42. Lloyd KC, Wang J, Aurang K, Gronhed P, Coy DH, Walsh JH. Activation of somatostatin receptor subtype 2 inhibits acid secretion in rats. Am J Physiol. 1995;268:G102–6.
43. Schubert ML, Edwards NF, Makhlouf GM. Regulation of gastric somatostatin secretion in the mouse by luminal acidity: a local feedback mechanism. Gastroenterology. 1988;94:317–22.
44. Chayvialle JA, Miyata M, Rayford PL, Thompson JC. Effects of test meal, intragastric nutrients, and intraduodenal bile on plasma concentrations of immunoreactive somatostatin and vasoactive intestinal peptide in dogs. Gastroenterology. 1980;79:844–52.
45. Inui T, Kinoshita Y, Yamaguchi A, Yamatani T, Chiba T. Linkage between capsaicin-stimulated calcitonin gene-related peptide and somatostatin release in rat stomach. Am J Physiol. 1991;261: G770–4.
46. Wu V, Sumii K, Tari A, Sumii M, Walsh JH. Regulation of rat antral gastrin and somatostatin gene expression during starvation and after refeeding. Gastroenterology. 1991;101:1552–8.
47. Kaneko H, Nakada K, Mitsuma T et al. *Helicobacter pylori* infection induces a decrease in immunoreactive-somatostatin concentrations of human stomach. Dig Dis Sci. 1992;37:409–16.
48. Moss SF, Legon S, Bishop AE, Polak JM, Calam J. Effect of *Helicobacter pylori* on gastric somatostatin in duodenal ulcer disease. Lancet. 1992;340:930–2.
49. Odum L, Petersen HD, Andersen IB, Hansen BF, Rehfeld JF. Gastrin and somatostatin in *Helicobacter pylori* infected antral mucosa. Gut. 1994;35:615–18.
50. Gotz JM, Veenendaal RA, Biemond I, Muller ES, Veselic M, Lamers CB. Serum gastrin and mucosal somatostatin in *Helicobacter pylori*-associated gastritis. Scand J Gastroenterol. 1995; 30:1064–8.
51. Haruma K, Sumii K, Okamoto S et al. *Helicobacter pylori* infection is associated with low antral somatostatin content in young adults. Implications for the pathogenesis of hypergastrinemia. Scand J Gastroenterol. 1995;30:550–3.
52. Queiroz DM, Moura SB, Mendes EN, Rocha GA, Barbosa AJ, de Carvalho AS. Effect of *Helicobacter pylori* eradication on G-cell and D-cell density in children. Lancet. 1994;343: 1191–3.
53. Graham DY, Lew GM, Lechago J. Antral G-cell and D-cell numbers in *Helicobacter pylori* infection: effect of H. pylori eradication. Gastroenterology. 1993;104:1655–60.

54. Gibbons AH, Legon S, Calam J. Effect of gastrin releasing peptide (GRP) infusions on the mRNAs encoding gastrin and somatostatin in patients with and without *H. pylori* infection. Gastroenterology. 1995;108:A100.
55. Park J, Chiba T, Yokotani K, DelValle J, Yamada T. Somatostatin receptors on canine fundic D-cells: evidence for autocrine regulation of gastric somatostatin. Am J Physiol. 1989;257:G235–41.
56. Sipponen P. Natural history of gastritis and its relationship to peptic ulcer disease. Digestion. 1992;51(Suppl. 1):70–5.
57. Beales ILP, Post L, Srinivasan S, Calam J, Yamada T, Del Valle J. Tumour necrosis factor-alpha (TNFa) decreases somatostatin release and somatostatin content of cultured canine D-cells. Gut. 1995;37(Suppl. 1):A84.
58. Vuyyuru L, Schubert ML, Harrington L, Arimura A, Makhlouf GM. Dual inhibitory pathways link antral somatostatin and histamin secretion in human, dog, and rat stomach. Gastroenterology. 1995;109:1566–74.
59. Queiroz DM, Mendes EN, Rocha GA *et al.* Histamine concentration of gastric mucosa in *Helicobacter pylori* positive and negative children. Gut. 1991;32:464–6.
60. Courillon-Mallet A, Launay JM *et al. Helicobacter pylori* infection: physiopathologic implication of N alpha-methyl histamine. Gastroenterology. 1995;108:959–66.
61. Prinz C, Neumayer N, Classen M, Schepp W. Functional impairment of isolated rat enterochromaffin-like cells by interleukin-1 beta. Gastroenterology. 1996;110:A234.
62. Bado A, Hervatin F, Lewin MJ. Pharmacological evidence for histamine H3 receptor in the control of gastric acid secretion in cats. Am J Physiol. 1991;260:G631–5.
63. Bado A, Moizo L, Laigneau JP, Lewin MJ. Pharmacological characterization of histamine H3 receptors in isolated rabbit gastric glands. Am J Physiol. 1992;262:G56–61.
64. Prinz C, Kajimura M, Scott DR, Mercier F, Helander HF, Sachs G. Histamine secretion from rat enterochromaffin-like cells. Gastroenterology. 1993;105:449–61.
65. Preiss DU, Code CF. Effect of the H2-receptor antagonists (burimamide and metiamide) on gastric secretion stimulated by histamine and its methyl derivatives. J Pharmacol Exp Ther. 1975; 193:614–20.
66. Huang LL, Cave DR, Gilbert JV, Wright A. Cloning and sequencing of the gene encoding an acid-inhibitory protein in *Helicobacter pylori*. Gastroenterology. 1996;110:A927.
67. Beil W, Birkholz C, Wagner S, Sewing KF. Interaction of *Helicobacter pylori* and its fatty acids with parietal cells and gastric H+/K+ ATPase. Gut. 1994;35:1176–80.
68. Beales ILP, Calam J. Interleukin-1beta and tumor necrosis factor-alpha inhibit aminopyrine accumulation in cultured rabbit parietal cells by multiple pathways. Gastroenterology. 1996; 110:A62.
69. Beales ILP, Calam J. Effect of N-alpha methylhistamine on acid secretion in cultured rabbit parietal cells: implications for hypergastrinaemia and acid secretion. Gut. 1996;38(Suppl. 1):A37.
70. Kuipers EJ, Uyterlinde AM, Pena AS *et al.* Long-term sequelae of *Helicobacter pylori* gastritis. Lancet. 1995;345:1525–8.
71. Graham DY, Alpert LC, Smith JL, Yoshimura HH. Iatrogenic *Campylobacter pylori* infection is a cause of epidemic achlorhydria. Am J Gastroenterol. 1988;83:974–80.
72. Kovaks TOG, Sytnik B, Calam J, Walsh JH. *Helicobacter pylori* infection impairs pH inhibition in non-duodenal ulcer subjects. Gastroenterology. 1993;104:A123.
73. Katelaris PH, Seow F, Lin BP, Napoli J, Ngu MC, Jones DB. Effect of age, *Helicobacter pylori* infection, and gastritis with atrophy on serum gastrin and gastric acid secretion in healthy men. Gut. 1993;34:1032–7.
74. Rademaker JW, Hunt RH. *Helicobacter pylori* and gastric acid secretion: the ulcer link? Scand J Gastroenterol Suppl. 1991;187:71–7.
75. Haruma K, Kawaguchi H, Yoshihara M *et al.* Relationship between *Helicobacter pylori* infection and gastric acid secretion in young healthy subjects. J Clin Gastroenterol. 1994;19:20–2.
76. Chandrakumaran K, Vaira D, Hobsley M. Duodenal ulcer, *Helicobacter pylori*, and gastric secretion [see comments]. Gut. 1994;35:1033–6.
77. Finlayson NDC, Girdwood RH, Samson RR, Shearman DJC. Gastric secretion, gastric antibody status and pernicious anaemia in carcinoma of the stomach. Digestion. 1969;2:338–46.
78. El-Omar E, Oien H, Wirz A, McColl KEL. Divergent effects of *H. pylori* on acid secretion. Gastroenterology. 1996;110:A102.
79. Moss SF, Calam J. Acid secretion and sensitivity to gastrin in patients with duodenal ulcer: effect of eradication of *Helicobacter pylori*. Gut. 1993;34:888–92.

80. Chittajallu RS, Howie CA, McColl KE. Effect of *Helicobacter pylori* on parietal cell sensitivity to pentagastrin in duodenal ulcer subjects. Scand J Gastroenterol. 1992;27:857–62.
81. Jacobson K, Chiba N, James C, Armstrong D, Barrientos M, Hunt RH. Protracted gastric acid secretion in *H. pylori* positive DU patients following eradication. Gastroenterology. 1995;108: A122.
82. Harris AW, Gummett PA, Misiewicz JJ, Baron JH. The effect of eradication of *Helicobacter pylori* on gastric acid output in patients with duodenal ulcers. Gastroenterology. 1995;108:A109.
83. Fontham ET, Ruiz B, Perez A, Hunter F, Correa P. Determinants of *Helicobacter pylori* infection and chronic gastritis. Am J Gastroenterol. 1995;90:1094–101.
84. Correa P. Is gastric carcinoma an infectious disease? [editorial; comment]. N Engl J Med. 1991; 325:1170–1.
85. Beales ILP, Davey N, Scunes D, Pusey C, Lechler R, Calam J. HLA Class II type and *H. pylori*-induced gastric atrophy. Gut. 1994;35(Suppl. 5):S45.
86. Bechi P, Romagnoli P, Panula P *et al.* Enterochromaffin-like cells and the 'gastrin link' between *Helicobacter pylori* and duodenal ulcer. Gastroenterology. 1996;110:A62.
87. Moss SF, Calam J. Acid secretion and sensitivity to gastrin in duodenal ulcer patients: effect of eradication of *H. pylori*. Gut. 1993;34:888–92.
88. el Omar E, Penman I, Dorrian CA, Ardill JE, McColl KE. Eradicating *Helicobacter pylori* infection lowers gastrin mediated acid secretion by two thirds in patients with duodenal ulcer. Gut. 1993;34:1060–5.
89. Verhulst ML, Hopman WP, Tangerman A, Jansen JB. Eradication of *Helicobacter pylori* infection in patients with non-ulcer dyspepsia. Effects on basal and bombesin-stimulated serum gastrin and gastric acid secretion. Scand J Gastroenterol. 1995;30:968–73.
90. Hamlet A, Dalenback L, Fandriks L, Olbe L. *Helicobacter pylori* infection interferes with the regulation of gastrin release and acid secretion. Acta Gastro-Enterol Belg. 1993;56(Suppl. 111).
91. El-Omar E, Penman I, Dorrian CA, Ardill JES, McColl KEL. Eradicating *Helicobacter pylori* infection lowers gastrin-mediated acid secretion by two-thirds in duodenal ulcer patients. Gut. 1993;34:1060–5.
92. Bojko JB, Burage M, Erdag S *et al.* Novel GRP/CCK test exqluates D–G interaction and parietal cell secretion in H.P.-positive duodenal ulcer patients. Gastroenterology. 1996;110:A67.
93. Hamlet A, Olbe L. Gastric emptying, duodenal acid load and duodenal bulb acidity in *Helicobacter pylori*-infected subjects. Am J Gastroenterol. 1994;89:1325.

12
Helicobacter pylori gastritis and gastric acid secretory function – an integrated approach

K. E. L. McCOLL, D. GILLEN, E. EL-OMAR, K. OIEN and S. DAHILL

INTRODUCTION

There is evidence of a two-way relationship between gastric acid secretory function and *H. pylori*-associated gastritis. Gastric acid secretory function influences the density of *H. pylori* colonization, its distribution within the stomach and the severity of the mucosal inflammatory response to the infection. In addition, *H. pylori* gastritis alters gastric acid secretion. In subjects with a predominant antral gastritis it increases acid secretion predisposing to duodenal ulcers (DU), whereas in others, with predominant body gastritis, acid secretion is impaired and the subjects have an increased risk of gastric cancer. In this chapter we discuss the interaction between gastric acid secretory function and *H. pylori* gastritis and its importance in determining disease outcome.

CHRONIC *H. PYLORI* GASTRITIS AND DISTURBANCES OF GASTRIC ACID SECRETORY FUNCTION IN DUODENAL ULCER PATIENTS

In DU patients *H. pylori* infection is usually found densely colonizing the mucosa of both the antrum and body of the stomach. In the antrum the infection is accompanied by a marked gastritis with infiltration of the mucosa with acute and chronic inflammatory cells. In contrast, there is relatively little inflammation of the body mucosa.

In addition to the above histological changes, the infection also induces alterations in gastric physiology. *H. pylori*-positive subjects have increased basal, meal-stimulated and gastrin releasing peptide-stimulated gastrin levels[1-6]. This increase in gastrin is predominantly due to a rise in gastrin 17, which is the main form synthesized by the G cells within the antral mucosa[7]. Several studies have shown depletion of antral somatostatin concentrations, and the increased gastrin

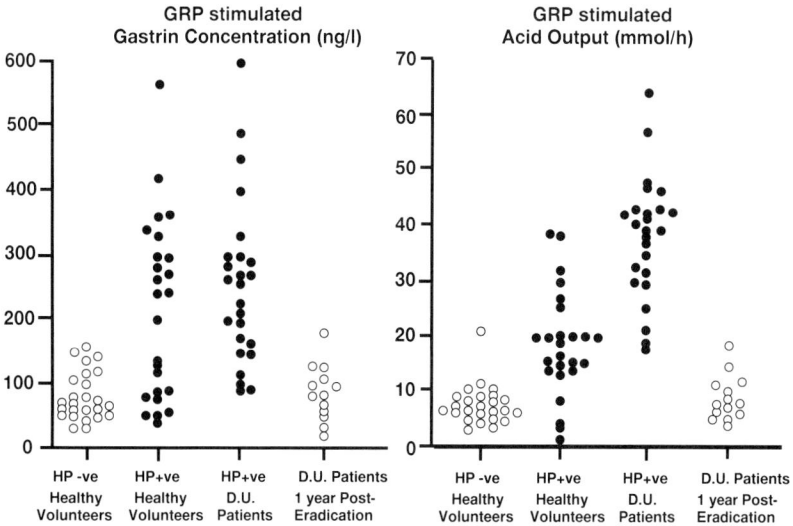

Figure 1 Gastrin and acid response to stimulation with gastrin releasing peptide in subjects of different *H. pylori* status

levels are likely to be secondary to failure of the physiological inhibition of gastrin release exerted via somatostatin[8–12]. The degree of elevation of serum gastrin associated with *H. pylori* infection is similar in DU patients and non-ulcer subjects who are infected[5,6,13]. Eradication of the infection results in early resolution of the hypergastrinaemia[14].

There has been considerable debate concerning the effect of the increased gastrin on acid secretion. However, in DU patients it is accompanied by increased basal acid secretion and increased acid secretion in response to stimulation with gastrin-releasing peptide (GRP)[5,6,15,16]. This increased acid secretory response normalizes following eradication of the infection, indicating that it is a consequence of the infection[5,6,16]. Though *H. pylori*-induced hypergastrinaemia is associated with markedly increased acid secretion in DU patients, this is not usually so in *H. pylori*-infected non-ulcer subjects (Figure 1). In most of the latter, basal acid output is normal, and GRP-stimulated acid output either normal or only slightly increased[5,6,16].

H. pylori infection thus induces a similar degree of elevation of gastrin in subjects with and without DU disease, but the associated increase in acid secretion is much more marked in the ulcer subjects (Figure 1). This increased acid response to gastrin stimulation, which is characteristic of the ulcer patients, is likely to be a key factor in determining the development of the ulceration. The increased acid response, characteristic of the DU patients, could be due to either the body of the stomach having an increased total acid secretory capacity and/or being more sensitive to stimulation by gastrin. In order to investigate this we have measured maximal acid output and sensitivity to stimulation with increasing doses of gastrin 17 in *H. pylori*-negative healthy volunteers, *H. pylori*-positive healthy volunteers and *H. pylori*-positive DU patients[17].

These studies indicate that DU patients have slightly increased maximal acid secretory capacity compared to both *H. pylori*-positive healthy volunteers and *H. pylori*-negative healthy volunteers. The degree of increase in maximal acid secretory capacity is insufficient to explain fully the increased acid secretory response to gastrin stimulation either basally or during stimulation with GRP. The studies of sensitivity to gastrin reveal more marked differences between *H. pylori*-positive ulcer subjects and *H. pylori*-positive healthy volunteers, with the former being twice as sensitive to gastrin stimulation.

What is the cause of the increased maximal acid output and sensitivity to gastrin in the DU patients?

The cause of the increased maximal acid secretory capacity in the DU patients is unclear. Gastrin exerts trophic effects on the oxyntic mucosa and thus the increased parietal cell mass could be due to a long-term trophic influence of *H. pylori*-induced hypergastrinaemia. If this were the case eradication of the infection and resolution of the hypergastrinaemia should result in a fall in the maximal acid output. Patients with Zollinger–Ellison syndrome have an increased parietal cell mass due to the trophic effects of the gastrin produced by their gastrinoma. Resolution of the hypergastrinaemia by curative resection of the gastrinoma produces resolution of their increased parietal cell mass within 6 months[18]. One study has shown a significant fall in maximal acid output following eradication of *H. pylori* in DU patients[16], but most others have not[5,2,19]. An alternative or additional explanation is that the increased parietal cell mass is a host factor predisposing to DU, and evidence supporting this is the observation that some true normal controls (i.e. *H. pylori*-negative healthy volunteers) can have maximal acid output values equivalent to those of DU patients[17].

The cause of the increased sensitivity to gastrin in the DU patients is also unclear. However, the high sensitivity to gastrin seen in the DU patients is also seen in some true normal controls, and this is again consistent with it being a host factor rather than a consequence of the *H. pylori* infection. Another observation supporting the sensitivity being a host factor is the observation that it does not change following eradication of the infection[15].

An alternative explanation for the *H. pylori*-positive DU patients having a higher maximal acid output and higher sensitivity to gastrin than the *H. pylori*-positive non-ulcer subjects is that the latter have abnormally low values, possibly due to them having *H. pylori*-induced body gastritis. However, this does not appear to be the case, as the maximal acid output and sensitivity to gastrin in the *H. pylori*-positive non-ulcer patients is similar to that of the true normal volunteers without *H. pylori* infection. However, a small subgroup of *H. pylori*-positive non-ulcer subjects do have markedly reduced acid secretion due to the infection, and they will be discussed in more detail below.

In summary, therefore, *H. pylori* infection and the accompanying antral gastritis stimulates increased gastrin release while the degree of acid hypersecretion associated with the hypergastrinaemia is variable. The acid hypersecretion is most pronounced in subjects who develop DU, and this can be explained by the combination of their increased maximal acid secretory capacity and their increased

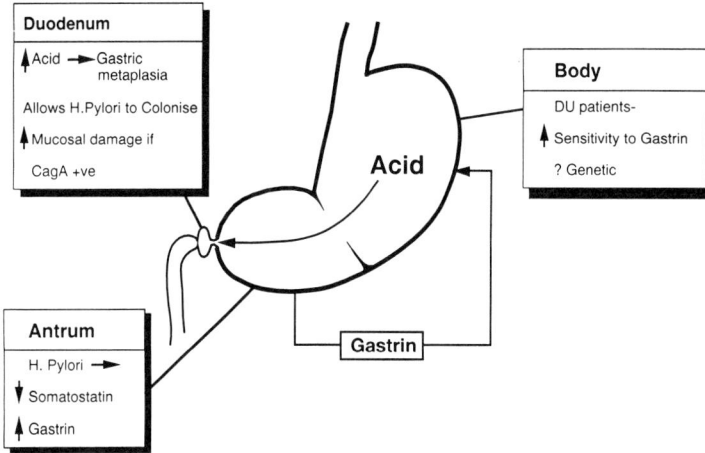

Figure 2 Sequence of events involved in the development of *H. pylori*-associated duodenal ulceration

sensitivity to gastrin. This high sensitivity to gastrin in the DU patients is probably a host characteristic, and is likely to be a key factor in determining the development of ulcer disease.

The importance of gastric acid hypersecretion in development of duodenal ulceration

This marked hypersecretion of acid induced by *H. pylori* infection in the subjects with high sensitivity to gastrin will increase their duodenal acid load and result in damage to the duodenal mucosa. Recent studies have shown a strong direct correlation between the degree of gastric acid hypersecretion induced by *H. pylori* infection and the extent of gastric metaplasia within the duodenal bulb[20,21]. The development of gastric metaplasia within the duodenum will further contribute to the development of duodenal ulcer disease by allowing *H. pylori* to colonize the duodenum and produce direct local mucosal damage. This local bacterial damage to the mucosa will be more pronounced with CagA-positive strains due to the associated cytotoxin production. Damage to the mucosa by the combination of increased acid load and local bacterial toxins will eventually result in breakdown of the mucosa and ulceration (Figure 2).

CHRONIC *H. PYLORI* INFECTION AND GASTRIC ACID HYPOSECRETION

As discussed above, the majority of subjects in the Western world with chronic *H. pylori* infection have either normal or increased gastric acid secretion. However, in a subgroup of subjects with chronic *H. pylori* infection there is a marked lowering of gastric acid secretion or complete achlorhydria[22–24]. We have recently studied 15 such subjects with a mean age of 55 years[24]. Six of them were completely achlorhydric to supramaximal doses of pentagastrin, and the others produced only minimal acid secretion. The chronic nature of the hypochlorhydria was confirmed by repeating the acid secretion measurement in 50% of the subjects after a 1-year period, and this showed no spontaneous return of acid secretion. None of the subjects had antibodies to intrinsic factor or parietal cells, thus excluding an autoimmune basis for their achlorhydria.

Histological examination of the gastric mucosa of these subjects showed distinct differences between those with *H. pylori* infection and hypochlorhydria and subjects with *H. pylori* and DU who have markedly increased acid secretion. The antral mucosa of the duodenal ulcer patients showed both more dense colonization with *H. pylori* and more marked inflammation than the acid hyposecretors. The prevalence of intestinal metaplasia and atrophy of the antral mucosa was similar in the DU patients and hypersecretors. Histological examination of the body of the stomach again showed that the colonization with *H. pylori* was slightly more dense in the DU patients than in the acid hyposecretors. However, the degree of inflammation of the body of the stomach was much more marked in the acid hyposecretors than in the DU patients. It thus appeared that, within the body of the stomach, the degree of inflammation relative to the density of *H. pylori* infection was much more marked in the acid hyposecretors. The majority of the acid hyposecretors had intestinal metaplasia and atrophy of the body mucosa, whereas these findings were rare in the DU patients.

Eradication of *H. pylori* infection in the acid hyposecretors resulted in a return of gastric acid secretion. The median gastric acid output increased from 0 to 12.6 mmol/h (normal > 15). The degree of recovery of acid secretion was variable, and was least in those with the most profound atrophy. Eradication of *H. pylori* infection resulted in a marked improvement in the degree of body gastritis, but this was not associated with any discernible resolution of the atrophy.

In this subgroup, chronic *H. pylori* infection is resulting in a marked inhibition of gastric acid secretion. The acid hyposecretion is partly due to atrophy of the oxyntic mucosa. However, it is also due to functional inhibition of acid secretion which resolves with eradication of the infection. The mechanism of this functional inhibition of acid secretion is unclear. It cannot be explained merely by the increased density of *H. pylori* infection within the body mucosa, as the density of colonization is more marked in DU patients than in the patients with acid hyposecretion. However, it may be explained by the inflammation of the body mucosa, as this is much more pronounced in the hyposecretors.

Relevance of *H. pylori*-induced hypochlorhydria to gastric cancer

The subgroup with chronic *H. pylori* infection and marked hyposecretion of acid is likely to be important in explaining the association between *H. pylori* infection and the subsequent development of gastric cancer[25-27]. It has been shown that subjects with *H. pylori* infection have a three-fold increased risk of developing gastric cancer. However, it has also been shown that patients with *H. pylori* infection and a history of DU disease have a significantly reduced risk of developing gastric cancer compared to the general population, with an odds ratio of 0.2[25]. It therefore appears that patients with *H. pylori* infection and duodenal ulcer disease have a similar risk of gastric cancer to patients without *H. pylori* infection. This therefore suggests that *H. pylori* infection, when associated with increased acid secretion, is not a risk factor for gastric cancer. It has been recognized for many years that gastric cancer tends to develop against a background of low or absent acid secretion. It therefore seems likely that it is this subgroup of subjects with *H. pylori* and hypochlorhydria who will have the increased risk of gastric cancer. In addition to this subgroup having the functional abnormality associated with gastric cancer they also have the histological changes, namely predominant body gastritis with accompanying atrophy and intestinal metaplasia.

WHAT DETERMINES THE FORM OF ACID SECRETORY RESPONSE AND PATTERN OF GASTRITIS IN CHRONIC *H. PYLORI* INFECTION?

It is clear that *H. pylori* infection has divergent effects on the gastric secretory function and the patterns of gastritis. In some subjects it results in a markedly increased acid secretion associated with a predominant antral gastritis. In other subjects it results in a profound inhibition of acid secretion associated with a severe body gastritis. The pattern of response is important as it determines the disease outcome. Our studies in DU patients suggest that their pattern of hypersecretion of acid may be a consequence of the host's pre-existing high sensitivity to the acid-stimulatory effects of gastrin. The hosts' natural high acid output may therefore predetermine their histological and functional response to the *H. pylori* infection. This has previously been postulated by Lee and Dickson *et al.*[28]. There is also indirect evidence that a host with low acid secretion will develop a predominant body gastritis in response to *H. pylori* infection and a consequent further fall in acid secretion. This evidence comes from observing the effects of proton pump inhibitor therapy in subjects with *H. pylori* infection.

When *H. pylori*-positive DU patients are treated with proton pump inhibitor therapy, they develop a histological picture which is identical to that we have observed in our chronic hyposecretors. They develop a predominant body gastritis relative to the severity of colonization of the body mucosa with *H. pylori* infection[29-31]. In addition, the subjects develop intestinal metaplasia and atrophy of the body mucosa[32-34]. The efficacy of the antisecretory effect of the proton pump inhibitor therapy is also greater in *H. pylori*-positive subjects[35,36] and this may be explained by the body gastritis inhibiting acid secretion and thus augmenting the antisecretory effect of the drug. It therefore appears likely that the hosts' acid secretory status and, in particular, their sensitivity to the acid-stimulatory effects of gastrin, may determine the pattern of gastritis and disturbance of acid secretion associated with chronic *H. pylori* infection. Those with a naturally high acid secretion and high sensitivity to gastrin will develop a predominant antral gastritis and high acid secretion, and be at risk of developing DU. In contrast, those with a natural low acid secretion and with a low sensitivity to gastrin will develop a marked body gastritis and associated hyposecretion of acid, and an increased risk of subsequent gastric cancer.

Why do subjects with low gastric acid secretion develop a severe body gastritis in response to *H. pylori* infection?

Subjects with low acid secretion due to antisecretory therapy develop a severe body gastritis in response to *H. pylori* infection. This cannot be explained simply by more marked *H. pylori* colonization of their gastric body mucosa by *H. pylori*, as the intensity of colonization of their body mucosa is less than in DU patients who show little body gastritis. The overall picture may be explained by the high acid output somehow providing protection from developing body gastritis. This protection is thus absent in subjects with low acid secretion, and such patients develop body gastritis. It may thus be more appropriate to regard the pattern of gastritis in DU patients as body-sparing rather than antral-predominant. Several mechanisms could explain the sparing of the body mucosa from gastritis in acid hypersecretors. Ammonia is toxic to epithelial cells only in its un-ionized form. At acid pH it is all ionized and therefore in subjects with normal or high acid output any ammonia produced by *H. pylori* in the acid-secreting body mucosa will be immediately ionized and thus rendered non-toxic. In contrast, in subjects with low acid secretion more of the ammonia may remain un-ionized and thus exert damage on the epithelium with a consequent inflammatory reaction. It is also possible that toxins produced by *H. pylori* may be denatured by acid and thus prevented from damaging the body mucosa in high acid secretors. In addition to having a higher pH in the region of their body mucosa, acid hyper-secretors also secrete a much larger volume of gastric juice than acid hyposecretion. The former, therefore, will tend to dilute and to flush out a variety of toxic products produced by *H. pylori*, and thus prevent them from damaging the mucosa.

TWO-WAY INTERACTION BETWEEN *H. PYLORI* GASTRITIS AND GASTRIC ACID SECRETORY FUNCTION

It thus appears that there are complex interactions between *H. pylori* gastritis and gastric acid secretory function, and that these are important in determining the clinical outcomes of the infection (Figure 3). The patients' natural acid secretory status will determine the pattern of gastritis they develop in response to the infection, and this, in turn, will lead to further alterations in acid secretory function which will then predispose to the different disease outcomes.

In subjects with a high sensitivity to gastrin, the infection will result in a marked antral gastritis with increased antral gastrin release. Due to their high sensitivity to the acid-stimulatory effects of gastrin, their highly acidic body mucosa will be protected from the development of body gastritis in spite of the presence of bacteria, and consequently will remain healthy and fully functioning. This combination of increased gastrin and a healthy body mucosa will result in a marked hypersecretion of acid. These subjects will be at risk to go on to develop duodenal ulceration due to the increased duodenal acid load.

Subjects with a low sensitivity to the acid-stimulatory effects of gastrin will also develop antral gastritis and increased antral gastrin release. However, their low sensitivity to the acid-stimulatory effects of gastrin will result in a less acidic

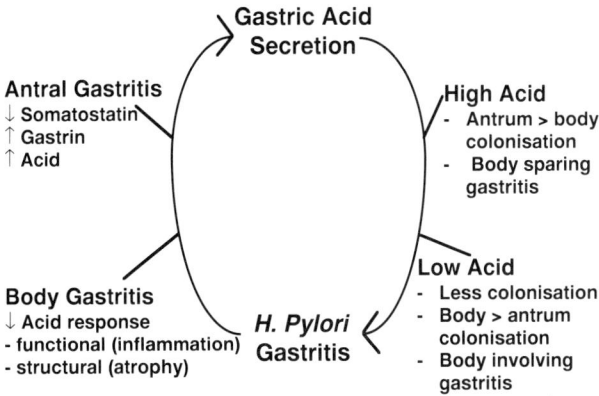

Figure 3 The two-way interaction between gastric acid secretory function and *H. pylori* gastritis

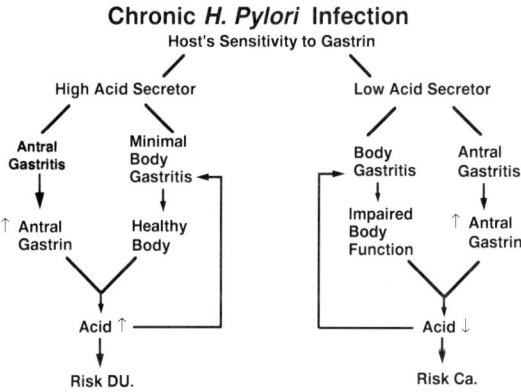

Figure 4 Sensitivity to gastrin may be a key factor in determining the clinical outcome of *H. pylori* infection

oxyntic mucosa and they will therefore not be protected from the development of body gastritis. This body gastritis will impair their gastric acid secretory function leading to acid hyposecretion. This further lowering of acid secretion will result in even more marked body gastritis and consequently more marked reduction of acid secretion. Such patients may then develop a profound reduction of acid secretion and many will be achlorhydric. These patients are likely to be at risk of developing gastric cancer.

The host's pre-existing acid secretory status and sensitivity to gastrin are thus likely to play a key role in determining the outcome of *H. pylori* infection (Figure 4). The determinants of a subject's natural acid secretory status at the time of development of *H. pylori* infection are unclear, but could include genetic factors, dietary or other environmental factors and the age of acquisition of infection.

CLINICAL IMPORTANCE OF DIVERGENT RESPONSE TO *H. PYLORI* INFECTION

There are two practical implications to the recognition of this divergent response to *H. pylori* infection. The first is the possibility of identifying the subgroup who are progressing down the hyposecretory pathway, and targeting them for *H. pylori* eradication therapy. Treatment of such patients will be particularly important as current information suggests that they are the ones at greatest risk of subsequently developing gastric cancer. Treatment of this cancer, once it presents clinically, is very unsatisfactory and prevention is the best strategy. Another important observation is that proton pump inhibitor therapy in *H. pylori*-positive patients produces the histological and functional picture of patients recognized to have an increased risk of gastric cancer, i.e. predominant body gastritis and profound inhibition of acid secretion. While many other factors are clearly important to the development of gastric cancer, it would seem advisable to ensure that patients are *H. pylori*-negative prior to the commencement of long-term proton pump inhibitory therapy.

References

1. Graham DY, Opekum A, Lew GM, Evans DJ, Klein PD, Evans DG. Ablation of exaggerated meal-stimulated gastrin release in duodenal ulcer patients after clearance of *Helicobacter (Campylobacter) pylori* infection. Am J Gastroenterol. 1990;85:394–8.
2. Levi S, Beardshall K, Desa LA, Calam J. *Campylobacter pylori*, gastrin, acid secretion and duodenal ulcers. Lancet. 2;613.
3. Smith JTL, Pounder RE, Nwokolo CU *et al*. Inappropriate hypergastrinaemia in asymptomatic healthy subjects infected with *Helicobacter pylori*. Gut. 1990;31:522–5.
4. McColl KEL, Fullarton GM, Chittajallu R *et al*. Plasma gastrin, daytime intragastric pH, and nocturnal acid output before and at 1 and 7 months after eradication of *Helicobacter pylori* in duodenal ulcer subjects. Scand J Gastroenterol. 1991;26:339–46.
5. El-Omar E, Penman ID, Ardill JES, Chittajallu RS, Howie C, McColl KEL. *Helicobacter pylori* infection and abnormalities of acid secretion in patients with duodenal ulcer disease. Gastroenterology. 1995;109:681–91.
6. El-Omar E, Penman I, Dorrian CA, Ardill JES, McColl KEL. Eradicating *Helicobacter pylori* infection lowers gastrin mediated acid secretion by two thirds in patients with duodenal ulcer. Gut. 1993;34:1060–5.
7. Mulholland G, Ardill JES, Fillmore D, Chittajallu RS, Fullarton GM, McColl KEL. *Helicobacter pylori* related hypergastrinaemia is the result of a selective increase in gastrin 17. Gut. 1993; 34:757–61.
8. Kaneko H, Nakada K, Mitsuma T *et al*. *Helicobacter pylori* infection induces a decrease in immunoreactive-somatostatin concentrations of human stomach. Dig Dis Sci. 1992;37:409–16.
9. Moss SF, Legon S, Bishop AE, Polak JM, Calam J. Effect of *Helicobacter pylori* on gastric somatostatin in duodenal ulcer disease. Lancet. 1992;340:930–2.
10. Queiroz DMM, Mendes EN, Rocha GA *et al*. Effect of *Helicobacter pylori* eradication on antral gastrin- and somatostatin-immunoreactive cell density and gastrin and somatostatin concentrations. Scand J Gastroenterol. 1993;28:858–64.
11. Graham DY, Lew GM, Lechago J. Antral G-cell and D-cell numbers in *Helicobacter pylori* infection: effect of *H. pylori* eradication. Gastroenterology. 1993;104:1655–60.
12. Sumii M, Summi K, Tari A *et al*. Expression of antral gastrin and somatostatin mRNA in *Helicobacter pylori*-infected subjects. Am J Gastroenterol. 1994;89:1515–19.
13. Chittajallu RS, Ardill JES, McColl KEL. The degree of hypergastrinaemia induced by *Helicobacter pylori* is the same in duodenal ulcer patients and asymptomatic volunteers. Eur J Gastroenterol Hepatol. 1992;4:49–53.
14. Graham DY, Go MF, Lew GM, Genta RM, Rehfeld JF. *Helicobacter pylori* infection and

exaggerated gastrin release. Effects of inflammation and progastrin processing. Scand J Gastroenterol. 1993;28:690–4.

15. Moss SF, Calam J. Acid secretion and sensitivity to gastrin in patients with duodenal ulcer: effect of eradication of *Helicobacter pylori*. Gut. 1993;34:888–92.

16. Harris AW, Gummett PA, Misiewicz JJ, Baron JH. Eradication of *Helicobacter pylori* in patients with duodenal ulcer lowers basal and peak acid outputs to gastrin releasing peptide and pentagastrin. Gut. 1996;38:663–8.

17. Gillen D, El-Omar E, McColl KEL. Parietal cell sensitivity to gastrin distinguishes *H. pylori* D.U. patients from *H. pylori* infected healthy volunteers. Gastroenterology. 1996;110:A116.

18. Pisegna JR, Norton JA, Slimak GG *et al*. Effect of curative gastrinoma resection on gastric secretory function and antisecretory drug requirement in the Zollinger–Ellison syndrome. Gastroenterology. 1992;102:767–78.

19. Montbriand JR, Appelman HD, Cotner EK, Nostrant TT, Elta GH. Treatment of *Campylobacter pylori* does not alter gastric acid secretion. Am J Gastroenterol. 1989;84:1513–16.

20. Harris AW, Gummett PA, Walker MM, Misiewicz JJ, Baron JH. The relationship between gastric acid output, *Helicobacter pylori* and gastric metaplasia in the duodenal bulb. Gut. 1996 (in press).

21. Khulusi S, Badve S, Patel P *et al*. Pathogenesis of gastric metaplasia of the human duodenum: role of *Helicobacter pylori*, gastric acid, and ulceration. Gastroenterology. 1996;110:452–8.

22. Tucci A, Poli L, Paparo GF *et al*. Effect of *Helicobacter pylori* (*HP*) eradication in patients with fundic atrophic gastritis. Gut. 1994;35(Suppl. 4):1514.

23. Yasunaga Y, Shinomura Y, Kanayam S *et al*. Improved fold width and increased acid secretion after eradication of the organism in *Helicobacter pylori* associated enlarged fold gastritis. Gut. 1994;35:1571–4.

24. El-Omar E, Oien K, Wirz A, Mccoll KEL. Divergent effects of *H. pylori* on acid secretion. Gastroenterology. 1996;110:A102.

25. Parsonnet J, Friedman GD, Vandersteen DP *et al*. *Helicobacter pylori* infection and the risk of gastric carcinoma. N Engl J Med. 1991;325:1127–31.

26. Forman D, Newell DG, Fullerton F *et al*. Association between infection with *Helicobacter pylori* and risk of gastric cancer: evidence from a prospective investigation. Br Med J. 1991;302:1302–5.

27. Nomura A, Stemmermann GN, Po-Huang C, Kato I, Perez-Perez GI, Blaser MJ. *Helicobacter pylori* infection and gastric carcinoma among Japanese Americans in Hawaii. N Engl J Med. 1991;325:1132–6.

28. Lee A, Dixon MF, Danon SJ *et al*. Local acid production and *Helicobacter pylori* – a unifying hypothesis of gastroduodenal disease. Eur J Gastroenterol Hepatol. 1995;7:461–5.

29. Logan RPH, Walker MM, Misiewicz JJ, Gummett PA, Karim QN, Baron JH. Changes in the intragastric distribution of *Helicobacter pylori* during treatment with omeprazole. Gut. 1995;36:12–16.

30. Kuipers EJ, Uyterlinde AM, Pena AS *et al*. Increase of *Helicobacter pylori*-associated corpus gastritis during acid suppressive therapy: implications for longterm safety. Am J Gastroenterol. 1995;90:1401–6.

31. Solcia E, Villani L, Fiocca R *et al*. Effects of eradication of *Helicobacter pylori* on gastritis in duodenal ulcer patients. Scand J Gastroenterol. 1994;29(Suppl. 201):28–34.

32. Solcia E, Fiocca R, Havu N, Dalvag A, Carlsson R. Gastric endocrine cells and gastritis in patients receiving long-term omeprazole treatment. Digestion. 1992;5(Suppl. 1):82–92.

33. Kuipers EJ, Uyterlinde AM, Pena AS *et al*. Increase of *Helicobacter pylori*-associated corpus gastritis during acid suppressive therapy: implications for longterm safety. Am J Gastroenterol. 1995;90:1401–6.

34. Kuipers EJ, Lee A, Klinkenberg-Knol EC, Meuwissen SGM. Review article: The development of atrophic gastritis – *Helicobacter pylori* and the effects of acid suppressive therapy. Aliment Pharmacol Ther. 1995;9:331–40.

35. Verdu EF, Armstrong D, Fraser R *et al*. Effect of *Helicobacter pylori* status on intragastric pH during treatment with omeprazole. Gut. 1995;36:539–43.

36. Verdu EF, Armstrong D, Idstrom J-P *et al*. Effect of curing *Helicobacter pylori* infection on intragastric pH during treatment with omeprazole. Gut. 1995;37:743–8.

13
Nitric oxide, bacteria and ulcer healing

S. N. ELLIOTT and J. L. WALLACE

INTRODUCTION

While there is a firmly established link between gastric colonization by *Helicobacter pylori* and recurrent peptic ulcer disease, the mechanisms through which this bacterium alters mucosal defence, leading to injury, are not fully understood. Likewise, pathogenesis of the ulceration associated with the use of non-steroidal anti-inflammatory drugs (NSAIDs), while apparently linked to the ability of these drugs to suppress mucosal prostaglandin synthesis, has not been completely elucidated. The fact that eradication of *H. pylori* leads to accelerated healing of ulcers suggests that the bacterium is capable of interfering with the ulcer healing process. This may be related to elevated acid secretion in patients infected with *H. pylori*. On the other hand, NSAIDs can delay the healing of ulcers and can increase the risk of bleeding from pre-existing ulcers[1]. This effect of NSAIDs presents a dilemma in terms of the treatment of arthritis in a patient who develops an ulcer. The delaying effect of the NSAID on ulcer healing, and the possibility that this could lead to life-threatening haemorrhage, usually requires the patient to cease taking the NSAID. On the other hand, the patient may have few therapeutic options in terms of management of the pain and inflammation associated with the arthritis.

A number of strategies have been employed to develop anti-inflammatory and analgesic drugs that do not cause gastrointestinal damage. One such strategy is the linking of a nitric oxide-releasing moiety to standard NSAIDs[2,3]. The rationale behind this strategy is that the nitric oxide released from the compounds will exert beneficial effects on the mucosa by maintaining gastrointestinal blood flow and inhibiting neutrophil adherence and activation within the gastrointestinal microcirculation[2,3]. Reduced blood flow and neutrophil adherence/activation have been implicated in the pathogenesis of NSAID gastropathy[4]. As the NO-NSAIDs suppress prostaglandin synthesis in the gastrointestinal tract as effectively as the parent NSAIDs[2,3,5], and since the delaying effect of NSAIDs on ulcer healing is thought to be attributable to suppression of prostaglandin synthesis[6,7], it is conceivable that these 'NO-NSAIDs' may impair ulcer healing. On the other hand, nitric oxide may exert beneficial effects in terms of ulcer healing. Konturek *et al.*[8] recently reported that a nitric oxide donor, glyceryl trinitrate, significantly accelerated the healing of experimental gastric ulcers in the rat, while inhibitors of endogenous nitric oxide synthesis retarded ulcer healing. Interestingly, a nitric oxide donor (glyceryl trinitrate) has recently been reported to be effective, when applied topically, at accelerating the healing of anal fissures and ulcers[9].

EXPERIMENTAL GASTRIC ULCER

There are numerous models of gastric ulcer that can be used in experimental animals, such as the rat. In terms of studies of factors affecting rates of ulcer healing, probably the best model is that developed by Okabe and Pfeiffer[10]. This model involves the brief application of acetic acid to the serosal wall of the stomach. While this model clearly has little if any relevance in terms of the pathogenesis of *H. pylori*- or NSAID-associated gastric ulceration, its main value is in the fact that it reproducibly elicits ulceration of a fixed size. Moreover, the ulcers bear marked histological similarity to gastric ulcers in humans. Once induced, experimental treatments can be administered to the animals to evaluate their effects on ulcer healing rates. We have utilized the 'Okabe' ulcer model in these studies[11].

NITRIC OXIDE AND ULCER HEALING

In preliminary studies we observed considerable variability in the size of ulcers over the first 7 days after serosal application of acetic acid to the rat stomach. However, by day 7 the ulcer size was consistent. For this reason, studies of the effects of various drugs on ulcer healing were started on the 7th day after induction of ulcers. The rats were given one of the following drugs orally, once a day for 7 days: diclofenac (5 mg/kg), nitrofenac (7.5 mg/kg, equimolar to the dose of diclofenac), or vehicle. These doses of the test drugs have previously been shown to exhibit anti-inflammatory effects in the rat[3]. At the end of the treatment period the rats were sacrificed and the stomach was removed and pinned out on a wax block. The ulcer area was then determined by planimetry, by an observer who was 'blind' as to the treatment the rats had received. Haematocrit was determined at the beginning and end of the study period.

In order to determine if a standard nitric oxide-generating compound would alter the healing of gastric ulcers, we tested the effects of daily oral administration of glyceryl trinitrate from day 7 to day 14 post-induction of ulcers. Glyceryl trinitrate was tested at doses of 0.1, 1 and 10 mg/rat. In other rats glyceryl trinitrate was administered intraperitoneally at doses of 1, 10 and 50 mg/rat. Ulcer area and haematocrit were measured as above.

Since any suppression of acid secretion can accelerate ulcer healing in this animal model[12,13], as it can in humans, we evaluated the effects of the test drugs on acid secretion in rats with gastric ulcers, in comparison to rats without ulcers[11].

Serosal application of acetic acid resulted in the formation of spherical ulcers which persisted for several weeks. Histologically, the ulcers observed 7–14 days after acetic acid administration were characterized by a thick layer of granulation

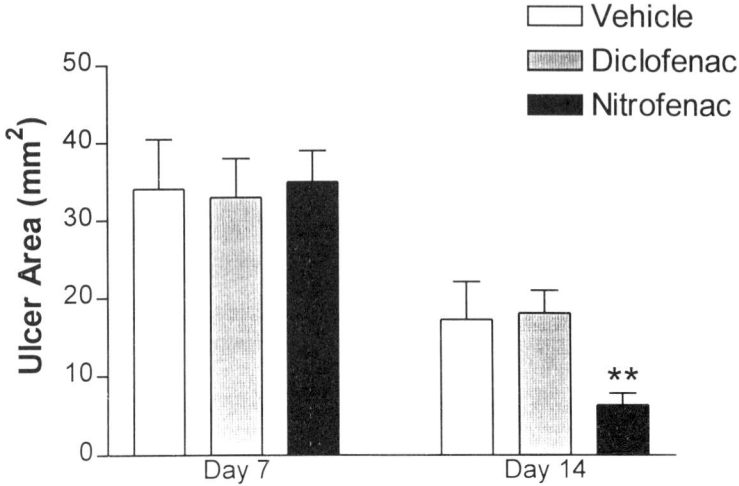

Figure 1 Area (in mm^2) of gastric ulcers induced by serosal acetic acid before and after 7 days oral treatment with vehicle, diclofenac (5 mg/kg) or an equimolar dose of nitrofenac (7.5 mg/kg). Each group consisted of 10 (nitrofenac and diclofenac) or 20 (vehicle) rats. **$p < 0.01$ compared to vehicle-treated group

tissue, with evidence of glandular disorganization at the ulcer margins. Interestingly, there appeared to be a considerable number of bacteria present within the ulcer bed, but not on adjacent healthy tissue. The ulcers involved the full thickness of the mucosa, and penetrated through the muscularis mucosae and sometimes to the muscularis propria. The average area of ulceration at day 7 after application of acetic acid was 34.1 ± 6.4 mm^2 ($n = 10$). Spontaneous healing was observed over the following 7 days, with the mean ulcer area on day 14 being 22.5 ± 2.5 mm^2 ($n = 40$).

Daily administration of diclofenac from days 7 to 14 after ulcer induction did not significantly alter ulcer area (Figure 1), although it did markedly suppress body weight gain, and caused a decrease in haematocrit from 42.5% to 28.6% ($p < 0.001$). In contrast, daily treatment with nitrofenac resulted in a significant acceleration of ulcer healing ($p < 0.05$; Figure 1), and had no effect on haematocrit. A similar acceleration of ulcer healing was observed when rats were treated orally with the nitric oxide donor glyceryl trinitrate (Figure 2). However, when this drug was administered intraperitoneally it had no effect on ulcer healing. This suggests that the nitric oxide released from this drug acts topically to accelerate ulcer healing, perhaps by elevating mucosal blood flow or by promoting angiogenesis.

The acceleration of ulcer healing observed with nitrofenac and glyceryl trinitrate was not attributable to effects of these drugs on acid secretion. Indeed, rats with gastric ulcers secreted acid in quantities that exceeded those in rats without ulcers (Figure 3), if one considers that a considerable portion of the acid-secreting mucosa was damaged (therefore non-functional) in the former group.

It is now well established that nitric oxide is an important mediator of gastric mucosal defence, promoting both mucosal blood flow[14] and mucus secretion[15]. It

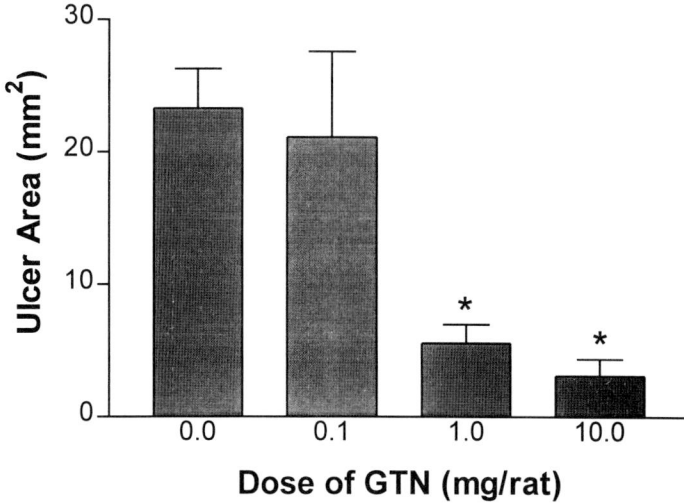

Figure 2 Dose-dependent acceleration of ulcer healing by orally administered glyceryl trinitrate (GTN). *$p < 0.05$ compared to the vehicle-treated group. Each group consisted of at least five rats

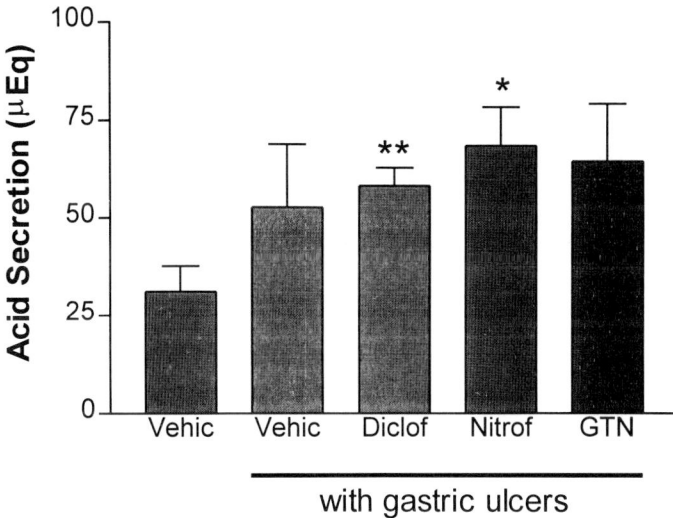

Figure 3 Effects of the presence of a gastric ulcer and of treatment with diclofenac, nitrofenac or glyceryl trinitrate, on gastric acid secretion in rats. *$p < 0.05$; **$p < 0.01$ compared to the vehicle-treated group without pre-existing ulcers. Diclofenac was administered at a dose of 5 mg/kg, nitrofenac at an equimolar dose (7.5 mg/kg) and glyceryl trinitrate at a dose of 10 mg/kg. Each group consisted of at least five rats

is therefore possible that nitric oxide accelerates ulcer healing by elevating the resistance of the mucosa at the ulcer margin to further damage. It has been demonstrated previously that agents which reduce blood flow at the ulcer margin, such as nicotine, delay healing[16]. Another possibility is that nitric oxide modulates the production of growth factors that are implicated in ulcer healing. Growth factors such as epidermal growth factor and fibroblast growth factor have been shown to modulate ulcer healing[17,18], and the receptors for some growth factors (e.g. epidermal growth factor) are expressed in much greater numbers at sites of ulceration[19].

BACTERIA AND ULCER HEALING

As mentioned above, histological examination of acetic acid-induced gastric ulcers revealed the presence of considerable numbers of bacteria within the ulcer bed. Subsequent studies involving culturing of gastric tissue confirmed this observation. At day 7 after ulcer induction, up to 10^9 colony-forming units per gram of tissue were found at the ulcer site, compared to $\sim 10^4$ c.f.u./g in healthy control rats or at adjacent sites of normal tissue in the rats with ulcers. The most common bacterium in these cultures was *E. coli*, with smaller quantities of *Enterococcus* spp. and *Lactobacillus* spp. By day 14, bacterial numbers had decreased to levels not significantly different from those seen in healthy rats. This decrease in bacterial numbers paralleled the spontaneous healing observed in this model.

Given the association between *H. pylori* infection and recurrence of peptic ulcers, it seemed possible that the bacteria colonizing gastric ulcers in the rat model might interfere with the healing process. To test this hypothesis, rats with gastric ulcers were treated with a combination of streptomycin (140 mg/kg) and penicillin (70 mg/kg) twice daily for 7 days. This treatment resulted in a significant reduction in the numbers of bacteria colonizing the ulcers. Moreover, ulcer healing was significantly accelerated, with the mean ulcer size at the end of a 7-day course of the antibiotics being 3.5 ± 0.6 mm^2, versus 23.0 ± 3.0 mm^2 in rats treated with the vehicle ($p < 0.005$).

Nitric oxide is released by macrophages when appropriately stimulated, and is a major contributor to the bactericidal arsenal of these cells. Therefore, it seemed possible that the ulcer-healing properties of nitrofenac and glyceryl trinitrate might be related to bactericidal effects of the nitric oxide released from these drugs. However, when bacterial cultures were prepared from rats treated with these nitric oxide donors, no significant effect was observed, despite the fact that the drugs accelerated ulcer healing. Moreover, addition of nitrofenac to the cultures of bacteria harvested from the ulcer beds did not interfere with the growth of the bacteria. It therefore seems highly unlikely that the beneficial effects of nitrofenac and glyceryl trinitrate on ulcer healing were attributable to effects on the bacteria that colonize the ulcer site.

SUMMARY AND CONCLUSIONS

While NSAIDs have well-characterized retarding effects on ulcer healing, nitric oxide-releasing NSAID derivatives are capable of significantly accelerating the healing of experimental ulcers in rats. As a structurally unrelated nitric oxide donor, glyceryl trinitrate, also caused a dose-dependent acceleration of ulcer healing, it would appear that nitric oxide is responsible for the observed effects. The recently reported ability of a nitric oxide donor to accelerate the healing of anal ulcers and fissures[9] is consistent with the notion that nitric oxide accelerates tissue repair. It is important to note that, in order for glyceryl trinitrate to accelerate gastric ulcer healing in our rat model, it was necessary for this drug to be given orally, suggesting that the nitric oxide acted topically.

Induction of gastric ulcers in rats resulted in a rapid colonization of the stomach, with the vast majority of the bacteria localized within the ulcer bed. The observation that eradication of these bacteria with antibiotics resulted in a highly significant acceleration of ulcer healing strongly suggests that the bacteria delay ulcer healing. In this regard our observations are similar to what has been observed in humans infected with *H. pylori*. Whether or not there are similarities between the bacteria that colonize ulcers in rats, and the *H. pylori* that colonize the stomach in humans, in terms of their mechanism of action in retarding ulcer healing, remains to be determined. However, the rat model may prove useful for studies of these mechanisms. This model may also prove useful for studies of the mechanisms underlying alterations in gastric acid secretion in individuals infected with *H. pylori*.

Acknowledgements

This work was supported by a grant from the Medical Research Council of Canada (MRC). Dr Wallace is an MRC Senior Scientist and an Alberta Heritage Foundation for Medical Research (AHFMR) Scientist. Ms Elliott is supported by an AHFMR Studentship.

References

1. Armstrong HP, Blower AL. Non-steroidal anti-inflammatory drugs and life-threatening complications of peptic ulceration. Gut. 1987;28:527–32.
2. Wallace JL, Reuter B, Cicala C, McKnight W, Grisham MB, Cirino G. Novel nonsteroidal anti-inflammatory drug derivatives with markedly reduced ulcerogenic properties in the rat. Gastroenterology. 1994;107:173–9.
3. Wallace JL, Reuter B, Cicala C, McKnight W, Grisham M, Cirino G. A diclofenac derivative without ulcerogenic properties. Eur J Pharmacol. 1994;257:249–55.
4. Wallace JL, Cirino G. The development of gastrointestinal-sparing nonsteroidal anti-inflammatory drugs. Trends Pharmacol Sci. 1994;15:405–6.
5. Mitchell JA, Cirino G, Akarasereenont P, Wallace JL, Flower RJ, Vane JR. Flurbinitroxybutylester: a novel anti-inflammatory drug devoid of ulcerogenic activity, inhibits cyclo-oxygenase-1 and cyclo-oxygenase-2. Can J Physiol Pharmacol. 1994;72:270.
6. Penney AG, Andrews FJ, O'Brien PE. Effects of misoprostol on delayed ulcer healing induced by aspirin. Dig Dis Sci. 1994;39:934–9.
7. Stadler P, Armstrong D, Margalith D et al. Diclofenac delays healing of gastroduodenal mucosal lesions. Double-blind, placebo-controlled endoscopic study in healthy volunteers. Dig Dis Sci. 1991;36:594–600.
8. Konturek SJ, Brzozowski T, Majka J, Pytko-Polonczyk J, Stachura J. Inhibition of nitric oxide synthase delays healing of chronic gastric ulcers. Eur J Pharmacol. 1993;239:215–17.
9. Gorfine SR. Topical nitroglycerine therapy for anal fissures and ulcers. N Engl J Med. 1995;333:1156–7.
10. Okabe S, Pfeiffer CJ. Chronicity of acetic acid ulcer in the rat stomach. Am J Dig Dis. 1972;17:619–29.
11. Elliott SN, McKnight W, Cirino G, Wallace JL. A nitric oxide-releasing nonsteroidal anti-inflammatory drug accelerates gastric ulcer healing in rats. Gastroenterology. 1995;109:524–30.

12. Wang JY, Yamasaki S, Takeuchi K, Okabe S. Delayed healing of acetic acid-induced gastric ulcers in rats by indomethacin. Gastroenterology. 1989;96:393–402.
13. Schmassmann A, Tarnawski A, Peskar BM, Varga L, Flogerzi B, Halter F. Influence of acid and angiogenesis on kinetics of gastric ulcer healing in rats: interaction with indomethacin. Am J Physiol. 1995;268 (In press).
14. Pique JM, Whittle BJR, Esplugues JV. The vasodilator role of endogenous nitric oxide in the rat gastric microcirculation. Eur J Pharmacol. 1989;174:293–6.
15. Brown JF, Keates AC, Hanson PJ, Whittle BJR. Nitric oxide generators and cGMP stimulate mucus secretion by rat gastric mucosal cells. Am J Physiol. 1993;265:G418–22.
16. Iwata F, Leung FW. Tobacco smoke aggravates gastric ulcer in rats by attenuation of ulcer margin hyperemia. Am J Physiol. 1995;268:G153–60.
17. Konturek SJ, Dembinski A, Warzecha Z, Brzozoski T, Gregory H. Role of epidermal growth factor in healing of chronic gastroduoenal ulcers in rats. Gastroenterology. 1988;94:1300–7.
18. Szabo S, Folkman J, Vattay P, Morales RE, Pinkus GS, Kato K. Accelerated healing of duodenal ulcers by oral administration of a mutein of basic fibroblast growth factor in rats. Gastroenterology. 1994;106:1106–11.
19. Tarnawski A, Stachura J, Durbin T, Sarfeh IJ, Gergely H. Increased expression of epidermal growth factor receptor during gastric ulcer healing in rats. Gastroenterology. 1992;102:695–8.

14
Effects of infection with *Helicobacter pylori* on gastric epithelium

S. E. CROWE, X. FAN, S. BEHAR and G. YE

INTRODUCTION

There is growing evidence to support a key role for the gastric epithelium in the pathogenesis of *Helicobacter pylori*-associated gastroduodenal disorders. *H. pylori* is largely regarded as a non-invasive pathogen, yet is capable of inducing a significant inflammatory response. The concept that the epithelium could play an active role in *H. pylori*-associated inflammation has been substantiated over the past few years by work from several laboratories (reviewed by others in refs 1 and 2). In these studies gastric epithelial production of interleukin-8 (IL-8), a cytokine with potent neutrophil chemotactic and activating properties[3,4], was significantly increased during *H. pylori* infection[5–9]. More recent data suggest that other chemokines including members of the C-C family that stimulate lymphocytes and monocytes/macrophages, are also expressed by gastric epithelial cells in response to *H. pylori* infection. Gastric epithelial cells are also capable of interacting with immune and inflammatory cells through adhesion or immune accessory molecules including Class II MHC, invariant chain (Ii), intracellular adhesion molecule (ICAM)-1, lymphocyte function antigen (LFA)-3, and B7. Expression of such molecules is increased by *H. pylori* infection with both direct and indirect events involved in the enhanced expression. Together, this information provides a basis to establish potential mechanisms whereby the epithelium can signal immune cells to establish the gastritis associated with *H. pylori* infection. In turn, immune or inflammatory cells may mediate alterations of the gastric epithelium that occur during *H. pylori* infection.

The gastric epithelium is a target of the inflammatory response elicited in *H. pylori* infection, with the most notable changes ranging from an absence of epithelium (erosions or ulceration), to metaplasia of the gastric epithelium (intestinal metaplasia) and neoplasia (gastric adenocarcinoma). While such distinct changes are not evident in most infected individuals, alterations of gastric epithelial structure and function are being increasingly recognized. Parietal cell acid secretion and the factors regulating this function are affected by *H. pylori* infection, although the mechanisms of these changes remain uncertain. Other gastric epithelial

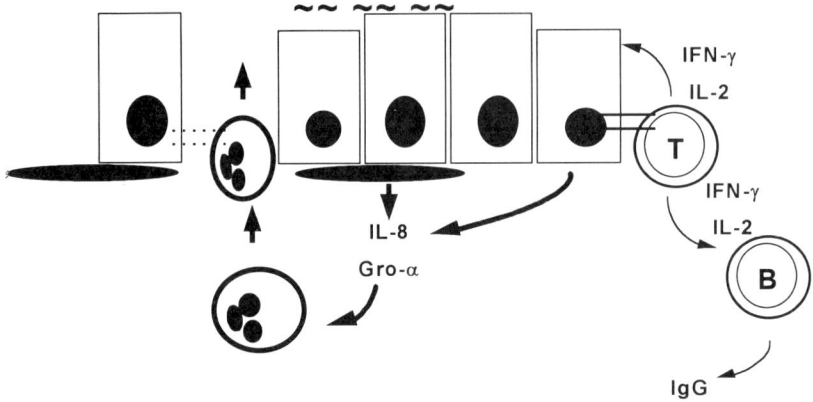

Figure 1 Immune–epithelial cell interactions during infection with *H. pylori*. Subsequent to infection with *H. pylori*, several inflammatory processes are concomitantly initiated. The earliest change is probably the stimulation of epithelial cells to produce chemokines including IL-8 and Gro-α. These chemokines will lead to the recruitment and activation of neutrophils that can bind to the epithelial cells via adhesion molecules and then migrate across the epithelium and into the lumen. The release of inflammatory mediators, including reactive oxidative metabolites, will alter epithelial cell structure and function. In addition to these changes, T cells can be activated. Gastric epithelial cells appear to express the necessary MHC and accessory molecules for T cell activation. Through the production of cytokines such as IFNγ and IL-2, T cells can modulate gene expression in adjacent epithelial cells and fibroblasts, including the induction of additional amounts of IL-8 as well as an increase in the expression of MHC and accessory molecules. T cell cytokines can also modulate immune and inflammatory cells in the lamina propria which, in turn, can impact on epithelial cell proliferation and apoptosis, as well as physiological functions

functional properties including mucus secretion and barrier function are also altered by *H. pylori* infection. Examination of how *H. pylori* affects epithelial proliferation, differentiation, cell death, and injury and repair mechanisms, has yielded information relevant to our understanding of the development of peptic ulcer disease and gastric cancer. This chapter will review studies employing human gastric tissues, as well as those involving gastric epithelial cell lines, to summarize current knowledge concerning the effects of *H. pylori* on the gastric epithelium.

GASTRIC EPITHELIAL CYTOKINE EXPRESSION

H. pylori infection is associated with increased mucosal levels of certain cytokines including IL-1, IL-6, IL-8, and tumour necrosis factor alpha (TNFα). Of these, the neutrophil-activating and chemoattractant chemokine, IL-8, has been shown to be produced by epithelial cells as well as other cells within the gastric mucosa. Using immunohistochemistry Crabtree and colleagues have shown increased epithelial staining for IL-8 in gastric biopsies from *H. pylori*-infected patients compared to uninfected subjects[5,10]. *In-vitro* studies from a number of laboratories, including our own, that employed gastric epithelial cell lines have demonstrated enhanced IL-8 mRNA and protein expression after *H. pylori* infection[11–14]. This expression is dependent on the adherence of live organisms[12,13] and is increased by strains with the cagA-positive phenotype[11,13], although cagA⁻ mutants are still able to induce IL-8[13,15]. More recently expression of other members of the chemokine family of cytokines has been shown to be increased by *H. pylori*. mRNA for Gro-α, another C-X-C chemokine which also activates and recruits neutrophils[16], was increased in biopsies from patients with *H. pylori* infection compared to uninfected samples[17]. While non-epithelial cell sources for mRNA could account for this finding, we and others have found increased levels of immunoreactive Gro-α after *H. pylori* infection of gastric epithelial cell lines[18]. Preliminary reports suggest that MCP-1, RANTES, and other members of the C-C family of chemokines may also be enhanced during *H. pylori* infection[17,19]. Since C-C chemokines exert their actions on cells other than neutrophils, these findings substantiate a role for the epithelium in initiating the inflammatory response with lymphocytes, monocytes, and eosinophils, as well as the better-established epithelial relationship with neutrophils.

Much less is known about the expression of other cytokines in gastric epithelial cells. One preliminary report describes up-regulation of IL-1α/β and GM-CSF mRNA in cultured gastric epithelial cells after *H. pylori* infection[19]. It is not clear that IL-1 protein is expressed by gastric epithelial cells since intestinal epithelial cells that express similar cytokine profiles to their gastric counterparts do not secrete significant amounts of IL-1[20]. In contrast, GM-CSF protein is produced by intestinal epithelial cells and along with IL-8, MCP-1, GM-CSF expression is increased by bacterial infection of enterocytes[21]. Thus, it is likely that further studies will confirm enhanced gastric epithelial expression of GM-CSF in *H. pylori* infection.

IMMUNE ACCESSORY MOLECULES EXPRESSED BY GASTRIC EPITHELIUM

Gut epithelial cells express a number of molecules that are involved in interactions with neutrophils and lymphocytes. The basic understanding of immune adhesion or accessory molecules has come primarily from studies in immune and endothelial cells, but findings in gastrointestinal epithelial cells are comparable. There is some suggestion that gastric epithelial cells bear a greater resemblance to classical antigen-presenting cells than to intestinal epithelial cells which, until recently, have been studied more than gastric epithelial cells.

Class II major histocompatibility complex (MHC) molecules are involved in the presentation of exogenous antigen to CD4+ T lymphocytes. Many cell types express Class II MHC, including B cells, endothelial cells, and a variety of epithelia. Like intestinal epithelial cells[22], gastric epithelial cells have been shown to express Class II MHC in native tissues as well as in cultured cells[23-27]. Gastrointestinal inflammatory conditions are associated with enhanced epithelial expression of Class II MHC. Engstrand and colleagues reported increased epithelial Class II MHC in gastric biopsies from patients with gastritis[23]. It is not clear that infection directly stimulates Class II MHC expression. Work from our laboratory indicates that *H. pylori* alone does not consistently increase Class II MHC (unpublished observations). However, Class II MHC expression is increased by interferon gamma (IFNγ) and TNFα[27], cytokines known to be increased during *H. pylori* infection[6,28-30]. We have also shown that invariant chain (Ii), a molecule which regulates Class II MHC function, is expressed by gastric epithelial cells and that this expression is increased in cell lines as well as native tissues during *H. pylori* infection (Victor Reyes *et al.*, unpublished observation).

ICAM-1 (CD54) the counter-receptor for the β-integrin molecules found on neutrophils and T lymphocytes, mediates immune adhesion to the various cell types expressing this molecule, including respiratory tract epithelial cells[31]. ICAM-1 has also been demonstrated in gastrointestinal epithelial cell lines, but it is not clear that this molecule is expressed in native gut epithelium. Immuno-histochemical staining for ICAM-1 was reported in epithelial cells in intestinal biopsies from patients with graft-versus-host disease[32], but the majority of studies, including one involving gastric tissues, do not describe ICAM-1 expression by the epithelium[26,33]. In contrast, cultured cells derived from human gastrointestinal carcinomas express ICAM-1, expression that is up-regulated by cytokines and other factors[12,34,35]. The discrepancy between native and cultured gut epithelial cells may reflect the neoplastic origin of the cell lines, or alternatively, the limitation of current methods to detect the native gastrointestinal epithelial form(s) of ICAM-1. The latter hypothesis is supported by a study in which only a pro-portion of a panel of antibodies detected Class II MHC in the intestinal epithelium, while Class II MHC was consistently detected in classical antigen-presenting cells using the same reagents[36]. We have shown that cytokines that are increased during *H. pylori* infection, such as IFNγ and TNFα, enhanced ICAM-1 expression in gastric epithelial Kato III cells, while *H. pylori* infection had no effect[12]. In another study employing AGS cells, *H. pylori* alone did increase ICAM-1 expression[35]. Since gastric epithelial cells recruit and activate immune cells through the secretion of IL-8, gastric epithelial ICAM-1 expression may be an additional mechanism by which the inflammatory response is focused in the gastric mucosa during *H. pylori* infection. A similar role for intestinal epithelial ICAM-1 expression has been proposed as a pathogenic mechanism in intestinal inflammation[37,38] although clearly there are limitations in extrapolating from *in-vitro* data.

LFA-3 (CD58), the counter-receptor for CD2 (LFA-2) on T cells, is an accessory molecule known to be involved in antigen presentation to T cells[31]. This function has been demonstrated for epithelial cells in the intestine as well as classical antigen-presenting cells[39]. LFA-3 is presumed to have a similar role in the stomach, although this has not been confirmed. Using fluorescent antibodies to LFA-3 we have shown increased staining in freshly isolated gastric epithelial cells from biopsies obtained from *H. pylori*-infected patients compared to levels in uninfected control samples. When this was examined in gastric epithelial cell lines, *H. pylori* infection alone had no effect on basal LFA-3 while a combination of IFNγ and TNFα stimulated its expression (H. Haberle, manuscript in preparation).

B7-related co-stimulatory molecules (including B7.1, CD80 and B7.2, CD86) are required in conventional Class II MHC-mediated T cell responses[40,41]. Unlike the other accessory molecules discussed above, B7 expression has not been well substantiated in intestinal epithelial cells. In contrast, we have demonstrated B7 in isolated human gastric epithelial cells as well as gastric epithelial cell lines (G. Ye *et al.*, manuscript in preparation). These studies showed that B7 expression is increased in isolated gastric epithelial cells from patients with *H. pylori* infection compared to uninfected controls. Studies with cell lines indicate that B7 mRNA and protein are increased by crosslinking Class II MHC, although cytokines themselves had no effect.

Together, these studies indicate that immune accessory molecules are expressed by gastric epithelial cells. Data from our laboratory confirm the functional significance of this expression since the proliferative response of CD4⁺ T cells to allogeneic gastric epithelial cells, reflecting stimulation by Class II MHC, is blocked by antibodies to ICAM-1, to LFA-3, or to B7 (Helene Haberle and Gang Ye, manuscripts in preparation). Except for ICAM-1, epithelial expression of these molecules is increased in *H. pylori*-infected gastric tissues. Studies with cell lines suggest that bacteria and their products may act directly or indirectly on epithelial cells to stimulate accessory/adhesion molecule expression. Inflammatory cytokines released from non-epithelial cells during *H. pylori* infection represent a likely mechanism (indirect) whereby Class II MHC and LFA-3 expression are increased.

GASTRIC EPITHELIAL FUNCTION

Acid secretion is a major function of the gastric epithelium that is highly regulated by a variety of neural, endocrine and immune factors. Elevated fasting and meal-stimulated or hormonally stimulated levels of gastrin are well documented in *H. pylori* infection. Expression of somatostatin, an acid-inhibitory peptide, is diminished in infected individuals. The effect of *H. pylori* infection on acid secretion is complex and varies depending on the presence of duodenal ulcer disease, duration of infection and presence of mucosal atrophy. It is beyond the scope of this chapter to discuss acid secretion and the alterations that have been reported during *H. pylori* infection in any detail. Instead, the reader is referred to chapters in this book by Adrian Lee, David Graham, John Calam, and Kenneth McColl, as well as recent reviews of this topic[42,43].

Secretion of mucus is another important function of the gastric epithelium that appears to be affected by *H. pylori* infection. Initial studies noted that carbohydrates in secreted and intracellular gastric mucus were altered in antral biopsies from *H. pylori*-infected patients. *In-vitro* studies employing an intestinal epithelial cell line demonstrated a small decrease in basal mucus secretion 24h after *H. pylori* infection, while responses to secretory agonists were strongly inhibited[44]. Work from the laboratories of Lichtenberger and of Northfield have demonstrated reduced gastric mucosal hydrophobicity in *H. pylori* individuals with reversal of this abnormality after eradication of infection[45–47], while another study suggests this may be an *in-vitro* artifact[48]. A more detailed review of this aspect of gastric function and the alterations associated with *H. pylori* infection are presented in this text in the chapter by Dr Lichtenberger.

In contrast to other gastric epithelial properties, epithelial barrier function, its regulation, and the changes that may occur during *H. pylori* infection are less well understood. Enhanced gastric uptake of macromolecules reflecting altered epithelial permeability has been reported in allergic reactions, NSAID gastropathy, corticosteroid administration, and lymphocytic gastritis[49–51]. Initial studies from Graham and colleagues demonstrated normal sucrose permeability test results in *H. pylori*-infected subjects, while a recent report from this group describes a small but statistically significant reduction of sucrose excretion after *H. pylori* eradication, suggesting that *H. pylori* may have an effect on gastric permeability[52]. As has been shown with intestinal permeability, these *in-vivo* studies of gastric permeability indicate that a large number of conditions will alter gut epithelial barrier function. *In-vitro* studies employing polarized intestinal epithelial cell lines have greatly enhanced our understanding of the mechanisms regulating the intestinal epithelial barrier[53,54]. The lack of polarized gastric cell models has precluded parallel advancements of knowledge concerning the stomach, although it is likely that similar regulatory factors are involved. Of particular interest, relevant to *H. pylori*-associated inflammation, are the findings of increased intestinal epithelial permeability induced by certain cytokines, including IFNγ and TNFα, and by the transmigration of neutrophils or eosinophils[55-59]. In a preliminary study conducted in primary rabbit gastric epithelial cells cultured on membranes with $3\,\mu$m pores, IL-8-stimulated transmigration of neutrophils was associated with increased back-diffusion of sodium ion, suggesting some modification of gastric epithelial permeability[60]. In another preliminary study, *H. pylori* infection of a polarized intestinal epithelial cell line was accompanied by an increase in transcellular macromolecular transport (J.-F. Desjeux and F. Megraud, personal communication). While both of these studies have their limitations, they provide certain insights into alterations of gastric barrier function in *H. pylori* infection.

GASTRIC EPITHELIAL GROWTH AND REPAIR

Proliferation of the gastric epithelium has been shown to be altered in *H. pylori* infection in both gastric tissues and cell lines, although the results differ markedly in these two groups. In general, studies of biopsy samples obtained from *H. pylori*-infected subjects indicate that gastric epithelial proliferation is increased with a return to normal growth after eradication of infection[61]. In contrast, most studies with cell lines demonstrate an inhibitory effect of *H. pylori* on epithelial cell growth with delayed restitution, although one study reported increased growth of AGS[62]. Direct effects of the bacteria as well as secreted products have been proposed to alter epithelial growth during *H. pylori* infection. Smoot and co-workers have reported that both live organisms and bacterial extracts reduced AGS cell growth (personal communication). Other workers describe a bacterial factor unrelated to cagA or vacA that inhibited gastric epithelial growth[63]. In other *in-vitro* studies, NH_2Cl and NH_4Cl inhibit rat mucosal growth and epithelial cell migration[64,65]. It is likely that factors released from other cell types within the gastric mucosa also play a role, and may explain differences in proliferation found in tissue samples and in cultured cells. Potential stimulatory factors include certain cytokines and growth factors, although others may reduce growth. One can speculate that the balance of inhibitory or stimulatory influences on epithelial growth may mediate epithelial outcomes that include ulceration, intestinal metaplasia, and gastric neoplasia.

EPITHELIAL CELL DEATH

Cell death represents another mechanism whereby epithelial growth can be regulated. In contrast to necrosis, apoptosis is a programmed form of cell death in which accumulation of DNA fragments consisting of multiples of 180 base-pairs forms the basis of several assays to detect apoptosis. Apoptosis is rarely detected in normal intestinal epithelium but is increased in melanosis coli, graft-versus-host disease, NSAID-induced enteropathy, HIV infection, and with chemotherapy or radiation[66]. Defective apoptosis is thought to play a role in carcinogenesis, since certain genes that are associated with the development of colorectal cancer (*c-myc*, *p53*, and *bcl-2*) regulate apoptosis. Apoptosis has not been as well studied in the stomach, but several reports suggest *H. pylori* infection is associated with increased apoptosis. Recently, Moss and colleagues have published that apoptotic cells were rare in uninfected gastric tissue samples with a mean of 2.9% of epithelial cells, located in the most superficial aspect of the gastric glands[67]. In infected tissues, apoptotic cells were located throughout the depth of the gastric glands and increased in mean numbers (16.8%), a value that fell to 3.1% after *H. pylori* eradication. A preliminary study by Jones *et al.* has confirmed increased epithelial apoptosis in gastric biopsies from *H. pylori*-infected patients that also decreased after successful eradication therapy[68]. The frequency of epithelial apoptosis was found to be significantly lower in other forms of gastritis or non-inflamed mucosa in this study. Another initial report also describes increased apoptosis of epithelial cells in the neck region of the gastric glands of *H. pylori*-infected subjects that decreased after eradication therapy[69]. Immuno-histochemical staining for inducible nitric oxide synthase (iNOS) expression, and for a marker of peroxynitrite formation, was also increased before *H. pylori* treatment in this study. While these three studies support the concept that *H. pylori* infection is associated with increased epithelial apoptosis, Peek and colleagues suggest that this effect may be due to cagA$^-$ strains, since their data show increased apoptosis in biopsies from patients infected with cagA$^-$ strains. In contrast, cagA$^+$ strains were associated with increased epithelial proliferation but apoptosis was not different from uninfected controls[70].

Other recent studies of gastric epithelial apoptosis have employed human carcinoma-derived cell lines of primary rabbit cultures to study *H. pylori* infection and potential mediators of apoptosis. Initial results from our laboratory indicate that *H. pylori* induces apoptosis in gastric epithelial cell lines and that the combination of *H. pylori* infection and IFNγ has a synergistic effect (X.J. Fan, manuscript in preparation). Additional studies will be needed to examine the role of cagA expression in this *in-vitro* system given the findings discussed above. Several reports describe NH_2Cl to increase apoptosis in cultured rabbit gastric epithelial cells while $HOCl$, NH_3, or NH_4Cl did not induce DNA strand breaks[65,71]. Nitric oxide was shown to induce apoptosis in another study employing isolated rabbit gastric mucus-secreting cells[72]. While much of the information concerning gastric epithelial apoptosis is preliminary, there is substantial support for implicating *H. pylori* and products of the associated inflammatory response in the regulation of cell growth and death. This is an important area for future research since it is clearly relevant to an understanding of *H. pylori*-associated disease pathogenesis.

CONCLUSION

It is well established that gastric epithelial cells express chemotactic cytokines and immune accessory molecules, providing a mechanism whereby the epithelium can initiate and localize mucosal inflammation. Since these properties are up-regulated in *H. pylori* infection, the gastric epithelium has a potentially greater role as an effector cell in the inflammatory response. In turn, recruited and activated immune cells may alter the gastric epithelium, as may bacteria and their products. Effects on the epithelium include altered epithelial function, as well as growth and repair. Yet unrecognized host and microbial factors determine the net effect of these events and the associated disease manifestation. One can conclude that gastric epithelial cells play a pivotal role in *H. pylori* infection. It would appear, however, that gastric epithelial cells themselves are responsible for their own fate, and may indirectly contribute to their demise in this important infection.

References

1. Dixon MF. Pathophysiology of *Helicobacter pylori* infection. Scand J Gastroenterol. 1994;29: 7–10.
2. Ernst PB, Crowe SE, Reyes VE. The immunopathogenesis of gastroduodenal disease associated with *Helicobacter pylori* infection. Curr Opin Gastroenterol. 1995;11:512–18.
3. Oppenheim JJ, Zachariae COC, Mukaida N, Matsushima K. Properties of the novel proinflammatory supergene 'intercrine' cytokine family. Annu Rev Immunol. 1991;9:617–48.
4. Bagglioni M, Walz A, Kunkel SL. Neutrophil-activating peptide/interleukin 8, a novel cytokine that activates neutrophils. J Clin Invest. 1989;84:1045–9.
5. Crabtree JE, Wyatt JI, Trejdosiewicz LK *et al*. Interleukin-8 expression in *Helicobacter pylori* infected, normal, and neoplastic gastroduodenal mucosa. J Clin Pathol. 1994;47:61–6.
6. Moss SF, Legon S, Davies J, Calam J. Cytokine gene expression in *Helicobacter pylori* associated antral gastritis. Gut. 1995;35:1567–70.
7. Peek RM, Miller GG, Tham KT *et al*. Heightened inflammatory response and cytokine expression *in vivo* to cagA$^+$ *Helicobacter pylori* strains. Lab Invest. 1995;71:760–70.
8. Fan XG, Chua A, Fan XJ, Keeling PW. Increased gastric production of interleukin-8 and tumour necrosis factor in patients with *Helicobacter pylori* infection. J Clin Pathol. 1995;48:133–6.
9. Crabtree JE, Lindley IJD. Mucosal interleukin-8 and *Helicobacter pylori*-associated gastroduodenal disease. Eur J Gastroenterol Hepatol. 1995;6:S33–8.
10. Crabtree JE, Peichl P, Wyatt JI, Stachl U, Lindley IJD. Gastric interleukin-8 and IgA IL-8 auto-antibodies in *Helicobacter pylori* infection. Scand J Immunol. 1993;37:65–70.
11. Crabtree JE, Farmery SM, Lindley IJD, Figura N, Peichl P, Tompkins DS. CagA/cytotoxic strains of *Helicobacter pylori* and interleukin-8 in gastric epithelial cell lines. J Clin Pathol. 1994;47:945–50.
12. Crowe SE, Alvarez L, Dytoc M *et al*. Expression of interleukin-8 and CD54 by human gastric epithelium after *Helicobacter pylori* infection *in vitro*. Gastroenterology. 1995;108:65–74.
13. Sharma SA, Tummuru MKR, Miller GG, Blaser MJ. Interleukin-8 response of gastric epithelial cell lines to *Helicobacter pylori* stimulation *in vitro*. Infect Immun. 1995;63:1681–7.
14. Huang J, O'Toole PW, Doig P, Trust TJ. Stimulation of interleukin-8 production in epithelial cell lines by *Helicobacter pylori*. Infect Immun. 1995;63:1732–8.
15. Crabtree JE, Xiang Z, Lindley IJD, Tompkins DS, Rappuoli R, Covacci A. Induction of interleukin-8 secretion from gastric epithelial cells by a *cagA* negative isogenic mutant of *Helicobacter pylori*. J Clin Pathol. 1995;48:967–9.
16. Geiser T, Dewald B, Ehrengruber MU, Clark-Lewis I, Baggiolini M. The interleukin-8-related chemotactic cytokines GROα, GROβ, and GRO activate human neutrophil and basophil leukocytes. J Biol Chem. 1993;268:15419–24.
17. Yamaoka Y, Kita M, Kodama T, Sawai N, Kashima K, Imanishi J. Expression of chemokine mRNA in gastric mucosa with *Helicobacter pylori* infection. Gastroenterology. 1996;110: A1049(abstract).

18. Takizawa H, Azuma A, Aihara M *et al*. *Helicobacter pylori*-induced chemokines production in human gastric carcinoma cell lines: effects of rebapimide. Gastroenterology. 1996;110:A272 (abstract).
19. Jung HC, Kim JM, Song IS, Kim CY. Increased motility of *Helicobacter pylori* by methyl-cellulose could upregulate the expression of proinflammatory cytokines in human gastric epithelial cells. Gastroenterology. 1996;110:A146(abstract).
20. Eckmann L, Jung HC, Schurer-Maly C, Panja A, Morzycka-Wroblewska E, Kagnoff MF. Differential cytokine expression by human intestinal epithelial cell lines: regulated expression of interleukin 8. Gastroenterology. 1993;105:1689–97.
21. Jung HC, Eckmann L, Yang S-K *et al*. A distinct array of proinflammatory cytokines is expressed in human colon epithelial cells in response to bacterial invasion. J Clin Invest. 1995;95:55–65.
22. Mayer L, Eisenhardt D, Salomon P, Bauer W, Plous R, Piccinini L. Expression of class II molecules on intestinal epithelial cells in humans. Differences between normal and inflammatory bowel disease. Gastroenterology. 1991;100:3–12.
23. Engstrand L, Scheynius A, Pathlson C, Grimelius L, Schwan S. Association of *Campylobacter pylori* with induced expression of class II transplantation antigens on gastric epithelial cells. Infect Immun. 1989;57:827–32.
24. Valnes K, Huitfeldt HS, Brandtzaeg P. Relation between T cell number and epithelial HLA class II expression quantified by image analysis in normal and inflamed human gastric mucosa. Gut. 1990;31:647–52.
25. Chiba M, Ishii N, Ishioka T *et al*. Topographic study of *Helicobacter pylori* and HLA-DR antigen expression on gastric epithelium. J Gastroenterol. 1995;30:149–55.
26. Scheynius A, Engstrand L. Gastric epithelial cells in *Helicobacter pylori*-associated gastritis express HLA-DR but not ICAM-1. Scand J Immunol. 1991;33:237–41.
27. Sakai K, Takiguchi M, Mori S *et al*. Expression and function of class II antigens on gastric carcinoma cells and gastric epithelia: differential expression of DR, DQ, and DP antigens. J Natl Cancer Inst. 1987;79:923–32.
28. Noach LA, Bosma NB, Jansen J, Hoek FJ, van-Deventer SJ, Tytgat GN. Mucosal tumor necrosis factor-alpha, interleukin-1 beta and interleukin-8 production in patients with *Helicobacter pylori*. Scand J Gastroenterol. 1994;29:425–9.
29. Karttunen R, Karttunen T, Ekre H-PT, Macdonald TT. Interferon gamma and interleukin 4 secreting cells in the gastric antrum in *Helicobacter pylori* positive and negative gastritis. Gut. 1995;36:341–5.
30. Yamaoka Y, Kita M, Kodama T, Sawai N, Imanishi J. *Helicobacter pylori cagA* gene and expression of cytokine messenger mRNA in gastric mucosa. Gastroenterology. 1996;110:1744–52.
31. Springer TA. Adhesion receptors of the immune system. Nature. 1990;346:425–34.
32. Norton J, Sloane JP, Al-Saffar N, Haskard DO. Expression of adhesion molecules in human intestinal graft-versus-host disease. Clin Exp Immunol. 1992;87:231–6.
33. Nakamura S, Ohtani H, Watanabe Y *et al*. *In situ* expression of the cell adhesion molecules in inflammatory bowel disease. Evidence of immunologic activation of vascular endothelial cells. Lab Invest. 1993;69:77–85.
34. Kaiserlian D, Rigal D, Abello J, Revillard J-P. Expression, function and regulation of the inter-cellular adhesion molecule-1 (ICAM-1) on human intestinal epithelial cell lines. Eur J Immunol. 1991;21:2415–21.
35. Fan XG, Fan XJ, Xia HX, Keeling PWN, Kelleher D. Up-regulation of CD44 and ICAM-1 expression on gastric epithelial cells by *H. pylori*. APMIS. 1995;103:744–8.
36. Vidal K, Samarut C, Magaud J-P, Revillard J-P, Kaiserlian D. Unexpected lack of reactivity of allogeneic anti-Ia monoclonal antibodies with MHC class II molecules expressed by mouse intestinal epithelial cells. J Immunol. 1993;151:4642–50.
37. Kelly CP, O'Keana JC, Orellana J *et al*. Human colon cancer cells express ICAM-1 in vivo and support LFA-1-dependent lymphocyte adhesion in vitro. Am J Physiol. 1992;263:G864–70.
38. Parkos CA, Colgan SP, Madara JL. Interactions of PMN with epithelial cells: lessons from the intestine. J Am Soc Nephrol. 1994;5:138–52.
39. Kvale D, Krajci P, Brandtzaeg P. Expression and regulation of adhesion molecules ICAM-1 (CD54) and LFA-3 (CD 58) in human intestinal epithelial cell lines. Scand J Immunol. 1992;35:669–76.
40. Bluestone JA. New perspectives of CD28-B7-mediated T cell costimulation. Cell. 1995;81:555–9.

41. Hagerty DT, Evavoid BD, Allen PM. Regulation of the costimulatory B7, not class II major histocompatibility complex, restricts the ability of murine kidney tubule cells to stimulate CD4+ T cells. J Clin Invest. 1994;93:1208–15.
42. Lee A, Dixon MF, Danon SJ *et al.* Local acid production and *Helicobacter pylori*: a unifying hypothesis of gastroduodenal disease. Eur J Gastroenterol Hepatol. 1995;7:461–5.
43. McGowan CC, Cover TL, Blaser MJ. *Helicobacter pylori* and gastric acid: biological and therapeutic implications. Gastroenterology. 1996;110:926–38.
44. Micots I, Augeron C, Laboisse CL, Muzeau F, Megraud F. Mucin exocytosis: a major target for *Helicobacter pylori*. J Clin Pathol. 1993;46:241–5.
45. Goggin PM, Marrero JM, Spychal RT, Jackson PA, Corbishley CM, Northfield TC. Surface hydrophobicity of gastric mucosa in *Helicobacter pylori* infection: effect of clearance and eradication. Gastroenterology. 1992;103:1486–90.
46. Go MF, Lew GM, Lichtenberger LM, Genta RM, Graham DY. Gastric mucosal hydrophobicity and *Helicobacter pylori*: response to antimicrobial therapy. Am J Gastroenterol. 1993;88:1362–5.
47. Lichtenberger LM, Romero JJ. Effect of ammonium ion on the hydrophobic and barrier properties of the gastric mucus gel layer: implications on the role of ammonium in *H. pylori*-induced gastritis. J Gastroenterol Hepatol. 1994;9:S13–19.
48. Markesich DC, Anand BS, Lew GM, Graham DY. *Helicobacter pylori* infection does not reduce the viscosity of human gastric mucus gel. Gut. 1995;36:327–9.
49. Hatz RA, Bloch KJ, Harmatz PR *et al.* Divalent hapten-induced intestinal anaphylaxis in the mouse enhances macromolecular uptake from the stomach. Gastroenterology. 1990;98:894–900.
50. Catto-Smith AG, Patrick MK, Scott RB, Davison JS, Gall DG. Gastric response to mucosal IgE-mediated reactions. Am J Physiol. 1989;257:G704–8.
51. Sutherland LR, Verhoef M, Wallace JL, Van Rosendaal G, Crutcher R, Meddings JB. A simple, non-invasive marker of gastric damage: sucrose permeability. Lancet. 1994;343:998–1000.
52. Graham DY, Malaty HM, Goodgame R, Ou CN. Effect of cure of *H. pylori* infection on the gastric mucosal permeability. Gastroenterology. 1996;110:A122(abstract).
53. Madara JL. Loosening tight junctions: lessons from the intestine. J Clin Invest. 1989;83:1089–94.
54. Madara JL. Pathobiology of the intestinal epithelial barrier. Am J Pathol. 1990;137:1273–81.
55. Madara JL, Stafford J. Interferon-γ directly affects barrier function of cultured intestinal epithelial monolayers. J Clin Invest. 1989;83:724–7.
56. Colgan SP, Resnick MB, Parkos CA *et al.* IL-4 directly modulates function of a model human intestinal epithelium. J Immunol. 1994;153:2122–9.
57. Parkos CA, Colgan SP, Delp C, Arnaout MA, Madara JL. Neutrophil migration across a cultured epithelial monolayer elicits a biphasic resistance response representing sequential effects on transcellular and paracellular pathways. J Cell Biol. 1992;117:757–64.
58. Nash S, Stafford J, Madara JL. Effects of polymorphonuclear leukocyte transmigration on the barrier function of cultured intestinal epithelial monolayers. J Clin Invest. 1987;80:1104–13.
59. Resnick MB, Colgan SP, Patapoff TW *et al.* Activated eosinophils evoke chloride secretion in model intestinal epithelia primarily via regulated release of 5′-AMP. J Immunol. 1993;151:5716–23.
60. Fujiwara Y, Sasaki E, Ikeda Y *et al.* Interleukin-8 stimulates polymorphonuclear leukocyte migration across a cultured monolayer of rabbit gastric epithelial cells and impairs their barrier function. Gastroenterology. 1996;110:A110(abstract).
61. Cahill RJ, Xia H, Kilgallen C, Beattie S, Hamilton H, O'Morain C. Effect of eradication of *Helicobacter pylori* infection on gastric epithelial cell proliferation. Dig Dis Sci. 1995;40:1627–31.
62. Fan XG, Kelleher D, Fan XJ, Xia HX, Keeling PWN. *Helicobacter pylori* increases proliferation of gastric epithelial cells. Gut. 1996;38:19–22.
63. Wagner S, Beil W, Nietart M *et al.* Antiproliferative effect of *Helicobacter pylori* on human gastric epithelial cells *in vitro*. Gastroenterology. 1996;110:A1040(abstract).
64. Dekigai H, Murakami M, Saita H *et al.* Monochloramine and ammonia produced by *Helicobacter pylori* infection inhibit restitution of gastric epithelial cell. Gastroenterology. 1996;110:A92(abstract).
65. Naito Y, Yoshikawa T, Yagi N *et al.* Cell growth inhibition and apoptosis induced by monochloramine in a gastric mucosal cell line. Gastroenterology. 1996;110:A205(abstract).
66. Watson AJM. Necrosis and apoptosis in the gastrointestinal tract. Gut. 1995;37:165–7.
67. Moss SF, Calam J, Agarwal B, Wang S, Holt PG. Induction of gastric epithelial apoptosis by *Helicobacter pylori*. Gut. 1996;38:498–501.

68. Jones NL, Yeger H, Cutz E, Sherman PM. *Helicobacter pylori* induces apoptosis of gastric antral epithelial cells *in vivo*. Gastroenterology. 1996;110:A933.
69. Bravo LE, Mannick EE, Zhang X-J, Ruiz B, Correa P, Miller MJS. *H. pylori* infection is associated with inducible nitric oxide synthase expression, nitrotyrosine and DNA damage. Gastroenterology. 1995;108:A63(abstract).
70. Peek RM, Moss SF, Tham KT *et al*. Infection with *H. pylori* cagA⁺ strains dissociates gastric epithelial proliferation from apoptosis. Gastroenterology. 1996;110:A575(abstract).
71. Mori M, Suzuki M, Suzuki H, Akiba Y, Miura S, Ishii H. Extensive oxidative DNA damage is induced by ammonia-related oxidant, monochloramine, in cultured gastric epithelial cell. Gastroenterology. 1996;110:A201(abstract).
72. Fukuda T, Arakawa T, Fujiwara Y *et al*. Nitric oxide induces apoptosis in gastric mucosal cells. Gastroenterology. 1996;110:A110(abstract).

15
Is the Th1/Th2 lymphocyte balance upset by *Helicobacter pylori* infection?

P. B. ERNST, V. E. REYES, W. R. GOURLEY, H. HÄBERLE and
K. B. BAMFORD

INTRODUCTION

Since *H. pylori* became recognized as a gastric pathogen, many people have felt that antibiotics would expedite the eradication of, or at least the decrease in, gastric diseases associated with this infection. However, history reminds us that antibiotics have been relatively ineffective at eradicating other bacterial infections. In the case of *H. pylori* the infection is widespread on a global basis. Although the rate of infection with *H. pylori* is slow, our understanding of the epidemiology of the spread of this pathogen is incomplete, thereby limiting the success of interventions to decrease the incidence of infection. Furthermore, antibiotic regimens may be too expensive for some individuals or societies, and resistance to antibiotics is emerging. Thus, it is essential to understand the immunopathogenesis of gastric disease associated with *H. pylori* infection and to counter these processes through vaccines that may shift the host response away from chronic inflammation and tissue destruction towards effective immunity. This review will summarize the means by which mucosal immune responses can confer protection to luminal flora without inducing disease. In addition, the current understanding of T-cell biology in *H. pylori* infection will be examined and contrasted with the T-cell responses that may be induced by the vaccines for *H. pylori* that are currently in the development stage.

GOAL OF MUCOSAL IMMUNITY

Mucosal immune responses in the digestive tract have evolved such that they are capable of conferring protection without inducing excessive amounts of inflammation. Current dogma suggests that secretion of IgA into the lumen is largely responsible for achieving immunity. This is based on the fact that more than 90%

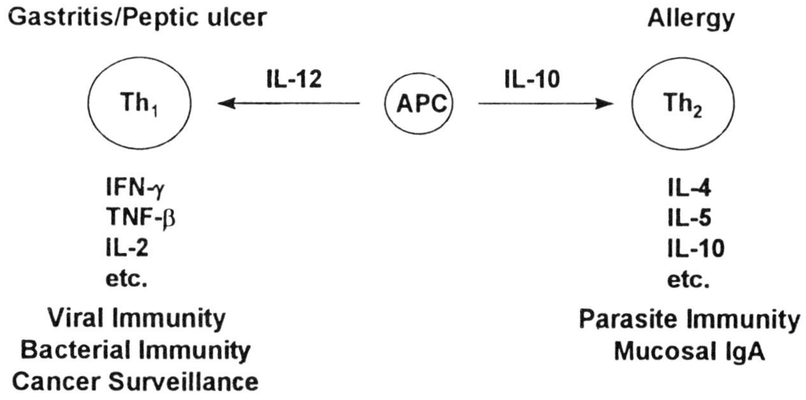

Gastritis/Peptic ulcer   **Allergy**

Figure 1   Characterization of Th1 and Th2 cells. Th1 and Th2 cells are characterized by their cytokine profile. After exposure to IL-12, Th1 cells are selected and produce IFNγ, TNFβ and IL-2 that can combine to increase cell-mediated immunity. They also can increase complement-fixing IgG and enhance phagocytosis of opsonized bacteria. However, Th2 cells have a decided advantage at inducing mucosal immune responses including IgA. Either subset can also contribute to disease. For example, Th2 cells are implicated in the pathogenesis of allergies and Th1 could contribute to epithelial damage in the stomach

of the B cells and plasma cells in healthy gastrointestinal tissue produce IgA. Moreover, IgA is secreted in the digestive tract as a dimer – a structure that permits it to be transported across the epithelium and into the lumen. IgA has been shown to be capable of neutralizing bacteria or their toxins. Despite this, IgA deficiency is the most common immunodeficiency in humans, and these individuals have little disadvantage in their ability to prevent infections. Thus, other mechanisms may contribute to protection, but IgA is likely to play a significant role.

HELPER T CELL HETEROGENEITY

Immunological effector mechanisms may be driven by antigen but the magnitude and type of immune response that develops is largely dictated by cytokines. Helper T cells can be functionally divided into subsets based on their cytokine profile. Through the production of interferon-γ (IFNγ), TNFα and IL-2, Th1 cells select for a rather specific panel of immune responses including cell-mediated immunity, while Th2 cells preferentially regulate mucosal IgA responses through the production of TGFβ, IL-4, IL-5, IL-6 and IL-10[1] (Figure 1). Since naive T cells retain the potential to differentiate into either subset, most antigens probably induce a mixture of T-cell responses. However, over time, some pathogens that are associated with chronic infection favour a response that is predominantly either Th1 or Th2 in nature. Both subsets have been shown to play a pivotal role in immunity and both also have been implicated in the immunopathogenesis of disease[2]. Thus, in order to maintain health the host must strike the correct balance between these subsets.

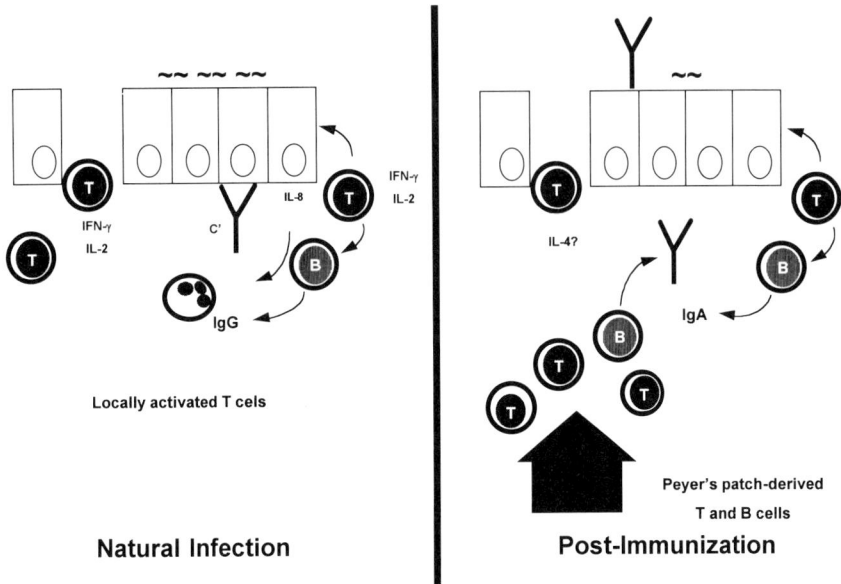

Figure 2 Induction of Th1 and Th2 cells. This figure contrasts T-cell selection after natural infection with live *H. pylori* versus immunization. Natural infection is focused in the stomach where local influences are probably responsible for the selection of Th1 cells. In turn, cytokines from these cells alone, or in combination with cytokines from other cells or products from *H. pylori* itself, can alter gene expression in the epithelium, induce apoptosis of the epithelium as well as selecting for immunological responses that may damage the tissue. In particular, the expansion of IgG-producing B cells by T cells may lead to the formation of autoantibodies, immune complex formation, complement activation (C′) and immune complex-mediated disease. In contrast, immunization strategies are believed to stimulate immune responses in the inductive sites such as the Peyer's patches. This is postulated to lead to the induction of Th2 cells and IgA-producing B cells that, in turn, migrate to other mucosal tissues, perhaps including the stomach. The effector mechanisms selected by Th2 cells are more protective and less inflammatory

INDUCTION OF IMMUNE AND INFLAMMATORY RESPONSES IN THE GASTROINTESTINAL TRACT

The induction of immune responses in the intestinal tract has been extensively reviewed elsewhere[3–5]. Briefly, lymphoid aggregates in the Peyer's patches are believed to be the primary inductive site for T- and B-cell responses in the intestine. Various cytokines have been shown to direct the differentiation of B cells into IgA-producing cells while others expand the number of IgA-producing cells and IgA secretion. These cytokines include TGFβ, IL-4, IL-5, IL-6 and IL-10. This panel of cytokines is produced by T cells associated with the Th2 subset of helper T cells. Stimulated T and B lymphoblasts are believed to exit the Peyer's patches and seed other areas of the intestine as well as more remote mucosal tissues including the salivary glands and the respiratory and urogenital tracts. This model implies that lymphocytes from Peyer's patches would also seed the stomach (Figure 2);

however, there is no direct evidence that this occurs. In fact, in the absence of gastric inflammation, very few T and B cells are found in the gastric mucosa.

Th2 cells satisfy the criterion of selecting for protective mucosal IgA responses while inhibiting cell-mediated immunity. The mucosal inflammation, in association with a persistent exposure to antigen, intimates that Th1 cells predominate in the inflamed stomach and subvert the strategy of developing protection without inflammation.

REGULATION OF Th CELL DIFFERENTIATION

Following exposure to infection, the host produces an acute inflammatory response that contributes to the recruitment and activation of cells that can present antigen to T cells. These antigen-presenting cells then stimulate adjacent T cells. *H. pylori* has been shown to be a modest T-cell mitogen *in vitro*; it may even inhibit some T-cell responses[6]. It is possible that one of several molecules expressed by *H. pylori*, including proteases, interfere with antigen presentation and T-cell activation. However, the striking accumulation of T cells in the gastric mucosa during infection with *H. pylori* speaks to the fact that T cells are recruited and activated *in vivo*. MHC-restricted, *H. pylori*-specific T-cell clones have been derived from both the peripheral blood and gastric mucosa of infected individuals[7]. Furthermore, *H. pylori* induces IFNγ production from peripheral blood leucocytes[8] as well as those isolated from the gut[6]. In addition, IFNγ-producing cells are increased in the gastric mucosa during infection[9]. This latter study also suggested that Th1 cells predominate in gastritis, since the number of IL-4-producing Th2 cells varied little in response to inflammation[9]. It should be noted that the increase in IFNγ-producing cells was also observed in gastritis due to aetiologies other than *H. pylori*[9]. Therefore, this response may reflect the influence of the gastric microenvironment on helper T cell selection.

The selection for Th1 and Th2 cells is largely controlled by their interaction with antigen-presenting cells. First, the production of IL-10 and IL-12 by antigen-presenting cells can select for Th2 and Th1 cells respectively (Figure 1). Preliminary data from our laboratory have shown that live *H. pylori* preferentially induces IL-12 and that IL-12 predominates over IL-10 in gastric biopsies. This would be consistent with the increase in IFNγ that was reported previously[8]. Secondly, interactions between antigen-presenting cells and T cells mediated via adhesion molecules can also control Th cell differentiation. Although these have yet to be defined in the stomach, the current view is that there is an expansion of IFNγ-producing T cells in the gastric mucosa in response to infection.

It is not clear if Th1 responses, which select for cell-mediated immunity, are in the best interest of the host in its attempt to clear an extracellular infection. Moreover, Th2 responses have been directly implicated in mucosal protection as well as split tolerance – that is, enhanced IgA responses in association with suppressed cell-mediated immunity. Th1 cells and the associated cell-mediated immunity may be tolerable but an overwhelming Th1 response, in combination with host genetics, specific strains of bacteria as well as other environmental factors, could combine to contribute to ulcerogenesis.

CONTRIBUTION OF Th1 CELLS TO AUTOIMMUNITY IN THE STOMACH

The immune response has evolved to protect the host from infection. In the case of the mucosal tissues the host further discriminates between pathogens and commensal flora. This is achieved by an apparent inhibition of immune responses to enteric commensal organisms. However, an inappropriate response in certain individuals to commensal flora may occur. Thus, a failure in immune regulation to flora that persist in the lumen, such as *H. pylori*, may lead to tissue damage on a scale equivalent to classical autoimmune diseases. This notion is supported by a report describing the development of colitis in mice following the ablation of the gene coding for IL-10, a cytokine which selects for Th2 responses[10]. This disease appears to be driven by luminal bacteria, as animals maintained in an environment free of commensal flora do not develop colitis. The evidence that Th1 cells may be increased relative to Th2 cells during *H. pylori* infection suggests that a marked skewing in this response may lead to disease as implicated in the pathogenesis of more classical autoimmune diseases[2]. These observations suggest that the difference in gastric disease associated with *H. pylori* infection may be partially attributed to the magnitude of the host response.

The first suggestion that *H. pylori* may cause a bona-fide autoimmune response was based on evidence that monoclonal antibodies directed against *H. pylori* could recognize an epitope on the gastric epithelium of mice and humans. Moreover, administration of these antibodies to mice resulted in gastritis and caused mild erosions[11]. More recently, IgM antibodies produced from immortalized B cells obtained from the gastric mucosa have been shown to recognize the gastric epithelium[12]. Other evidence suggests that B cells within a MALToma express a repertoire that recognizes a determinant shared by both IgA and IgM[13]. Thus, antibodies within the gastric mucosa may recognize epithelial cells or act as rheumatoid factors. This may lead to immune complex-mediated disease that could directly damage the epithelium. If this hypothesis is correct, then future studies may show activated complement adjacent to damaged epithelium.

The presence of Th1 cells and IFNγ production are likely to lead to immuno-physiological interactions that directly promote tissue damage. For example, IFNγ alters epithelial barrier function in intestinal cell lines[14]. Other cytokines, including TNFα, can collaborate with IFNγ to alter epithelial cell IL-8 gene expression[15]. Recent results also suggest that cytokines from Th1 cells can enhance apoptosis in gastric epithelial cells. Additional intercellular interactions between epithelial cells and T cells mediated by Fas–Fas ligand interactions may also contribute to apoptosis of epithelial cells. Apoptotic cells have also been observed to be increased in number in gastroduodenal epithelium during infection with *H. pylori*[16].

Through T-cell regulation, most luminal flora stimulate a balance among tolerance, inflammation and immunity, thereby limiting tissue damage. The failure to accomplish this during infection with *H. pylori* supports the hypothesis that an imbalance in Th-cell cytokines may shift the host response away from protective immunity and more towards chronic inflammation and tissue damage.

If peptic ulcer is in part due to an autoimmune response, it should be noted that there is apparently very little immunological memory, as cure of the infection effectively prevents recurrence of peptic ulcer. However, T cells from seropositive and seronegative donors can respond to stimulation with water-extractable *H. pylori* proteins[17]. This suggests that either seronegative donors have cleared an infection and retain T-cell memory or that these proteins crossreact with other antigens against which the host is sensitized. Despite this, there is no protective immunity as reinfection can occur. These observations are not inconsistent with the concept that at least some autoreactive T and B cells are activated during *H. pylori* infection since the immunological memory of *mucosal* lymphocytes appears to be very short. Indeed, most of the increase in T and B cells observed in the gastric mucosa is reversed after antibiotic treatment. In addition, the 'self' antigen may be present only during infection. For example, epithelial cells may express surface antigens in response to the stress of infection and the inflammatory milieu. Likewise, the loss of gastric B cells after treatment may permit rheumatoid factors to wane, and the absence of *H. pylori* itself may remove a luminal antigen to which the host has never established an immunological equilibrium.

STRATEGIES IN IMMUNOTHERAPY

We would propose that an excessive Th1 response driven by *H. pylori* would favour IFNγ production, the development of cell-mediated immunity and a set of conditions that contribute to the onset of epithelial damage. This damage may be direct, through the recognition of immunogenic peptides presented by the epithelial cells, or by the transient or permanent expression of epitopes that are recognized by antibodies produced during infection. If this model is correct, then immunological intervention that shifts the T cell response from Th1 to Th2 may favour the development of IgA responses and protective immunity in association with a decrease in tissue damage. This notion is supported since IgA antibodies recognizing urease are sufficient to provide protection in an animal model[18]. In addition, protective immunity can be achieved since immunization of mice with *H. pylori* antigens, in combination with cholera toxin as an adjuvant, provides protection against a challenge with *H. felis* or *H. pylori*[19–21] (reviewed in ref. 22). These data further support our hypothesis since cholera toxins boosts the Th2 cell response and IgA responses[1]. Thus, qualitatively changing the response through oral immunization provides a tremendous opportunity for prevention as well as a complement to therapy. Future experiments will have to determine the relative strength of the Th1- and Th2-cell responses in different stages of gastric disease versus the response induced by the numerous candidate oral vaccines that are being developed.

SUMMARY

Our understanding of the control of helper T-cell differentiation is in its infancy, but the general principles that are emerging appear to predict Th cell differentiation in response to *H. pylori* infection. *H. pylori* induces IL-12 leading to the production of IFNγ-producing T cells resembling Th1 cells. Work in progress is confirming the presence of these cells in the gastric mucosa. Since the infection is not invasive, cell-mediated responses selected by Th1 cells are ineffective at clearing the infection. Moreover, they can contribute to inflammation and epithelial damage. The increased turnover of epithelial cells may exceed cytoprotective mechanisms and the restorative powers of restitution. This could lead to ulceration as luminal acid and pepsin gain access to the underlying tissue. Since the T-cell response is so homogeneously biased towards Th1 cells, the successful induction of Th2 cells in the gastric mucosa provides a logical and probably highly successful approach to increase host immunity to *H. pylori*.

Acknowledgements

Results described in this review were obtained through support from the John Sealy Memorial Endowment Fund for Biomedical Research and the National Institutes of Health, DK 50669.

References

1. Xu-Amano BJ, Kiyono H, Jackson RJ *et al*. Helper T cell subsets for immunoglobulin A responses: oral immunization with tetanus toxoid and cholera toxin as adjuvant selectively induces Th2 cells in mucosa associated tissues. J Exp Med. 1993;178:1309–20.
2. Liblau RS, Singer SM, McDevitt HO. Th1 and Th2 CD4⁺ T cells in the pathogenesis of organ-specific autoimmune diseases. Immunol Today. 1995;16:34–8.
3. McGhee JR, Mestecky J, Dertzbaugh MT, Eldridge JH, Hirasawa M, Kiyono H. The mucosal immune system: from fundamental concepts to vaccine development. Vaccine. 1992;10:75–88.
4. Manganaro M, Ogra PL, Ernst PB. Oral immunization: turning fantasy into reality. Int Arch Allergy Appl Immunol. 1994;103:223–33.
5. Ernst PB, Crowe SE, Reyes VE. The immunopathogenesis of gastroduodenal disease associated with *Helicobacter pylori* infection. Curr Opin Gastroenterol. 1995;11:512–18.
6. Fan XJ, Chua A, Shahi CN, McDevitt J, Keeling PWN, Kelleher D. Gastric T lymphocyte response to *Helicobacter pylori* in patients with *H. pylori* colonisation. Gut. 1994;35:1379–84.
7. Di Tommaso A, Xiang Z, Bugnoli M *et al*. *Helicobacter pylori*-specific CD4⁺ T-cell clones from peripheral blood and gastric biopsies. Infect Immun. 1995;63:1102–6.
8. Tarkkanen J, Kosunen TU, Saksela E. Contact of lymphocytes with *Helicobacter pylori* augments natural killer cell activity and induces production of gamma interferon. Infect Immun. 1993;61:3012–16.
9. Karttunen R, Karttunen T, Ekre H-PT, MacDonald TT. Interferon gamma and interleukin 4 secreting cells in the gastric antrum in *Helicobacter pylori* positive and negative gastritis. Gut. 1995;36:341–5.
10. Kuhn R, Lohler J, Rennick D, Rajewsky K, Muller W. Interleukin-10-deficient mice develop chronic enterocolitis. Cell. 1993;75:263–74.
11. Negrini R, Lisato L, Zanella I *et al*. *Helicobacter pylori* infection induces antibodies cross-reacting with human gastric mucosa. Gastroenterology. 1991;101:437–45.
12. Vollmers HP, Dammrich J, Ribbert H *et al*. Human monoclonal antibodies from stomach carcinoma patients react with *Helicobacter pylori* and stimulate stomach cancer cells in vitro. Cancer. 1994;74:1525–32.
13. Greiner A, Marx A, Heesemann J, Leebmann J, Schmausser B, Muller-Hermelink HK. Idiotype identity in a MALT-type lymphoma and B cells in *Helicobacter pylori* associated chronic gastritis. Lab Invest. 1994;70:572–8.
14. Madara JL, Stafford J. Interferon-γ directly affects barrier function of cultured intestinal epithelial monolayers. J Clin Invest. 1989;83:724–7.
15. Yasumoto K, Okamoto S, Mukaida N, Murakami S, Mai M, Matsushima K. Tumor necrosis factor α and interferon γ synergistically induce interleukin 8 production in a human gastric cancer cell line through acting concurrently on AP-1 and NF-kappaB-like binding sites of the interleukin 8 gene. J Biol Chem. 1992;267:22506–11.

16. Moss SF, Calam J, Agarwal B, Wang S, Holt PG. Induction of gastric epithelial apoptosis by *Helicobacter pylori*. Gut. 1996;38:498–501.

17. Sharma SA, Miller GG, Perez-Perez GI, Gupta RS, Blaser MJ. Humoral and cellular immune recognition of *Helicobacter pylori* proteins are not concordant. Clin Exp Immunol. 1994;97: 126–32.

18. Blanchard TG, Czinn SJ, Maurer R, Thomas WD, Soman G, Nedrud JG. Urease-specific monoclonal antibodies prevent *Helicobacter felis* infection in mice. Infect Immun. 1995;63:1394–9.

19. Chen M, Lee A, Hazell S. Immunisation against gastric helicobacter infection in a mouse *Helicobacter felis* model. Lancet. 1992;339:1120–1.

20. Michetti P, Corthesy-Theulaz I, Davin C *et al*. Immunization of BALB/c mice against *Helicobacter felis* infection with *Helicobacter pylori* urease. Gastroenterology. 1994;107:1002–11.

21. Pappo J, Thomas WD, Kabok Z, Taylor NS, Murphy JC, Fox JG. Effect of oral immunization with recombinant urease on murine *Helicobacter felis* gastritis. Infect Immun. 1995;63:1246–52.

22. Ghiara P, Michetti P. Development of a vaccine. Curr Opin Gastroenterol. 1995;11:52–5.

16
What determines the vigour of the immune response to *Helicobacter pylori*?

K. CROITORU and D. SNIDER

INTRODUCTION

The term 'vigour' refers to both the 'active strength' and the 'effective force' of a response. This difference is exemplified by the quandary encountered when studying the immune response to *Helicobacter pylori* infection. Patients infected with *H. pylori* mount an antibody response and possibly even a cell-mediated or T cell response; yet the infection persists. This suggests that the vigour of the immune response, that is, strength of the antibody or cell-mediated immunity, is not paralleled by the effectiveness of the immune response, i.e. the ability to either prevent or eliminate the infection. It is in this context that we will consider the factors that contribute to the vigour of the immune response to *H. pylori*.

THE IMMUNE RESPONSE AT THE MUCOSA-ASSOCIATED LYMPHOID TISSUE

In an effort to understand the mechanisms controlling the strength and effectiveness of the immune response to *H. pylori* it is first necessary to review our understanding of the mucosal immune response and to compare what is known of the intestine with what is known of the stomach.

The mucosa-associated lymphoid tissue (MALT) of the small intestine is characterized by organized lymphoid structures such as the Peyer's patches (PP) or lymphoid follicles and mesenteric lymph nodes. In addition, other anatomical compartments of the intestine such as the epithelial layer and lamina propria contain immune cells[1]. Overlying the PP are specialized epithelial cells referred to as 'M cells', which are thought to serve as entry points for foreign antigens[2,3]. Antigens taken up by M cells are transported into the PP, where the inductive phase of the intestinal immune response is thought to occur. It is here that antigen-specific B cells are stimulated and undergo switching from IgM- to IgA-producing B cells[4,5]. These cells leave the PP via the lymphatics to enter the thoracic duct and travel to the systemic circulation to return selectively to mucosal sites, particularly the intestine[6]. This ability to recirculate has led to the notion of a 'common mucosal immune system', whereby immunization at one mucosal surface leads to immunity at other mucosal surfaces[7,8]. Although it would be reasonable to assume that the gastric mucosa is part of this common mucosal immune system, there is no direct evidence for this at this time.

The normal gastric mucosa has a paucity of immune cells; a consequence presumably of the fact that the acid conditions present in the normal stomach maintain a relatively sterile environment. On the other hand, the gastric mucosa in patients infected with *H. pylori* is characterized by a chronic active gastritis with neutrophil, lymphocyte and plasma cell infiltrates in the lamina propria and an increase in intra-epithelial lymphocytes[9–11]. In patients with a severely inflamed gastric mucosa, lymphoid aggregates and follicles develop in the lamina propria similar to that seen in the normal intestine. Under these conditions the stomach may acquire the ability to mount an immune response in a fashion similar to that seen in the intestine. A notable difference between this stomach-associated lymphoid tissue or SALT and the GALT is the absence of specialized M cells in the stomach. This raises the important question of whether an immune response can be initiated in the gastric mucosa and, if so, how antigen is taken up and presented to the local lymphocytes. In the small intestine, intestinal epithelial cells can be induced to express MHC Class II molecules and these cells can function as antigen-presenting cells *in vitro*[12,13]. In the *H. pylori* infected and inflamed stomach, epithelial cells can also acquire MHC Class II expression, suggesting that the gastric epithelial cell may function in a comparable way, although evidence for this is not yet available[14,15]. Therefore, the presence of elements of the immune system in the gastric mucosa of *H. pylori* infected individuals suggests some capacity to respond to the infection.

The notion that gastric mucosal immune cells contribute to the effector arm of the local immune response is based primarily on the detection of IgA antibody responses in gastric secretions. IgA is the predominant antibody isotype seen in the normal immune response at most mucosal surfaces. It has been argued that this is due to the fact that IgA, which is relatively resistant to protease digestion, is well suited to the hostile environment of the intestinal lumen. In addition, mechanisms have evolved to selectively transport secretory IgA (sIgA) from the tissue into the lumen via the polymeric Ig receptor or secretory component, expressed on intestinal epithelial cells[16,17]. In the intestine T cells preferentially drive B cells toward IgA production through the secretion of cytokines such as IL-4[18,19]. The ability of gastric T cells to contribute to gastric IgA responses is less well studied.

Therefore, although the normal uninflamed stomach lacks obvious organized lymphoid tissue, in response to *H. pylori* infection it is evident that immune effector cells accumulate and presumably participate in the local immune response to this organism.

IMMUNE ACTIVATION IN THE MUCOSA

The generation of antigen-specific T and B cell responses with IgA production and cytokine release could contribute to the prevention and possibly elimination of established infection. At the same time, however, release of inflammatory cytokines, production of IgG and activation of complement could contribute to inflammation and local tissue destruction. For example, cytokines such as IL-4 have a direct injurious effect on the gastric mucosa[20]. Further, immune activation of T cells can affect the normal physiological function of the intestine, and in the stomach may alter acid secretion and motility[21-23].

It is evident that in *H. pylori*-associated gastritis there is accumulation of both CD4 and CD8 T cells in the lamina propria, and there is an increase in CD8 expressing IEL, including a possible increase in γδ T cell receptor (TcR)-expressing T cells[24,25]. Whether this is a deleterious response contributing to mucosal damage seen in some patients with *H. pylori* infection, or whether this aids in controlling the infection, is not clear. There is evidence to suggest an element of autoimmune reactivity in *H. pylori*-associated gastritis[26,27].

In the intestine mechanisms have evolved to control the vigour of the mucosal immune response to prevent inflammatory damage and autoimmunity. Early observations that oral immunization can lead to specific non-reactivity or oral tolerance have led to extensive investigation[28-30]. T cells in the intestinal mucosa are unique in phenotype and function when compared to peripheral T cells[31]. In part, this is related to the influence of the mucosal microenvironment including the gut flora on T cell differentiation and repertoire selection. It is now apparent that, in the mouse, mucosal T cells include a lineage that can develop independent of normal thymic influences and the epithelial environment plays an important role in this process[32-34]. The selection of the TcR repertoire of mucosal T cells involves mechanisms of deletion through programmed cell death and the induction of anergy[35-37]. It is probable that such mechanisms are involved in the induction and/or maintenance of the oral tolerance response in the intestine. The ability of gastric T cells to undergo similar processes within the gastric mucosa has not been examined. Overcoming the processes responsible for oral tolerance is a major obstacle impeding the design of oral vaccines.

NATURE OF THE IMMUNE RESPONSE IN THE STOMACH

The nature of the immune response to antigens presented to the stomach in humans is not well understood. In animal models antigen introduced into the stomach of a sensitized animal can lead to an increase in serum gastrin, suggesting that local immune activation can occur, and further that normal physiological functions are altered as a result[38]. Few studies have examined directly the B and T cell responses to protein antigens in the stomach.

The fact that local production of IgA to *H. pylori*-related antigens does suggest a local component to this immune response[39]. The factors controlling these responses include those derived from the organism directly, or result from the interaction between *H. pylori* and the epithelial cells lining the gastric mucosa. Therefore, factors that influence the adhesion of *H. pylori* to enterocytes such as the Lewis antigen-type glycoproteins may be important[40,41]. Such interactions lead to epithelial cell activation and the induction of intracellular second signals with changes in function and the induction of surface molecules that are involved in the immune response. Furthermore, it has been shown that bacterial interaction with epithelial cells in the intestine and the stomach leads to the induction of cytokine production. For example, *H. pylori* can induce IL-8 production, which is important in the recruitment of neutrophils and possibly monocytes[42,43]. Other cytokines such as TNFα, TGFβ or IL-6 are increased in the gastric mucosa of *H. pylori*-infected patients, and can influence the nature of the gastric T cell response[44-47]. It is possible that these interactions actually deflect the T cell response toward the Th1 response, which may not favour elimination of the organisms but contributes to tissue damage (discussed further in Chapter X by Dr P Ernst).

Studies examining the ability of *H. pylori* to cause inflammation and mucosal damage have shown that the *H. pylori* strains carrying the *cagA* gene tend to show greater virulence[48]. Further studies have led to the identification of a genetic locus in the cagA region that contains genes that may contribute to the pathogenic ability of the organism. This area has been called the 'pathogenicity island', and includes such genes as the *PicB* gene which directly increases IL-8 production by epithelial cells[49]. Therefore, *H. pylori* has evolved mechanisms that allow it to communicate with, and influence, the immune system and the nature of its response.

In humans, studies of antibody responses have demonstrated serum and gastric IgG and gastric IgA specific to *H. pylori* and antigenic components such as urease[50,51]. Since the immune response to most extracellular bacteria is an MHC Class II-restricted CD4 T cell response, it is to be expected that *H. pylori* would generate an antibody response that at a mucosal site would favour IgA production. The nature of the *H. pylori*-specific cellular immune response is not well understood, primarily because of the technical difficulty in obtaining sufficient numbers of lymphocytes for *in-vitro* functional studies. Immunohistochemical studies have shown changes in T cell subsets in both lamina propria and epithelium. Several groups have examined the proliferative response and IFNγ production from lymphocytes cultured from gastric biopsies, with conflicting and sometimes confusing results. In fact, several groups have suggested that *H. pylori*-positive patients had a smaller response to *H. pylori* antigen than patients who are *H. pylori*-negative[24,52-55]. This may be due to the fact that, in bulk cultures, peripheral blood proliferative responses to whole bacteria are not specific, while at the clonal level one can demonstrate disease-specific responses[24]. *In-situ* studies indicate that both TNFα and IFNγ production occurs in *H. pylori*-associated gastritis, suggesting a local Th1 type response[56]. *H. pylori* also appears to increase NK activity *in vitro*[57]. More information is emerging as new techniques such as intracellular cytokine detection by flow cytometry and quantitative PCR are being used to address these issues. At this time, however, there is little insight into the factors controlling these responses in humans.

HELICOBACTER FELIS-INDUCED IMMUNE RESPONSES IN MICE

Studies in animal models provide the unique opportunity to gain insight in the factors that may control the local immune response to *Helicobacter* infection. The best examples for this are the studies of the immune response to *H. felis* infection in the mouse[58-60]. The nature of this bacterium and the character of the gastric inflammation that can develop in mice indicates that this is an important model of the human disease. Infection with *H. felis* results in an inflammatory infiltrate in some mice, and on occasion can lead to the emergence of gastric lymphoid follicles containing B220[+] cells surrounded by CD4[+] T cells. The B cells found in these inflamed stomachs included IgM[+] and IgA[+] cells. Anti-*H. pylori* IgM and IgG can be detected in serum for up to 50 weeks[61,62]. IgA responses can also be detected, and may in fact be protective[63]. The cellular immune response to *H. felis* infection in the mouse has also been characterized recently in mice. In a well-designed study, two types of response were detected: the first a *Helicobacter*-independent response directed against urease and heat-shock proteins; and the second a *Helicobacter*-dependent response characterized by a Th1 type of cytokine responses with IFNγ production but with little IL-4 production[64]. The ability of antibody to IFNγ to inhibit the inflammatory changes that occurred in these mice supports the notion that the immune response can be responsible for some of the mucosal damage.

ROLE OF THE HOST IN *HELICOBACTER*-INDUCED IMMUNE RESPONSE

Studies of peptic ulcer disease, that preceded the identification of *H. pylori*, suggested a strong genetic component to the development of duodenal ulceration[65]. The knowledge that *H. pylori* is the cause of the majority of peptic ulcers forces us to re-examine this issue. Clearly the immune competence of the host influences the immune response and the associated gastritis. Immunocompromised patients infected with the HIV virus appear to have a decreased incidence of *H. pylori* infection and associated gastritis. This is not thought to be related to the use of antibiotics[66,67]. In the mouse, *H. pylori* infection of SCID mice leads to gastritis that does not appear to be different from that seen in immunocompetent strains, yet these mice do not develop invasive disease[68].

Comparison of different genetic strains of immunocompetent mice suggests that the genetic background plays an important role[69]. For example, Balb/c mice have a decreased intensity of inflammation and perhaps a less severe infection than C57Bl/6 mice. The exact cause for this is not known; however, it was pointed out by the authors of this study that these mice differ in the character of their T cell response to other infections. Balb/c mice tend to produce a Th2-type response (increase IL-4, IL-5) while the C57Bl/6 mouse tends to produce a Th1-predominant response with increases in IFNγ. How this relates to differences in inflammation, or in the ability of the two strains to eliminate the infection, is not clear. Interestingly, treating the C57Bl/6 mice with anti-IFNγ diminished the gastritis, but with no significant effect on the severity or persistence of *H. felis* infection[64].

ORAL IMMUNIZATION IN ANIMAL MODELS

In spite of the difficulty of spontaneously eliminating *Helicobacter* infection once established, several studies have now shown that mice can be immunized to prevent infection with *H. felis*. This has been done using either whole bacterium or antigenic components such as urease. However, the immunization is effective only if the antigen is given with a mucosal adjuvant such as cholera toxin or *E. coli* heat-labile enterotoxin[59,63,70,71]. More recently, mice have been infected with fresh isolates of *H. pylori*, leading to inflammation and epithelial damage. Vaccination of these mice with a mucosal adjuvant is also effective at preventing infection[72]. Therefore, under the appropriate circumstances, an effective and vigorous immune response to *Helicobacter* can be generated in the stomach.

Even more intriguing is the finding that, in mice infected with *H. felis*, immunization with urease B in the presence of cholera toxin can lead to elimination of the established infection[73]. Therefore, it is possible to use immunotherapy to treat established infection. It is evident that understanding the mechanism by which mucosal adjuvants augment the vigour of the immune response inducing the elimination of an established infection, and protecting against primary infection, is important. Cholera toxin and the heat-labile enterotoxin are known to be strong oral immunogens and adjuvants[74–76]. These proteins can break oral tolerance that normally occurs when protein antigen is presented to the gastrointestinal-associated lymphoid tissue[76,77]. Both the adjuvant activity and possibly the mechanism that breaks oral tolerance are related to the ability of these toxins to activate cAMP via ADP ribosylation of G proteins in target cells[78]. CT also inhibits CD8 T cells and decreases IEL numbers in the mouse intestine[79]. The mucosal adjuvant effect of CT occurs in mice lacking CD8 T cells, suggesting that the mechanisms of action are independent of CD8 T cells[80]. The enhancement of mucosal immune response by CT can include selective enhancement of Th2-type cytokines, at least with repetitive immunization[81]. It is possible that shifting the T cell response to a IL-4, IL-5 predominant profile is beneficial to establishing protective immunity via stimulating local IgA antibody responses. Alternatively, shifting the T cell response away from IL-2 and IFNγ may help prevent inflammation that could directly damage the gastric mucosa. This effect of CT on Th1/Th2 cytokine balance is controversial[78,80], and these hypotheses and speculations require further study.

CONCLUSION

Helicobacter infection of the stomach in human or mouse therefore represents an enigma in that there is persistent infection in the face of an apparent immune response and an associated inflammatory response. On the other hand, oral vaccination, at least with mucosal adjuvants, can prevent infection, and may even be effective in eliminating established infection. The fact that the absence of an immune response, such as occurs in patients with AIDS or in mice with genetically engineered immunodeficiency, does not lead to a more severe clinical infection with *Helicobacter*, suggests that there are several mechanisms that protect the host from this organism. Understanding the factors that control the immune response and lead to prevention or elimination of infection with *Helicobacter* is critical to the design of future treatments.

References

1. Croitoru K, Bienenstock J. Characteristics and functions of mucosa-associated lymphoid tissue. In: Ogra PL, Strober W, Mestecky J, McGhee JR, Lamm ME, Bienenstock J, editors. Handbook of mucosal immunology. San Diego: Academic Press; 1994:141–9.

2. Neutra MR, Kraehenbuhl J-P. The role of transepithelial transport by M cells in microbial invasion and host defence. J Cell Sci. 1993;106(Suppl. 17):209–15.
3. Owen RL, Jones AL. Epithelial cell specialization within human Peyer patches: an ultrastructural study of intestinal lymphoid follicles. Gastroenterology. 1974;66:189–203.
4. Murray PD, McKenzie DT, Swain SL, Kagnoff MF. Interleukin 5 and interleukin 4 produced by Peyer's patch T cells selectively enhance immunoglobulin A expression. J Immunol. 1987;139: 2669–74.
5. Weinstein PD, Cebra JJ. The preference for switching to IgA expression by Peyer's patch germinal center B cells is likely due to the intrinsic influence of their microenvironment. J Immunol. 1991; 147:4126–35.
6. Reynolds JD, Kennedy L, Peppard J, Pabst R. Ileal Peyer's patch emigrants are predominantly B cells and travel to all lymphoid tissues in sheep. Eur J Immunol. 1991;21:283–9.
7. Bienenstock J, McDermott M, Befus D, O'Neill M. A common mucosal immunologic system involving the bronchus, breast and bowel. Adv Exp Med Biol. 1978;107:53–9.
8. McDermott MR, Bienenstock J. Evidence for a common mucosal immunologic system. I. Migration of B immunoblasts into intestinal, respiratory, and genital tissues. J Immunol. 1979;122: 1892–8.
9. Engstrand L, Scheynius A, Påhlson C. An increased number of γ/δ T-cells and gastric epithelial cell expression of the groEL stress-protein homologue in *Helicobacter pylori*-associated chronic gastritis of the antrum. Am J Gastroenterol. 1991;86:976–80.
10. Hood CJ, Lesna M. Immunocytochemical quantitation of inflammatory cells associated with *Helicobacter pylori* infection. Br J Biomed Sci. 1993;50:82–8.
11. Trejdosiewicz LK, Calabrese A, Smart CJ et al. Gamma/d T cell receptor-positive cells of the human gastrointestinal mucosa: Occurrence and V region gene expression in *Helicobacter pylori*-associated gastritis, coeliac disease and inflammatory bowel disease. Clin Exp Immunol. 1991; 84:440–4.
12. Bland PW, Kambarage DM. Antigen handling by the epithelium and lamina propria macrophages. Gastroenterol Clin N Am. 1991;20:577–96.
13. Mayer L. The role of epithelial cells as accessory cells. Adv Exp Med Biol. 1987;216A:209–18.
14. Papadimitrou CS, Ioachim-Velogianni EE, Tsianos EB, Moutsopoulos HM. Epithelial HLA-DR expression and lymphocyte subsets in gastric mucosa in type B chronic gastritis. Virchows Arch[A]. 1988;413:197–204.
15. Wee A, Teh M, Kang JY. Association of *Helicobacter pylori* with HLA-DR antigen expression in gastritis. J Clin Pathol. 1992;45:30–3.
16. Hanson LÅ, Brandtzaeg P. The discovery of secretory IgA and the mucosal immune system. Immunol Today. 1993;14:416–17.
17. Underdown BJ, Schiff JM. Immunoglobin A: strategic defense initiative at the mucosal surface. Annu Rev Immunol. 1984;4:389–417.
18. Vajdy M, Koscos-Vilbois MH, Kopf M, Kohler G, Lycke N. Impaired mucosal immune responses in interleukin 4-targeted mice. J Exp Med. 1995;181:41–53.
19. Cebra JJ, Logan AC, Weinstein PD. The preference for switching to expression of the IgA isotype of antibody exhibited by B lymphocytes in Peyer's patches is likely due to intrinsic properties of their microenvironment. Immunol Res. 1991;10:393–5.
20. Rubin JT, Lotze MT. Acute gastric mucosal injury associated with the systemic administration of interleukin-4. Surgery. 1992;111:274–80.
21. Collins SM, Croitoru K. The pathophysiology of inflammatory bowel disease: The effect of inflammation on intestinal function. In: Targan S, Shanahan F, editors. Inflammatory bowel disease: from bench to bedside. Baltimore: Williams & Wilkins; 1993:194–209.
22. McKay DM, Perdue MH. Intestinal epithelial function: The case for immunophysiological regulation. Cells and mediators [first of two parts]. Dig Dis Sci. 1993;38:1377–87.
23. Muller MJ, Padol I, Ernst PB, Croitoru K, Hunt RH. Interferon-gamma inhibits secretagogue-mediated acid secretion in isolated murine gastric glands. Gastroenterology. 1993;104:A151 (abstract).
24. Di Tommaso A, Xiang Z, Bugnoli M et al. *Helicobacter pylori*-specific CD4+ T-cell clones from peripheral blood and gastric biopsies. Infect Immun. 1995;63:1102–6.
25. Valnes K, Huitfeldt HS, Brandtzaeg P. Relation between T cell number and epithelial HLA class II expression quantified by image analysis in normal and inflamed human gastric mucosa. Gut. 1990;31:647–52.
26. Macchia G, Massone A, Burroni D, Covacci A, Censini S, Rappuoli R. The Hsp60 protein of

Helicobacter pylori: structure and immune response in patients with gastroduodenal diseases. Mol Microbiol. 1993;9:645–52.

27. Negrini R, Lisato L, Zanella I *et al. Helicobacter pylori* infection induces antibodies cross-reacting with human gastric mucosa. Gastroenterology. 1991;101:437–45.

28. Brandtzaeg P. History of oral tolerance and mucosal immunity. Ann NY Acad Sci. 1996;778:1–27.

29. Husby S, Mestecky J, Moldoveanu Z, Holland S, Elson CO. Oral tolerance in humans: T cell but not B cell tolerance after antigen feeding. J Immunol. 1994;152:4663–70.

30. Mowat AM. The regulation of immune responses to dietary protein antigens. Immunol Today. 1987;8:93–8.

31. Croitoru K, Ernst PB. Leukocytes in the intestinal epithelium: an unusual immunological compartment revisited. Regional Immunol. 1992;4:63–9.

32. Guy-Grand D, Cerf-Bensussan N, Malissen B, Malassis-Seris M, Briottet C, Vassalli P. Two gut intraepithelial CD8⁺ lymphocyte populations with different T cell receptors: a role for the gut epithelium in T cell differentiation. J Exp Med. 1991;173:471–81.

33. Lefrançois L. Extrathymic differentiation of intraepithelial lymphocytes: generation of a separate and unequal T-cell repertoire. Immunol Today. 1991;12:436–8.

34. Maric D, Kaiserlian D, Croitoru K. A murine intestinal epithelial cell line can induce *in vitro* T cell differentiation from T cell-depleted bone marrow. Cell Immunol. 1996 (In press).

35. Barrett TA, Tatsumi Y, Bluestone JA. Tolerance of T cell receptor γ/δ cells in the intestine. J Exp Med. 1993;177:1755–62.

36. Gramzinski RA, Adams E, Gross JA, Goodman TG, Allison JP, Lefrançois L. T cell receptor-triggered activation of intraepithelial lymphocytes *in vitro*. Int Immunol. 1993;5:145–53.

37. Croitoru K, Bienenstock J, Ernst PB. Phenotypic and functional assessment of intraepithelial lymphocytes bearing a 'forbidden' α/β T cell receptor. Int Immunol. 1994;6:1467–73.

38. Kramling HJ, Enders G, Teichmann RK, Demmel T, Merkle R, Brendel W. Antigen-induced gastrin release: an immunologic mechanism of gastric antral mucosa. Adv Exp Med Biol. 1987; 216A:427–9.

39. Crabtree JE, Taylor JD, Wyatt JI *et al.* Mucosal IgA recognition of *Helicobacter pylori* 120 kDa protein, peptic ulceration and gastric pathology. Lancet. 1991;338:332–5.

40. Boren T, Falk P, Roth KA, Larson G, Normak S. Attachment of *Helicobacter pylori* to human gastric epithelium mediated by blood group antigens. Science. 1993;262:1892–5.

41. Smoot DT, Resau JH, Naab T *et al.* Adherence of *Helicobacter pylori* to cultured human gastric epithelial cells. Infect Immun. 1993;61:350–5.

42. Crabtree JE, Covacci A, Farmery SM *et al. Helicobacter pylori*-induced interleukin-8 expression in gastric epithelial cells is associated with CagA positive phenotype. J Clin Pathol. 1995;48: 41–5.

43. Crowe SE, Alvarez L, Dytoc M *et al.* Expression of interleukin 8 and CD54 by human gastric epithelium after *Helicobacter pylori* infection *in vitro*. Gastroenterology. 1995;108:65–74.

44. Crabtree JE, Shallcross TM, Heatley RV, Wyatt JI. Mucosal tumour necrosis factor α and interleukin-6 in patients with *Helicobacter pylori* associated gastritis. Gut. 1991;32:1473–7.

45. Fan X-G, Chua A, Fan X-J, Keeling PWN. Increased gastric production of interleukin-8 and tumour necrosis factor in patients with *Helicobacter pylori* infection. J Clin Pathol. 1995;48: 133–6.

46. Gionchetti P, Vaira D, Campieri M *et al.* Enhanced mucosal interleukin-6 and -8 in *Helicobacter pylori*-positive dyspeptic patients. Am J Gastroenterol. 1994;89:883–7.

47. Noach LA, Bosma NB, Jansen J, Hoek FJ, Van Deventer SJH, Tytgat GNJ. Mucosal tumor necrosis factor-a, interleukin-1b, and interleukin-8 production in patients with *Helicobacter pylori* infection. Scand J Gastroenterol. 1994;29:425–9.

48. Peek RM Jr, Miller GG, Tham KT *et al.* Heightened inflammatory response and cytokine expression *in vivo* to cagA⁺ *Helicobacter pylori* strains. Lab Invest. 1995;73:760–70.

49. Tummuru MKR, Sharma SA, Blaser MJ. *Helicobacter pylori* picB, a homologue of the *Bordetella pertussis* toxin secretion protein, is required for induction of IL-8 in gastric epithelial cells. Mol Microbiol. 1995;18:867–76.

50. Cover TL, Cao P, Murthy UK, Sipple MS, Blaser MJ. Serum neutralizing antibody response to the vacuolating cytotoxin of *Helicobacter pylori*. J Clin Invest. 1992;90:913–18.

51. Perez-Perez GI, Dworkin BM, Chodos JE, Blaser MJ. *Campylobacter pylori* antibodies in humans. Ann Intern Med. 1988;109:11–17.

52. Tosi MF, Sorensen RU, Czinn SJ. Cell-mediated immune responsiveness to *Helicobacter pylori*

165

in healthy seropositive and seronegative adults. Immunol Infect Dis. 1992;2:133.

53. Karttunen R. Blood lymphocyte proliferation, cytokine secretion and appearance of T cells with activation surface markers in cultures with *Helicobacter pylori*. Comparison of the responses of subjects with and without antibodies to *H. pylori*. Clin Exp Immunol. 1991;83:396–400.
54. Sharma SA, Miller GG, Perez-Perez GI, Gupta RS, Blaser MJ. Humoral and cellular immune recognition of *Helicobacter pylori* proteins are not concordant. Clin Exp Immunol. 1994;97:126–32.
55. Fan XJ, Chua A, Shahi CN, McDevitt J, Keeling PW, Kelleher D. Gastric T lymphocyte responses to *Helicobacter pylori* in patients with *H. pylori* colonisation. Gut. 1994;35:1379–84.
56. Karttunen R, Karttunen T, Ekre HP, MacDonald TT. Interferon gamma and interleukin 4 secreting cells in the gastric antrum in *Helicobacter pylori* positive and negative gastritis. Gut. 1995;36:341–5.
57. Tarkkanen J, Kosunen TU, Saksela E. Contact of lymphocytes with *Helicobacter pylori* augments natural killer cell activity and induces production of gamma interferon. Infect Immun. 1993;61:3012–16.
58. Karita M, Kouchiyama T, Okita K, Nakzawa T. New small animal model of human gastric *Helicobacter pylori* infection: success in both nude and euthymic mice. Am J Gastroenterol. 1991;86:1596.
59. Michetti P, Corthésy-Theulaz I, Davin C et al. Immunization of BALB/c mice against *Helicobacter felis* infection with *Helicobacter pylori* urease. Gastroenterology. 1994;107:1002–11.
60. Enno A, O'Rourke JL, Howlett CR, Jack A, Dixon MF, Lee A. MALToma-like lesions in the murine gastric mucosa after long-term infection with *Helicobacter felis*: a mouse model of *Helicobacter pylori*-induced gastric lymphoma. Am J Pathol. 1995;147:217–22.
61. Lee A, Fox JG, Otto G, Murphy J. A small animal model of human *Helicobacter pylori* active chronic gastritis. Gastroenterology. 1990;99:1315.
62. Fox JG, Blanco M, Murphy JC et al. Local and systemic immune responses in murine *Helicobacter felis* active chronic gastritis. Infect Immun. 1993;61:2309–15.
63. Lee CK, Weltzin R, Thomas WD Jr et al. Oral immunization with recombinant *Helicobacter pylori* urease induces secretory IgA antibodies and protects mice from challenge with *Helicobacter felis*. J Infect Dis. 1995;172:161–72.
64. Mohammadi M, Czinn S, Redline R, Nedrud J. *Helicobacter*-specific cell-mediated immune responses display a predominant Th1 phenotype and promote a delayer-type hypersensitivity response in the stomachs of mice. J Immunol. 1996;156:4729–38.
65. Rotter JI, Sones JQ, Samloff IM et al. Duodenal-ulcer disease associated with elevated serum pepsinogen I: an inherited autosomal dominant disorder. N Engl J Med. 1979;300:63–6.
66. Blecker U, Keymolen K, Levy J, Vandenplas Y. Low prevalence of *Helicobacter pylori* in the acquired immunodeficiency syndrome. Am J Gastroenterol. 1993;88:1294.
67. Edwards PD, Carrick J, Turner J, Lee A, Mitchell H, Cooper DA. *Helicobacter pylori*-associated gastritis is rare in AIDS: antibiotic effect or a consequence of immunodeficiency? Am J Gastroenterol. 1991;86:1761–4.
68. Blanchard TG, Czinn SJ, Nedrud JG, Redline RW. *Helicobacter*-associated gastritis in SCID mice. Infect Immun. 1995;63:1113–15.
69. Mohammadi M, Redline R, Nedrud J, Czinn S. Role of the host in pathogenesis of *Helicobacter*-associated gastritis: *H. felis* infection of inbred and congenic mouse strains. Infect Immun. 1996;64:238–45.
70. Chen M, Lee A, Hazell S. Immunization against gastric helicobacter infection in a mouse/*Helicobacter felis* model. Lancet. 1992;339:1120–1 (letter).
71. Czinn SJ, Nedrud JG. Oral immunization against *Helicobacter pylori*. Infect Immun. 1991;59:2359–63.
72. Marchetti M, Arico B, Burroni D, Figura N, Rappuoli R, Ghiara P. Development of a mouse model of *Helicobacter pylori* infection that mimics human disease. Science. 1995;267:1655–8.
73. Corthésy-Theulaz I, Porta N, Glauser M et al. Oral immunization with *Helicobacter pylori* urease B subunit as a treatment against *Helicobacter* infection in mice. Gastroenterology. 1995;109:115–21.
74. Holmgren J, Lycke N, Czerkinsky C. Cholera toxin and cholera B subunit as oral-mucosal adjuvant and antigen vector systems. Vaccine. 1993;11:1179–84.
75. Lycke N, Holmgen J. Strong adjuvant properties of cholera toxin on gut mucosal immune responses to orally presented antigens. Immunology. 1986;59:301–8.
76. Clements JD, Hartzog NM, Lyon FL. Adjuvant activity of *Escherichia coli* heat-labile enterotoxin

and effect on the induction of oral tolerance in mice to unrelated protein antigens. Vaccine. 1988; 6:269–77.

77. Elson CO, Ealding W. Cholera toxin feeding did not induce oral tolerance in mice and abrogated oral tolerance to an unrelated protein antigen. J Immunol. 1984:133:2892–7.

78. Snider DP. The mucosal adjuvant activities of ADP-ribosylating bacterial enterotoxins. Crit Rev Immunol. 1995;15:317–48.

79. Elson CO, Holland SP, Dertzbaugh MT, Cuff CF, Anderson AO. Morphological and functional alterations of mucosal T cells by cholera toxin and its B subunit. J Immunol. 1995;154:1032–40.

80. Hörnquist E, Grdic KD, Mak T, Lycke N. CD8-deficient mice exhibit augmented mucosal immune responses and intact adjuvant effects to cholera toxin. Immunology. 1996;87:220–9.

81. Xu-Amano J, Kiyono H, Jackson RJ *et al*. Helper T cell subsets for immunoglobulin A responses: oral immunization with tetanus toxoid and cholera toxin as adjuvant selectively induces Th2 cells in mucosa associated tissues. J Exp Med. 1993;178:1309–20.

17
Theories of vaccination for *Helicobacter pylori*

W. F. DOE

INTRODUCTION

Successful eradication of *Helicobacter pylori* infection leading to cure of peptic ulceration has led to intensive antimicrobical therapy involving combinations of antibiotics on a very large scale. However, the failures of chemotherapy due to compliance, cost, development of resistant organisms, the very high global prevalence of *H. pylori* infection, and its association with gastric malignancy provide a compelling case for considering other preventive strategies. Recent insights into the nature of antigen uptake by mucosal surfaces and recognition by T cells have suggested new strategies for antigen delivery by oral vaccines, for overcoming oral tolerance and for enhancing mucosal immune responses. The concept of developing an oral vaccine to prevent *H. pylori* infection in humans however, poses several questions. Why doesn't the readily detected antibody response found in infected patients kill the organism? Why doesn't previous infection protect against reinfection? Given the finding that *H. pylori* infection occurs in infancy or early childhood in developing countries, will immunization of already-infected populations provide any therapeutic benefit? Are there concerns about the ability of *H. pylori* vaccines to eliminate all the *Helicobacter* strains?

WHY DEVELOP AN ORAL VACCINE?

The success of the live attenuated Sabin oral polio vaccine in protecting the host from infection, its capacity to induce both mucosal and systemic responses and to prevent the carrier state gave a powerful impetus to the development of oral vaccines[1]. Moreover, the high prevalence of *H. pylori* in developing countries demands a vaccine delivery system characterized by ease of mass administration, low costs, freedom from the public health risks associated with parenteral immunization and a vaccine that can cure, as well as protect, the host from *H. pylori* infection and its sequelae.

Mucosal immunity generates antigen-specific IgA antibodies highly adapted to function at the mucosal surface due to a peptide called secretory piece that protects dimeric IgA from proteolysis in the lumen of the gastrointestinal tract (GIT). Secretory IgA neutralizes viruses, prevents bacterial adherence and forms immune complexes with soluble protein antigens without activating the complement system. Particulate antigens, especially microorganisms, induce Th1 mucosal immune responses leading to cell-mediated immunity and to the generation of effector T cells.

Oral administration of proteins, however, can lead to systemic immunological hyporesponsiveness, a phenomenon called oral tolerance. While the development of systemic unresponsiveness to antigens present in the GIT provides protection for the host, it represents a significant barrier to oral immunization using proteins. This barrier, together with the need to protect the antigens from the low pH and proteolysis in the GIT, have made oral vaccines the most challenging route of vaccination against infectious microorganisms[2].

INEFFECTUAL NATURAL IMMUNITY TO *H. PYLORI*

Although serum antibodies to *H. pylori* epitopes are readily detectable in infected patients, the natural immune response appears unable to eradicate the organism[3]. In humans about 50% of those infected have no detectable serum antibody to urease, and less than 5% have serum IgA antibody. Salivary sIgA antibody is only sometimes detectable and *H. pylori* antibody-secreting cells are rare in the gastric mucosa. Studies of the gastric mucosal immune response to *H. felis* infection suggest that there is suppression of the Th2 response with low levels of specific sIgA-neutralizing antibodies in gastric juice[4]. Active and passive oral immunization of mice using sIgA-neutralizing antibodies is highly protective of germ-free mice exposed to *H. felis* infection[5] and mucosal immunization is ineffective in IL-4-deficient mice, indicating that the generation of Th2 immune responses is necessary for successful protection by oral vaccines against *Helicobacter* organisms[6]. In mice vaccinated by recombinant *H. pylori* urease particles and adjuvant, protection against virulent *H. felis* challenge correlated with the levels of specific faecal sIgA antibodies against urease[7].

The reasons for the apparent suppression of Th2 responses in the gastric mucosa are not clear. The unique ecological niche of *H. pylori* organisms adherent to gastric epithelial cells but rarely invading the epithelium, the relative lack of organized lymphoid tissue structures in the stomach, possible molecular mimicry involving shared epitopes with those present in the inflamed gastric mucosa such as hsp 60[8] and antigenic drift may contribute to the inability of natural immunity to eliminate the infection.

STRATEGIES FOR ORAL IMMUNIZATION

To date the success of oral *Helicobacter* vaccines has depended upon the use of immunological adjuvants to provide a mechanism for antigen persistence in the mucosa and enhancing the immune response to *H. pylori* immunogens by prolonging their release and their interaction with antigen-presenting cells. Some adjuvants also activate macrophages to release interleukin-1 (IL-1) which, combined with antigen, induce IL-2 release by T cells resulting in the generation of mediators that activate effector T cells (cell-mediated immunity) or antibody-forming B cells. Most of the successful oral vaccines for *Helicobacter* to date have used cholera toxin (CT), its B subunit or the heat-labile toxin (LT) of *E. coli*, which are closely similar molecules, as adjuvants. Both provide powerful adjuvant effects because CT-B binds to the ganglioside, GM_1, that is abundantly expressed on the surface of gastrointestinal epithelial cells, where LT binds to both GM_1 and GM_2. Both CT and LT are also highly immunogenic, carrying both the B and T cell epitopes required to elicit systemic immunity. Given orally, they may alter the regulatory environment of the gut-associated lymphoid tissue from overall suppression to responsiveness[9]. Only alum, however, is approved for use in humans, but it is not always effective, cannot be lyophilized and requires refrigerated storage[10]. There is a pressing need, therefore, to develop an effective non-toxic adjuvant for human use.

One approach to this requirement for oral immunization has been to use antigen delivery systems that have adjuvant properties such as liposomes or immune stimulating complexes (ISCOMs). Liposomes, vesicles comprising concentric bilayer membranes of phospholipids and other polar molecules that trap water and solutes, have been widely used in animals to deliver peptides successfully as oral vaccines. The liposome vesicle protects the peptide from luminal digestion and also acts as an immunological adjuvant to generate strong mucosal sIgA antibody responses to poorly immunogenic peptides, to overcome oral tolerance and to stimulate cell-mediated immunity[10]. Another established antigen carrier system with adjuvant properties is the ISCOM, which is a cage-like particle that forms spontaneously on mixing cholesterol and saponin, allowing the incorporation of proteins and phospholipids. Used as oral vaccine carriers, the mucosal adjuvant properties of ISCOMs provoke strong mucosal secretory antibody and cell-mediated immune responses to protein antigens[11,12].

The novel concept of introducing the naked DNA of the gene sequence for an antigen of interest incorporated into a non-replicating plasmid as a vaccine using direct injection of DNA or DNA-coated particle bombardment on the skin or the mucosa, has attracted great interest[13]. Naked DNA vaccines offer a radically new approach for the prevention of infectious disease that are potentially suitable for mass immunization in developing countries. DNA is very stable and is readily prepared on a large scale at high purity, providing the flexibility needed for working with a vaccine in impoverished areas of the world. The technology may be relevant to future development of *H. pylori* vaccines. To date the major mucosal immunization experiments have involved DNA vaccines for influenza using intranasal injection of a haemagglutinin DNA vaccine to produce protective immunization of mice against lethal challenge with live influenza virus[14]. The potential safety issues have not so far proven a problem in animal experiments. Neither the concerns over the potential integration of plasmid DNA into chromosomes nor concerns about the generation of anti-DNA antibodies has been realized.

Another exciting solution to the mass production of affordable oral vaccines suitable for use in the Third World on a large scale for *H. pylori* immunization is the development of genetically engineered plants. Initial success with oral immunization using transgenic plants suggests that it may be possible to build

Table 1   *H. pylori* immunogens

Generic	Virulence factors
Urease	CagA
Flagellum	VacA
Sod	IceA1
hsp 60	
Adhesin	

the vaccines into plants that are eaten as part of the normal diet[15]. There is the prospect of developing edible vaccines as transgenic plants grown domestically in developing countries. For example, potato tubers that have been genetically engineered to express the B subunit of the *E. coli* heat-labile exterotoxin (LT-B) gene have been fed to mice. The mice developed specific mucosal IgA antibodies that neutralized the enterotoxin in cell protection assays[16]. Bananas, the world's fourth most important food crop, also recently have been genetically engineered to provide another potential edible vaccine, possibly suitable for early oral immunization of children against *H. pylori*[15]. This early success using LT-B as an immunogen relates to its highly immunogenic nature and to its adjuvant properties. Future transgenic plant vaccines will need to introduce an adjuvant sequence and possibly interleukin (IL-6) as part of the transgene to ensure coexpression with the immunogen so as to enhance the mucosal sIgA response. Coexpression of IL-6 to augment primary mucosal IgA responses has been successful in enhancing mouse mucosal responses to influenza immunization using a live fowlpox virus as vector[17]. This strategy may also be applicable to the current generation of candidate *Helicobacter* vaccines and to edible vaccines involving transgenic plants.

WHAT IS THE OBJECTIVE OF AN ORAL VACCINE?

The design of an optimal oral vaccine for *H. pylori* requires responses to several of the questions posed in the introduction. If the purpose of the vaccine is to eliminate all strains of *H. pylori* organisms, the immunogens used must include one or more of the generic epitopes (Table 1). However, the global prevalence of *H. pylori*, its low morbidity, the evidence for its extraordinary 'success' as a persistent chronic gastric infection suggest that some benefits may accrue to the host at least from non-pathogenic infection such as that seen with the Type II strain. There may be a balanced polymorphism. Little is known, as yet, about the epidemiology of the pathogenic and non-pathogenic strains, and more research is needed to determine whether there are *H. pylori* strains that are symbiotic. In these circumstances the current developments of *H. pylori* vaccines for clinical use should focus on immunogens that are virulence factors. At least three of these factors are under active study for use in oral vaccines (Table 1).

THERAPEUTIC VACCINES

The progress in developing oral *Helicobacter* vaccines is discussed in Chapter 18. One aspect relevant to this chapter, however, is not only the question whether

Table 2 Therapeutic *Helicobacter* vaccination

Vaccine	Model	Weeks post-vaccine	Percentage cure	Reference
H. pylori urea-B	Mice	8	57	Corthesy-Theulaz et al.[19]
H. felis sonicate	Mice	12	94	Doidge et al.[20]
H. pylori urease	Ferrets	6	33	Cuenca et al.[21]

Helicobacter vaccines will protect naive hosts from subsequent exposure, but will oral vaccines also eliminate *H. pylori* from the stomach of people who are already infected? Given the very high prevalence of *H. pylori*, and the evidence that infection in the Third World develops in infancy, this question is important to the concept, expectations and use of oral vaccines for *H. pylori*.

In Gambia, where *H. pylori* infection is ubiquitous, most children are infected before the age of 5 years. Infants breast-fed for their first 2 years of life are protected against *H. pylori* infection if their mothers' breast milk contains significant levels of specific IgA antibody. All infants infected by 9 months of age were breast-fed by mothers whose milk contained very low titres of *H. pylori* antibody[18]. In developing countries, therefore, it is highly likely that an oral vaccine must be both therapeutic and protective if it is to be effective. Table 2 shows some of the preliminary evidence in experimental models to suggest that oral vaccines can both eliminate existing *H. pylori* infection and protect against subsequent reinfection[19–21]. However, these experiments have so far been conducted for brief periods of up to 3 months, and involve elimination of recent infection of *H. felis* in mice. Further research is needed into the duration of the therapeutic and protective effects. Moreover, it is not yet known whether an oral *Helicobacter* vaccine can eliminate *Helicobacter* organisms from the mucosal lesion of chronic gastritis.

CONCLUSION

The future of oral vaccination for *H. pylori* appears full of promise. Among the immediate concerns are the need to develop the non-toxic adjuvants that are essential to augment mucosal immune responses to the present generation of candidate vaccines. The question of directing vaccines at all *H. pylori* strains by using generic *Helicobacter* immunogens, or only at virulence factors, remains unresolved. Developments in molecular cell biology offer many new approaches to oral subunit vaccines, including novel carrier and targeting systems and the radically new opportunities presented by naked DNA vaccines and transgenic plant vaccines as part of the diet. The widespread use of oral vaccines providing both therapy and protection against *H. pylori* and suitable for mass administration in countries with almost 100% prevalence is a realistic future prospect.

References

1. Ogra PL, Karzon DT. Distribution of poliovirus antibody in serum, nasopharynx and alimentary tract following segmental immunization of lower alimentary tract with poliovaccine. J Immunol. 1969;102:1423–30.

2. Staats HF, Jackson RJ, Marinaro M, Takahashi I, Kiyono H, McGhee JR. Mucosal immunity to infection with implications for vaccine development. Curr Opin Immunol. 1994;6:572–83.

3. Jaskiewicz K, Loow JA, Marks IN. Local cellular and immune response by antral mucosa in patients undergoing treatment for eradication of *Helicobacter pylori*. Dig Dis Sci. 1993;38:937–43.

4. Blaser MJ. Hypothesis on the pathogenesis and natural history of *Helicobacter pylori*-induced inflammation. Gastroenterology. 1992;102:720–7.

5. Czinn SJ, Cai A, Nedrud JG. Protection of germ-free mice from infection by *Helicobacter felis* after active oral or passive IgA immunization. Vaccine. 1993;11:636–42.

6. Radcliff FJ, Ramsay AJ, Lee A. Failure of immunisation against *Helicobacter* infection in IL-4 deficient mice: evidence for a TH2 immune response as the basis for protective immunity. Gastroenterology. 1995;939:A3754.

7. Lee CK, Weltzin R, Thomas WD Jr *et al*. Oral immunization with recombinant *Helicobacter pylori* urease induces secretory IgA antibodies and protects mice from challenge with *Helicobacter felis*. J Infect Dis. 1995;172:161–72.

8. Goodwin S. *Helicobacters* shed new light on chaperonins. Lancet. 1995;346:653–5.

9. Dertzbaugh MT, Elson CO. Cholera toxin as a mucosal adjuvant. Topics Vaccine Adjuvant Res. 1991;11:119–31.

10. Gregoriadis G. Immunological adjuvants: a role for liposomes. Immunol Today. 1990;11:89–90.

11. Mowat A McI, Donachie AM. ISCOMS – a novel strategy for mucosal immunization? Immunol Today. 1991;12:383–5.

12. Mowat A McI, Maloy KJ, Donachie AM. Immune-stimulating complexes as adjuvants for inducing local and systemic immunity after oral immunization with protein antigens. Immunology. 1993;80:527–34.

13. Pardoll DM, Beckerieg AM. Exposing the immunology of naked DNA vaccines. Immunology. 1995;3:165–9.

14. Fynan EF, Webster RG, Fuller DH, Haynes JR, Santoro JC, Robinson HL. DNA vaccines: protective immunizations by parenteral, mucosal, and gene-gun inoculations. Proc Natl Acad Sci. 1993;90:11478–82.

15. Moffat AS. Exploring transgenic plants as a new vaccine source. Science. 1995;268:658–60.

16. Haq TA, Mason HS, Clements JD, Arntzen CJ. Oral immunization with a recombinant bacterial antigen produced in transgenic plants. Science. 1995;268:714–16.

17. Leong KH, Ramsay AJ, Boyle DB, Ramshaw IA. Selective induction of immune responses by cytokines coexpressed in recombinant fowlpox virus. J Virol. 1994;8125–30.

18. Thomas JE, Austin S, Dale A *et al*. Protection by human milk IgA against *Helicobacter pylori* infection in infancy. Lancet. 1993;342:121.

19. Corthesy-Theulaz I, Porta N, Glauser M *et al*. Oral immunization with *Helicobacter pylori* urease B subunit as a treatment against *Helicobacter* infection in mice. Gastroenterology. 1995;109:115–21.

20. Doidge C, Gust I, Lee A, Buck F, Hazell S, Manne U. Therapeutic immunisation against *Helicobacter* infection. Lancet. 1994;343:914–15.

21. Cuenca R, Blanchard T, Lee C *et al*. Therapeutic immunization against *Helicobacter mustelae* infection in naturally infected ferrets. Gastroenterology. 1995;108:A78.

18
Vaccines for the treatment and prevention of *Helicobacter pylori* infection

I. CORTHÉSY-THEULAZ, A. L. BLUM and J.-P. KRAEHENBUHL

INTRODUCTION

An immunological approach or a vaccine approach to clear chronic *Helicobacter pylori* infection was initially rejected by many investigators and clinicians, based on the observation that natural immunity was unable to cure or prevent *Helicobacter* infection and chronic atrophic gastritis. Recent animal studies, however, have established that immunization with *Helicobacter* whole cell extracts or purified components is efficient for the prevention of infection, and more importantly for the treatment of pre-existing infections. Therefore there is now considerable interest in the design of *Helicobacter* vaccines, which represent a promising alternative to conventional therapies, in which bad compliance and antibiotic resistance represent serious drawbacks[1].

Novel animal models (for review see ref. 2), in which *H. pylori* infection mimics the lesions seen in infected human stomachs[3–7], allowed the safety and efficacy of several candidate vaccines to be tested[8–13]. The immune effectors which mediate cure and/or prevention, however, have not been identified; nor is it understood how *Helicobacter* escapes the host immune system. The aim of this review is to evaluate critically the state of the art in *H. pylori* vaccination, and to summarize our current understanding of the immunological mechanisms mediating protection/treatment following vaccination.

VACCINE CANDIDATES

Several vaccines, including whole cell bacterial preparations, purified components, or recombinant proteins, have been tested with respect to tolerance and efficacy (Table 1) and some are in clinical trials. We shall describe briefly the properties of each candidate vaccine and outline its advantages and problems.

Table 1

Protective Immunogens

Antigen used for immunization	Animal model	Pathogen	
Whole cell extract ⟹	Mouse ⟹	*H. felis*	Chen et al 1992[9] Czinn et al 1993[8]
	⟹ Mouse	⟹ *H. felis*	Michetti et al 1994[10] Ferrero et al 1994[19] Lee et al 1995[20]
Urease		⟹ *H. pylori*	Marchetti et al 1995[13]
	⟹ Ferret ⟹	*H. mustelae*	Monath et al and results
HspA ⟹	Mouse ⟹	*H. felis*	Ferrero et al 1995[12]
Cytotoxin ⟹	Mouse ⟹	*H. pylori* cag+	Marchetti et al 1995[13]

Whole cell vaccines

Whole cell bacterial preparations, inactivated by sonication, were the first vaccines tested to show protection[8,14]. More recently oral immunization with whole cell preparations was shown to cure *Helicobacter* infection in mice[15]. Lipopoly-saccharides (LPS) of *H. pylori* express Lewis y, Lewis x and Lewis H type I blood group structures similar to those commonly found in gastric mucosa[16], which trigger in mice and humans cross-reactive antibodies[17]. When Lewis-specific monoclonal antibodies were injected into mice, they induced lesions similar to those seen in *Helicobacter* infection, suggesting a potential role of molecular mimicry for *H. pylori* LPS in autoimmunity. Therefore, there is a potential risk that vaccination with whole cell preparations can trigger auto-immunity in humans. This explains why major efforts have been directed towards the identification of *H. pylori* antigens as candidate vaccines.

Urease

Urease, a ~550 kDa hexameric molecule composed of two subunits (27 kDa UreA and 62 kDa UreB estimated from the amino-acid sequence), plays an essential role both in infection and the development of gastritis. The urease operon consists of nine accessory genes necessary for the proper assembly and function of the enzyme[18]. Immunization of mice with native or recombinant apoenzyme (structural A and B subunits), or UreB subunit in conjunction with a mucosal adjuvant pre-vented[10,19,20] or cured[11] *Helicobacter* infection. Recently we have shown that deleting the first 220 amino acids of the UreB subunit does not alter its protective or therapeutic potential, while removing the first 360 amino acids abolished protective activity[21]. Because of the high sequence conservation in all ureases[18], it is likely that these proteins adopt a similar tridimensional structure. The primary structure of *H. pylori* UreB, and part of that of UreA, was aligned on the crystal structure of *Klebsiella aerogenes* urease by Dr Manuel Peitsch (Glaxo, Geneva, Switzerland) and the UreB fragment that confers protection was mapped (Figure 1). This will facilitate the identification of the protective epitopes associated with UreB.

The safety of the enzymatically inactive recombinant urease has already been tested in *H. pylori*-infected adult volunteers in a double-blind, placebo-controlled phase I clinical trial[22]. Oral administration of urease was well tolerated by *H. pylori*-infected asymptomatic adults, and did not change the course of the infection as expected due to the absence of a mucosal adjuvant. A phase II trial to monitor the safety and efficacy of recombinant urease in the presence of *E. coli* heat-labile enterotoxin (LT) is under way (P. Michetti and T. Monath, unpublished data).

VacA

An ~87 kDa toxin (VacA) that induces vacuolization in several gastric cell lines is not expressed in all *H. pylori* isolates, although the gene is present in all *H. pylori* strains[23]. Cytotoxic activity is more prevalent in isolates from patients with peptic ulcers[24]. Orogastric immunization with purified *H. pylori* VacA, together with LT, protected mice against infection by CagA+ *H. pylori* strains[13]. Although cytotoxin produced in *E. coli* retained antigenicity, the recombinant protein appeared unable to prevent *H. pylori* infection in mice (P. Ghiara, meeting communication). VacA-based vaccines will not cure or prevent infection with CagA⁻ strains which retain their oncogenic potential.

Chaperones

Chaperones are conserved proteins that contribute to the proper folding of proteins and their assembly into oligomeric structures. They also bind to cellular proteins and protect them against denaturation during stress conditions. Two chaperones, HspA and HspB (heat-shock proteins) homologous to GroES and GroEL, respectively, have been identified in *H. pylori*[25]. HspA is involved in the oligomerization of urease. Recombinant *H. pylori* HspA was shown to confer protective immunity in the *H. felis* mouse model[12]. Combining *H. pylori* HspA and UreB with cholera toxin protected mice as efficiently as whole cell preparations. The use of heat-shock proteins, however, as vaccine candidates could induce adverse autoimmune reactions due to the high degree of conservation among the members of the heat-shock family, and to the expression of *H. pylori* chaperones in gastric epithelial cells[26]. Autoimmunity, however, has not been documented in animals immunized with HspA.

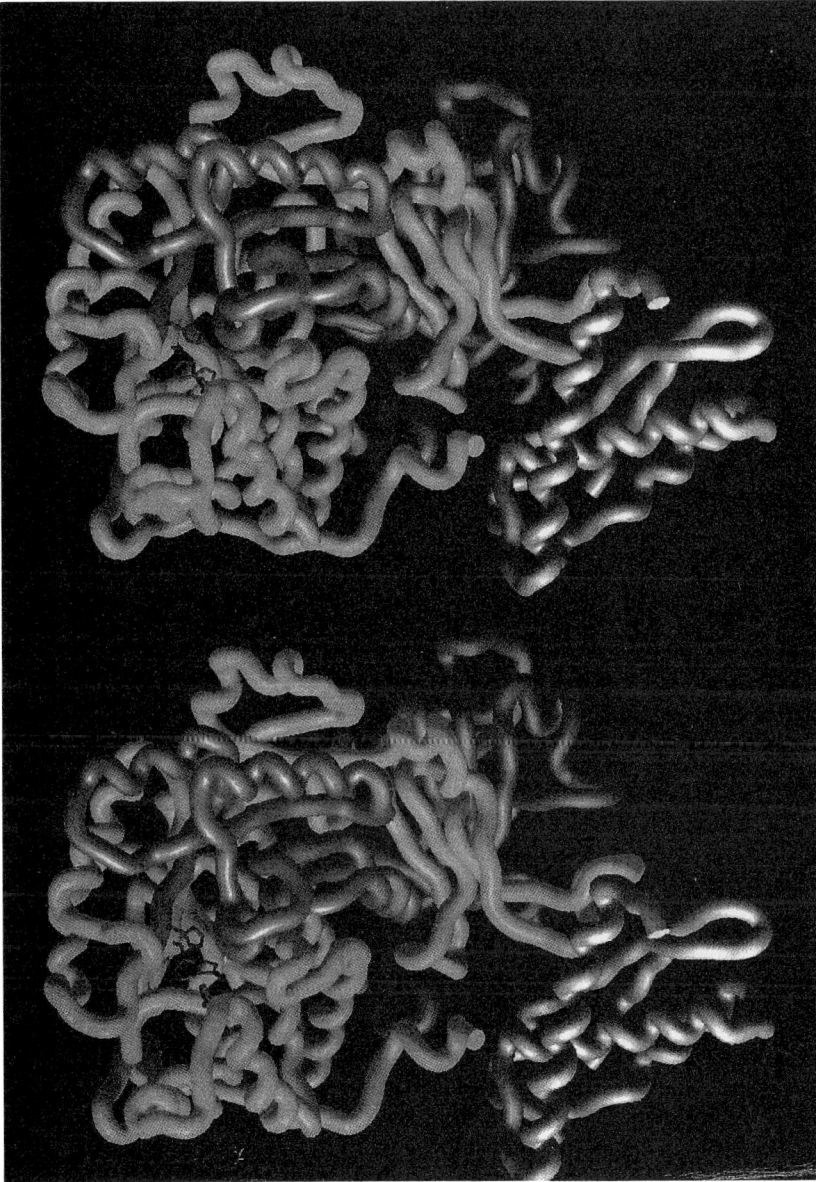

Figure 1 Stereo view of *H. pylori* urease B subunit. The three-dimensional structure of the UreB based on the experimentally obtained atomic coordinates of *Klebsiella aerogenes* urease was established by Dr Manuel Petisch, Glaxo, Geneva, Switzerland. In mid-grey the structure of UreB; in dark grey the fragment that confers protection when used as immunogens with cholera toxin, and in light grey part of the UreA subunit. The histidine residues that are involved in nickel binding are shown as thin structures

Table 2

Therapeutic Immunogens

Pathogen	Animal model	Antigen used for immunization	
H. felis	Mouse	Whole cell extract	Doidge et al 1994[15]
H. felis	Mouse	Urease	Corthésy-Theulaz et al 1995[11]
H. pylori	Mouse	Urease	Kleanthous et al 1995[52]
H. mustelae	Ferret	Urease	Cuenca et al 1995[38]
H. pylori	Cat	Urease	Batchelder et al 1996[37]

Novel vaccine candidates

Surface proteins, such as adhesins, or exported virulence factors, may represent alternatives to the existing vaccines. For instance, an 18 kDa *H. felis* outer membrane protein has recently been shown to confer protection against bacterial challenge[27]. Cloning strategies to selectively identify surface-exposed or secreted proteins have been developed that should facilitate the identification of novel vaccine candidates[28].

ROUTE AND ADMINISTRATION: ANTIGEN AND VACCINE SAMPLING

So far in all preclinical and clinical trials, *Helicobacter*-specific vaccines were administered by the oral or orogastric route. It is not yet known where the vaccines are sampled. All mucosal surfaces, including those of the airways, the gut and the genital tract, are able to sample antigens and take up vaccines[29] triggering both local and systemic immune responses. Two major sampling mechanisms have been identified. In stratified epithelia of the upper digestive and the lower genital tracts, intra-epithelial antigen-presenting cells, the dendritic or Langerhans cells, take up antigens and transport them to distant (vagina) or local (tonsils) organized lymphoid (for review see ref. 30). Dendritic cells are also present in simple epithelia, for instance in the colon[31] or in the lower respiratory tract[32]. In simple epithelia, specialized resident epithelial cells, the so-called M cells, in the follicle-associated epithelium (FAE) over mucosal-associated lymphoid tissue (MALT) are also able to take up and transport antigens and microorganisms into the underlying lymphoid tissue. The stomach corpus and antrum do not contain FAE and M cells, and hence probably do not sample antigens via M cells. Whether dendritic cells are present in the gastric epithelium and mediate antigen uptake is not yet known. In the *Helicobacter*-infected stomach, however, the bacteria induce MALT[33], and it is likely that the overlying epithelium contains M cells. The induction of MALT, FAE and M cells by microorganisms has been demonstrated in germfree mice, which contain only one or two Peyer's patches. The oral administration of a non-pathogenic microorganism (*Clostridium indolis*) to germfree mice restores within a few days the normal number of patches (Kernéis *et al.*, unpublished observation). We have recently shown in BALB/c mice that Peyer's patch lymphocytes, introduced into a mucosa site that lacks MALT, induce the formation of FAE with typical M cells. The conversion of differentiated human colonic enterocytes (Caco-2 cells) into cells that express many M cell features, including the loss of the brush border and its associated digestive enzymes and the gain of transepithelial transport activity, was shown to be mediated by Peyer's patch lymphocytes[34]. The three-way interaction of epithelium, lymphoid cells, and microorganisms seen in the FAE which controls the formation of MALT provides a dramatic demonstration of the phenotypic plasticity of the intestinal epithelium. Whether the same applies to the gastric mucosa remains to be established.

From these considerations it is conceivable that vaccine sampling in *H. pylori*-infected (therapeutic vaccine) or in non-infected stomach (prophylactic vaccine) is different. The identification of the sites where the antigens are taken up in infected compared to uninfected individuals, as well as the fate of the vaccines once transported across the gastric epithelium, might contribute to a better understanding of how mucosal vaccines mediate cure of chronic *H. pylori* infection.

IMMUNIZATION AND AUTOIMMUNITY: VACCINE SAFETY

Adverse reactions have been observed in inbred or outbred mice immunized with *H. felis* sonicates or *H. pylori* urease. The mice were protected against infection but an inflammatory infiltrate developed in the gastric corpus of immunized mice following *H. felis* challenge[10,19]. The inflammation consisted mainly of mononuclear leucocytes with scattered CD45R+ B cells and IgM+ and IgA+ B cells[35]. No anti-parietal cell reactivity and no H+,K+-ATPase-specific autoantibodies typical of type A autoimmune gastritis were observed, although the histopathological lesions were indistinguishable from those of autoimmune gastritis[36]. Post-immunization gastritis has not been observed in other animal models, including ferrets and cats[37]. In a recent study, however, proton pump (α and β subunit)-specific autoantibodies have been detected in a few *H. pylori*-infected patients (Claeys, D. *et al.*, manuscript in preparation). More work will be required to understand the relationship between infectious and autoimmune gastritis in mice and humans, and the role of the antigen and the mucosal adjuvants in post-immunization gastritis. Therapeutic vaccination of mice and ferrets with urease or UreB resulted in the resolution of the gastritic inflammation together with cure of the infection[11,38].

MUCOSAL ADJUVANTS

Cholera toxin (CT) or *E. coli* labile toxin (LT) bind to membrane glycolipids via their B pentameric subunit and activate adenylate cyclase via the APD ribosylating A subunit. The toxins are also known for their adjuvant activity in mucosal immunity[39], although their mode of action is only poorly understood. They have to be added to *H. pylori* antigens in order to induce successful vaccination. The B subunit of CT (CTB) is inefficient. The APD ribosylation activity of the two toxins, however, does not seem to be essential, since genetically detoxified toxins[40] retain their adjuvancy[41]. In humans, CT cannot be used because the toxic and pharmacological concentrations are too close. Thus clinical trials are conducted with low doses of LT. The success of therapeutic immunization in humans is likely to depend on the efficacy of the mucosal adjuvant. Improvement of existing, or the development of novel, mucosal adjuvants will require a better under-standing of their molecular and cellular mechanisms mediating adjuvancy. So far most studies were restricted to the effects of the toxins on immune cells. CT, however, when administered orally, binds first to the enterocytes of the intestinal mucosa. Which epithelial cytokines are released upon CT or LT interaction are not known, and the cellular targets of such cytokines have to be identified. The complex interaction between toxins, epithelial and immune cells may result in the activation of unresponsive immune cells which then become able to clear the infection. The toxins are known to break tolerance[42].

IMMUNOLOGICAL CORRELATES OF PROTECTION OR CURE

The immunological correlates of protection and/or cure of the vaccines described above have not been identified. Different immune effectors and mechanisms have been implicated in the protective or therapeutic activity of the vaccines. These include secretory IgA (sIgA) antibodies and/or T cells with Th2 helper activity. Alternatively the vaccines may trigger a break of tolerance. Since *H. pylori* is essentially a non-invasive pathogen, the immune effectors have to gain access to the gastric mucosal surface in order to mediate their function.

We shall now critically review experimental data supporting each of the mechanisms described above.

Humoral effectors: systemic and local *Helicobacter*-specific antibodies

H. pylori-specific secretory IgA antibodies are found in secretions of infected individuals, but they are inefficient to clear an established infection. The protective potential of sIgA is supported by studies in Gambia, in which babies breast-fed by *H. pylori*-infected mothers are protected against infection during the entire lactation period. Protection correlated with the presence of specific sIgA in milk[43]. A correlation between the presence of *Helicobacter*-specific IgA antibodies and protection was reported for outbred mice immunized with urease apoenzyme[20], but not for BALB/c mice immunized with UreB[10] or truncated UreB[21] recombinant proteins. Similarly, no correlation was found between sIgA titres and protection in mice immunized with heat-shock proteins[12]. In contrast, protection correlated with high levels of *H. pylori*-specific IgG1 antibodies.

A role for systemic humoral antibodies in protection was not supported by recent DNA vaccination studies. Following the intramuscular injection of urease B DNA, high titres of IgG of all isotypes were generated. The decreased colonization, however, did not correlate with urease-specific IgG titres, suggesting that cellular effectors are involved[44].

To analyse the potential role of sIgA in prevention and treatment, we vaccinated IL-6-deficient mice with urease and CT. These mice are known to have drastically reduced mucosal dimeric and secretory IgA antibody levels[45]. In wild-type C57/Bl6 mice from which the knockout mice were generated, *H. felis* induced more severe lesions when compared to BALB/c mice, and protection or treatment after urease apoenzyme immunization was only partial. Recombinant UreB was inefficient, suggesting that the UreB T helper epitopes were MHC Class II restricted and not recognized by C57Bl6 mice. In IL-6-deficient mice; however, no protection, reduced colonization, or cure was observed following urease apoenzyme immunization. Whether the loss of partial protection is due to a lack of mucosal IgA and sIgA, or to the absence of IL-6 is presently not known.

Mucosal antibodies probably play a role in protection or treatment of *H. pylori* infection, but whether they are sufficient for protection or cure remains to be established.

Th1 to Th2 switch

It has been speculated that following immunization of infected mice there is a shift from a T helper Th1 to a Th2 response which is able to clear the infection and the gastric inflammation, as reported for other infectious or parasitic diseases[46,47]. The cytokine profile of the infiltrating T cells before and after immunization recently has been analysed[48]. We have tested whether attenuated *Salmonella* expressing *H. pylori* urease under the control of a phase transition promotor[49] was able to confer protective immunity or mediate cure of the infection. *Salmonella* vaccines are known to initially trigger a Th1 response. Mice were orally immunized with recombinant *Salmonella* in the absence of CT or LT, as previously reported[29] for hepatitis B virus core antigen. Despite a strong systemic IgG response, and the presence of sIgA in local secretions, the animals were not protected; nor could they cure a pre-existing infection. In a recent study reported in abstract form, Radcliff and co-workers addressed more directly the role of a Th2 response in the prevention of *H. felis* infection. They used IL-4-deficient mice immunized with *H. felis* sonicates and CT. Protection was not completely lost in the knockout mice and one-fifth of the mice were protected, suggesting that other mechanisms are probably involved in protection or treatment[50].

Break of tolerance

In natural infection it has been proposed that *H. pylori* induces unresponsiveness, by inducing tolerance. The proliferation and cytokine profile of peripheral blood and gastric lymphocytes was analysed in *H. pylori*-infected patients[51]. *H. pylori* antigen stimulated peripheral blood lymphocyte proliferative responses both in *H. pylori*-positive and -negative patients, although the responses were much lower in infected patients. Similarly antigen-specific proliferative responses and interferon γ production by gastric lamina propria lymphocytes were also depressed in *H. pylori*-positive patients. It appears that antigen-specific responses to *H.*

pylori are lower in infected individuals, suggesting activation of antigen-specific suppression.

Cholera and labile toxins are known to break tolerance[39,42]. All the vaccine candidates described in this review require cholera or labile toxins to prevent or cure *Helicobacter* infection. Whether the toxins break the state of unresponsiveness induced by *H. pylori* remains to be established. Such studies will require a better understanding of the interaction between the gastric epithelial cells and the local immune cells, and of the modulating role of the toxins.

CONCLUSIONS AND PERSPECTIVES

Protective and/or therapeutic vaccines against *H. pylori* have now been tested successfully in several animal models. New animal models have been generated to test the safety and efficacy of the vaccines. Testing the vaccines in these animal models has also contributed to a better understanding of the host response to *Helicobacter*. To improve on existing vaccines it will be essential further to characterize the mechanisms which allow *Helicobacter* to escape immunity. New safer mucosal adjuvants have also to be developed, as well as efficient delivery systems. The vaccination studies go beyond mere preparation of new drugs; they help us understand why the *Helicobacter* can survive and induce chronic infection and inflammation in the stomach.

Acknowledgements

We are grateful to Pierre Michetti for his advice, suggestions and constructive criticisms. We thank Sally Hopkins for revising the manuscript. This work was supported by grants from the Swiss National Science Foundation (grants no. 31 37612.93 to J.P.K. and 31 43240.95 to A.B.).

References

1. Megraud F. Rationale for the choice of antibiotics for the eradication of *Helicobacter pylori*. Eur J Gastroenterol Hepatol. 1995;7(Suppl. 1):S49.
2. Engstrand L. Potential animal models for *Helicobacter pylori* infection in immunological and vaccine research. FEMS Immunol Med Microbiol. 1995;10:265.
3. Lee A, Fox JG, Otto G, Murphy J. A small animal model of human *Helicobacter pylori* active chronic gastritis. Gastroenterology. 1990;99:1315.
4. Fox JG, Otto G, Murphy HC, Taylor NS, Lee A. Gastric colonization of the ferret with *Helicobacter* species: natural and experimental infections. Rev Infect Dis. 1991;13(Suppl. 8P):S67.
5. Fox JG, Lee A, Otto G, Taylor NS, Murphy JC. *Helicobacter felis* gastritis in gnotobiotic rats: an animal model of *Helicobacter pylori* gastritis. Infect Immun. 1991;59:785.
6. Handt LK, Fox JG, Stalis IH *et al*. Characterization of feline *Helicobacter pylori* strains and associated gastritis in a colony of domestic cats. J Clin Microbiol. 1995;33:2280.
7. Dubois A, Fiala N, Heman-Ackah LM *et al*. Natural gastric infection with *Helicobacter pylori* in monkeys: a model for spiral bacteria infection in humans. Gastroenterology. 1994;106:1405.
8. Czinn SJ, Cai A, Nedrud JG. Protection of germ-free mice from infection by *Helicobacter felis* after active oral or passive IgA immunization. *Vaccine*. 1993;11:637–42.
9. Chen M, Lee A, Hazell S. Immunization against gastric *Helicobacter* infection in a mouse/ *Helicobacter felis* model [letter]. Lancet. 1992;339:1120.

10. Michetti P, Corthésy-Theulaz I, Davin C *et al*. Immunization of BALB/c mice against *Helicobacter felis* infection with *Helicobacter pylori* urease. Gastroenterology. 1994;107:1002.
11. Corthésy-Theulaz I, Porta N, Glauser M *et al*. Oral immunization with *Helicobacter pylori* urease as a treatment against *Helicobacter* infection. Gastroenterology. 1995;109:115.
12. Ferrero RL, Thiberge JM, Kansau I, Wuscher N, Huerre M, Labigne A. The GroES homolog of *Helicobacter pylori* confers protective immunity against mucosal infection in mice. Proc Natl Acad Sci USA. 1995;92:6499.
13. Marchetti M, Arico B, Buyrroni D, Figura N, Rappuoli R, Ghiara P. Development of a mouse model of *Helicobacter pylori* infection that mimics human disease. Science. 1995;267:1655.
14. Lee A, Chen M. Successful immunization against gastric infection with *Helicobacter* species: use of a cholera toxin b-subunit-whole-cell vaccine. Infect Immun. 1994;62:3594.
15. Doidge C, Crust I, Lee A, Buck F, Hazell S, Manne U. Therapeutic immunization against *Helicobacter* infection. Lancet. 1994;343:914.
16. Song W, Vaerman JP, Mostov KE. Dimeric and tetrameric IgA are transcytosed equally by the polymeric Ig receptor. Immunology. 1995;155:715.
17. Appelmelk BJ, Simoons-Smit I, Negrini R *et al*. Potential role of molecular mimicry between *Helicobacter pylori* liposaccharide and host Lewis blood group antigens in autoimmunity. Infect Immun. 1996;64:2031–40.
18. Labigne A, Cussac V, Courcoux P. Shuttle cloning and nucleotide sequences of *Helicobacter pylori* genes responsible for urease activity. J Bacteriol. 1991;173:1920.
19. Ferrero RL, Thiberge JM, Huerre M, Labigne A. Recombinant antigens prepared from the urease subunits of *Helicobacter* spp: evidence of protection in a mouse model of gastric infection. Infect Immun. 1994;62:4981.
20. Lee CK, Weltzin R, Thomas WD *et al*. Oral immunization with recombinant *Helicobacter pylori* urease induces secretory IgA antibodies and protects mice from challenge with *Helicobacter felis*. J Infect Dis. 1995;172:161.
21. Doré-Davin C, Michetti P, Saraga E, Blum AL, Corthésy-Theulaz I. 37 kDa fragment of UreB is sufficient to confer protection against *Helicobacter felis* infection in mice. Gastroenterology. 1996;110:A97 (abstract).
22. Kreiss C, Buclin T, Cosma M, Corthésy-Theulaz I, Michetti P. Safety of oral immunization with recombinant urease in patients with *Helicobacter pylori* infection. Lancet. 1996;347:1630–1.
23. Telford JL, Ghiara P, Dell'Orco M *et al*. Gene structure of the *Helicobacter pylori* cytotoxin and evidence of its key role in gastric disease. J Exp Med. 1994;179:1653.
24. Figura N, Guglielmetti P, Rossolini A *et al*. Cytotoxin production by *Campylobacter pylori* strains isolated from patients with peptic ulcers and from patients with chronic gastritis only. J Clin Microbiol. 1987;27:225.
25. Dunn BE, Roop RM, Sung CC, Sharma SA, Perez-Perez GI, Blaser MJ. Identification and purification of a cpn60 heat shock protein homolog from *Helicobacter pylori*. Infect Immun. 1992;60:1946.
26. Engstrand L, Scheynius A, Pahlson C. An increased number of gamma/delta T-cells and gastric epithelial cell expression of the GroEL stress-protein homologue in *Helicobacter pylori*-associated chronic gastritis of the antrum. Am J Gastroenterol. 1991;86:976.
27. Keenan J, Allardyce AR, Bagshaw P. *Helicobacter felis* surface antigens serve as protective targets in orally immunized mice. Gut. 1995;37:A93 (abstract).
28. Odenbreit S, Till M, Haas R. Identification of a *Helicobacter pylori* specific protein involved in adherence to gastric epithelial cells. Gut. 1995;37:A1 (abstract).
29. Hopkins S, Kraehenbuhl JP, Schödel F *et al*. A recombinant *Salmonella typhimurium* vaccine induces local immunity by four different routes of immunization. Infect Immun. 1995;63:3279.
30. Neutra MR, Pringault E, Kraehenbuhl JP. Antigen sampling across epithelial barriers and induction of mucosal immune responses. Annu Rev Immunol. 1996;14:275.
31. Maric I, Holt PG, Perdue MH, Bienenstock J. Class II MHC antigen (Ia)-bearing dendritic cells in the epithelium of the rat intestine. Immunology. 1996;1546:1408.
32. McWilliam AS, Nelson D, Thomas JA, Holt PG. Rapid dendritic cell recruitment is a hallmark of the acute inflammatory response at mucosal surfaces. J Exp Med. 1994;179:1331.
33. Stolte M, Eidt S. Lymphoid follicles in antral mucosa: immune response to *Campylobacter pylori*. J Clin Pathol. 1989;42:1269.
34. Kernéis S, Bogdanova A, Kraehenbuhl JP, Pringault E. Peyer's patch lymphocytes trigger the conversion of human enterocytes into M cells that transcytose inert particles. (Submitted).

35. Pappo J, Thomas WD, Kabok Z, Taylor NS, Murphy NS, Fox JG. Effect of oral immunization with recombinant urease on murine *Helicobacter felis* gastritis. Infect Immun. 1995;63:1246.
36. Claeys D, Corthésy-Theulaz I, Gaudin M *et al.* Absence of H,K-ATPase serum autoantibodies in mice immunized against *Helicobacter* infection. Gastroenterology. 1995;108:A797 (abstract).
37. Batchelder M, Fox JG, Monath TP *et al.* Oral vaccination with recombinant urease reduces gastric *Helicobacter pylori* colonization in the cat. Gastroenterology. 1996;110:A58 (abstract).
38. Cuenca R, Blanchard T, Lee CK *et al.* Therapeutic immunization against *Helicobacter mustelae* in naturally infected ferrets. Gastroenterology. 1995;108:A78 (abstract).
39. Holmgren J, Lycke N, Czerkinsky C. Cholera toxin and cholera B subunit as oral–mucosal adjuvant and antigen vector systems. Vaccine. 1993;11:1179.
40. Pizza M, Fontana MR, Giuliani MM *et al.* A genetically detoxified derivative of heat labile *Escherichia coli* enterotoxin induces neutralizing antibodies against the A subunit. J Exp Med. 1994;180:2147.
41. di Tommaso A, Saletti G, Pizza M *et al.* Induction of antigen-specific antibodies in vaginal secretions by using a nontoxic mutant of heat-labile enterotoxin as a mucosal adjuvant. Infect Immun. 1996;64:974–9.
42. Sun JB, Holmgarten J, Czerinsky C. Cholera toxin B subunit: an efficient transmucosal carrier-delivery system for induction of peripheral immunological tolerance. Proc Natl Acad Sci USA. 1994;91:10795.
43. Thomas JE, Austin S, Dale A *et al.* Protection by human milk IgA against *Helicobacter pylori* infection in infancy. Lancet. 1993;342:121 (letter).
44. Corthésy-Theulaz IB, Corthésy B, Bachmann D *et al.* Naked DNA immunization against *Helicobacter* infection. Gastroenterology. 1996;110:A889 (abstract).
45. Ramsay AJ, Husband AJ, Ramshaw IA *et al.* The role of interleukin-6 in mucosal IgA antibody responses in vivo. Science. 1994;264:561.
46. Locksley RM, Louis JA. Immunology of leishmaniasis. Curr Opin Immunol. 1992;4:413.
47. Nobentrauth N, Kropf P, Muller I. Susceptibility to leishmania major infection in interleukin-4-deficient mice. Science. 1996;271:987.
48. Mohammadi M, Czinn S, Redline R, Nedrud J. *Helicobacter*-specific cell-mediated immune responses display a predominant Th1 phenotype and promote a delayed-type hypersensitivity in the stomachs of mice. J Immunol. 1996;156:4729.
49. Yan ZX, Reuss F, Meyer TF. Construction of an invertible DNA segment for improved antigen expression by a hybrid *Salmonella* vaccine strain. Res Microbiol. 1990;141:1003.
50. Radcliffe FJ, Ramsay AJ, Lee A. Failure of immunization against *Helicobacter* infection in IL-4-deficient mice: evidence for a Th2 immune response as the basis for protective immunity. Gastroenterology. 1996;110: (abstract).
51. Fan XJ, Chua A, Shahi CN, McDevitt J, Keeling PW, Kelleher D. Gastric T lymphocyte responses to *Helicobacter pylori* in patients with *H. pylori* colonization. Gut. 1994;35:1379.
52. Kleanthous H, Tibbits T, Bakios T *et al.* In vivo selection of a highly adapted *Helicobacter pylori* mouse model for studying vaccine efficacy and attenuating lesion. Gut. 1995;37:A94 (abstract).

19
The epithelial changes associated with *Helicobacter pylori* infection: the biology of gastric and intestinal metaplasia

N. WRIGHT

INTRODUCTION

It is now abundantly clear that *Helicobacter pylori* has an aetiological role in the pathogenesis of chronic gastritis and peptic ulcer in both the stomach and the duodenum[1,2], and highly likely that it is incriminated in the induction of carcinoma of the stomach[3] and low-grade gastric (MALT) lymphoma[4]. However, the actual mechanisms by which this organism exerts its effects have not yet been elucidated. What is clear is that colonization and adhesion of the bacteria to the mucosal surface, followed either by the production of toxin(s) and/or mucosal invasion, are the prerequisites for induction of tissue damage. This implies that adhesion of the organism to the epithelial cells of the gastroduodenal mucosa is an extremely important step. The organism maintains a microenvironment with a more neutral pH immediately adjacent to the mucosa[5], with direct adhesion of the organism to the apical plasma membrane of the epithelial cell to form the characteristic adhesion pedestal[6], with some authors suggesting a preference for intercellular junctions[7].

H. pylori is very selective in its preferences for colonizing epithelial cells, and will generally colonize only the gastric epithelium; it will not colonize epithelial cells of the small intestine; however, the appearance of a cell lineage in the duodenum, with the phenotype of mucus-secreting gastric foveolar cells – so-called gastric metaplasia – can be colonized by *H. pylori*[8], and this is considered by many to be an essential first event in the pathogenesis of duodenal ulcer disease (see below). The factors which may affect the adhesion of *H. pylori* to epithelial cells have been well reviewed by Sherman[9]; these include specific characteristics of the organism and of the epithelial cells. Factors considered important include hydrophobicity, conferred by the overlying gastric mucus glycoprotein, to which *H. pylori* adheres, and carbohydrate and glycolipids present on the epithelial cell membrane. It is not known, however, which specific characteristic of gastric epithelial or metaplastic cells makes it open to coloniz-ation by *H. pylori* but, whatever it is, it is a property not shared by small intestinal enterocytes. Morphological studies might suggest that it is the nature of the apical surface membrane which is most important, rather than the local mucus micro-environment. It is a common observation in *H. pylori*-associated duodenitis that a gastric metaplastic epithelial cell heavily colonized with *H. pylori* coexists with an adjacent enterocyte bearing no organisms.

A corollary of this proposal is that a change in the nature of the gastric epithelium will affect the ability of *H. pylori* to colonize the gastric mucosa. This occurs as the end-result of chronic gastritis where the epithelium undergoes a phenotypic change to a small intestinal format, the well-known phenomenon of intestinal metaplasia, where the enterocytes cannot be colonized. Consequently, the development and natural history of these two epithelia – 'gastric metaplasia' and 'intestinal metaplasia', become critical in understanding the relationship between *H. pylori* and gastroduodenal disease.

GASTRIC METAPLASIA

This is the term usually applied to the presence of cells with the phenotype of foveolar-pit cells apparently in the surface epithelium of the duodenal mucosa, replacing the indigenous small intestinal cell lineages. Perhaps the best way of distinguishing these cells is by their characteristic positive staining with the periodic acid Schiff/Alcian blue method, which stains the neutral mucin magenta while the local goblet cells, with their acidic mucin, are coloured blue (Figure 1). There are probably two contrasting hypotheses which attempt to explain the histogenesis of these cells: first, that they represent a true metaplasia, presumably of stem cells in the underlying crypts[10], although some authors have assumed that villus cells are capable of metaplasia. This proposal has the support of the observation of cells apparently intermediate between enterocytes and gastric mucus-secreting cells, which exhibit only partial development of the gastric phenotype[10]. A second, contrasting, theory proposes that gastric metaplasia is not a metaplasia at all, but represents an overgrowth of cells from the ducts of the underlying Brunner's glands[11].

This rather strange suggestion has considerable observational support, and explains several previously puzzling facts about gastric metaplasia:

1. It is difficult to explain the restricted occurrence of gastric metaplasia, which occurs only in the duodenum, but if it is recalled that this is where Brunner's glands are selectively found, an origin from the ducts explains this.
2. Three-dimensional studies, using reconstruction from serial sections, are revealing[11]: ribbons of cells are seen streaming up from the base of the villus to meet towards the top, explaining the frequent observations of an apparent concentration of these cells at the tips of the villi. The ribbons of cells can be followed downwards through the crypt population into the Brunner's gland ducts.
3. Analysis of the trefoil peptide gene expression pattern in surface gastric metaplasia shows appearances which are consistent with Brunner's gland duct epithelium[12,13].

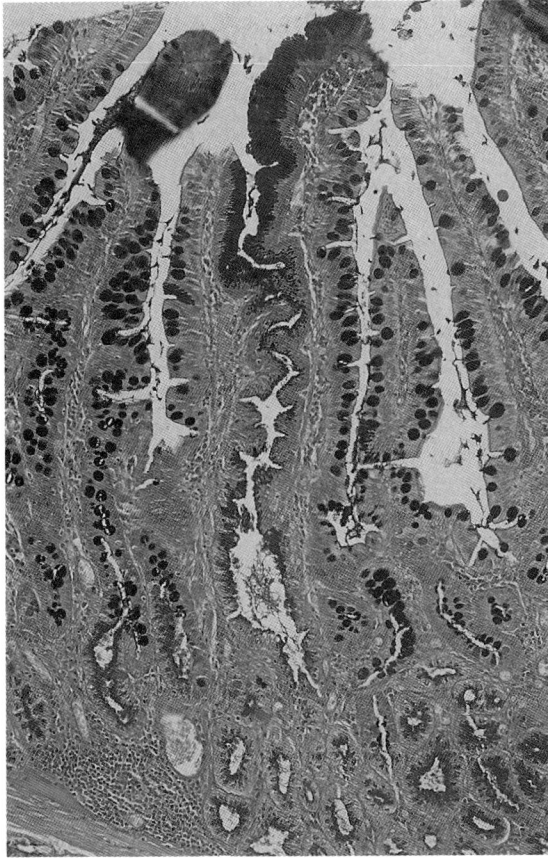

Figure 1 Duodenal mucosa showing gastric metaplasia stained with the periodic acid Schiff/Alcian blue method

4. There are subtle differences in the lectin-binding profile between gastric metaplastic epithelial cells and foveolar pit epithelial cells[14], and a detailed analysis favours the view that surface gastric metaplasia and Brunner's duct epithelium share a very similar lectin-binding profile[15].
5. There are intrinsic similarities between the way in which surface gastric epithelial cells clothe the villi and a similar phenomenon elsewhere in the small intestine. Chronic inflammation, for example in the ileum in Crohn's disease, induces the new growth of buds from the bases of intestinal crypts, which give rise to the tubules of a new gland which ramifies in the lamina propria adjacent to the ulcer[16]. Once formed, the gland develops a duct, which grows up the core of the nearest villus and fuses with the surface epithelium and creates an orifice. What follows is interesting and most germane to the histogenesis of gastric metaplasia. Cells from the duct migrate onto the surface and replace the villus cells, often totally covering the villus with cells similar in phenotype (but not in gene expression) to those seen in surface gastric metaplasia. The histogenetic programme of this so-called

ulcer-associated cell lineage (UACL) is intrinsically similar to that of Brunner's glands in embryonic life[17], with buds and then acini growing out of the early duodenal crypts. The fact that the UACL donates cells onto the surface, and has the same histogenesis as Brunner's glands, is at least circumstantial evidence that surface gastric epithelial cells emanate from the ducts of Brunner's glands. The stimulus for this overgrowth, and indeed the reasons for the development of the UACL in chronic inflammation, are as yet unknown.

6. There are similarities in growth factor gene expression between surface gastric metaplastic cells and Brunner's gland duct epithelium: epidermal growth factor/urogastrone (EGF/URO) is expressed in both lineages, and Ahnen and colleagues[18] have pointed out the common expression of a further type I growth factor, transforming growth factor alpha (TGFα) also.

It thus appears that the evidence favours an origin of gastric metaplasia from the Brunner's gland duct. Arguing teleologically, it would perhaps be common sense that, in the presence of incipient mucosal damage, possibly caused by excess acid secretion caused by antral colonization by *H. pylori*[19], the mucosa might respond by an overgrowth of cells which have the capacity to secrete mucus and bicarbonate to buffer the mucosa against acid, and produce EGF/URO and TGFα with their powerful growth-promoting properties[20], and trefoil peptides, which stimulate cell migration[21]. The presence of these cells in the duodenal mucosa would be expected to advance both cytoprotection and healing, but at what cost? The cost is the creation of a niche which *H. pylori* can then occupy, and once the surface is colonized by these organisms a duodenal ulcer can well result[22].

Usually only the surface component of the gastric metaplasia is seen, although occasionally true gastric heterotopia is seen in the form of mucosal nodules and, microscopically, groups of oxyntic glands are present; these are generally assumed to be of congenital origin[23]. However, other authors have drawn attention to groups of parietal cells in the deep crypts or superficial Brunner's gland ducts in chronic duodenitis, which could represent a true metaplasia and contribute to local acid production[24,25]; however, these parietal cells may not contribute to the hypersecretion of acid in *H. pylori* infection[25].

While there is a consensus that gastric metaplastic epithelial cells can indeed be colonized by *H. pylori* there is no general agreement about its relationship to duodenitis and duodenal ulceration[26]. While gastric metaplasia is uncommon in childhood, it is found in some 7% of endoscoped individuals less than 20 years of age[27], and in as many as 22% of a biopsied asymptomatic population[28]. There is, however, no real dispute that gastric metaplasia is a component part of duodenitis; duodenitis is also accepted as a precursor of duodenal ulcer. There is considerable evidence that excess acid reaching the duodenum is a primary cause of gastric metaplasia; experimentally-induced hyperchlorhydria produces gastric metaplasia[29,30], and in humans there is a correlation between the presence and extent of gastric metaplasia and acid output[31]; moreover, in duodenal ulcer patients with *H. pylori* infection the extent of gastric metaplasia is related to the gastric acid output[32]. However, it is clear that, at least in children, infection with *H. pylori per se* is not sufficient to cause gastric metaplasia[33].

However, once present, there is no doubt that gastric metaplastic cells are prone to colonization by *H. pylori*[34], although the recognition of duodenal gastric metaplasia may be problematic because of there being few cells and also because here the organism may adopt a coccoid form which makes identification difficult[26]. A combination of histology, culture and a rapid urease test markedly increases prevalence rates for the colonization of gastric metaplasia in duodenal ulcer and duodenitis patients[35].

The hypothesis of hypersecretion of acid induced by antral colonization with *H. pylori*, with resultant gastric acid hypersecretion followed by the induction of gastric metaplasia and duodenal colonization, duodenitis and duodenal ulcer formation[36], has received considerable attention. This predicts that gastric metaplasia, induced by acid, and *H. pylori* infection are both required for duodenitis and ulceration. In epidemiological studies[37], in which individuals with antral *H. pylori* infection were compared with others with gastric metaplasia, the predicted prevalence of duodenal disease in those with both markers agreed excellently with that determined by endoscopy. In duodenal ulcer patients, gastric metaplasia is seen very frequently in biopsies taken from the margins of the lesion, although *H. pylori* is seen less frequently[26].

Another important point in the biology of duodenal gastric metaplasia is the question of its reversibility, and this has evoked considerable debate[26]. If indeed the change is mediated through overgrowth of the Brunner's gland duct epithelium, as proposed above, it might be anticipated that eradication of *H. pylori* infection, and reduction in gastric acid secretion, would lead to regression of the gastric metaplasia. However, evidence for this point is mixed; healing of duodenal ulcers is not usually associated with regression of gastric metaplasia[38,39], although there have been claims that vagotomy[36] and omeprazole[40,41] are associated with regression. It would be anticipated that, because of the fact that increased acid secretion is reduced by eradication of *H. pylori*, the amount of duodenitis and therefore gastric metaplasia would be reduced by successful eradication: while some studies have indeed found this[42]; others[43] have not confirmed this observation. In the interpretation of these studies there must be major concern both about the effects of sampling error and the methods used to measure the amount of gastric metaplasia in the duodenal biopsies. It would appear from the available evidence that gastric metaplasia is not reversible, but further studies are evidently needed to settle the important point – as to whether the change is reversible, and also if the regression of gastric metaplasia is a realistic end-point for assessing if the duodenal mucosa is now normal.

INTESTINAL METAPLASIA

Compared with the comparatively detailed knowledge we now have about the histogenesis of gastric metaplasia, it is rather surprising that, notwithstanding its importance, we do not know a great deal about the origins and nature of intestinal metaplasia (IM). However, it is worth noting that IM is different from gastric metaplasia in that it shows multilineage differentiation, into enterocytes, goblet cells and endocrine cells, all characteristics of a fully fledged intestinal epithelium, unlike gastric metaplasia in which the predominant differentiation pathway is towards one lineage only. Thus IM is a complete change from the gastric pheno-

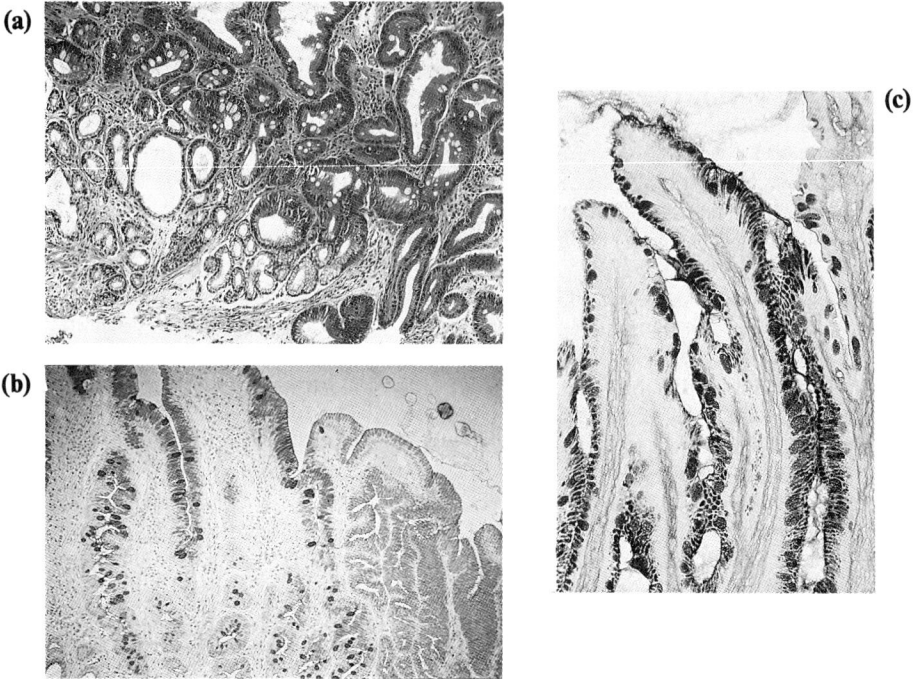

Figure 2 (a) An area of intestinal metaplasia of the complete type (Type 1); haematoxylin and eosin; (b) stained with Alcian blue DPAS, showing the characteristic goblet cells with alcianophilic mucin; (c) Type 2a or 3 IM, stained with the high iron diamine/Alcian blue method, showing that many of the cells contain brown-staining sulphomucin

type towards that of intestinal epithelium, which is more in keeping with classical ideas of metaplasia.

IM is important in gastric pathology for two main reasons: first, during the progression of chronic atrophic gastritis, caused by whatever means (but directly relevant here is that caused by *H. pylori*) IM is usually an invariant feature. Second, there is little doubt that IM is associated with the evolution of carcinoma of the stomach; indeed Morson[45], *inter alia*, noted that many earlier observers believed that gastric carcinoma arose from areas of IM.

The morphology of IM is quite distinctive (Figure 2): it appears as sharply defined islands of small intestinal epithelium, usually in the antral mucosa. Several types are recognized: perhaps the commonest is where typical small bowel crypts appear, complete with Paneth cells, enterocytes complete with brush border, and goblet cells which contain alcianophilic mucus in typical thecae (Figure 2a,b); this appearance is usually called type 1; a second type does not show Paneth cell differentiation, lacks typical enterocyte differentiation, and all the cells contain mucin (Figure 2c). This type is further divided depending on the type of mucin expressed: if sulphomucins are present, usually demonstrated by the high iron–diamine method, it is usually referred to as Type 2b (or Type 3); the importance of this distinction is that this is the type regarded by many (but not all, see below) as that which is associated with the development of dysplasia and carcinoma.

While it usually averred that the phenotype of intestinal metaplasia, particularly Type 1, is that of the small bowel, there are significant differences. For example, Paneth cells are not always present (usually in the distal stomach) and often lack their characteristic position in the crypt base, being found more superficially. Hybrid cells, intermediate between Paneth cells and mucous cells, are seen, and it is claimed that 'active' DNA synthesis occurs in Paneth cells in IM[45]. A rather strange feature of IM is the presence of ciliated cells, seen in cystically dilated glands in the basal portions of the metaplastic mucosa; some of these cells contain pepsinogen II, usually found in antral chief cells, indicating that they are remnants of the original mucosa. It is interesting to note that cilia are not normally found in any part of the intestinal mucosa, and that the cilia can be dysmorphic in their doublet structure; the microvilli of these cells are long and branched, as seen in microvilli in the epididymis, and in tumours such as mesotheliomas and ovarian cystadenomas (see ref. 45 for review). Additionally, there may be intracytoplasmic cysts into which microvilli project, as seen in malignant epithelial cells[45]. The stroma surrounding areas of IM may contain abundant inflammatory cells, especially where there is focal metaplastic change in active gastritis associated with *H. pylori* infection, and show areas of fibromuscular hyperplasia, but the organisms are not found on the metaplastic cells.

There is considerable variation in the distribution of glycocalyceal enzymes in IM, with individual adjacent cells often showing differences in expression, and of course the expression of these enzymes in areas of Type 1 or complete IM is markedly different from that shown in Type 2[46]. We have already noted that the expression of mucin may vary between the various subtypes of IM: because of this some authors have preferred the terms 'small intestine' and 'colonic' for Type 1 and Type 2 IM respectively (for example see ref. 47). However, it is worth noting that both large and small intestinal antigens are found in IM, and the same cells that produce the 'colonic' mucus can express small intestinal enzymes[45,48]; consequently it cannot be concluded that the subtypes of IM represent such tissue-specific differentiation[45].

The histogenesis of IM has certainly not received the attention it deserves; however, most authors conclude that it represents a true mutation in the stem cells of the gastric gland, which are thought to be housed in the isthmus-neck region in the fundic glands, although the location of stem cells in the antral gastric glands is obscure[49]. The genes which are thought to determine anteroposterior differentiation patterns are a large group of transcription factors which share a common, highly conserved domain, the homeodomain, and these genes are thus called the *homeobox* genes or *Hox* genes. It has been suggested that damage induced by inflammation causes inappropriate expression or mutation of such a gene[49], possibly induced by nitrosative deamination of DNA by nitric oxide produced by the inflammatory infiltrate induced by *H. pylori* infection[45]. In *Drosophila*, damage to an antenna can sometimes result in regeneration of a foreleg in that site: such 'heteromorphic transformation' has led Slack[49] to suggest that epithelial metaplasias are due to such genetic changes. This is certainly a very attractive hypothesis, and now that mammalian and indeed human *Hox* gene homologues are being isolated, is certainly worth pursuing.

The relationship between intestinal metaplasia and carcinoma of the stomach is well established[45], and some authors favour a selective association with Type 2b or 3. However, there have been a few reports of suggestive genetic changes in IM in the absence of metaplasia, but Soman *et al.*[50] have reported an *H-ras* mutation in an area of IM associated with gastric carcinoma, although search for other mutations, such as p53, has been unsuccessful[45]. However, it has been claimed that IM shows telomere reduction, compared with the length of telomere repeat arrays in normal gastric mucosa[51]; such telomere reduction is also found in colorectal adenomas, and is closely correlated with ageing of blood DNA[52]. These changes could lead to genetic instability, and favour the later mutations which occur in the progression of IM to gastric carcinoma[53].

While there has been considerable debate in the past about the association of *H. pylori* infection with the development of IM, most workers now accept that chronic atrophic gastritis associated with the organism can develop areas of IM[54]. This raises the question of whether there is reversibility of IM, a concept with which some have had difficulties, since IM is firmly embedded in a pathway which leads, apparently inexorably, to gastric carcinoma. However, notwithstanding the problems associated with sampling error, we might note on theoretical grounds that IM should be reversible: if the homeotic transformation merely involves a difference in gene expression, on the reduction in inflammation normal gene expression could result. If, however, there is a mutation involved, presumably there would have to be regrowth of the mucosa and recolonization with gastric glands at the expense of the intestinal-type crypts.

CONCLUSION

It might be thought strange that *H. pylori* infection is associated with the change from intestinal to gastric phenotype in the duodenum, and *vice-versa* in the stomach. However, the discussion above sets the scene for further studies which will not only cast light on the nature and mechanism of these changes, but might also explain why the gastrointestinal mucosa has evolved these adaptive mechanisms to protect itself.

References

1. Henschel E, Bradstatter G, Dragosics B *et al.* Effect of ranitidine and amoxycillin plus metranidazole on the eradication of *H. pylori* and the recurrence of duodenal ulcer. N Engl J Med. 1993;328:308–12.
2. Moss SJ. *Helicobacter pylori* and peptic ulcers: the current position. Gut. 1992;33:289–92.
3. Eurogast Study Group. An international association between *Helicobacter pylori* infection and gastric cancer. Lancet. 1993;341:1359–62.
4. Wotherspoon AC, Ortiz-Haldago C, Falzon MR *et al. Helicobacter pylori*-associated gastritis and primary B-cell gastric lymphoma. Lancet. 1991;338:1175–6.
5. Marshall BJ, Barrett LJ, Prakash C *et al.* Urea protects *Helicobacter pylori* from the bactericidal effects of acid. Gastroenterology. 1990;99:697–702.
6. Dytoc M, Gold B, Louie M *et al.* Comparison of *Helicobacter pylori* and attaching–effacing *Escherichia coli* adhesion to eukaryotic cells. Infect Immun. 1993;61:448–56.
7. Kazi JL, Sinniah R, Zaman V *et al.* Ultrastructural study of *Helicobacter pylori*-associated gastritis. J Pathol. 1990;16:65–70.

8. Wyatt JI, Rathbone BJ, Sobola GM *et al*. Gastric epithelium in the duodenum: its association with *Helicobacter pylori* and inflammation. J Clin Pathol. 1990;43:981–6.

9. Sherman PM. Adherence and internalisation of *H. pylori* by epithelial cells. In: Hunt R, Tytgat G, editors. *Helicobacter pylori*; basic mechanisms to clinical cure. London: Kluwer; 1994:148–62.

10. Gregory MA, Spitaels JM. Variation in the morphology of villus epithelial cells within 8 mm of untreated duodenal ulcers. J Pathol. 1987;153:109–19.

11. Lui KC, Wright NA. The migration pathway of epithelial cells on human duodenal villi: the origin and fate of 'gastric metaplastic' cells on duodenal villi. Epith Cell Biol. 1992;1:53–8.

12. Hanby AW, Poulsom R, Elia G *et al*. The expression of the trefoil peptides pS2 and human spasmolytic polypeptide (hSP) in gastric metaplasia of the proximal duodenum; implications for the nature of gastric metaplasia. J. 1993;169:355–60.

13. Khulusi S, Hanby AM, Marrers JM *et al*. Expression of trefoil peptides pS2 and human spasmolytic polypeptide in gastric metaplasia at the margins of duodenal ulcers. Gut. 1995;37:205–9.

14. Kuhl P, Naczaco K, Malfertheimer P. How does gastric metaplasia in the duodenum differ from gastric epithelium? Gut. 1995;37(Suppl.):A29.

15. Robert IS, Stoddart RW. The ulcer-associated cell lineage in Crohn's disease: a lectin histo-chemical study. J Pathol. 1993;171:13–19.

16. Wright N, Pike C, Elia G. Induction of a novel epidermal growth factor-secreting cell lineage by mucosal ulceration in gastrointestinal stem cells. Nature. 1990;343:82–5.

17. Ahnen D, Poulsom R, Stamp GWH *et al*. The ulceration-associated cell lineage (UACL) reiterates the Brunner's gland differentiation programme but acquires the proliferative organisation of the gastric gland. J Pathol. 1994;173:317–26.

18. Ahnen D, Gullick W, Wright NA. Expression of multiple growth factors by the ulcer-associated cell lineage in Crohn's disease. Gastroenterology. 1991;100:A512.

19. Levi S, Beardshall K, Haddad G *et al*. *Campylobacter pylori* and duodenal ulcers: the gastrin link. Lancet. 1989;1:1167–8.

20. Heitz P, Kasper M, Van Noorden S *et al*. Immunohistochemical localisation of urogastrone to human duodenal and submandibular glands. Gut. 1978;19:408–13.

21. Playford RJM, Marshbank T, Chinery R *et al*. Human spasmolytic polypeptide is a cyto-protective agent which stimulates cell migration. Gastroenterology. 1995;108:108–16.

22. Steer HW. Ultrastructure of cell migration through the gastric epithelium and its relationship to bacteria. J Clin Pathol. 1975;28:639–45.

23. Dixon MF. *Helicobacter pylori* and peptic ulceration: histopathological aspects. J Gastroenterol Hepatol. 1991;6:125–30.

24. Carrick J, Lee A, Hazell D *et al*. *Campylobacter pylori*, duodenal ulcer and gastric metaplasia: possible role of functional heterotopic tissue in ulcerogenesis. Gut. 1989;30:790–07.

25. Harris AW, Walker HM, Smotka A *et al*. Parietal cells in the duodenal bulb: the relation to *Helicobacter pylori* infection. J Clin Pathol. 1996;40:309–12.

26. Walker MM, Dixon MF. Gastric metaplasia: its role in duodenal ulceration. Aliment Pharmacol Ther. 1996;10(Suppl. 1):119–28.

27. Wyatt JL, Rathbone BJ, Sobola GM *et al*. Gastric epithelium in the duodenum: its association with *Helicobacter pylori* and inflammation. J Clin Pathol. 1990;43:981–6.

28. Fitzgibbons PL, Dooley CP, Cohen H *et al*. Prevalence of gastric metaplasia, inflammation, and *Campylobacter pylori* in the duodenum in members of a normal population. Am J Clin Pathol. 1988;90:711–14.

29. Rhodes J. Experimental production of gastric epithelium in the duodenum. Gut. 1964;5:454–8.

30. Tatsuta M, Ishii H, Yamamura H *et al*. Enhancement by tetragastrin of experimental induction of gastric epithelium in the duodenum. Gut. 1989;30:311–15.

31. Kruning J, van der Wal JM, Kuiper G *et al*. Chronic non-specific duodenitis: a multiple biopsy study of the duodenal bulb in health and disease. Scand J Gastroenterol. 1989;24(Suppl. 167): 16–20.

32. Harris AW, Gummett PA, Waller JM *et al*. The relationship between gastric acid output and gastric metaplasia of the duodenal bulb. Gut. 1994;34(Suppl. 5):S49.

33. Shahib SM, Cutz E, Drumm B *et al*. Association of gastric metaplasia and duodenitis with *Helicobacter pylori* infection in children. Am J Clin Pathol. 1994;102:188–91.

34. Marshall BJ, McCechie DB, Rogers PA *et al*. Pyloric *Campylobacter* infection and gastro-duodenal disease. Med J Aust. 1985;142:439–44.

35. Yang HT, Dixon MF, Zuo JS *et al*. *Helicobacter pylori* infection and gastric metaplasia in China. J Clin Gastroenterol. 1995;20:100–12.

36. Wyatt JL, Rathbone BJ, Dixon MF *et al*. *Campylobacter pyloridis* and acid-induced gastric metaplasia in the pathogenesis of duodenitis. J Clin Pathol. 1987;40:841–8.
37. Dixon MF, Sobala GM, Wyatt JL *et al*. Gastric metaplasia and *H. pylori* associated gastritis as predictors of the duodenal ulcer diathesis. Irish J Med Sci. 1992;161(Suppl. 10):11.
38. Fullman W, Van Deventer G, Schneidmann D *et al*. Healed duodenal ulcers are histologically ill. Gastroenterology. 1985;88:1390.
39. Moshal MC, Gregiry MA, Pillay D *et al*. Does the duodenal cell ever return to normal? A comparison between treatment with Cemitidine and Denol. Scand J Gastroenterol. 1979;14(Suppl. 54): 48–51.
40. Noach LA, Rolf TM, Bosma NB *et al*. Acid and gastric metaplasia in the duodenum. Gut. 1995;36(Suppl. 1):A51.
41. Khulusi S, Patel P, Badve S *et al*. Pathogenesis of gastric metaplasia in duodenal ulcer disease. Gut. 1995;36(Suppl. 1):A51.
42. Khulusi S, Mendall MA, Badve S *et al*. Effect of *Helicobacter pylori* eradication on gastric metaplasia of the duodenum. Gut. 1995;36:193–7.
43. Harris AW, Walker MM, Waller JM *et al*. Gastric metaplasia in the duodenal bulb before and six months after eradication of *Helicobacter pylori*. Gastroenterology. 1995;108:A108.
44. Morson BC. Carcinoma arising from areas of intestinal metaplasia in the gastric mucosa. Br J Cancer. 1955;9;377–85.
45. Stemmermann GN. Intestinal metaplasia of the stomach: a status report. Cancer. 1994;74:356–62.
46. Matsukara M, Suzuki K, Kawachi *et al*. Distribution of marker enzymes and mucin in intestinal metaplasia of the stomach and relation of complete and incomplete types of metaplasia to minute gastric cancer. J Natl Cancer Inst. 1980;65:231–6.
47. Segura DI, Montero C. Histochemical characterisation of different types of intestinal metaplasia in the gastric mucosa. Cancer. 1983;52:498–503.
48. Ma J, De Boer W, Nayman J. Intestinal mucinous substances in gastric intestinal metaplasia and carcinoma studied by immunofluorescence. Cancer. 1982;49:1664–7.
49. Slack J. From egg to embryo, 2nd edn. Cambridge: Cambridge University Press; 1993.
50. Soman NR, Correa P, Ruiz BA. The TYR-MET oncogenic rearrangement is present and expressed in human gastric and precursor lesions. Proc Natl Acad Sci USA. 1991;88:4892–6.
51. Taher E. Molecular mechanism of stomach carcinogenesis. J Cancer Res Clin Oncol. 1993; 119:265–72.
52. Hastie ND, Dempster M, Dunlop MG *et al*. Telomere reduction in human colorectal carcinoma and with aging. Nature. 1990;346:866–8.
53. Tahar E. Molecular biology of gastric cancer. World J Surg. 1995;19:484–90.
54. Sipponen P, Kekki M, Seppala K *et al*. The relationship between chronic gastritis and gastric acid secretion. Aliment Pharmacol Ther. 1996;10(Suppl. 1):103–18.

20
Cell regulation, differentiation and their sequelae in the *Helicobacter pylori* inflamed and eradicated stomach

R. H. RIDDELL

The issues of cell regulation and turnover in the stomach are of critical importance as they impact directly on the important lesions of erosions, ulcers and cancer, the major complications of *H. pylori* disease. In uncomplicated *H. pylori*-associated gastritis and duodenitis an erosion or ulcer results from the inability of the epithelial dynamics adequately to maintain or repair the epithelium at an adequate rate. Further, a persistent long-term increase in epithelial turnover in many organs may predispose to neoplastic sequelae, and in this regard the stomach is no exception. The theory is that increased cell turnover results from increased mitotic activity, and this in turn provides greater opportunities for the production of abnormal cells from which clones may arise, and from which neoplasms may ultimately develop. Further, it is increasingly apparent that while regular cell turnover is associated with a 3–5-day turnover at the surface, and a turnover time measured in months in the pits, that there is a second method of cell degeneration that must be taken into account in epithelial dynamics, which is that of cell apoptosis. Further, the relationships between cell turnover, the inflammatory response and *H. pylori* itself need to be separated as far as possible. Because *H. pylori* infection in humans is always associated with at least some degree of chronic inflammatory infiltrate, some of these data necessarily come from animal sources.

Cell differentiation must be kept in mind; just because cells look similar does not mean that they behave similarly under similar conditions. Explanations have to be found for:

1. The distribution of *H. pylori* within the stomach and why *H. pylori* changes its distribution with time.
2. Why gastric surface-like cells in the duodenum and stomach behave so differently with regard to their interaction with *H. pylori* and other noxious substances such as bile.

In this chapter the evidence that *H. pylori*-associated inflammation does modulate cell turnover, and that cell differentiation may be involved, will be examined. Some of these issues will also have been touched upon in previous chapters. Finally, some of the myths surrounding gastric cancer will be touched upon, particularly regarding their implications in *H. pylori* infection.

Gastric surface cells (or cells with this morphology) function differently in different locations, or why do cells that look the same behave differently?

Stomach

Cells identical to gastric mucous cells are found throughout the stomach superficially and also throughout the duodenum. Yet in the stomach initial infection by *H. pylori* is followed by localization of the organism maximally in the antrum, but with time both the organism and the accompanying inflammation spread proximally to involve increasingly the oxyntic mucosa. Subsequently there is gradual atrophy of oxyntic mucosa with, in some patients, development of intestinal metaplasia, dysplasia and carcinoma. One can argue that this is the result of differential expression of *H. pylori* receptors that are maximal in the antrum, but other mechanisms must be considered, bearing in mind, particularly, the mechanism by which proximal spread occurs.

1. The most likely is a creeping inflammation up the lesser curve to the incisura and beyond, aided by a similar creeping around the remainder of the circumference of the stomach over the transitional mucosa which contains gradually increasing numbers of parietal cells. This could result in inflammation and atrophy, gradually extending proximally and circumferentially, but with a predominance for the lesser curve which contains fewest specialized cells. This is also the area most subject to intestinal metaplasia and dysplasia.
2. There is also a second potential mechanism, which is that *H. pylori* is a pangastritis with antral predominance. The low-grade oxyntic inflammation probably gradually extends into the mucous neck region, possibly affecting the production of specialized cells, but slowly also resulting in pit inflammation followed by the destruction of specialized cells.

However, this also requires a second hypothesis to explain this selective distribution of infection, which is that *H. pylori* survives less well in a full acid environment, and survives better in a lower acid milieu. This is supported by:

1. Cultural characteristics.
2. The hypochlorhydria following initial infection. Therefore there seems to be a two-stage process, the first associated with at least one acid-inhibiting protein (AIF1)[1] which renders the patient hypochlorhydric and allows the organism to establish itself. However, this protein is probably only transcribed or active for a short period of time (weeks or a few months), which is time for the organism to establish itself in the antrum.
3. The redistribution of organisms within the antrum where there is copious non-acidic mucus in which to survive until the more proximal gastric mucosa

slowly undergoes creeping atrophy, allowing gradual proximal spread of organisms. This whole process can be stopped only with intestinal metaplasia, but at the cost of an increased risk of dysplasia and carcinoma.
4. The proximal shift in *H. pylori* colonization with increasing proximal inflammation and atrophy in patients taking proton pump inhibitors[2,3].

Thus, in this case, the distribution of *H. pylori* within the stomach may be entirely unrelated to cell differentiation and the differential expression of receptors to which *H. pylori* attaches, than to the ability of *H. pylori* to survive and multiply better in a pH milieu that does not have to bear the full brunt of gastric acidity.

Duodenum

Yet what happens in the duodenum? Similar gastric surface cells are readily found in the normal duodenum, and increase in area under conditions of increased acid output as is seen in *H. pylori*-associated duodenal ulcer patients, while this is partially reversible following eradication of the organism. However, although *H. pylori* are well described in the duodenal mucosa, they are far more difficult to detect than in the adjacent gastric antrum. These cells may differ in the number of receptors to which *H. pylori* can attach, but again there are local differences that may need to be considered, including the local effects of bile and activated pancreatic secretions, both of which are highly toxic to *H. pylori*. Further, there are parietal cells scattered throughout the duodenum, often in clusters resembling oxyntic mucosa. *H. pylori* are averse to dwelling in a milieu with a high local acid output. The ducts of all of the glands entering the duodenum such as Brunners, metaplastic and heterotopic gastric mucosa, and the greater and lesser papillae, are lined by epithelium indistinguishable from gastric surface mucosa. Yet surprisingly, although duodenogastric reflux into the stomach is associated with the typical appearances of reactive (chemical) gastropathy, these changes are virtually never found in the duodenal mucosa, where it is highly likely that they are regularly exposed to these agents. This probably represents the production of different kinds of mucus that are much more resistant to these substances.

Mechanisms of epithelial turnover

Is epithelial turnover unequivocally increased in H. pylori *gastritis*?

There are numerous studies in the literature that vary tremendously in their design, e.g. antrum or corpus biopsies but not both, and variously using human or rodent tissue, and utilizing flow cytometry, BRDU incorporation, Ki-67 (Mib-1) or PCNA staining, which arrive at the almost unanimous conclusion that, compared to normal, there is increased cell proliferation in the *H. pylori*-infected stomach[4–11]. This involves both the length of and number of cells in the proliferative compartment[4]. There is also evidence that following therapy this returns to normal, often irrespective of whether eradication had occurred[4,7,9–11]. This probably correlates with the marked reduction in the number of organisms during therapy. However, if eradication is successful, the hyperproliferative state recurs, with recovery of the organism and its associated inflammatory response.

Which cells are involved and how?

While it is reasonable to think that all studies have been directed at the entire gastric mucosa, they are actually directed at only the most superficial part, and it is unclear whether there is also increased turnover in the oxyntic mucosa, pyloric glands or endocrine cells. Some degree of linear hyperplasia can be found in the latter, associated with atrophic gastritis[12]. Endocrine cells appear to be relatively spared in this process and may accumulate in the base of the mucosa. There is a paradox to the increase in cell turnover in the superficial part of the mucosa, that is simultaneously accompanied by destruction of the mucous neck cells, for if it is unable to keep up with the turnover required to prevent its own destruction, the entire pit unit may be lost. However, unlike destruction at the surface that produces an erosion, epithelial destruction in the mucous neck cells is characterized by a neutrophilic infiltrate (pit abscess) but one never actually sees crypt destruction. This therefore raises the issue of the mechanism of pit destruction, for if it is not overtly visible then presumably it is much more subtle. In all likelihood it may well involve cell loss by apoptosis, to the point where the apoptotic rate either matches or exceeds the ability of the pit to produce cells. In this case the pit is lost, or may reach the point of equilibrium where cell production equals cell loss, possibly to the point that specialized cells stop being produced, and there is downward extension of mucous cells, producing what is called (pseudo)pyloric metaplasia. The alternative may be the drive to produce intestinal metaplasia, which affords relief as the inflammatory infiltrate is much reduced even though the cell turnover remains increased.

What drives cell turnover?

The two major players are a direct effect of *H. pylori* on the epithelium, or an effect through the immune response, or a combination of both.

Direct effect of H. pylori. Because *H. pylori* attaches directly to the surface epithelium, there is almost certainly a direct effect of *H. pylori*[13]. Because of the closeness of the relationship between *H. pylori* and inflammation, the direct effect of the organism alone can only be investigated in cell lines, a highly artificial system. Evidence suggests that *H. pylori* is probably directly toxic to epithelial cells and reduces the turnover rate[14], and may be most marked if attachment has occurred. Moreover, ammonia itself may cause arrest in the S-phase of the cycle[15].

Effect of inflammation. The question therefore becomes: What controls the intensity of inflammation? There is general agreement that the number of organisms overall correlates with the intensity of the inflammatory reaction, but there is also the suggestion that the inflammatory response is particularly intense when organisms are found attached to, or even between, epithelial cells. This is only a generalization, and some biopsies have numerous organisms and surprisingly little inflammation; others have heavy acute and chronic inflammation in which it is difficult to find organisms, which may mean that there is another cause of the inflammation. If the direct effect of *H. pylori* is to be given credence, then the increased cell turnover is related to the inflammation, which more than compensates for this effect. This must be the result of substances produced by the

epithelium: pre and post eradication indices of proliferating cell nuclear antigen. Am J Gastroenterol. 1993;88:1870–5.

12. Solcia E, Villani L, Luinetti O, Fiocca R. Proton-pump inhibitors, enterochromaffin-like cell growth, and *Helicobacter pylori* gastritis. Aliment Pharmacol Ther. 1993;7(Suppl. 1):29–31.

13. Taniguchi Y, Ido K, Kimura K *et al*. Morphological aspects of the cytotoxic action of *Helicobacter pylori*. Eur J Gastroenterol Hepatol. 1994;6(Suppl. 1):S17–21.

14. Chang K, Fujiwara Y, Wyle F, Tarnawski A. *Helicobacter pylori* toxin inhibits growth and proliferation of cultured gastric cancer cells-Kato II. J Physiol Pharmacol. 1993;44:17–22.

15. Matsui T, Matsukawa Y, Sakai T, Nakamura K, Aoike A, Kawai K. Effect of ammonia on cell cycle progression of human gastric cancer cells. Eur J Gastroenterol Hepatol. 1995;7(Suppl. 1): S79–81.

16. Crabtree JE, Farmery SM. *Helicobacter pylori* and gastric mucosal cytokines: evidence that CagA-positive strains are more virulent. Lab Invest. 1995;73:742–5.

17. Peek RM Jr, Miller GG, Tham KT *et al*. Heightened inflammatory response and cytokine expression *in vivo* to *cagA+ Helicobacter pylori* strains. Lab Invest. 1995;73:760–70.

18. Husson MO, Gottrand F, Vachee A *et al*. Importance in diagnosis of gastritis of detection by PCR of the *cagA* gene in *Helicobacter pylori* strains isolated from children. J Clin Microbiol. 1995;33: 3300–3.

19. Kuipers EJ, Pérez-Pérez GI, Meuwissen SGM, Blaser MJ. *Helicobacter pylori* and atrophic gastritis: importance of the cagA status. J Natl Cancer Inst. 1995;87:1777–80.

20. Weel JFL, Van der Hulst RWM, Gerrits Y *et al*. The interrelationship between cytotoxin-associated gene A, vacuolating cytotoxin, and *Helicobacter pylori*-related diseases. J Infect Dis. 1996;173: 1171–5.

21. Ching CK, Wong BCY, Kwok E, Ong L, Covacci A, Lam SK. Prevalence of CagA-bearing *Helicobacter pylori* strains detected by the anti-CagA assay in patients with peptic ulcer disease and in controls. Am J Gastroenterol. 1996;91:949–53.

22. Tee W, Lambert JR, Dwyer B. Cytotoxin production by *Helicobacter pylori* from patients with upper gastrointestinal tract disease. J Clin Microbiol. 1995;33:1203–5.

23. Murakita H, Hirai M, Ito S, Azuma T, Kato T, Kohli Y. Vacuolating cytotoxin production by *Helicobacter pylori* isolates from peptic ulcer, atrophic gastritis and gastric carcinoma. Eur J Gastroenterol Hepatol. 1994;6(Suppl. 1):S29–31.

24. Sipponen P, Kimura K. Intestinal metaplasia, atrophic gastritis and stomach cancer: trends over time. Eur J Gastroenterol Hepatol. 1994;6(Suppl. 1):S79–83.

25. Sharp R, Babyatski R, Takagi H *et al*. Transforming growth factor alpha disrupts the normal program of cellular differentiation in the gastric mucosa of transgenic mice. Development. 1995; 121:149–61.

26. Tsuji M, Kawano S, Tsuji S *et al*. Cell kinetics of mucosal atrophy in rat stomach induced by long-term administration of ammonia. Gastroenterology. 1993;104:796–801.

27. Li H, Helander HF. Hypergastrinemia increases proliferation of gastroduodenal epithelium during gastric ulcer healing in rats. Dig Dis Sci. 1996;41:40–8.

28. Jones NL, Yeger H, Cutz E, Sherman PM. *Helicobacter pylori* induces apoptosis of gastric antral epithelial cells *in vivo*. Gastroenterology. 1996;110:A933.

29. Zhu GH, Ching CK, Lam SK, Sheng JZ, Wong TM, Ding SZ. Sialic acid dependent *H. pylori* lectin as an activator of calcium signal in cultured epithelial cells. Gastroenterology. 1996;110:A307.

30. Fukuda T, Arakawa Y, Fujiwara Y *et al*. Nitric oxide induces apoptosis in gastric mucosal cells. Gastroenterology. 1996;110:A111.

31. Naito Y, Yoshikawa T, Yagi N *et al*. Cell growth inhibition and apoptosis induced by monochloramine in a gastric mucosal cell line. Gastroenterology. 1996;110:A205.

32. Kato K, Sasano H, Ohara S *et al*. DNA damages caused by ammonia administration in rat stomach. Gastroenterology. 1996;110:A150.

33. Higashide S, Gomez G, Rajaraman S, Thompson JC, Townsend CM Jr. The effects of gastrin and bombesin on apoptosis induced by fasting in the rat stomach. Gastroenterology. 1996;110:A529.

34. Saegusa M, Takano Y, Okayasu I. Bcl-2 expression and its association with cell kinetics in human gastric carcinoma and intestinal metaplasia. J Cancer Res Clin Oncol. 1995;121:357–63.

35. Lauwers GY, Scott GV, Hendricks J. Immunohistochemical evidence of aberrant bcl-2 expression in gastric epithelial dysplasia. Cancer. 1994;73:2900–4.

36. Okuyama S, Yokota K, Yuki M. Cell proliferation and cell death (apoptosis) in epithelial tumors of the stomach – analysis of tumor tissues by the endoscopic mucosal resection. Jpn J Gastroenterol. 1995;92:130–9.

37. Uemura M, Mukai T, Okamoto S *et al. Helicobacter pylori* eradication inhibits the growth of intestinal type of gastric cancer in initial stage. Gastroenterology. 1996;110:A282.

38. O'Connor E, Buckley M, O'Morain C. Intestinal metaplasia and the gastric cancer cascade. Gastroenterology. 1996;110:A214.

39. Khulusi S, Mendall MA, Badve S, Finlayson C, Northfield TC. Effect of *Helicobacter pylori* eradication on gastric metaplasia in the duodenum. Gut. 1995;36:193–7.

40. Hansson LE, Engstrand L, Nyrén O, Lindgren A. Prevalence of *Helicobacter pylori* infection in subtypes of gastric cancer. Gastroenterology. 1995;109:885–8.

41. Huang JQ, Sridhar S, Chen Y, Wilkinson J, Hunt RH. Do younger patients with *Helicobacter pylori* have a higher risk of gastric cancer? A meta-analysis between *Hp* seropositivity and gastric cancer. Gastroenterology. 1996;110:A532.

21
The gastric lymphomas and the role of *Helicobacter pylori* in tumour development: have criteria been set for diagnosis?

M. F. DIXON

INTRODUCTION

Gastric lymphomas account for only a small proportion of gastric malignancies, between 1% and 7% depending on the geographical area[1], but their incidence is increasing[2]. Almost all are B-cell lymphomas, a proportion of which recapitulate the appearances of mucosa-associated lymphoid tissue (MALT) and are similar to low-grade B-cell lymphomas arising in the lung, thyroid and salivary gland[3]. As with these latter two sites, the stomach has no intrinsic lymphoid tissue. It is now clear that the appearance of a lymphoid infiltrate in the gastric mucosa is largely a consequence of *H. pylori* infection. Thus it can be anticipated that *H. pylori* gastritis is a major precursor of gastric lymphoma, and evidence to this effect has accumulated over recent years.

A seroepidemiological study[4] has revealed a 6-fold increased risk for the ultimate development of gastric lymphoma in individuals with *H. pylori* antibodies compared to uninfected controls, while there was no significant difference in prior *H. pylori* infection between individuals with extragastric non-Hodgkin's lymphoma and controls. Most persuasive, however, have been the studies of Isaacson's group[5] showing that eradication of *H. pylori* leads to regression of gastric lymphoma. In this chapter I shall review the tissue changes that precede gastric B-cell lymphoma, give possible explanations for their development, and discuss the criteria currently employed in making a diagnosis of lymphoma.

INFLAMMATION VERSUS IMMUNITY

As with any acute bacterial infection the initial response to *H. pylori* is mounted by neutrophil polymorphs. The bacteria release a number of directly acting chemotactic moieties which penetrate through the damaged surface epithelium and induce polymorph emigration into the lamina propria and epithelium[6]. Bacterial products also activate mast cells and their degranulation releases other acute inflammatory mediators which increase vascular permeability, up-regulate expression of leucocyte adhesion molecules on endothelial cells and increase polymorph emigration[7]. *H. pylori* stimulates the gastric epithelium to produce a potent neutrophil chemokine, interleukin 8, whose production is up-regulated by tumour necrosis factor α (TNFα) and interleukin 1 (IL-1) released by macrophages in response to bacterial lipopolysaccharide[6].

After a few days the innate acute response to infection is augmented by a specific immune reaction which results in the synthesis of anti-*H. pylori* antibodies. Antigens which gain access to the lamina propria are taken up and processed by macrophages and dendritic cells which serve as antigen-presenting cells for naive T-helper (CD4[+]) lymphocytes. Antigen fragments are presented at the cell surface, bound to major histocompatibility complex (MHC) class II antigens, and activate T-helper cells. These in turn promote activation of an appropriate memory B cell by releasing stimulatory cytokines such as IL-2, IL-4 and IL-5, or by direct intercellular contact[8]. B-cell proliferation and subsequent plasma cell differentiation results in the synthesis of IgM and possibly IgE antibodies, which activate complement or trigger mast-cell degranulation to further amplify the acute inflammatory response. However, this vigorous inflammatory response fails to eliminate infection and the continued presence of *H. pylori* leads to the development of a second arm of the immune response more specifically aimed at preventing the damaging effects of intraluminal pathogens. This second-line response involves the recruitment of primed B cells into lymphoid follicles with the production of plasma cells largely committed to the synthesis of 'mucosally protective' IgA antibodies. The fact that, even when augmented by IgA, the response is insufficient to eradicate *H. pylori* in the great majority of cases, means that antigenic stimulation persists and the formation of follicles becomes a consistent feature of chronic *H. pylori* gastritis.

While the two arms of the reaction to *H. pylori*, the acute 'inflammatory' and the chronic 'immune', are both interrelated and to a large degree inseparable, they do not necessarily run in parallel. Although the typical histological picture of active chronic gastritis with lymphoid follicles reflects the overlap of these two processes, down-regulation of the acute 'active' inflammatory component can result in a picture of inactive chronic gastritis, i.e. one in which there is no polymorph component, with lymphoid follicles. In human *H. pylori* infection this disparity is most evident in children in whom the lymphofollicular pattern is dominant, and is sufficient to give rise to a characteristic nodularity of the mucosa, yet polymorph activity is minimal or absent. The dissociation between 'inflammatory' and 'immune' (follicular) lymphoid infiltration reaches its ultimate expression in some animal models. For example, in the Balb-C mouse infected with *H. felis*, no gastritis is observed for most of the animal's lifespan. However, aged infected mice may develop a pronounced follicular lymphoid infiltrate in the corpus mucosa which in some animals progresses to lymphoma[9]. These findings indicate the importance of host factors in determining the balance between inflammation and immunity, but bacterial (strain) factors should not be overlooked. Thus, genotypic differences in *cag*A and *vac*A genes appear to be important in determining inflammatory activity. On the other hand, follicle formation seems to be a universal response to *H. pylori* irrespective of the infecting strain[10], and there is no difference in the frequency of *cag*A and *vac*A S1-positive strains between cases of MALT lymphoma and *H. pylori* chronic gastritis[11].

The follicular lymphoid element that arises on the background of 'inflammatory' lymphocytic infiltration in chronic *H. pylori* gastritis is a classic example of an 'acquired' mucosa-associated lymphoid tissue or MALT.

THE NATURE OF MALT

Mucosa-associated lymphoid tissue has been defined as 'a specially adapted component of the immune system that has evolved to protect the freely permeable surface of the gastrointestinal tract and other mucosae directly exposed to the external environment'[12]. The archetypal MALT of the intestinal tract is found in the ileum as Peyer's patches, and these will serve as a model for all such tissue. Peyer's patches are non-encapsulated organized collections of lymphoid tissue characterized by the presence of follicle (germinal) centres and a consistent arrangement of surrounding B and T lymphocytes into zones containing certain predominant cell types[13].

The intestinal epithelium overlying Peyer's patches (dome epithelium) is structured to allow the passage of antigens, or antigenic fragments, into the under-lying lymphoid tissue. This particular function resides in specialized epithelial cells, termed M cells because they have numerous microfolds in their surface membranes. M cells are able to absorb, transport and (possibly) process and present antigens. However, certain intact antigens may also be able to traverse the dome epithelium directly.

The follicle centre consists of a 'dark' zone at its base containing principally centroblasts, and a 'light' zone towards its apical (luminal) aspect mostly made up of centrocytes. Admixed with these cells are the follicular dendritic cells (FDC) which specialize in binding antibody–antigen immune complexes and in inducing B-cell proliferation and differentiation. The follicle centres arise from the proliferation of one, or a very few, B-cell blasts. Following direct or T-cell-mediated antigenic activation of a specifically primed B cell, the resultant B-cell blast proliferates at a high rate to form an expansile collection of centroblasts devoid of surface immunoglobulin. Centroblasts mature into centrocytes and, following stimulation by antigen presented on FDC, the variable region immuno-globulin genes of the centrocytes undergo somatic hypermutation to increase their affinity for antigen. Then follows a process of selection in which the centrocytes, now bearing surface immunoglobulin, are 'interrogated' by FDC. Successful interaction of centrocytes bearing high-affinity receptors for antigen presented by the FDC gives rise to secondary B-cell blasts which proliferate and leave the apical light zone as either long-lived plasma cell precursors or primed memory B cells[14]. Centrocytes which fail to interact with an FDC are 'rejected' and undergo programmed cell death by apoptosis. Interaction between the FDC and the centrocytes is facilitated by numerous ligands and receptors, but an important component is the CD40 ligand on the FDC. Crosslinking between the two cells not only prevents apoptosis but also promotes immunoglobulin class switching, predominantly from IgM to IgA and IgG[8]. Karyorrhectic nuclear debris derived from the apoptotic centrocytes is taken up by phagocytes within the follicle centre, forming the so-called 'tingible body' macrophages.

The follicle centre is surrounded by a narrow 'mantle' zone of B cells which express surface IgM and IgD. This in turn is surrounded by a 'marginal' zone in which most of the cells are small to intermediate-sized B lymphocytes, while others have moderately abundant cytoplasm, so-called monocytoid B cells. The cell nuclei resemble those of centrocytes. These cells produce IgM but not IgD. The marginal zone extends towards the surface of the mucosa and some B lymphocytes may enter the dome epithelium. Thus, a B-cell 'lympho-epithelium' is a normal characteristic of MALT. Outside the marginal zone in the deeper parts of the Peyer's patch is a T-cell rich zone in which high endothelial venules are prominent.

One feature which serves to illustrate the distinctive nature of MALT is the selectivity of its cellular recirculation[15]. The plasma cell precursors leaving the follicle centres pass into the lamina propria, where many are retained locally while others enter lymphatics to reach the mesenteric lymph nodes and via the thoracic duct gain access to the blood stream. These circulating cells have a strong tendency to localize in other sites of MALT elsewhere in the gastro-intestinal tract or in other organs. Such recirculation involves lamina propria lymphocytes as well as plasma cell precursors, and appears to be governed by specific receptors on lymphoid cells which recognize *adressins* on high endothelial venules in the lamina propria of MALT. Thus, antigen stimulation at one mucosal site elicits an antibody response restricted to MALT, but not confined to the site of origin.

H. PYLORI GASTRITIS AS MALT

The normal stomach is virtually devoid of lymphocytes and plasma cells. A few small basally situated collections of lymphocytes may be found in the corpus, but never with germinal centres. One explanation for their absence is the protected state of the gastric mucosa. The viscid mucous layer minimizes contact with luminal contents, and the high acid content destroys most bacteria and may denature other potential antigens. However, a more important factor could be the absence from the gastric epithelium of cells equivalent to the M cell of the small intestine and a consequent lack of antigen presentation.

Following *H. pylori* infection large numbers of CD4+ lymphocytes and B cells arrive in the lamina propria, initially to augment the acute response but later to mount an IgA-predominant immune response. Just as in the Peyer's patch, antigen presentation is followed by T-cell activation and B-cell proliferation with follicle formation. Antigen-presenting cells (APC) may also migrate to local lymph nodes where a similar B-cell response is evoked and plasma-cell precursors and memory cells will pass via lymphatics and the blood stream to populate the lamina propria of the gastric mucosa. At first antigen presentation is by conventional macrophages or dendritic cells, but it is later enhanced by changes in the epithelium. Cytokine effects on the surface epithelium largely mediated by interferon γ and TNFα induce expression of MHC Class II antigen sites, thus rendering the epithelial cells capable of antigen processing and presentation. Cell-

H.pylori
infection   APC

                                  ‖   Antigen presentation

                              CD4⁺ T-cell

                                  │   Activation/induction

Lymphoid
infiltration   T-cell expressing CD40 L

                                  ‖   Cell - cell contact

Organised   Normal B cell
MALT

                                  │   Follicle centre
                                                        response

                              Plasma cell
                                 ╱ ╲
                                ╱   ╲
                               ↙   ↘
                             IgA   IgG

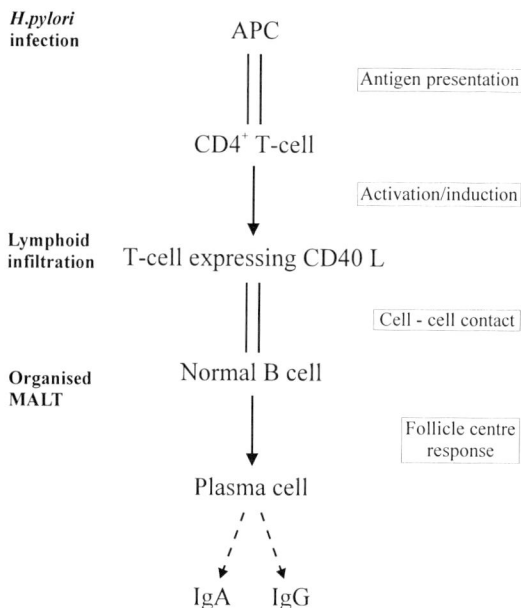

Figure 1 Diagram illustrating the steps involved in mounting a B-cell response in the acquired MALT of *H. pylori* gastritis. APC = antigen presenting cell; (CD40) L = ligand

to-cell contact between the antigen-presenting cell and a CD4⁺ T lymphocyte up-regulates the expression of the CD40 ligand (CD40L) on the T-cell surface[8]. CD40 is present on the surface of B cells, and crosslinking is a necessary requirement for B-cell activation by T cells. Resting T cells that lack CD40L cannot help B cells. Interaction between an activated (CD40L+) T lymphocyte and a normal memory B cell promotes B-cell activation and proliferation, leading to formation of a B-cell follicle. The resulting plasma cells produce large quantities of anti-*H. pylori* antibodies of predominantly IgA, but also of IgG1 and IgM types (Figure 1).

In keeping with the lymphoid cell migration, re-circulation and 'homing' characteristics of MALT, anti-*H. pylori* antibody-producing plasma cells are detectable in the regional lymph nodes[16], and secretory IgA antibodies are detected in saliva[17].

In chronic *H. pylori* infection the gastric mucosa acquires lymphoid follicles complete with mantle and marginal zones. Small numbers of marginal zone B lymphocytes can be seen within the surface or, more usually, foveolar epithelium. There are intervening T-cell rich zones and small numbers of intra-epithelial CD8⁺ (suppressor) T lymphocytes appear. Large numbers of plasma cells are found in the superficial lamina propria between the foveolae. Thus, chronic *H. pylori* gastritis recapitulates all the components of MALT.

THE ORIGINS OF B-CELL LYMPHOMA

Gastric B-cell lymphoma of marginal zone type (low-grade MALToma) consists of cells similar to those in the normal marginal zone of the MALT lymphoid

Lymphoid
infiltration   T-cell expressing CD40 L

                      | | | [Cell - cell contact]

Organised
MALT   "Growth-promoted" B cell

                                               CD40 stimulation
                                               ? Autoantigens

                      B-cell proliferation

                                               [T-cell stimulation]

Low-grade
MALToma   Monoclonal proliferation

                                               ? Autocrine
                                               stimulation

High-grade
MALToma   Blast cell proliferation

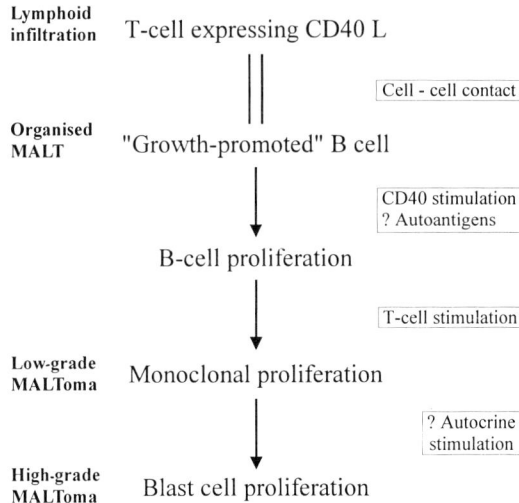

Figure 2 Hypothetical series of events in the development of MALT lymphoma. Following the initial interaction between an antigen-presenting cell and a CD4+ T cell, the activated T cell bearing the CD40 ligand binds to a B cell with an abnormal potential for uncontrolled proliferation. This gives rise to a clone of centrocyte-like B cells constituting a marginal zone (low-grade) lymphoma. Further genetic changes allied to abnormal growth factor stimulation lead to large B-cell (high-grade) lymphoma

follicle. In a series of experiments by Isaacson and co-workers[18,19] the principal functional characteristics of gastric B-cell lymphomas have been elucidated. Using *in-vitro* measures of B-cell proliferation they have shown that lymphoma cells will respond to extracts of *H. pylori*, and that such responses are strain-specific. They have also established that B-cell proliferation is dependent upon the presence of non-neoplastic T cells, and that such proliferation requires cell-to-cell contact from *H. pylori*-activated T cells mediated via CD40 ligand–receptor interactions. Thus, the stimulatory influences at work in lymphoma also recapitulate those that initiate gastric MALT development and its specific plasma cell response. Another interesting finding relates to the possible role of auto-antigens in the promotion of lymphomagenesis. Studies have shown that the immunoglobulin expressed by lymphoma cells recognizes epitopes on FDC and other normal tissue components, including plasma cells in gastric and small intestinal mucosa, but showed no reactivity with *H. pylori* itself[20–22].

The nature of the abnormal response to antigenic stimulation responsible for lymphomagenesis is the subject of speculation. Crabtree and Spencer[23] have proposed that T-cell activation of a 'growth-promoted B cell' could bring about its uncoordinated proliferation with clonal expansion of centrocyte-like cells. In so far as neoplasia arises through an accumulation of genetic alterations, which allows cells to escape from normal control mechanisms, the preneoplastic B cell has presumably undergone some genetic change which endows it with a growth advantage (Figure 2).

GENETIC CHANGES IN B-CELL LYMPHOMA

The elucidation of genetic abnormalities in gastric lymphoma is in its infancy. Nevertheless, some interesting and potentially important findings have emerged.

Using chromosome specific α-satellite probes and *in situ* hybridization, Wotherspoon *et al.*[24] found trisomy 3 in 18/29 (62%) cases of gastric marginal zone lymphoma. In so far as the putative proto-oncogene *bcl*-6 has been mapped to 3q27[25] and rearrangements of this band have been found in extranodal B-cell lymphomas, the authors speculate that *bcl*-6 might play a significant role in MALT lymphoma development. However, the significance of trisomy 3 in terms of clinical behaviour is presently unknown, and further work is required on the genes of chromosome 3 before its role in lymphomagenesis can be validated.

The *bcl*-2 gene rearrangement, which reflects a t(14;18) chromosomal translocation, is the most frequent karyotypic abnormality in non-Hodgkin's lymphomas of follicle centre cell lineage, but is uncommon in gastric MALT lymphomas[26]. However, this rearrangement is not infrequently found in normal lymphoid tissue and peripheral blood, so that its occasional finding in gastric tissue showing MALT lymphoma is not unexpected. Nevertheless, its low frequency does suggest that MALT lymphomas do not arise from follicle centre cells. As opposed to the gene rearrangement, *bcl*-2 protein expression is heterogeneous among MALT lymphomas and is independent of the presence or absence of the t(14;18) translocation[27]. It is possible that the 'growth-promoted' B-cell subset from which the lymphomas arise have higher levels of endogenous *bcl*-2 than normal B cells. Recently Nakamura *et al.*[27] have demonstrated that immunochemical expression of the anti-apoptotic *bcl*-2 protein in primary gastric lymphomas diminishes with advancing histological grade. Other translocations, namely t(1;14) and t(11;18), have also been observed in a small proportion of MALT lymphomas[28,29].

Oncogene activation has so far been limited to the demonstration of abnormalities in c-myc; c-myc gene point mutations were detected in 9/54 MALT lymphomas at sites critical to the negative regulation of the c-myc protein p64, indicating a possible role for this oncogene product in their development[30].

More interest has centred on the inactivation of tumour suppressor genes as determinants of lymphomagenesis. Our group looked at six tumour suppressor genes in a small number of gastric lymphomas using a highly sensitive fluorescent PCR technique to detect allelic imbalance[31]. Allelic imbalance was found in five of 12 cases at either the DCC or APC locus, but none showed imbalance at the p53 locus. In a subsequent study, however, p53 mutations were detected in 11/40 (27.5%) MALT lymphomas from various sites[32].

Most recently, the identification of microsatellite instability as a reflection of defective DNA mismatch repair has become an area of considerable interest in oncogenesis. Defects in mismatch repair genes lead to variations in the length of short-repeat motifs of bases distributed throughout the genome, so-called microsatellite sequences. Using polymorphic microsatellites as allele markers, extra allele bands can be demonstrated in some tumour DNA when compared with DNA from normal tissue, a phenomenon known as microsatellite instability. Peng *et al.*[32] found the replication error phenotype – defined as cases with microsatellite alterations at two or more of the five loci examined – in 21/40 (52.5%) MALT lymphomas from various sites, but the interpretation of such findings is a matter of debate. Studies in which large numbers of microsatellite loci have been examined point to low levels of instability as a frequent finding in neoplasia, and alterations in as few as five loci could be attributed to 'background'[33,34]. Indeed, instability can also be found in non-neoplastic disorders and alterations in two or more of five loci have been found in 2/14 (14%) cases of chronic gastritis[35].

Whichever genetic change or changes are eventually invoked in the development of MALT lymphoma, it is clear that the early stages of the disease are capable of reversal by withdrawal of antigenic stimulation. It will be interesting to document the sequence of genetic abnormalities in MALT lymphoma, because it seems likely that the transition from marginal zone type to diffuse large-cell-type lymphomas corresponds to a point of escape from antigen dependency. It appears that diffuse large B-cell gastric lymphoma (high-grade MALToma) has taken on the attributes of an autonomous growth, a property more in keeping with our conventional views of malignant neoplasia, concepts which have been challenged by the antigen-dependency and reversibility of most low-grade gastric MALTomas.

DIAGNOSTIC CRITERIA IN MARGINAL ZONE LYMPHOMA (LOW-GRADE MALTOMA)

Given the persuasive evidence that gastric B-cell lymphomas have their origin in the acquired MALT of *H. pylori* gastritis and, in particular, that normal marginal zone B cells and lymphoma cells share many phenotypic characteristics, the histological distinction between chronic gastritis and lymphoma is invariably difficult. The diagnosis rests on the identification of an atypical cellular infiltrate, evidence of destruction of the micro-architecture by this infiltrate, and (hitherto) its monoclonal nature.

The atypical infiltrate

In marginal zone lymphoma the infiltrate consists of cells that are slightly larger than normal lymphocytes with round or oval, irregularly shaped or cleaved nuclei, with small nucleoli and pale cytoplasm. These have been termed 'centrocyte-like (CCL) cells' by Isaacson[3]. A second cell type has abundant, clearer cytoplasm with well-defined borders, and these have been termed monocytoid B cells, but the cells are somewhat larger than those described in a 'true' monocytoid lymphoma[36]. The CCL cells are interspersed with B immunoblasts of the same clone. In some cases cells contain large intranuclear inclusions composed of immunoglobulins, so-called Dutcher bodies. Plasma cells are usually abundant, and are concentrated in a zone between the gastric foveolae; these may also be identifiable as part of the same clone[1]. Multifocal involvement throughout the stomach is characteristic of low grade B-cell lymphomas[37]. Typically, the infiltrate replaces parts of the mucosal glandular layer as a dense sheet which can also include occasional follicles (Figure 3). In *H. pylori* gastritis the glands are occasionally separated or pushed apart by follicles, but rarely widely destroyed, and in uncomplicated severe atrophic gastritis there is usually a substantial decline in the chronic inflammatory cell infiltrate. Nevertheless, it must be emphasized

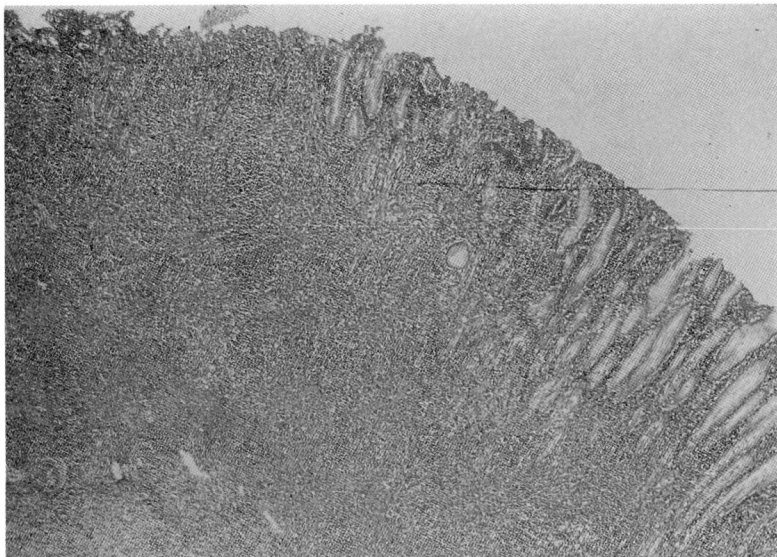

Figure 3 Low-power photomicrograph showing replacement of glands by a dense sheet of lymphoid cells in an example of a marginal zone lymphoma (low-grade MALToma)

that MALT lymphomas develop on a background of long-standing gastritis so that pre-existing glandular atrophy and intestinal metaplasia are to be expected[38]. If the lymphoid infiltrate extends through the muscularis mucosae then suspicion of lymphoma is greatly increased.

Destruction of micro-architecture

Apart from the 'wipe-out' of glands, more subtle indicators of the invasive nature of the atypical infiltrate are the finding of lympho-epithelial lesions and replacement of follicle centres.

Lympho-epithelial lesions are the cardinal feature of MALToma. Essentially they consist of glandular epithelium showing invasion by CCL cells with destruction of glandular structure and reactive changes in the residual epithelium (Figure 4). The epithelial reaction can be an impressive feature; the cells are enlarged with eosinophilic finely granular cytoplasm[39]. On occasion they appear to be forming small confluent clusters marking the last remnants of a destroyed gland. Such glandular remnants are easily overlooked in haematoxylin and eosin sections, but are readily picked out in sections stained for cytokeratins. The importance of destruction and epithelial reactive changes, in making a diagnosis of lymphoma, cannot be overemphasized. As indicated above, infiltration of epithelium by marginal zone B cells is a normal property of MALT and is an occasional finding in uncomplicated *H. pylori* gastritis. However, in chronic gastritis the glandular outline is preserved and there are no reactive changes in the epithelium (Figure 5).

Residual reactive follicles are a frequent finding in low-grade MALToma. Eidt *et al.*[40] found follicles in 79% of their low-grade gastric lymphoma cases. Such

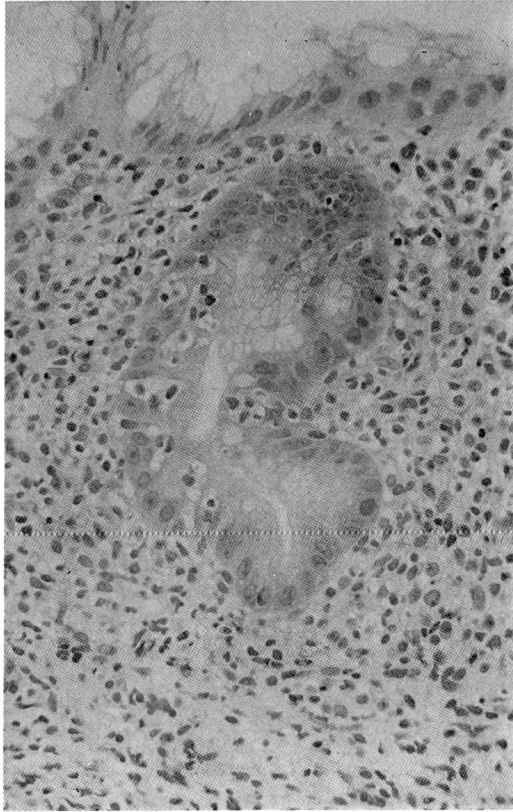

Figure 4   Lympho-epithelial lesions from a case of marginal zone lymphoma. The foveolar epithelium is infiltrated by small clusters of atypical lymphoid (centrocyte-like) cells. At this stage there is no destruction of the epithelial structures and such lesions have to be carefully distinguished from similar appearances in chronic *H. pylori* gastritis (see Figure 5)

follicles can become secondarily infiltrated by the CCL or monocytoid cells. This 'colonization' of follicles is an important diagnostic hallmark of MALT lymphomas and can take a variety of forms[41]. Most commonly the follicle is overrun and almost replaced by the CCL cells. Residual FDC can be demonstrated in paraffin sections using immunostains for CD21 or CD35; otherwise the ill-defined follicles may be missed with routine stains. Other follicles may show selective replacement of their germinal centres by CCL cells, with consequent loss of the light and dark zones characteristic of reactive centres, and in some cases the intrafollicular CCL cells may exhibit striking blast transformation. On occasion the intrafollicular CCL cells show uniform plasma cell differentiation.

Monoclonality

While histological criteria distinguishing between 'florid' chronic gastritis and low-grade lymphoma have been well defined[42,43], the demonstration of mono-

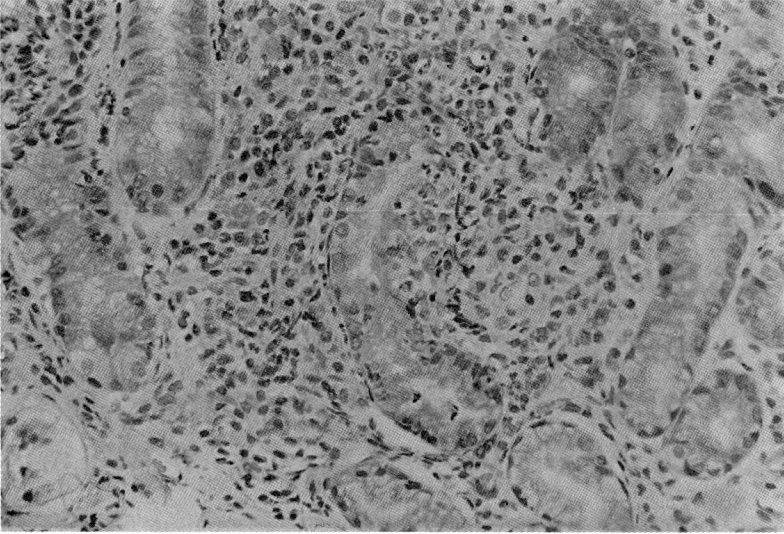

Figure 5   *H. pylori*-associated chronic gastritis in which very occasional foci of epithelial infiltration by mature B lymphocytes mimic the lympho-epithelial lesions of low-grade lymphoma

clonality is currently considered to be an essential requirement for lymphoma diagnosis. Monoclonality implies the origin of a neoplastic population from a single lymphoid cell, so that all the cells comprising a neoplastic B-cell clone will synthesize the same immunoglobulin (Ig) molecule. In addition to having a specific Ig gene rearrangement, any B-cell will produce only one of two Ig light chains, either κ or λ chains. Thus monoclonality is indicated by the finding that all the cells in a B-cell population exhibit the same light chain in cytoplasmic or surface Ig using immunohistochemistry as opposed to the mixture of κ and λ chains in reactive lymphoid populations[44]. Such demonstration of light-chain restriction using anti-κ or anti-λ antibodies can be valuable in reaching a diagnosis, but immunostaining of sIg is difficult in paraffin sections and convincing proof of monoclonality is sometimes difficult to obtain in biopsies compared with resection specimens, even if fresh frozen tissue is used[12]. A major source of difficulty is the range of κ:λ ratios found in normal reactive populations. While the 'normal' ratio is stated to be 2:1, a ratio of 7:1 or 8:1 can be seen in some benign reactive infiltrates, making the decision regarding light-chain 'restriction' particularly hazardous.

In putative B-cell lymphomas that fail to express sufficient Ig light chain for immunocytochemistry, clonality can be investigated only by molecular biological techniques[45]. Immunoglobulin heavy-chain gene rearrangements essential for immunological diversity bring about differences in the length of DNA sequences between restriction endonuclease sites. Therefore, if fresh tissue is available, long segment DNA can be extracted and subjected to restriction enzyme digestion and Southern blotting. If only paraffin-embedded material is available short, specific sequences that span the junctions between the variable and diversity segments of the Ig gene can be amplified using a polymerase chain reaction (PCR).

Table 1 Monoclonality in B-cell lymphoma – PCR-based findings

Reference	n	Monoclonal	Percentage
Fend et al. (1994)[48]	5 (untreated)	4	80
Inagaki et al. (1995)[49]	10	7	70
Savio et al. (1996)[50]	13	9	69
Calvert et al. (1996)[51]	12	8	67

Table 2 Monoclonality in chronic H. pylori gastritis – PCR-based findings

Reference	n	Monoclonal	Percentage
Fend et al. (1994)[48]	12	0	0
Savio et al. (1996)[50]	53	2	4
Hsi et al. (1996)[52]	41	6	15
Calvert et al. (1996)[51]	28	3	11

In either event, monoclonality within the test tissue is revealed by the finding of a single dominant band on blotting or in the PCR gel. Polyclonality is characterized by multiple gene rearrangements in different cells giving rise to a multiplicity of DNA segments which are individually in such low concentration that they fail to appear on a gel or produce a ladder or 'smear' effect. These techniques have displaced immunocytochemical tests for the determination of monoclonality in specialist centres, although even in such centres there is claimed to be a PCR 'failure' rate of about 20–30% in paraffin-processed tissue[46,47]. More recent studies[48–51] have given a similar frequency for monoclonality of between 67% and 80% (Table 1). Negative results have been attributed to the poor-quality DNA retrieved from paraffin-processed material, but some 'false-negative' results may be caused by chromosomal abnormalities involving the immunoglobulin locus leading to failure of primer binding. Of equal importance from a diagnostic viewpoint is the finding of monoclonality in biopsies showing chronic H. pylori gastritis with no features suspicious of lymphoma (Table 2). An early study claimed there were no instances of monoclonality in chronic gastritis, but three histologically 'inconclusive' cases showed a clonal gene rearrangement[48]. The authors stated that they 'favour a diagnosis of malignant lymphoma in such cases of clonal proliferations'. Likewise, Savio et al.[50] found two instances of monoclonality among 53 cases with reactive lymphoid infiltrates and concluded that 'The significance of PCR detected clonality in the absence of histological evidence of lymphoma is uncertain but may represent a stage of tumor progression or regression when the clonal population is insufficient to be detected by conventional histology'. The two most recent studies[51,52] have found the prevalence of monoclonality in straightforward cases of H. pylori chronic gastritis to be 11–15%. This frequency of monoclonality in random cases of gastritis cannot possibly equate to incipient lymphoma, and must point to the existence of 'benign' clonal gene rearrangements as a response to infection. This challenges the conventional view that monoclonality is a characteristic of neoplasia, and emphasizes that a diagnosis of lymphoma should not rest on this finding alone. Others have acknowledged that PCR-detected monoclonality occurs in chronic gastritis[53], but eschew the problem by concluding that Southern blotting should remain the gold standard. The authors state 'Current (PCR) techniques are too sensitive, detecting minute populations of clonal and oligoclonal lymphocytes that occur in benign diseases as well as larger populations of clonal lymphocytes..., associated with gastric MALToma'. In other words we should abandon the PCR technique, which is capable of detecting small clones of cells, in favour of Southern blotting in order to achieve more specificity for the diagnosis of lymphoma. Southern blotting, with its requirement for frozen tissue and its technical difficulty, is not practicable in most diagnostic situations, and the proposal is scientifically unsatisfactory. The development of quantitative PCR methods, hopefully in the near future, will be helpful in resolving this problem.

DIFFUSE LARGE B-CELL LYMPHOMA (HIGH-GRADE MALTOMA)

Formerly large-cell type (high-grade) gastric lymphomas were claimed to be much more common than low-grade tumours, but the prevalence rates have been radically revised in the light of new diagnostic criteria regarding MALT lymphomas. In the past many low-grade lymphomas have been interpreted as 'follicular gastritis' or 'pseudolymphoma'. In two recent series in which current criteria have been applied[1,40] high-grade lymphomas constituted 49% and 56% of B-cell lymphomas respectively, but the relative incidence in a particular population will depend on the lead-time to diagnosis. In countries with good health-care provision there is a greater chance that early, even asymptomatic, low-grade lesions will be detected, whereas in other populations advanced, ulcerated high-grade lesions are more likely to be found at clinical presentation. Most large B-cell lymphomas are assumed to have arisen from an initial marginal zone lymphoma, but evidence of residual low-grade features can be found in only one-third of cases even in resection material[1,40]. Where marginal zone type and diffuse large B-cell components coexist, the neoplastic cells exhibit the same class of immunoglobulin light chain[54]. Those cases which do not exhibit any low-grade component could be large B-cell lymphomas *ab initio*; certainly their relationship to marginal zone lymphomas is speculative. It is interesting, however, that the majority (88%) of lymphomas in the sero-epidemiological study referred to above[4], which linked them with previous *H. pylori* infection, were of the high-grade type. Likewise, although the prognosis of large B-cell lymphomas is significantly worse than marginal zone lymphomas, there is no difference in survival between those patients with and without concomitant low-grade elements[1].

Diffuse large B-cell lymphomas are composed of sheets of cells resembling centroblasts (large non-cleaved cells) or immunoblasts, and in the latter immunocytochemistry reveals abundant intracytoplasmic Ig. In some cases bizarre and multinucleated cells, which may resemble Reed–Sternberg cells, are seen. Fewer follicles are seen than in marginal zone lymphomas, and occasional lympho-epithelial lesions may be the only evidence of residual low-grade components in lymphomas with extensive, diffuse large-cell transformation. The centroblasts or immunoblasts of large-cell lymphoma rarely, if ever, infiltrate the epithelium to give rise to lympho-epithelial lesions, but their destructive capacity is demonstrated by the presence of ulceration in most cases[55].

Pure diffuse large B-cell lymphomas can present diagnostic confusion with undifferentiated carcinoma in routinely stained sections. The problem is resolved by immunostaining for cytokeratins and common leucocyte antigen (CD45).

CONCLUSION

The major thrust of this chapter has been the role of *H. pylori* in the development of B-cell lymphoma and the diagnostic criteria to be applied in the distinction of chronic gastritis and low-grade B-cell lymphoma. The diagnosis of lymphoma rests on the recognition of an atypical infiltrate, destruction of the micro-architecture reflecting the 'aggressive' nature of the infiltrate and the demonstration of monoclonality which, until recently, pointed to its neoplastic origins. In reaching this diagnosis there is considerable scope for misinterpretation. Typical chronic *H. pylori* gastritis can contain non-destructive 'lympho-epithelial lesions'[56] which, although distinguishable from the characteristic lesions of lymphoma, have overlapping features which can trap the unwary. Equally, the previous certainty which accompanied the finding of monoclonality as a marker of neoplasia has been challenged by its presence in a substantial proportion of otherwise unremarkable cases of *H. pylori* gastritis.

This diagnostic uncertainty is matched by reservations surrounding the true nature of marginal zone or low-grade B-cell lymphoma. Most definitions of neoplasia include the words 'uncoordinated' and 'autonomous'. While B-cell proliferation in low-grade lymphoma is certainly uncoordinated, some would argue that its regression after *H. pylori* eradication is strong evidence against such proliferation being a neoplastic process. Yet its biological characteristics, namely a destructive cellular infiltrate whose cells exhibit multiple genetic abnormalities, are properties associated with malignancy. Perhaps other established lymphoid malignancies will prove in due course to be 'antigen-dependent'. However, these are largely semantic issues. It is my belief that the careful application of the criteria outlined above will lead to a correct diagnosis. The main challenge is to develop tests which will allow us to predict which lymphomas will regress completely on antigen withdrawal (*H. pylori* eradication) and those which demand conventional anti-lymphoma chemo- or radiotherapy to achieve a potential cure.

Acknowledgements

I am grateful to my colleague Dr Andrew Jack for his constructive comments, to Jacquie Fearnley for secretarial help and to Stephen Toms for photographic assistance.

References

1. Cogliatti SB, Schmid U, Schumacher FE *et al.* Primary B-cell gastric lymphoma: a clinicopathological study of 145 patients. Gastroenterology. 1991;101:1159–70.
2. Severson RK, Davis S. Increasing incidence of primary gastric lymphoma. Cancer. 1990;66: 1283–7.

3. Isaacson PG. Lymphomas of mucosa-associated lymphoid tissue (MALT). Histopathology. 1990; 16:617–19.

4. Parsonnet J, Hansen S, Rodriguez L *et al*. *Helicobacter pylori* and gastric lymphoma. N Engl J Med. 1994;330:1267–71.

5. Wotherspoon AC, Doglioni C, Diss TC *et al*. Regression of primary low-grade B-cell gastric lymphoma of mucosa associated lymphoid tissue after eradication of *Helicobacter pylori*. Lancet. 1993;342:575–7.

6. Crabtree J. Gastric mucosal inflammatory responses to *Helicobacter pylori*. Aliment Pharmacol Ther. 1996;10(Suppl. 1):29–37.

7. Yoshida N, Granger DN, Evans DJ *et al*. Mechanisms involved in *Helicobacter pylori*-induced inflammation. Gastroenterology. 1993;105:1431–40.

8. Clark EA, Ledbetter JA. How B and T cells talk to each other. Nature. 1994;367:425–8.

9. Enno A, O'Rourke JL, Howlett CR, Jack A, Dixon MF, Lee A. MALT-oma-like lesions in the murine gastric mucosa after long-term infection with *Helicobacter felis*. A mouse model of *Helicobacter pylori*-induced gastric lymphoma. Am J Pathol. 1995;147:217–22.

10. Genta RM, Hamner HW, Graham DY. Gastric lymphoid follicles in *Helicobacter pylori* infection: frequency, distribution, and response to triple therapy. Hum Pathol. 1993;24:577–83.

11. Miehlke S, Lehn N, Bayerdörffer E, Meining A, Graham DY, Go MF. Are specific vacA subtypes of *Helicobacter pylori* associated with primary gastric lymphoma? Gastroenterology. 1996;110: A196.

12. Isaacson PG. Gastrointestinal lymphomas and lymphoid hyperplasias. In: Knowles DM, editor. Neoplastic haematopathology. Baltimore: Williams & Wilkins; 1992:953–78.

13. Isaacson PG, Norton AJ. Extranodal lymphomas. London: Churchill Livingstone; 1994:5–14.

14. Lydyard P, Grossi C. Secondary lymphoid organs and tissues. In: Roitt I, Brostoff J, Male D, editors. Immunology, 4th edn. London: Mosby; 1996:3.1–3.11.

15. Quiding-Järbrink M, Lakew M, Norström I *et al*. Human circulating specific antibody-forming cells after systemic and mucosal immunizations: differential homing commitments and cell surface differentiation markers. Eur J Immunol. 1995;25:322–7.

16. Newell DG, Stacey AR. Isotype and specificity of local and systemic anti-*Helicobacter pylori* antibodies. In: Menge H, Gregor M, Tytgat GNJ *et al.*, editors. *Helicobacter pylori*. Berlin: Springer-Verlag; 1991:83–9.

17. Patel P, Mendall MA, Khulusi S *et al*. Salivary antibodies to *Helicobacter pylori*: screening dyspeptic patients before endoscopy. Lancet. 1994;344:511–12.

18. Hussell T, Isaacson PG, Crabtree JE, Spencer J. The response of cells from low-grade B-cell gastric lymphomas of mucosa associated lymphoid tissue to *Helicobacter pylori*. Lancet. 1993; 342:571–4.

19. Hussell T, Isaacson PG, Crabtree JE, Spencer J. *Helicobacter pylori* specific tumour infiltrating T cells provide contact dependent help for the growth of malignant B cells in low grade gastric lymphoma of mucosa associated lymphoid tissue. J Pathol. 1996;178:122–7.

20. Spencer J, Diss TC, Isaacson PG. A study of the properties of a low-grade mucosal B-cell lymphoma using a monoclonal antibody specific for the tumour immunoglobulin. J Pathol. 1990; 160:231–8.

21. Greiner A, Marx A, Heesemann J, Leebmann J, Schmausser B, Müller-Hermelink HK. Idiotype identity in a MALT-type lymphoma and B cells in *Helicobacter pylori*-associated chronic gastritis. Lab Invest. 1994;70:572–8.

22. Greiner A, Marx A, Schmausser B, Müller-Hermelink HK. The pivotal role of the immuno-globulin receptor of tumor cells from B cell lymphomas of mucosa associated lymphoid tissue (MALT). Adv Exp Med Biol. 1994;355:189–93.

23. Crabtree JE, Spencer J. Immunologic aspects of *Helicobacter pylori* infection and malignant transformation of B cells. Sem Gastrointest Dis. 1996;7:30–40.

24. Wotherspoon AC, Finn TM, Isaacson PG. Trisomy 3 in low grade B cell lymphomas of mucosa associated lymphoid tissue (MALT). Blood. 1995;85:2000–4.

25. Ye BH, Rao PH, Chaganti RSK, Dalla-Favera R. Cloning of bcl-6, the locus involved in chromosome translocations affecting band 3q27 in B-cell lymphoma. Cancer Res. 1993;53:2732–5.

26. Pan L, Diss TC, Cunningham D, Isaacson PG. The bcl-2 gene in primary B cell lymphoma of mucosa-associated lymphoid tissue (MALT). Am J Pathol. 1989;135:7–11.

27. Nakamura S, Akazawa K, Kinukawa N, Yao T, Tsuneyoshi M. Inverse correlation between the expression of *bcl*-2 and p53 proteins in primary gastric lymphoma. Hum Pathol. 1996;27:225–33.

28. Wotherspoon AC, Pan L, Diss TC, Isaacson PG. Cytogenetic study of B-cell lymphoma of mucosa-associated lymphoid tissue. Cancer Genet Cytogenet. 1992;58:35–8.
29. Horsman D, Gascoyne R, Klasa R, Coupland R. t(11;18) (q21;q21.1): a recurring translocation in lymphomas of mucosa-associated lymphoid tissue (MALT). Genes Chromosom Cancer. 1992; 4:183–6.
30. Peng HZ, Diss TC, Isaacson PG, Pan LX. C-myc gene abnormalities in lymphomas arising in mucosa-associated lymphoid tissue (MALT). Lab Invest. 1996;74:120A.
31. Calvert R, Randerson J, Evans P *et al.* Genetic abnormalities during transition from *Helicobacter pylori*-associated gastritis to low-grade MALToma. Lancet. 1995;345:26–7.
32. Peng H, Chen G, Du M, Singh N, Isaacson PG, Pan L. Replication error phenotype and p53 gene mutation in lymphomas of mucosa-associated lymphoid tissue. Am J Pathol. 1996;148:643–8.
33. Gleeson CM, Sloan JM, McGuigan JA, Ritchie AJ, Weber JL, Russell SEH. Ubiquitous somatic alterations at microsatellite alleles occur infrequently in Barrett's-associated esophageal adeno-carcinoma. Cancer Res. 1996;56:259–63.
34. Gleeson CM, Sloan JM, McGuigan JA, Ritchie AJ, Weber JL, Russell SEH. Ubiquitous somatic alterations at microsatellite alleles occur infrequently in adenocarcinoma of the oesophagus and gastric cardia. Gut. 1996;38(Suppl. 1):A32.
35. Bronner MP, Crispin DA, Hueffed R *et al.* Microsatellite instability in non-neoplastic gastro-intestinal disorders. Lab Invest. 1996;74:55A.
36. Nizze H, Cogliatti SB, von Schilling C *et al.* Monocytoid B-cell lymphoma: morphological subtypes and relationship to the low-grade B-cell lymphoma of the mucosa associated lymphoid tissue. Histopathology. 1991;18:403–14.
37. Wotherspoon AC, Doglioni C, Isaacson PG. Low grade gastric B-cell lymphoma of mucosa-associated lymphoid tissue (MALT): a multifocal disease. Histopathology. 1992;20:29–34.
38. Anton RC, Steinbach G, Pugh W *et al.* Primary gastric lymphomas: strong correlation with *Helicobacter pylori* infection and atrophic gastritis. Lab Invest 1996;74:54A.
39. Papadaki L, Wotherspoon AC, Isaacson PG. The lymphoepithelial lesion of gastric low-grade B-cell lymphoma of mucosa-associated lymphoid tissue (MALT): an ultrastructural study. Histo-pathology. 1992;21:415–21.
40. Eidt S, Stolte M, Fischer R. *Helicobacter pylori* gastritis and primary gastric non-Hodgkin's lymphomas. J Clin Pathol. 1994;457:436–9.
41. Isaacson PG, Wotherspoon AC, Diss T, Pan L. Follicular colonization in B-cell lymphoma of mucosa-associated lymphoid tissue. Am J Surg Pathol. 1991;15:819–28.
42. Zuckerberg LR, Ferry JA, Southern JF, Harris NL. Lymphoid infiltrates of the stomach. Evaluation of histologic criteria for the diagnosis of low-grade gastric lymphoma on endoscopic biopsy specimens. Am J Surg Pathol. 1990;14:1087–99.
43. Arista-Nasr J, Jimenez A, Keirns C, Larraza O, Larriva-Sahd J. The role of endoscopic biopsy in the diagnosis of gastric lymphoma. Hum Pathol. 1991;22:339–48.
44. Spencer J, Diss TC, Isaacson PG. Primary B cell gastric lymphoma. A genotypic analysis. Am J Pathol. 1989;135:557–64.
45. Williams GT, Wynford-Thomas D. How may clonality be assessed in human tumours? Histo-pathology. 1994;24:287–92.
46. Algara P, Martinez P, Sanchez L *et al.* The detection of monoclonal B-cell populations by polymerase chain reaction: accuracy of approach and application in gastric endoscopic biopsy specimens. Hum Pathol. 1993;24:1184–8.
47. Diss TC, Pan L, Peng H *et al.* Sources of DNA for detecting B cell monoclonality using PCR. J Clin Pathol. 1994;47:493–6.
48. Fend F, Schwaiger A, Weyrer K *et al.* Early diagnosis of gastric lymphoma: gene rearrangement analysis of endoscopic biopsy samples. Leukemia. 1994;8:35–9.
49. Inagaki H, Nonaka M, Nagaya S, Tateyama H, Sasaki M, Eimoto T. Monoclonality in gastric lymphoma detected in formalin-fixed, paraffin-embedded endoscopic biopsy specimens using immunohistochemistry, *in situ* hybridization, and polymerase chain reaction. Diag Molec Pathol. 1995;4:32–8.
50. Savio A, Franzin G, Wotherspoon AC *et al.* Diagnosis and posttreatment follow-up of *Helicobacter pylori*-positive gastric lymphoma of mucosa-associated lymphoid tissue: histology, polymerase chain reaction or both? Blood. 1996;87:1255–60.
51. Calvert RJ, Evans PAS, Randerson JA *et al.* The significance of B-cell clonality in gastric lymphoid infiltrates. J Pathol. 1996 (In press).

52. Hsi ED, Greenson JK, Singleton TP, Siddiqui J, Schnitzer B, Ross CW. Detection of immuno-globulin heavy chain gene rearrangement by polymerase chain reaction in chronic active gastritis associated with *Helicobacter pylori*. Hum Pathol. 1996;27:290–6.
53. Banerjee SK, Weston AP, Horvat RT, Campbell DR, Cherian R, Makdisi WF. Determination of specificity of PCR monoclonality for the diagnosis of gastric lymphoma: direct comparison to Southern blot gene rearrangement. Gastroenterology. 1996;110:A487.
54. Chan JKC, Ng CS, Isaacson PG. Relationship between high grade lymphoma and low-grade B-cell mucosa-associated lymphoid tissue lymphoma (MALToma) of the stomach. Am J Pathol. 1990;136:1153–64.
55. Eidt S, Stolte M, Fischer R. Factors influencing lymph node infiltration in primary gastric malignant lymphoma of the mucosa-associated lymphoid tissue. Pathol Res Prac. 1994;190: 1077–81.
56. Wotherspoon AC, Ortiz-Hidalgo C, Falzon MR, Isaacson PG. *Helicobacter pylori*-associated gastritis and primary B-cell gastric lymphoma. Lancet. 1991;338:1175–6.

22
Clinical presentation, diagnosis and treatment of *Helicobacter pylori*-related gastric lymphoma

M. STOLTE, A. MORGNER, A. MEINING, C. THIEDE, A. NEUBAUER, E. SEIFERT and E. BAYERDÖRFFER

INTRODUCTION

Until the beginning of the 1980s, gastric lymphoma was categorized in accordance with the endoscopic classification suggested by Palmer in 1950[1]. At that time the lymphomas which pathologists examined were, for the most part, large advanced tumours, with involvement of all layers of the gastric wall. Often there was also infiltration of neighbouring tissue and involvement of the regional lymph nodes.

The lymphomas found in biopsy material were frequently wrongly diagnosed as carcinomas, and for further diagnostic work-up gastric resection was often recommended. The histological classification was, simply and undifferentiatedly, 'lymphosarcoma'.

Over the past 10 years or so this unsatisfactory state of diagnosis and therapy has improved considerably. Today, lymphomas are often detected endoscopically at an early stage[2,3]. New information concerning their pathogenesis has led to new histological classifications[4,5]. This has made their histological diagnosis in biopsy material more reliable, and in many cases it is now possible to diagnose low-grade lymphomas[6]. The high point of this rapid positive development is the initiation of a revolution in the treatment of low-grade mucosa-associated lymphoid tissue (MALT) lymphomas solely by *Helicobacter pylori* eradication.

MILESTONES IN GASTRIC LYMPHOMA

In 1983 and 1984 three important events heralded the beginning of this positive development. Isaacson developed the MALT concept of gastric lymphomas[7], Warren and Marshall described *H. pylori*[8], and from Japan came – in analogy to the early carcinomas – the first reports on early lymphomas, in which the depth of infiltration is limited to the mucosa and submucosa[9]. Thereafter, during the

1980s, the percentage of early lymphomas among gastric lymphomas increased rapidly. The figure in Vienna[10] between 1974 and 1978 was 21.7%; it increased in Tokyo[11] between 1977 and 1986 to 40.9%; and in our own material between 1983 and 1989 to 49.6%.

CHARACTERISTICS OF EARLY LYMPHOMAS

In an earlier publication we showed that early lymphomas did not differ in diameter from advanced lymphomas, and that they can be recognized macroscopically by a group of coincident findings – thickened folds, erosions and ulcerations caused by destructive tumour infiltration[2]. These lesions, like the early gastric carcinomas, undergo a malignant cycle[12], healing and reappearing again, with the result that a variegated picture including thickened folds, erosions, ulcers, scars and regenerative mucosa is seen (Figure 1).

The recognition of the early lymphoma was a step forward, as shown by the following data: the depth of infiltration correlates with the involvement of the regional lymph nodes and with the degree of malignancy of the tumour[13]; the deeper the infiltration, the greater the number of cases with lymph node involvement, and the more cases with high-grade malignancy (Figures 2 and 3). Early lymphomas, therefore, have significantly fewer cells expressing the Ki67 antigen, and fewer apoptotic bodies than advanced lymphomas, and the expression of p53 increases with the increasing depth of infiltration, while the expression of bcl2 decreases.

This means that the depth of infiltration is the major prognostic factor, as was shown by the Viennese working group headed by Dragosics and Radaskiewicz[10].

IMPROVED HISTOLOGICAL DIAGNOSIS

Knowledge of the variegated picture of the early lymphoma has resulted in an improved biopsy technique involving the removal of multiple large forceps specimens from the different areas.

The first good histological classification of the MALT lymphomas was proposed by Isaacson *et al.* in 1988[4]. Primary T-cell lymphomas of the stomach are very rare. Among our 220 surgical specimens with gastric lymphoma, only two were T-cell lymphomas. The high-grade lymphomas are predominantly centroblastic, polymorphous and easy to diagnose. Immunohistochemical confirmation is only rarely necessary. The site of tumour origin is the parafollicular marginal cells. For this reason, in the revised European-American classification of lymphoid neoplasms (REAL) the lymphoma is also termed a marginal B-cell lymphoma[5]. The decisive advance in the biopsy diagnosis of low-grade malignant lymphomas was the establishment of the following criteria by Isaacson and co-workers[14,15]:

1. replacement of glands by uniform infiltrates comprising centrocytoid cells, and
2. clear evidence of lymphoid destruction of the glands or foveolae.

The most important criterion is unequivocal evidence of lymphoepithelial destruction.

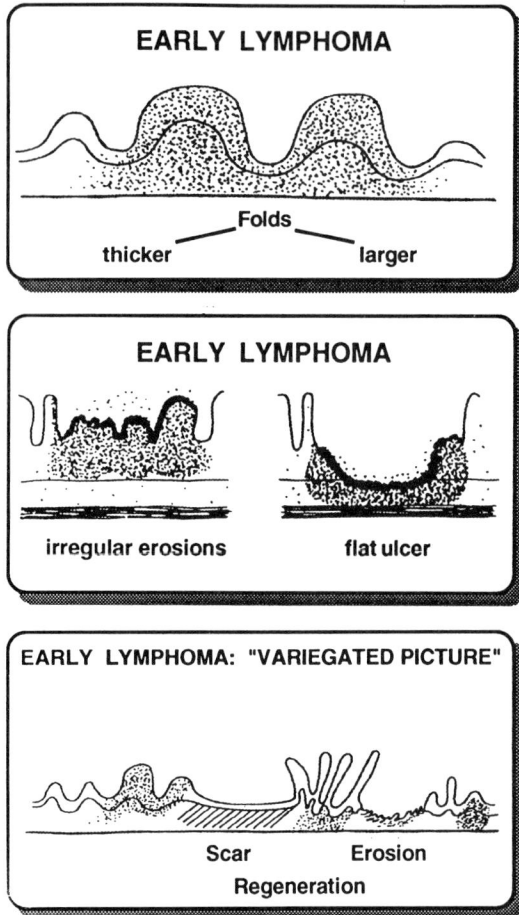

Figure 1 Typical macroscopic appearance of early gastric lymphoma: thickened folds (above), irregular erosions and shallow ulcers (centre) in combination with depressed scar areas following the malignant cycle and polypoid regenerative mucosa (below)

The diagnosis of low-grade MALT lymphoma of the stomach should be made only when invasive and destructive tumour growth is proven. That is when foveolae and/or glands are partially or almost completely destroyed by the lymphoid cell infiltrate.

In doubtful cases the destruction of the glands by lymphoma infiltrates can be well seen immunohistochemically with epithelial antibodies and B-cell antibodies (CD 20). Distinguishing between an infiltration by low-grade B-cell lymphoma from active autoimmune gastritis of the corpus mucosa and focal autoaggressive destruction of corpus glands may be difficult. The additional use of monoclonal antibodies recognizing T-cell antigen epitopes may be necessary, since the infiltrate associated with active type A gastritis without atrophy[16] usually comprises T lymphocytes (own unpublished data).

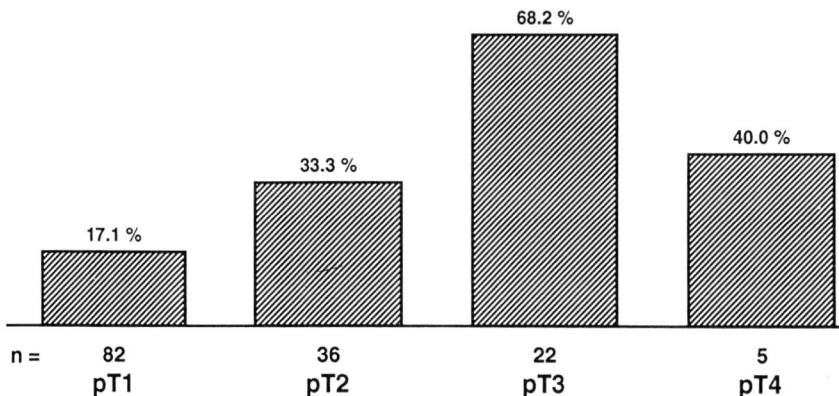

Figure 2 Incidence of lymphoma involvement of the perigastric lymph nodes as a function of pT stage

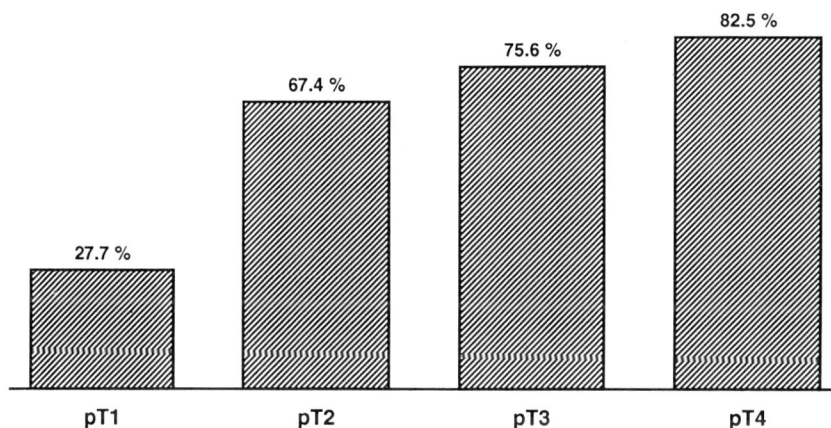

Figure 3 Incidence of high-grade lymphoma of the stomach as a function of pT stage

POLYMERASE CHAIN REACTION UNDER THE SCIENTIFIC MICROSCOPE

Presently undergoing scientific testing is the additional diagnostic examination using PCR. Investigations we carried out on 31 of our cases of low-grade gastric lymphoma revealed demonstrable gene rearrangements in 87%. Also, in cases of histologically suspected lymphoma with no definitive signs of lympho-epithelial lesions, PCR appears to enable an earlier diagnosis of lymphoma.

In principle our comparative investigation of bioptic histology and PCR allows three 'patterns' of findings to be differentiated[17]:

1. In the case of the histological diagnosis being 'reactive lymphatic infiltration', *H. pylori* eradication is followed by regression of the infiltration and PCR is polyclonal before and after eradication.

2.   In the case of the histological diagnosis being 'suspected lymphoma', PCR detected monoclonal B cells *before* histology revealed lymphoma.
3.   A problem are those cases in the third group: infiltrates classified histologically as reactive disappear following *H. pylori* eradication, PCR is initially positive and becomes negative after eradication.

A scientific problem still awaiting clarification is the histological diagnosis of a B-cell MALT lymphoma in biopsy material obtained from an endoscopically and endosonographically normal-appearing stomach. Histology reveals lymphatic infiltrates with only a few B lymphocytes infiltrating gland epithelial cells, but PCR indicates gene rearrangement of the heavy chain locus and monoclonality. Further studies will be needed to establish whether this monoclonality provides real evidence for the presence of an initial, autonomous and progressive neoplasia.

HELICOBACTER PYLORI AND MALT

The paths of MALT lymphoma and *H. pylori* research crossed for the first time in 1988 with the recognition that the cause of acquired gastric MALT is chronic infection with *H. pylori*[18,19]. The next logical question asked was whether MALT lymphoma arises against the background of *H. pylori* gastritis.

The first piece of the puzzle that helped clarify this relationship was the epidemiological comparative study performed by Doglioni *et al.*, which showed the dependence of the incidence of MALT lymphoma on the *H. pylori* infection rate[20]. The second was the fact that the early lymphomas – like acquired MALT – are located mainly in the gastric antrum.

Analysis of surgical specimens containing MALT lymphoma of the stomach showed *H. pylori* gastritis in 92% of the cases in London, and in 98.3% of those in Bayreuth[13,21]. The case–control study reported by Parsonnet *et al.*[22], revealing statistically significantly higher *H. pylori* infection rates among MALT lymphoma patients long before the development of the lymphoma, and experiments in the mouse, showed a lymphoma incidence of 26% after life-long infection with *H. felis* that produced only a mild form of gastritis[23]. In a further study the group headed by Lee transplanted gastric lymphoma cells subcutaneously or intra-peritoneally in young mice[24]. Only those animals infected with *H. pylori* developed lymphomas, while the control animals with no *H. pylori* infection did not. However, the lymphomas were not located at the sites of the subcutaneous or intra-peritoneal transplantation, but in the stomach! Over a lengthy follow-up period, some of these lymphomas underwent transformation from low-grade to high-grade lymphomas[24].

In another strain of mice, in contrast, the life-long infection with *H. felis* led to a severe form of gastritis with atrophy, but no lymphomas. Experimental lymphoma induction in BALB/C mice is also possible using *H. heilmannii*, but with differing frequencies – from 14% to 89% – depending on the host of the infection[25].

These animal experiments suggest that the factors (so far unknown) necessary to induce development of a gastric lymphoma in acquired MALT are probably to be sought among different bacterial and host factors.

That such factors may also be involved in the pathogenesis of human MALT lymphoma was shown in our material by the varying incidence of cytotoxin production in the strains of *H. pylori* from patients with gastric carcinoma and gastric lymphoma. There was a statistically significantly lower cytotoxin production found in the patients with gastric MALT lymphomas. These differences in cytotoxin production also led to a differing expression of gastritis. A matched control study of our material showed that, in patients with MALT lymphoma, gastritis is of lower grade in comparison with other *H. pylori* diseases, and that there is no difference between the antrum and corpus[26].

Our relatively frequent detection of low-grade MALT lymphomas in patients with *H. heilmannii* gastritis (eight out of 220 patients) in comparison with *H. pylori* gastritis, is evidence of an increased development of lymphomas in those harbouring relatively weakly pathogenic organisms that give rise to only mild gastritis[27].

It is thus possible that special antigens, arising either directly from weakly pathogenic strains of *Helicobacter* or indirectly via T lymphocytes, result in a positive selection of tumour cells via the antigen receptor. This is shown by findings in a new study reported by the group of Müller-Hermelink, showing that MALT-type lymphoma B cells are hypermutated postgerminal centre lymphocytes that have undergone antigen selection[28].

Isaacson's group has recently been able to show that changes to the p53 suppressor gene are involved in the development and transformation of MALT lymphomas; partial inactivation apparently leads to the development of low-grade MALT lymphomas, and complete inactivation to high-grade transformation[29].

TREATMENT OF MALT LYMPHOMA BY *H. PYLORI* ERADICATION

The discovery that low-grade gastric MALT lymphomas could be made to disappear by eradicating *H. pylori* was the fortuitous result of an attempt to establish whether *H. pylori* eradication could aid the differential diagnosis of lymphoma.

We then wondered whether the eradication of *H. pylori* might be capable of improving the differential diagnosis of reactive lymphatic infiltration from low-grade MALT lymphoma[30]. Our basic hypothesis was that *H. pylori* eradication should be associated with a disappearance of the reactive infiltrates, while lymphoma infiltrates would persist. To our great surprise our first analysis of 32 patients studied in 1992 showed that the MALT lymphomas could also disappear: in six out of 10 cases with low-grade MALT lymphomas follow-up revealed regression of lymphoma. Two of these six patients were submitted to surgery, and in both cases we found an empty lamina propria with small remnants of T lymphocytes, indicating regression of the tumour – a picture once seen only after successful chemotherapy of gastric MALT lymphomas.

In 1993 Isaacson's group reported regression of low-grade gastric MALT lymphomas in five out of six patients[31]. They investigated the proliferation behaviour of tumour cells from low-grade MALT lymphomas in cell cultures with and without *H. pylori*, and with and without T lymphocytes. It was found that

Table 1 Results obtained by treating MALT lymphomas with *H. pylori* eradication alone as a function of tumour stage, endoscopic appearance and tumour size (median follow-up: 15.5 months)

	Complete remission	*Partial remission*	*No change*
No. of patients	67 (79.7%)	6 (7.1%)	11 (13%)
Tumour stage	EI 1:67	EI 1:6	EI 1:4
	>EII:–	>EII:–	>EII:7
Endoscopic appearance			
Tumour	32	3	4
Ulcer	22	3	4
Erosion	2	0	0
Atypical mucosal relief	11	0	3
Tumour size			
Median	3.0 cm	4.0 cm	5.5 cm
Range	0.5–10.0 cm	1.0–7.0 cm	2.0–9.0 cm
Localization			
Antrum	38	1	7
Body	29	5	4
Period after *H. pylori* eradication			
Median	5.0 months	12.5 months	6.0 months
Range	0.5–26.0 months	4.0–28.0 months	2.0–22.0 months
Age			
Median	62.0 years	70.0 years	54.5 years
Range	31.0–84.0 years	60.0–86.0 years	35.0–86.0 years
Sex			
Male	32	3	5
Female	35	3	6

both *H. pylori* and T lymphocytes were needed for the proliferation of the tumour cells[32].

Encouraged by these initial results, we in Germany began a study of the treatment of low-grade B cell MALT lymphomas of the stomach consisting solely of eradication of *H. pylori*. Our first analysis of the results obtained after treating 33 patients in this manner revealed complete regression of the tumour in 70% of the cases[33]. Our study now involves 84 patients (median follow-up 15.5 months; range: 2–36 months). The present complete remission rate is 79.7%, while partial remission was achieved in 7.2%. In 11 of the 84 patients, neither endoscopy nor histology revealed any signs of remission. (The relevant data of these patients are shown in Table 1.) In 50 of our cases the follow-up period now exceeds 24 months; among these patients there has been complete remission in 74%, and partial remission in 10%. In 16% no change has been found.

If we summarize all the reports to date on the results of treatment of gastric lymphoma by *H. pylori* eradication (see Table 2), we find a complete regression figure of 74.3% in 171 patients. Further studies with longer follow-up periods are necessary, to show whether this regression is long-lasting. An initial case of recurrence has been reported in the literature; here, however, reinfection with *H. pylori* had also occurred[35]. In one of our patients, histological investigation revealed recurrent lymphoma 13 months after complete remission, despite the fact that no reinfection with *H. pylori* had occurred, and the endoscopic picture was unremarkable. On the other hand, the literature also reports on a recurrence-free case that had been followed up for as long as 7 years[36].

Table 2   Complete remission rates of low-grade MALT lymphomas so far reported after *H. pylori* eradication (see refs 31, 37, 38; other data: personal communication and our own material)

	n	Complete remission (%)
Stolte (1992)	10	60.0
Wotherspoon (1993)[31]	6	83.3
Dragosics (1995)	10	60.0
Fischbach (1995)	10	80.0
Savio (1995)[38]	14	92.8
Roggero (1995)[37]	37	59.4
Bayerdörffer (1996)	84	79.7
Totals	171	74.3

CONCLUSION AND OPEN QUESTIONS

The diagnosis and therapy of MALT lymphoma of the stomach have finally evolved after decades of stagnation. The past decade has seen major progress in this area, including improvement of biopsy diagnosis, a better histological classification, new information concerning the pathogenesis, and the start of a revolution in the treatment of low-grade gastric MALT lymphomas by eradication of *H. pylori* infection.

However, with the wealth of new information, numerous questions have also arisen, and these will need to be answered in the coming years:

1. What additional factors are needed to transform a reactive lymphocytic proliferation into a MALT lymphoma?
2. What *H. pylori* or T-lymphocyte products influence the proliferation of lymphoma cells, and via what receptors on the tumour cells?
3. Why do some low-grade MALT lymphomas regress, while others do not?
4. Is there a molecular–genetic point of no return?
5. Can we develop better diagnostic methods?
6. Is complete remission long-lasting, and how high is the local recurrence rate?
7. Will a molecular–genetic subclassification of the lymphomas be forthcoming?
8. Are there antigen-responsive tumours other than the low-grade MALT lymphomas of the stomach?

There is still a great deal of work to be done.

References

1. Palmer E. The sarcoma of the stomach. Am J Dig Dis. 1950;17:186–95.
2. Stolte M, Eidt S. The diagnosis of early gastric lymphoma. Z Gastroenterol. 1991;29:6–10.
3. Weismüller J, Seifert E, Goronzy R, Stolte M. Das maligne Lymphom des Magens - Fortschritte in der Frühdiagnostik. Schweiz Rundschau Med (Praxis). 1986;75:1531–2.
4. Isaacson PG, Spencer J, Wright DH. Classifying primary gut lymphomas. Lancet. 1988;2:1148–9.
5. Harris NL, Jaffe ES, Stein H *et al*. A revised European–American classification of lymphoid neoplasms. A proposal from the international lymphoma study group. Blood. 1994;84:1361–92.
6. Weismüller J, Seifert E, Schulte F, Lütke A, Stolte M. Endoskopisch-bioptische Diagnostik des malignen Lymphomes des Magens und des Magenfrühlymphomes. Leber Magen Darm. 1989; 19:258–68.

7. Isaacson PG, Wright DH. Malignant lymphoma of mucosa-associated lymphoid tissue: a distinctive type of B cell lymphoma. Cancer. 1983;52:1410–16.
8. Warren JR, Marshall BJ. Unidentified curved bacilli on gastric epithelium in active chronic gastritis. Lancet. 1983;330:1273–5.
9. Murayama H, Kikuchi M, Eimoto T, Doki I, Doki K. Early lymphoma coexisting with reactive lymphoid hyperplasia of the stomach. Acta Pathol Jpn. 1984;34:679–86.
10. Rawicz T, Dragosics B, Bauer P. Gastrointestinal malignant lymphomas of the mucosa-associated lymphoid tissue: factors relevant to prognosis. Gastroenterology. 1992;102:1628–38.
11. Mohri N. Primary gastric non-Hodgkin's lymphomas in Japan. Virchow Arch A. 1987;411: 459–66.
12. Eidt S, Stolte M. Evidence of a malignant cycle in early gastric lymphoma. Endoscopy. 1994;26: 295–8.
13. Eidt S, Stolte M, Fischer R. *Helicobacter pylori* gastritis and gastric non-Hodgkin's lymphoma. J Clin Pathol. 1994;47:436–9.
14. Isaacson PG, Spencer J. Malignant lymphoma of mucosa-associated lymphoid tissue. Histo-pathology. 1987;11:445–62.
15. Isaacson PG, Norton AJ. Extranodal lymphomas. Edinburgh: Churchill Livingstone; 1994.
16. Stolte M, Baumann H, Bethke B, Lauer E, Ritter M. Active autoimmune gastritis without total atrophy of the glands. Z Gastroenterol. 1992;30:729–53.
17. Rudolph B, Bayerdörffer E, Neubauer A *et al.* PCR improves the differential diagnosis between *Helicobacter pylori* infection induced lymphoid cell infiltration and early gastric MALT-lymphoma. Gastroenterology. 1995;108:A531.
18. Wyatt JI, Rathbone BJ. Immune response of the gastric mucosa to *Campylobacter pylori*. Scand J Gastroenterol. 1988;23(Suppl. 142):44–9.
19. Stolte M, Eidt S. Lymphoid follicles in the antral mucosa: immune response to *Campylobacter pylori*. J Clin Pathol. 1989;42:1269–71.
20. Doglioni C, Wotherspoon AC, Moschini A, de Boni M, Isaacson PG. High incidence of primary gastric lymphoma in northeastern Italy. Lancet. 1992;339:1175–6.
21. Wotherspoon AC, Ortiz-Hidalgo C, Falzon MR, Isaacson PG. *Helicobacter pylori*-associated gastritis and primary B-cell gastric lymphoma. Lancet. 1991;338:1175–6.
22. Parsonnet J, Hansen S, Rodriquez L *et al. Helicobacter pylori* infection and gastric lymphoma. N Engl J Med. 1994;330:1267–71.
23. Enno A, O'Rourke J, Lee A, Dixon MF. MALToma-like lesions in the stomach resulting from long-standing *Helicobacter* infection in the mouse. Am J Gastroenterol. 1994;89:1357.
24. Enno A, O'Rourke J, Howlett CR, Lee A. Mouse to mouse resuscitation of low-grade MALT lymphoma induced by prolonged *Helicobacter* infection. A preliminary study of transplanted tumors. Gastroenterology. 1996;110:A536.
25. O'Rourke JL, Enno A, Dixon MF, Lee A. Gastric B-cell lymphomas induced in the single mouse strain by various isolates of *Helicobacter heilmannii*. Similarities and differences. Gut. 1995; 37(Suppl. 1):A7.
26. Meining A, Stolte M, Lehn N *et al.* Differing expression of gastritis in *Helicobacter pylori*-associated diseases. Gastroenterology. 1996;110(In press).
27. Stolte M, Wellens E, Bethke B, Ritter M, Eidt H. *Helicobacter heilmanni* (formerly *Gastro-spirillum hominis*) gastritis: an infection transmitted by animals? Scand J Gastroenterol. 1994; 29:1061–4.
28. Qin Y, Greiner A, Trunk MJF, Schmausser B, Ott MM, Müller-Hermelink HK. Somatic hyper-mutation in low-grade mucosa-associated lymphoid tissue-type B-cell lymphoma. Blood. 1995; 86:3528–34.
29. Du M, Peng H, Singh N, Isaacson PG, Pan L. The accumulation of p53 abnormalities is associated with progression of mucosa-associated lymphoid tissue lymphoma. Blood. 1995;86:4587–93.
30. Stolte M. *Helicobacter pylori* and MALT-lymphoma. Lancet. 1992;339:745–7.
31. Wotherspoon AC, Doglioni C, Diss TC *et al.* Regression of primary low-grade B-cell gastric lymphoma of mucosa-associated lymphoid tissue type after eradication of *Helicobacter pylori*. Lancet. 1993;342:575–7.
32. Hussell T, Isaacson PG, Crabtree JE, Spencer J. The response of cells from low-grade B-cell gastric lymphomas of mucosa-associated lymphoid tissue to *Helicobacter pylori*. Lancet. 1993; 342:571–4.
33. Bayerdörffer E, Neubauer A, Rudolph B *et al.* MALT lymphoma study group. Regression of

primary gastric lymphoma of mucosa-associated tissue type after cure of *Helicobacter pylori* infection. Lancet. 1995;345:1591–4.

34. Bayerdörffer E, Morgner A, Neubauer A *et al*. Regression of primary gastric MALT-lymphoma after cure of *Helicobacter pylori* infection: a two-year follow-up report of the German MALT-lymphoma trial. Gastroenterology. 1996;110:A526.
35. Horstmann M, Erttmann R, Winkler K. Relapse of MALT lymphoma associated with *Helicobacter pylori* after antibiotic treatment. Lancet. 1994;1098–9.
36. Blecker U, McKeithan TW, Hart J, Kirschner BS. Resolution of *Helicobacter pylori*-associated gastritic lymphoproliferative disease in a child. Gastroenterology. 1995;109:973–7.
37. Roggero E, Zucca E, Pinotti G *et al*. Eradication of *Helicobacter pylori* infection in primary low-grade gastric lymphoma of mucosa associated lymphoid tissue. Ann Intern Med. 1995;122:767–9.
38. Savio A, Franzin G, Wotherspoon AC *et al*. Long-term effect of anti-*Helicobacter pylori* therapy on gastric MALT-lymphoma. Histological and molecular evaluation of 15 cases. Gut. 1995; 37:A246.

23
Mechanisms of paralysis and apoptosis of the inflammatory cells in *Helicobacter pylori* infection

K. DEUSCH

INTRODUCTION

It is well established that *Helicobacter pylori* is implicated as a causal agent of active chronic gastritis and peptic ulcer disease in humans[1-4]. However, although *H. pylori* is clearly pathogenic, most of those infected are clinically silent or asymptomatic subjects. To this end, the basis for the differing clinical manifestations in those affected with *H. pylori*, including gastric and duodenal ulceration, atrophic gastritis and clinically silent superficial gastritis, is unclear. Hence, it has been hypothesized that individuals vary in their immune recognition and effector mechanisms directed towards this organism. Thus, a vigorous inflammatory response mediated by activated neutrophils, macrophages and CD4+CD25+ T cells may result in substantial mucosal injury[5,6]. In contrast, down-regulation of inflammation mediated by CD8+ cells[7], antigen-induced anergy[8] or apoptosis[9] may diminish the acute and chronic inflammatory response to the organism and result in less mucosal damage. To test the hypothesis whether apoptosis plays a role in the limitation of the gastric mucosal immune response in *H. pylori* infection it is first necessary to establish that T cells residing in the gastric epithelium and lamina propria are subjected to regulation by the molecules governing apoptosis. A central pathway leading to cellular apoptosis in lymphocytes is initiated by Fas, a ~50 kDa widely distributed surface receptor belonging to the TNF receptor family[10]. In T lymphocytes, Fas is preferentially expressed late, following cellular activation[11], and its crosslinking results in rapid triggering of apoptotic programmes[12]. Fas crosslinking at the cell surface is mediated by fas ligand[13] expressed transiently soon after activation of T lymphocytes. Fas/fas-ligand interactions are therefore intimately related to the process of lymphocyte activation, and perhaps crucial for its control and termination by mediating apoptotic cell death of activated lymphocytes[13]. However, whether or not Fas/fas-ligand interaction leads to cell death is influenced by intracellular levels of bcl-2. In lymphocytes, high levels of this molecule due to an accidental gene translocation or experimental gene transfer have been shown to correlate with prolonged cell survival leading to lymphoma[14,15]. Therefore, in this study we investigated the expression of Fas, fas-ligand and bcl-2 in intraepithelial lymphocytes residing in the gastric epithelium in individuals chronically infected with *H. pylori*.

MATERIALS AND METHODS

Isolation, flow cytometric staining, apoptosis and culturing of epithelial lymphocytes (IEL) from the gastric mucosa

Gastric IEL were isolated according to a modified protocol adopted from Bull and Bookman[16,17]. For surface phenotyping cells were reacted with anti-CD3 antibodies (Becton Dickinson, Heidelberg) and either anti-Fas (CD95), anti-fas-ligand, or anti-bcl-2 antibodies and analysed for dual-colour fluorescence employing flow cytometry (FacsScan, Becton Dickinson, Heidelberg). For the analysis of intracellular bcl-2, cells were permeabilized employing a commercially available kit (Hölzel Diagnostica, Köln). For the detection of apoptosis in IEL, the TUNEL reaction was performed employing a commercially available kit (Boehringer-Mannheim, Mannheim). IEL were cultured in RPMI 1640 medium containing 10% FCS (Gibco, Eggenstein), 3 mmol/L glutamine, penicillin (100 IU/ml), streptomycin (100 μg/ml) and amphotericin B (0.25 μg/ml) in coated 96-well round-bottom microtitre plates (Costar, Bodenheim).

RESULTS

Fas expression on gastric IEL isolated from *H. pylori*-infected mucosa

Freshly isolated gastric IEL were stained with CD3 and anti-Fas antibodies and the fraction of CD3+/Fas+ cells determined employing dual-colour fluorescence. Moreover, cells were cultured for 48 h in the presence or absence of anti-CD3 antibodies and subsequently analysed for Fas expression. It could be observed that the majority of gastric IEL (93%) expressed Fas constitutively with an increase of Fas+ cells after 48 h incubation in culture medium (98%) and anti-CD3 antibodies (99%).

Fas-ligand expression on gastric IEL isolated from *H. pylori*-infected mucosa

Freshly isolated gastric IEL were stained with CD3 and fas-ligand antibodies and the fraction of CD3+/fas-ligand+ cells determined, employing dual-colour fluorescence. Moreover, cells were cultured for 48 h in the presence or absence of anti-CD3 antibodies and subsequently analysed for fas-ligand expression. Only a minute fraction of gastric IEL isolated from *H. pylori*-infected mucosa expressed fas-ligand constitutively (1.1%). However, incubation of these cells in culture medium or the presence of anti-CD3 antibodies led to a substantial increase of fas-ligand+ gastric IEL, i.e. 22% and 27%.

Bcl-2 expression on gastric IEL isolated from *H. pylori*-infected mucosa

Freshly isolated gastric IEL were stained with CD3 and anti-bcl-2 antibodies and the fraction of CD3+/bcl-2+ cells determined, employing dual-colour fluorescence. Moreover, cells were cultured for 48 h in the presence or absence of anti-Fas antibodies and subsequently analysed for bcl-2 expression. The vast majority of gastric IEL (99%) constitutively expressed bcl-2. Incubation in culture medium for 48 h did not alter significantly the fraction of bcl-2+ cells. In contrast, cross-linking the Fas receptor with the fas-ligand led to substantial reduction of the fraction of bcl-2+ cells. Moreover, the bcl-2 content of the bcl-2 staining cells was markedly reduced.

Apoptosis of gastric IEL

Freshly isolated gastric IEL were assessed for apoptosis employing the TUNEL reaction and subsequent flow cytometric analysis. Only a small fraction of freshly isolated IEL were observed to be undergoing apoptosis (2.8%). In contrast, incubation in culture medium led to an increase in the fraction of apoptosing cells (21%), with a further increase when anti-Fas antibodies were added at the beginning of the incubation (27%).

DISCUSSION

The molecular basis for the various clinical pictures that can be observed in *H. pylori* infection is at present poorly understood. Clearly, the cytotoxin-producing strains of *H. pylori* (CagA+) cause destruction of the epithelial layer and thereby contribute to the ulcerative disease manifestations but, surprisingly, their presence does not correlate with the occurrence of gastric malignancy. Therefore, it has become apparent that the host's immune response towards this organism may be relevant for the entire disease course. This has become particularly relevant since it has been shown that T lymphocytes and their secreted products can alter basic gastric functions such as acid secretion, mucus production and motility. Hence, it might very well be that the nature of the host's immune response, which may be governed by environmental and genetic factors, influences the clinical outcome of *H. pylori* infection. Therefore, it is evident that the study of the mechanisms regulating the local immune response may be critical for understanding the pathogenesis of *H. pylori*-induced gastric pathology. Next to the study of inflammatory cell-associated cytokines involved in the development of gastric lesions is the understanding of the mechanisms that may aid in down-regulating the host's immune response, i.e. anergy, active suppression and apoptosis, all of which are critically important. In particular, the latter mechanism bears relevance, not only

I. Active Suppression

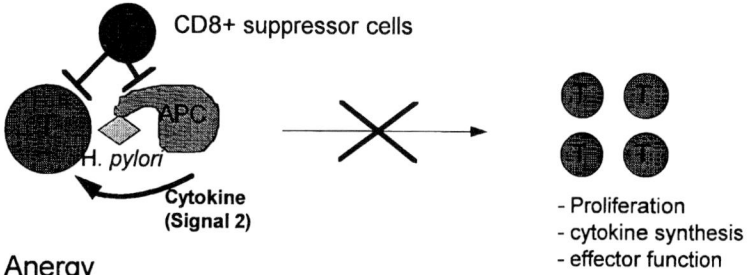

II. Anergy

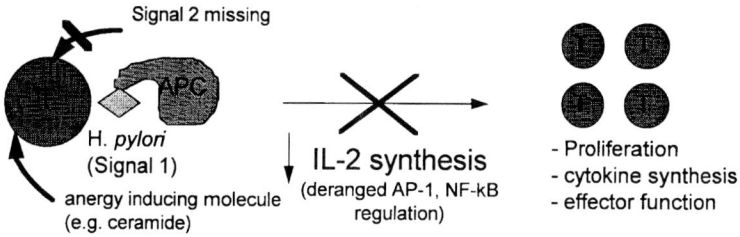

III. Apoptosis

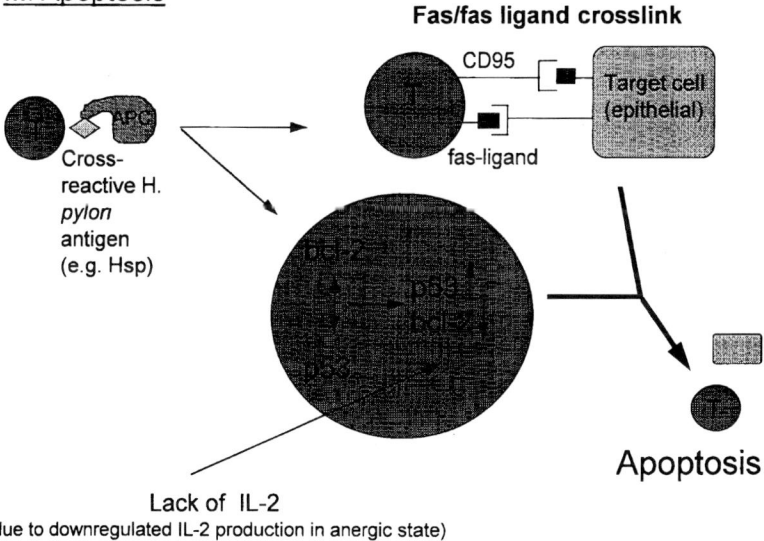

Figure 1 Mechanisms thought to confer immunological tolerance in the gastric mucosa

in controlling potential autoreactivity, but also to the development of lymphoid malignancy. Therefore, in this study we analysed, in gastric T lymphocytes, the expression and content of molecules believed to play a major role in regulating apoptosis. As a result we could demonstrate that the vast majority of gastric IEL constitutively express Fas and bcl-2 during *H. pylori* infection. The fas-ligand was expressed on a very minor fraction of gastric IEL (<2%) but could be induced following stimulation with anti-CD3 antibodies *in vitro*. Moreover, freshly isolated IEL were not found to apoptose immediately, but were found to do so after a period of 48 h *in vitro*. Moreover, crosslinking the Fas molecules employing monoclonal anti-Fas antibodies increased the fraction of apoptosing cells.

These results are comparable to those observed in IEL isolated from normal intestinal mucosa and those obtained from inflamed intestinal mucosa in patients with Crohn's disease. In addition, the fraction of T lymphocytes isolated from the peripheral blood (PBL) that express the Fas molecule was found to be much smaller. More importantly, PBL were not found to apoptose during a 48-h culture period *in vitro*. Therefore, we conclude that the regulation of apoptosis in gastric IEL appears to be comparable to that observed for intestinal IEL. The observed expression of Fas on the vast majority of IEL (>95%) underlines the concept that these cells are activated *in vivo* and can be induced to apoptose upon reception of the appropriate signal. At this point it can only be speculated that apoptosis may serve to prevent an immune response in *H. pylori* infection that may otherwise lead to autoimmune disease. We hypothesize that, in individuals chronically infected with *H. pylori*, the cellular immune system is not equipped to eradicate the organism. Teleologically, this may be due to the fact that a more efficient immune response would be detrimental to the host, i.e. causing inappropriate tissue destruction or autoimmunity. Hence, it could be assumed that the local immune response is modified or down-regulated by mechanisms such as active suppression, anergy and apoptosis. In fact, in bacterial superantigen-induced down-regulation of the immune response, anergy and apoptosis work in concert. Here the T cell receptor V-beta segment specific staphylococcal superantigen SEB leads to massive stimulation with enormous production of cytokines that is followed by apoptosis of the majority of cells. The remaining cells fail to proliferate and secrete IL-2 upon repeated stimulation[8]. Transformed to the situation in *H. pylori*-infected patients initial massive colonization with *H. pylori* may induce potent T cell activation with subsequent reduced responsiveness. It is conceivable that cells specific for bacterial heat-shock protein (Hsp60) may crossreact with autologous human p60, and are therefore deleted and subsequently anergized. The failure to find human p60 heat-shock protein-specific cells in the peripheral blood of *H. pylori*-infected individuals underscores this point[18]. To this end, peripheral deletion of antigen-reactive T cells has been demonstrated in animal models for oral tolerance[19]. However, despite these mechanisms, genetic variability or other factors may allow some *H. pylori*-specific T cells exhibiting crossreactivity with autoantigens, or others that belong to the physiological luminal microbial or food antigens, to persist, and may subsequently be responsible for autoimmune gastric disease such as food intolerance or autoimmune chronic atrophic gastritis. Further studies will be necessary to determine the exact nature of the immunoregulatory mechanisms that mediate either tolerance to *H. pylori* or autoreactivity due to *H. pylori* infection. Most importantly, these critical issues have to be clarified prior to the design of vaccination strategies, since potentially an inappropriate choice of vaccine may cause more harm than benefit, by inducing an unfavourable imbalance of immunological homeostasis in the gastric mucosa.

References

1. Blaser MJ. Epidemiology and pathophysiology of *Campylobacter pylori* infections. Rev Infect Dis. 1990;12(Suppl.):S99–106.
2. Warren JR, Marshall BJ. Unidentified curved bacilli on gastric epithelium in active chronic gastritis. Lancet. 1983;1:1273–5.
3. Marshall BJ, Warren JR. Unidentified curved bacilli in the stomach of patients with gastritis and peptic ulceration. Lancet. 1984;1:1311–14.
4. Graham DY. *Campylobacter pylori* and peptic ulcer disease. Gastroenterology. 1989;96:615–25.
5. Seifarth C, Deusch K, Reich K, Classen M. Local and cellular immune response in *Helicobacter pylori* associated Type B gastritis – selective increase of CD4+ but not of gamma/delta T cells in the immune response to *H. pylori* antigens. Z Gastroenterol. 1996;34:215–24.
6. Ernst PB, Jin Y, Reyes VE, Crowe SE. The role of the local immune response in the pathogenesis of peptic ulcer formation. Scand J Gastroenterol. 1994;29(Suppl. 205):22–8.
7. Fan XJ, Chua A, Shahi CN, McDevitt J, Keeling PWN, Kelleher D. Gastric T lymphocyte responses to *Helicobacter pylori* in patients with *H. pylori* colonisation. Gut. 1994;35:1379–84.
8. Sundstedt A, Sigvardsson M, Leandersson T, Hedlung G, Kalland T, Dohlsten M. In vivo anergized CD4+ T cells express perturbed AP-1 and NF-kappaB transcription factors. Proc Natl Acad Sci USA. 1996;93:979–84.
9. Nagata S, Golstein P. The Fas death receptor. Science. 1995;267:1449–56.
10. Krammer PH, Dhein H, Walzak I et.al. The role of APO-1-mediated apoptosis in the immune system. Immunol Rev. 1994;142:175–91.
11. Miyawaki T, Uehara T, Nibu R et al. Differential expression of apoptosis related Fas-antigen on lymphocyte subpopulations in human peripheral blood. J Immunol. 1992;149:3753–8.
12. Klas C, Debatin KM, Jonker R, Krammer PH. Activation interferes with the APO-1 pathway in mature human T cells. Int Immunol. 1993;5:625–30.
13. Alderson MR, Tough TW, Davis-Smith T et al. Fas ligand mediates activation-induced cell death in human T lymphocytes. J Exp Med. 1995;181:71–7.
14. Akbar AN, Salmon M, Savill J, Janossy G. A possible role for bcl-2 in regulating T-cell memory – a 'balancing act' between cell death and survival. Immunol Today. 1993;14:526–32.
15. Reed JC, Miyashita T, Krajewski S et al. Location and modulation of the bcl-2 protein: Implications for the regulation of programmed cell death. In: Tsuchiya M et al., editors. Current topics in mucosal immunology. Amsterdam: Elsevier; 1992:83–87.
16. Bull DM, Bookman MA. Isolation and functional characterization of human intestinal mucosal lymphoid cells. J Clin Invest. 1977;59:966–74.
17. Deusch K, Lüling F, Reich K, Flassen M, Wagner H. A major fraction of human intraepithelial lymphocyte simultaneously express the gamma/delta T cell receptor, the CD8 accessory molecule and preferentially uses the V-delta-1 gene segment. Eur J Immunol. 1991;21:1053–9.
18. Sharma SA, Miller GG, Perez-Perez GI, Gupta RS, Blaser MJ. Humoral and cellular immune recognition of *Helicobacter pylori* proteins are not concordant. Clin Exp Immunol. 1994;97:126–32.
19. Chen Y, Inobe Jun-Ichi, Marks R, Gonella P, Duchroo Vlay K, Weiner HL. Peripheral deletion of antigen-reactive T cell in oral tolerance. Nature. 1995;376:177–80.

24
Lessons from the epidemiology of *Helicobacter pylori* and cancer

J. PARSONNET

INTRODUCTION

In 1994 the International Agency for Research on Cancer (IARC) declared *Helicobacter pylori* to be a type I carcinogen, a definite cause of cancer in humans[1]. The strongest support for this assertion came from epidemiological studies solidly linking infection with the later development of malignancy. Bolstering these epidemiological findings are a series of laboratory studies demonstrating credible mechanisms for *H. pylori*-induced carcinogenesis, including: enhanced cell proliferation, induction of reactive oxygen species and intraepithelial formation of mutagenic oxidative DNA adducts[2-4]. Similarities between gastric inflammation and other inflammatory precursors to cancer at other sites (e.g. schistosomiasis and hepatitis B infection) reinforce the likelihood for an *H. pylori* – gastric cancer link. Yet the IARC statement remains controversial, largely because epidemiological studies have not been completely consistent across all populations and because statistical associations are often viewed with some scepticism. In the years before and since the IARC statement, papers have been published refuting a role for *H. pylori* in adenocarcinoma[5,6]. While some negative studies (particularly those presented as abstracts) are of dubious quality, others are well conducted and contain few obvious sources of bias. In this chapter, I will address the question: if *H. pylori* is so critical to gastric carcinogenesis, why do not all studies show an association?

GASTRIC CANCER: THE END OF MANY PATHS

Cancer is virtually always a multifactorial process. To address this, Kenneth Rothman, a renowned epidemiologist, conceptualized pie charts for sufficient cause. For any given disease there are many combinations of factors that are sufficient to cause disease (Figure 1)[7]. Each individual pie, in turn, is composed of slices representing specific risk factors. Some factors may be found in all pies – these would be considered 'necessary' causes. Necessary causes, however, may

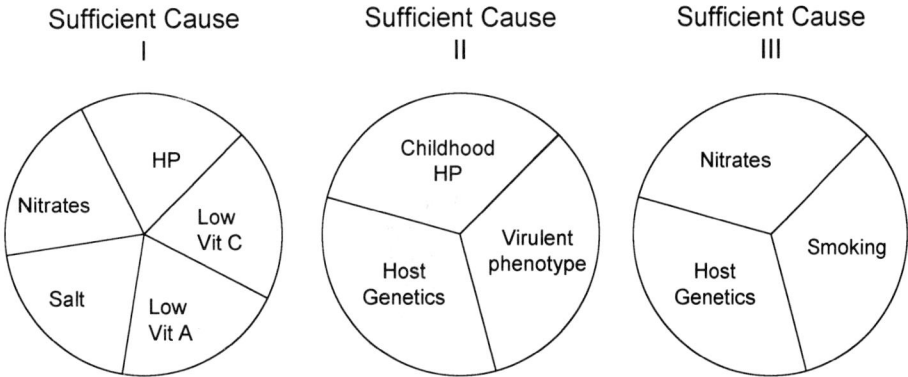

Figure 1 Rothman proposes modelling disease using pie charts of sufficient cause[7]. Each pie represents one pathway to disease. In this figure are hypothetical pies for gastric carcinogenesis. These pies should not be considered factual but rather a model for conceptualizing multifactorial carcinogenesis. One can develop cancer by having all of the elements in one of these pies. In pies I and II *H. pylori* is a required component of the sufficient cause pathway. Because *H. pylori* prevalence may be far more common than other elements in the pie, however, it may not be the element that determines disease incidence. Generally, the rarest wedge in the pie is the one that is critical. In pie III *H. pylori* is not a factor; this pie represents one pathway for cancer not attributable to infection

be of dubious help in disease prevention. This is because factors that are necessary for a disease are often omnipresent in healthy persons as well. As an extreme example, breathing could be considered a necessary factor for cancer, but is certainly not remediable nor, consequently, important. Also, if a necessary cause is found in all persons, it cannot be epidemiologically identified as a disease risk factor. For a risk factor to be statistically recognized it must be unevenly distributed between cases and non-cases.

Rarely, a sufficient cause pie will consist of only one factor. For instance, sickle-cell disease is caused by the lack of a normal haemoglobin gene. More commonly, however, diseases reflect an aggregation of factors, none necessary and none sufficient. Within each pie the least common element will be the one that determines the actual incidence of disease. Thus, if one factor is found in only a tiny minority of people, this pie will rarely be complete and disease will rarely occur by this pathway. It will be even more unlikely if two rare factors are required to complete a pie.

Gastric cancer, like other diseases, is undoubtedly the consequence of a number of different pathways. Hypothetical examples of Rothman pies for gastric cancer are shown in Figure 1. In this model *H. pylori* is involved in some, but not all, pies. Within each pie the prevalence of *H. pylori* infection may not be the determining factor for disease. *H. pylori* is very common. Since only a minority of infections results in cancer, the distributions of other pie elements must be critical in determining ultimate disease incidence. Thus, cancer incidence may depend more on rare cofactors than on the most common cause. In some populations the distribution of pie elements may foster non-*H. pylori* related pathways to malignancy. All depends upon the frequencies and distributions of the many aetiological factors in disease.

The Rothman pies are helpful in conceptualizing disease since, without question, *H. pylori* is not a causal factor in all gastric adenocarcinomas. Most studies reveal little association between *H. pylori* and cancers of the cardia or gastro-oesophageal junction[8-11]. Even for distal cancers the proportion of tumours attributable to *H. pylori* has been calculated to be only 50–60%[8,9]. While these values for attributable risk, computed from nested case–control studies, may underestimate the true risk (see below), a substantial proportion of distal gastric cancers would still occur if *H. pylori* did not exist. In the United States, gastric cancer occurs at a rate of approximately 8/100000 per year[12]. In recent years only 50% of these malignancies affected the distal stomach and are potentially associated with *H. pylori*[13]. If one assumes an attributable proportion in distal cancer of 50% then, excluding proximal malignancies, only one-fourth of cancers are related to *H. pylori* and three-fourths are not. This being the case, one can easily envision populations in which *H. pylori* might not be identified as a risk factor for cancer.

The absence of infection in some cases of cancer indicates the complexity of cancer causation; it does not refute a real risk, particularly given the weight of existing evidence.

EPIDEMIOLOGICAL STUDIES CONTAIN INHERENT BIAS

In addition to the recognition of multiple causal pathways to cancer, there are other ways to explain the absence of significant findings in studies of *H. pylori* and gastric cancer. Epidemiological studies suffer from some inherent sources of bias. Specifically, misclassification of exposure and/or outcome is an unavoidable problem. This is especially true in case–control studies in which measures of past exposure are often inaccurate.

Misclassification bias can be of two types: differential or non-differential. In seroepidemiological studies of *H. pylori* infection, non-differential misclassification occurs when cases and controls are equally misclassified as infected or uninfected due to imperfect serological assays. Non-differential misclassification can also occur if cancer outcome is misdiagnosed in persons with and without infection. In either case misclassification is non-differential only if it occurs proportionately in all exposure and outcome groups. Non-differential misclassification bias is an element in all epidemiological studies, because no diagnostic test is perfect. Almost always it tends to favour the null hypothesis, lowering the risk estimate. An example of how non-differential misclassification bias might affect a study is shown in Figure 2.

Differential misclassification is a bigger problem because it can impact study results either towards or away from the null. Differential misclassification occurs when either cases or controls are disproportionately misclassified. A potential source of differential misclassification in *H. pylori* studies is varying sensitivity of serology in cases and controls. It is widely believed that *H. pylori* infection is lost with advancing preneoplasia and that serum titres correspondingly drop. Because cases are more likely to have advanced preneoplasia than are controls, misclassification is more likely to occur in cases. In Figure 2 the effects of differential misclassification of *H. pylori* infection can be observed. Combining

A.

	Infected	Uninfected	
Cases	70	30	100
Controls	60	40	100

No adjustment for misclassification
OR = 1.6, 95% CI = 0.8 - 2.9

B.

	Infected	Uninfected	
Cases	75	25	100
Controls	63	37	100

Sensitivity and specificity of HP assay = 90%
OR = 1.8, 95% CI = 1.0 - 3.2

C.

	Infected	Uninfected	
Cases	79	21	100
Controls	62	38	100

Specificity of cancer diagnosis = 80%
Sensitivity and specificity of HP assay = 90%
OR = 2.3, 95% CI = 1.2 - 4.5

D.

	Infected	Uninfected	
Cases	71	29	100
Controls	46	54	100

Specificity of cancer diagnosis = 80%
Sensitivity HP assay (cases) = 80%
Specificity HP assay (cases) = 90%
Sensitivity and specificity of HP assay (controls)= 90%
OR = 4.0, 95% CI = 2.1 - 8.0

Figure 2 Misclassification of exposure and/or outcome can have important impacts on study results. In section **A** are numbers from a hypothetical case–control study of *H. pylori* and gastric cancer. The proportions of cases and controls infected with *H. pylori* are similar to those reported in several negative studies. Note that the odds ratio of 1.6 is not significant. The serological tests for *H. pylori*, however, are imperfect. If the serological assay is 90% sensitive and specific (**B**), then the adjusted odds ratio is 1.8 and borderline significant. If, in addition, the diagnosis of cancer in cases is not confirmed (the pathology is not reviewed or cardiac/gastro-oesophageal cancers are included in the analysis), the odds ratio rises even further and is strongly significant (**C**). Finally, if there is differential misclassification and the serology works better in controls than in cases, the odds ratio becomes strongly significant (**D**). This is likely to occur in retrospective studies since preneoplasia appears to cause loss of both infection and anti-*H. pylori* antibodies (Methods of adjustment for misclassification from ref. 27)

all forms of misclassification the relative risk for cancer given *H. pylori* infection, in this example, rises from 1.6 to 4.0. The attributable proportion more than doubles from 26% to 58%. Thus, understanding of the tools used and biases intrinsic to epidemiological studies is critical in interpreting research findings. When one incorporates adjust-ments for misclassification, both differential and non-differential, it is rare to find studies that do not link *H. pylori* infection to malignancy.

BACTERIAL DIVERSITY

H. pylori exhibits great genetic diversity[14–17]. Approximately 50% of organisms express the CagA protein while the remainder do not[18,19]. Fortunately, the CagA protein is highly immunogenic and persons infected with CagA-positive strains will have detectable serum antibodies. From an epidemiological perspective this has been helpful in classifying *H. pylori* infection and its relationship to disease[20,21]. One prospective study found that persons with CagA-expressing *H. pylori* infection were more likely to progress to atrophic gastritis than those infected with CagA-negative strains[22]. Two nested case–control studies have indicated that CagA antibodies are more common in infected persons who develop malignancy than in infected persons without malignancy[23,24]. In one of these studies, infection with CagA-negative *H. pylori* strains only weakly increased the risk for cancer, whereas the CagA-positive phenotype was strongly associated with the disease[24]. While the mechanisms by which the CagA phenotype produces excess disease have not yet been elucidated, CagA antibodies have proved to be an important epidemiological tool.

Variation in CagA prevalence among population groups could explain some of the discrepancies observed in case–control studies of *H. pylori* infection and gastric cancer[25]. In populations in which CagA-positive *H. pylori* infection is rare, *H. pylori* would be less likely to be identified as a disease risk factor. In fact, data are accumulating to show that the CagA phenotype is not uniformly distributed between regions or even among ethnic/racial groups. In one study, *H. pylori*-infected Europeans had a substantially higher proportion of CagA-positive strains than an African-born comparison group (95.3% vs. 35.3%)[25]. In a second study *H. pylori*-infected US blacks had a substantially higher proportion of CagA-positive strains than demographically similar whites[26]. These differences, in turn, could strongly influence gastric cancer incidence. Until broader ecological studies are conducted, however, the contribution of CagA to the 'African enigma' of low gastric cancer incidence will remain unknown.

SUMMARY

Epidemiological studies strongly link *H. pylori* infection to gastric cancer. Because of biases intrinsic to these studies the true association is undoubtedly underestimated to a substantial degree. The amount of underestimation is dependent on three factors: the accuracy of the diagnostic tests for the presence of *H. pylori* infection, the accuracy of the cancer diagnosis, and the extent of preneoplasia with gastric atrophy in the cases and controls at the time of *H. pylori* diagnosis. In the light of these myriad biases the statistical associations must be considered extremely strong. Yet for statistical data to have credibility they must have physiological plausibility. The association between *H. pylori* and gastric cancer is eminently plausible. The many parallels with other inflammation-related cancers merely strengthen its probability.

The time has come to stop debating a role of *H. pylori* in gastric carcinogenesis. As the IARC confirmed, the evidence is there. If we wait for even more definitive proof of cause (such as long-term intervention studies) before interceding, we will be doing our patients a disservice. While intervention studies have great merit, they will take years to complete and may, in the end, be technically impractical. Furthermore, it is likely that more than one such study will be necessary before a clear picture emerges. In the meantime we must not forget those who will die of gastric cancer before long-term studies are complete.

We must focus our attention now on how *H. pylori* causes gastric cancer, on identifying cofactors that mediate this outcome, and on developing prevention strategies for infected patients in developing, transitional and developed countries. With these tools we may not only prevent a considerable proportion of gastric cancers, but may also gain valuable insights into the pathogenesis of other inflammation-related malignancies.

References

1. IARC Working Group on the Evaluation of Carcinogenic Risks to Humans. *Helicobacter pylori*. In: Anonymous. Schistosomes, liver flukes and *Helicobacter pylori*: views and expert opinions of an IARC Working Group on the Evaluation of Carcinogenic Risks to Humans. Lyon: IARC; 1994:177–240.
2. Davies GR, Simmonds NJ, Stevens TRJ et al. *Helicobacter pylori* stimulates antral mucosal reactive oxygen metabolite production in vivo. Gut. 1994;35:179–85.
3. Lynch DA, Mapstone NP, Clarke AM et al. Cell proliferation in *Helicobacter pylori* associated gastritis and the effect of eradication therapy. Gut. 1995;36:346–50.
4. Baik S, Youn H, Chung M et al. Increased oxidative DNA damage in *Helicobacter pylori*-infected human gastric mucosa. Cancer Res. 1996;56:1279–82.
5. Estevens J, Fidalgo P, Tendeiro T et al. Anti-*Helicobacter pylori* antibodies prevalence and gastric adenocarcinoma in Portugal: report of a case–control study. Eur J Cancer Prev. 1993;2:377–80.
6. Rudi J, Muller M, von Herbay A et al. Lack of association of *Helicobacter pylori* seroprevalence and gastric cancer in a population with low gastric cancer incidence. Scand J Gastroenterol. 1995;30:958–63.
7. Rothman KJ. Modern epidemiology. Boston: Little, Brown; 1996:2–21.
8. Parsonnet J, Friedman GD, Vandersteen DP et al. *Helicobacter pylori* infection and the risk of gastric carcinoma. N Engl J Med. 1991;325:1127–31.
9. Nomura AMY, Stemmerman GN, Chyou P, Kato I, Perez-Perez GI, Blaser MJ. *Helicobacter pylori* infection and gastric carcinoma in a population of Japanese–Americans in Hawaii. N Engl J Med. 1991;325:1132–6.
10. Fukuda H, Saito D, Hayashi S et al. *Helicobacter pylori* infection, serum pepsinogen level and gastric cancer. a case control study in Japan. Jpn J Cancer Res. 1995;86:64–71.
11. Hansson LR, Engstrand L, Nyren O, Lindgren A. Prevalence of *Helicobacter pylori* infection in subtypes of gastric cancer. Gastroenterology. 1995;109:885–8.
12. Gloeckner Ries LA, Hankey BF, Miller BA, Hartman AM, Edwards BK. Cancer statistics review. National Cancer Institute. NIH Publ. No. 91-2789; 1991.
13. Salvon-Harmon JC, Cady B, Nikulasson S, Khettry U, Stone MD, Levin P. Shifting proportions of gastric adenocarcinomas. Arch Surg. 1994;129:381–8 (discussion 388–9).
14. Cover TL, Tummuru MK, Cao P, Thompson SA, Blaser MJ. Divergence of genetic sequences for the vacuolating cytotoxin among *Helicobacter pylori* strains. J Biol Chem. 1994;269:10566–73.
15. Takami S, Hayashi T, Tonokatsu Y, Shimoyama T, Tamura T. Chromosomal heterogeneity of *Helicobacter pylori* isolates by pulsed-field gel electrophoresis. Int J Med Microbiol Virol Parasitol Infect Dis. 1993;280:120–7.
16. Desai M, Linton D, Owen RJ, Cameron H, Stanley J. Genetic diversity of *Helicobacter pylori* indexed with respect to clinical symptomatology, using a 16S rRNA and a species-specific DNA probe. J Appl Bacteriol. 1993;75:574–82.
17. Taylor DE, Eaton M, Chang N, Salama SM. Construction of a *Helicobacter pylori* genome map and demonstration of diversity at the genome level. J Bacteriol. 1992;174:6800–6.
18. Cover TL, Glupczynski Y, Lage AP et al. Serologic detection of infection with cagA+ *Helicobacter pylori* strains. J Clin Microbiol. 1995;33:1496–500.
19. Xiang Z, Censini S, Bayeli PF et al. Analysis of expression of CagA and VacA virulence factors in 43 strains of *Helicobacter pylori* reveals that clinical isolates can be divided into two major types and that CagA is not necessary for expression of the vacuolating cytotoxin. Infect Immun. 1995;63:94–8.
20. Telford JL, Covacci A, Ghiara P, Montecucco C, Rappuoli R. Unravelling the pathogenic role of

Helicobacter pylori in peptic ulcer: potential new therapies and vaccines. Trends Biotechnol. 1994;12:420–6.

21. Xiang Z, Censini S, Bayeli PF *et al.* Analysis of expression of CagA and VacA virulence factors in 43 strains of *Helicobacter pylori* reveals that clinical isolates can be divided into two major types and that CagA is not necessary for expression of the vacuolating cytotoxin. Infect Immun. 1995;63:94–8.

22. Kuipers EJ, Perez-Perez GI, Meuwissen SG, Blaser MJ. *Helicobacter pylori* and atrophic gastritis: importance of the cagA status [see comments]. J Natl Cancer Inst. 1995;87:1777–80.

23. Blaser MJ, Perez-Perez GI, Kleanthous H *et al.* Infection with *Helicobacter pylori* strains possessing cagA is associated with an increased risk of developing adenocarcinoma of the stomach. Cancer Res. 1995;55:2111–15.

24. Parsonnet J, Friedman GD, Orentreich N, Vogelman JH. Infection with the Type 1 phenotype of *H. pylori* increases risk for gastric cancer independent of corpus atrophy. Gastroenterology. 1996; 110:A221(abstract).

25. Fauconnier A, Burette A, Goutier S, Butzler JP, Bollen A, Glupczynski Y. Frequency of *cagA* in *Helicobacter pylori* strains isolated from Belgian and Moroccan patients. Gut. 1995;37: A69(abstract).

26. Parsonnet J, Replogle ML, Yang S, Hiatt RA. Prevalence of the type 1 *H. pylori* phenotype differs among ethnic/racial groups in the San Francisco Bay area. Gastroenterology. 1996;110: A221(abstract).

27. Kleinbaum DG, Kupper LL, Morgenstern H. Epidemiologic research. New York: Van Nostrand Reinhold; 1982:221–41.

25
Helicobacter pylori, acid, gastritis, atrophy and progression to cancer: a critical view

J. W. FRESTON

INTRODUCTION

The risk of developing gastric cancer is now generally recognized to be strongly influenced by the presence of *H. pylori* gastritis. The World Health Organization's International Agency for Research on Cancer recently classified *H. pylori* as a Group 1, or definite carcinogen[1]. This classification resulted largely from epidemiological studies that showed an increased cancer risk in people infected with *H. pylori*. The rate of *H. pylori* infection parallels that of gastric adenocarcinoma in different countries[2]. Three serological cohort studies have demonstrated an increased risk for gastric cancer in *H. pylori*-infected people[3-5]. The odds ratio for gastric adenocarcinoma in *H. pylori*-infected individuals in these prospective studies of different populations ranged from 1.2 to 6.0, with the highest figure found in Japanese Americans living in Hawaii[3].

Moreover, it was recently established that the increased cancer risk is associated with infection with a cagA-positive strain[6]. The way in which *H. pylori* infection contributes to carcinogenesis is a subject of intense investigation. Current studies are concentrating on the relationship of gene products of *H. pylori* and mediators of tissue injury and repair, and on the relationship between the stages of gastritis and the final transformation of cells to cancer. Suppression of gastric acidity recently has been demonstrated to accelerate the progression of chronic gastritis to stages of atrophy and intestinal metaplasia[7], presumably increasing the risk of subsequent progression to cancer if left unchecked. This discovery has significant implications for the way we view the relationship of acid suppression and *H. pylori* infection over time, on the one hand, and the mechanism whereby *H. pylori* infection enhances gastric cancer risk, on the other.

The purpose of this chapter is to describe and examine selective aspects of the relationship of *H. pylori* to the progression of chronic gastritis through its evolution to cancer, focusing on new information that implicates disturbed mucosal regulation of apoptosis, or programmed cell death, in promoting proliferation while

H.p. infection

      ↘

   chronic gastritis

          ↘

           gastric atrophy

                ↘

                  intestinal metaplasia

                        ↘

                        dysplasia

                              ↘

                              adenocarcinoma

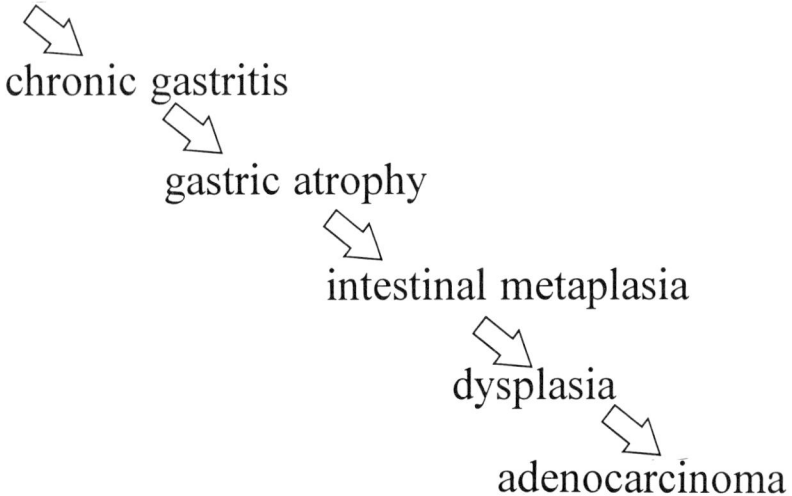

Figure 1   Multistep process of gastric carcinogenesis proposed by Correa[8]. Actual progression through gastric atrophy and intestinal metaplasia has recently been established in a prospective long-term study[7]

inducing atrophy, thus explaining a vexing contradiction in terms of gastric epithelial behaviour under the influence of *H. pylori* infection. Finally, the proposed role of inducible nitric oxide synthase on proliferation and atrophy will be addressed in light of very recent studies of this enzyme and its product, nitric oxide.

GASTRITIS AND ITS PROGRESSION TO CANCER

The sequence of events from infection to cancer is presumed to include the development of acute gastritis, followed by progression to chronic gastritis, intestinal metaplasia, dysplasia and adenocarcinoma (Figure 1)[8]. This presumed sequence is based on earlier observations linking chronic gastritis to cancer in stages that inevitably include a stage of atrophic gastritis[9,10]. A recent case–control study showed that *H. pylori* infection was strongly associated with gastric atrophy and intestinal metaplasia, and that both conditions increased in prevalence with age[11]. Intake of antioxidant micronutrients was negatively associated with the risk of atrophy after adjustment for *H. pylori* infection.

While *H. pylori* infection has been described at each stage, actual *progression* through all stages has not been reported. In fact, progression of gastritis to chronic atrophic gastritis was documented recently by Kuipers and colleagues (Table 1)[7,12]. They prospectively studied 49 *H. pylori*-negative and 58 *H. pylori*-positive subjects for a mean of 11.5 years (range 10–13 years). Sera for *H. pylori* IgG antibodies were sampled and gastric biopsies were obtained for assessment of *H. pylori* infection and histology at the beginning and end of the study[7].

Progression to atrophic gastritis occurred in 16 infected subjects (28%) and

Table 1 *H. pylori*, atrophic gastritis and intestinal metaplasia (from ref. 7)

Mean follow-up	11.5 years
Prospective evaluation of natural history of gastritis	49 *H. pylori*-negative 58 *H. pylori*-positive
Atrophic gastritis with intestinal metaplasia	28% *H. pylori*-positive 4% *H. pylori*-negative
Development of atrophic gastritis associated with *H. pylori*	OR = 9.0 *p* = 0.014

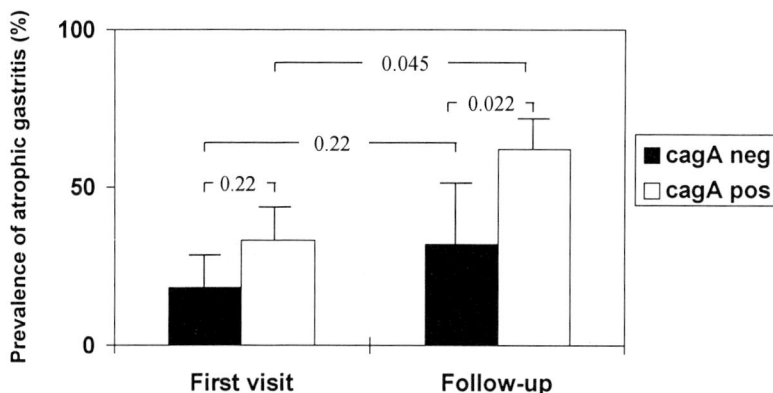

Figure 2 Prevalence of atrophic gastritis in *H. pylori*-infected subjects at first visit and follow-up visit after 10–13 years (mean 11.5 years). Seropositivity for cagA–vacA-positive strains, but not negative strains, was associated with a significant increase in prevalence of atrophic gastritis. From Kuipers *et al.*[12], with permission

intestinal metaplasia developed in six. Only two patients (4%) developed atrophic gastritis and one of these, who was found to have pernicious anaemia, developed intestinal metaplasia. This landmark study proved that *H. pylori* infection significantly increases the risk of developing atrophic gastritis and intestinal metaplasia.

A subsequent report by the same group[12] addressed the relationship of cagA status and the development of atrophic gastritis and intestinal metaplasia in the same cohort of subjects. *H. pylori* strains differ with respect to the difference of *cagA* (cytotoxin-associated gene A), a gene encoding a high molecular weight immunodominant antigen. While the *cagA* gene is no longer believed to express a cytotoxic product, the *cagA* gene and its protein, together with the gene for vacuolating cytotoxin (*vacA*), define the type I, or more virulent strain, of *H. pylori*[13,14].

Kuipers *et al.*[12] found that 24 of the 58 (41%) *H. pylori*-infected subjects had serum antibodies against cagA, while 34 (60%) did not. At the beginning of the study, moderate to severe atrophic gastritis was observed in eight (33%) of the cagA-positive subjects and in six (18%) of the cagA-negative subjects. There was no significant relationship at that time between positive cagA status and gastric atrophy. At the end of the observation period, 16 (36%) of the 44 individuals who initially had no atrophy had developed atrophic gastritis, which was accompanied by the development of intestinal metaplasia in six (Figure 2). One of these 16 subjects had developed an early gastric cancer. Eight of the 16 subjects, including

Table 2 Development of atrophic gastritis in populations with specific entry criteria (from ref. 23)

Reference	Country	n	Follow-up (years)	Annual increase in atrophy prevalence
Ihamaki, 1978[15]	Finland	137	25	1.3
Correa, 1990[16]	Colombia	1422	5	3.3
Villako, 1991[17]	Estonia	142	6	1.2
Kuipers, 1995[7]	Netherlands	115	11.5	1.2

Table 3 Development of atrophic gastritis in low-acid states (modified from ref. 23)

Reference	Country	n	Follow-up (years)	Condition	Annual increase in atrophy prevalence
Maaroos, 1985[18]	Estonia	39	7	Gastric ulcer	7.4
Jonsson, 1988[19]	Sweden	23	3	Vagotomy	8.7
Solcia, 1992[20]	Italy	195	1.75	Omeprazole Rx	7.0
Lamberts, 1993[21]	Germany	74	5	Omeprazole Rx	3.8
Klinkenberg-Knol, 1994[22]	Netherlands	89	4	Omeprazole Rx	5.0
Freston, 1994	USA	416	1.25	Lansoprazole Rx	1.4

the one with cancer, were cagA-positive. After accounting for subjects with apparent regression of atrophic gastritis (possibly a sampling artifact), the final tabulation showed atrophic gastritis in 15 (62%) of the 24 cagA-positive subjects and in 11 (32%) of the 34 cagA-negative subjects, a statistically significant difference ($p = 0.022$). The increase in prevalence of atrophic gastritis reached statistical significance in the cagA-positive ($p = 0.045$), but not in the cagA-negative group ($p = 0.22$). The development of atrophy was observed in eight of 16 subjects (50%) who were cagA-positive versus eight of 28 (29%) who were cagA-negative ($p = 0.20$). Finally, intestinal metaplasia developed in 31% of the cagA-positive subjects versus 4% of the cagA-negative subjects ($p = 0.02$).

RATE OF DEVELOPMENT OF ATROPHY

Since the development of atrophic gastritis plays a central role in the multistep progression to gastric cancer, the rate at which atrophy develops has been addressed by investigators in several different countries[7,15-22], and has been summarized recently by Kuipers[23] (Tables 2 and 3). A now-classical Finnish study in 1978 found an annual increase in prevalence of 1.3% based on follow-up for a mean of 25 years[15]. A large Colombian study reported an annual increase in the prevalence of atrophic gastritis of 3.3%[16]. The *H. pylori* status of subjects in these studies was unknown. An Estonian study in 1991, reporting an annual increase in the prevalence of atrophic gastritis of 1.2%, was the first to address *H. pylori* status: nearly all subjects were infected[17]. A Netherlands' study composed of nearly equal numbers of infected and non-infected subjects reported annual increased prevalence of 1.2%[7]. Thus, these studies establish a range of 1.2–3.3% for the annual rate of development of atrophic gastritis in populations that presumably differ with respect to other factors that might bear on atrophic gastritis, such as genetics, diet and the prevalence of *H. pylori* infection. These studies also provide a basis for comparisons of the rate of development of atrophic gastritis in low-acid states.

Conditions characterized by low rates of gastric acid secretion that are documented to develop atrophic gastritis include gastric ulcer disease, vagotomy and treatment with acid-inhibiting drugs. With the exception of the short-term lansoprazole experience (J. Freston, presentation of lansoprazole safety and efficacy to US Food and Drug Administration, 1 December 1994), all studies show annual rates of development of atrophic gastritis that exceed the upper bound of the range for conditions not associated with low-acid secretion (Table 3). The lansoprazole study was of short duration (1.25 years) and contained fewer than 20% of H. pylori-infected subjects, which may explain its low rate of progression to atrophic gastritis. The definitive study of progression to atrophy was in two groups of patients with gastro-oesophageal reflux disease, one treated long-term with omeprazole and the other by fundoplication[24]. The patients with H. pylori infection who were in the omeprazole-treated group developed significantly more atrophic gastritis than did the fundoplication-treated group.

The high rate of progression to atrophy in low-acid states is an important observation, given the fact that acid suppression fosters H. pylori colonization of the gastric corpus and the development of corpus gastritis[22–25]. Thus, acid suppression not only promotes the migration of H. pylori to the corpus but also accelerates the transition of chronic active gastritis to atrophic change. It is not known if acceleration also occurs in the rate of transition from atrophy to dysplasia and then to neoplasia, as no studies have directly addressed this issue. Moreover, prospective studies in humans have not yet documented the progression to dysplasia, although a recent preliminary report demonstrated progression to dysplasia in mice infected with H. felis[26]. Several studies have examined the gastric cancer risk in duodenal ulcer patients, most of whom can be presumed to be infected with H. pylori, after vagotomy or long-term treatment with acid-suppressing drugs[27–32]. A study of 7198 vagotomized patients had a relative incidence rate of gastric cancer of only 1.33 during an average follow-up of 10 years[27]. However, this result must be interpreted cautiously, because neither the H. pylori status nor the acid-secretory status was measured in these patients, and some vagotomized patients are known to regain acid-secretory status[33,34]. Other large series of vagotomized patients provide data of limited value because they have usually contained a significant number of patients who also had undergone partial gastric resection, thus introducing the variable of duodenogastric reflux. The behaviour of the gastric epithelium in such patients cannot be compared directly to that of H. pylori gastritis.

Long-term acid suppression by H_2-receptor antagonists has not demonstrated an increased risk of gastric cancer[28–32], although two studies showed a trend towards increased risk after 7–10 years of continuous treatment with cimetidine[28,30]. There has as yet been no comprehensive, long-term study of gastric cancer risk during continuous treatment with proton pump inhibitors.

THE PARADOX OF COEXISTING ATROPHY AND PROLIFERATION

A critical question to resolve in understanding the progression of gastritis to cancer is the relationship of atrophy to proliferation. In fact, the *role* of atrophy itself, as

CagA – VacA-positive
H. pylori gastritis
⇓
iNOS
⇓
NO

neck region of   superficial
gastric glands   epithelium
⇓   ⇓

apoptosis   DNA damage
⇓   ⇓

atrophy   proliferation

neoplasia

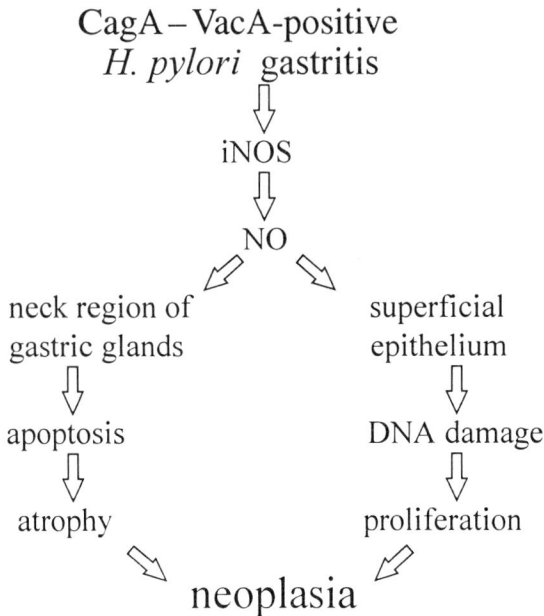

Figure 3 Hypothesis for relationship between cagA – vacA-positive strains of *H. pylori*, inducible nitric acid synthase, apoptosis, proliferation and neoplasia. NO activity in gastric glands fosters apoptosis and atrophy, while NO induces DNA damage and proliferation in superficial epithelium[35]

opposed to its presence in the transition to neoplasia, is not understood, apart from the fact that atrophy appears to be an essential step in the progression to cancer. How can atrophy be essential in carcinogenesis, a condition of unregulated hyper-proliferation?[35] Hyperproliferation has been documented in *H. pylori*-infected gastric mucosa[36–38], particularly in superficial cells[38]. Thus it is possible that *H. pylori*-induced hyperproliferation, under the influence of proinflammatory cytokines[39] and mutagenic reactive oxygen and nitrogen species[35], determines the extent of DNA damage and point mutations. As indicated by Correa and Miller[35], however, this does not explain why atrophy appears to be essential in the precancerous process. They and Moss *et al.*[40] have postulated that apoptosis (non-necrotic, programmed death of individual cells) may explain the paradox.

A cell with damaged DNA may arrest its reproductive cycle and repair the DNA or, if the damage is more severe, it may undergo apoptosis, thereby eliminating the risk of replicating mutated DNA. Severe DNA damage can also cause cell death by necrosis, a non-apoptotic process. The various means of dealing with DNA damage may coexist in gastric mucosa, and each may operate simul-taneously in different cells. Apoptosis could explain the loss of glands in gastric atrophy, while proliferating cells may be characterized by failure of apoptosis of transformed cells, thereby allowing the process to enter the next stage towards cancer (Figure 3)[35].

Increased antral mucosal apoptosis has been demonstrated in *H. pylori*-infected individuals[40–42], and eradication of the organism was found to restore the frequency of apoptosis to that found in normal subjects[40]. A preliminary study recently found that *H. pylori* infection caused gastric antral hyperproliferation, but increased apoptosis occurred only with cagA-negative strains[42]. Patients infected with cagA-positive strains exhibited hyperproliferation without increased apoptosis, a situation that would disrupt the normal balance between cell growth and death. If confirmed, this could be a highly relevant observation because colorectal cancer is characterized by uncoupled apoptosis and hyperplasia[43,44]. It should not be inferred that apoptoses and hyperproliferation are dissociated through the evolution of gastritis to neoplasia. Sustained hyperproliferation appears to produce cells that are resistant to apoptosis, leading to decreased apoptosis over time, which, in the face of sustained hyperproliferation, promotes tissue growth and neoplasia, as described in colorectal carcinogenesis[44]. Supporting this sequence is the observation that bcl-2, an anti-apoptosis protein, was increased in the presence of gastric epithelial dysplasia[45].

iNOS, NITRIC OXIDE AND APOPTOSIS

The way in which apoptosis is influenced in chronic gastritis is unknown; recent studies have focused on the possible role of iNOS[35,38,46–49]. iNOS catalyses the oxidation of arginine to citrulline and releases the messenger molecule NO, which acts as a mediator of endothelial relaxation and neurotransmission and also induces cytotoxicity and DNA damage. iNOS immunoreactivity was found in the antral mucosa of individuals infected with *H. pylori*[46–49]. Bravo *et al.*[46] found iNOS to be expressed particularly in neutrophils and macrophages in the neck region of gastric glands where cell replication normally takes place. Rieder *et al.*[48] found increased transcription and expression of iNOS in *H. pylori*-infected patients. The iNOS-positive cells were in the lamina propria close to the bottom of the crypts and between epithelial cells at the villus tips. While NO exerts a mild antimicrobial effect, few patients spontaneously clear their *H. pylori* infection. Rieder *et al.*[48] speculated that constant NO production over years, together with other radicals and mediators, might enhance the development of cancer.

Overall, there is a pattern of reports of iNOS expression in samples from *H. pylori*-infected gastric mucosa, and preliminary evidence that NO may be linked to apoptosis, but considerably more evidence is needed before concluding that NO is more or less important than other mediators in altering apoptosis.

SUMMARY

The 'Correa sequence' of carcinogenesis has been proved through the steps of atrophic gastritis and intestinal metaplasia. Preliminary studies of *H. felis*-induced gastritis suggest that the dysplasia step will also soon be established. The rate of progression to atrophic gastritis clearly is accelerated in low-acid states, but it is unknown if accelerated development of dysplasia also occurs; no convincing evidence of such has been found in long-term follow-up of patients subjected to vagotomy or to chronic treatment with acid-suppressing drugs. Changes in apoptosis and its relationship to hyperproliferation in the gastric mucosa are evident in *H. pylori* infection, although it is, as yet, unclear if increased apoptosis occurs early but then decreases in response to apoptotic resistance induced by sustained hyperproliferation, as occurs in colorectal cancer. The role of iNOS and its product NO in apoptosis is suggested by preliminary studies, but confirmation is needed.

References

1. IARC Working Group on the Evaluation of Carcinogenic Risks to Humans, Schistosomes, Liver Flukes and *Helicobacter pylori*. Vol. 61 of IARC monographs on the evaluation of carcinogenic risks to humans. Lyon: International Agency for Research on Cancer; 1994.
2. Eurogast Study Group. An international association between *Helicobacter pylori* infection and gastric cancer. Lancet. 1993;341:1359–62.
3. Nomura A, Stemmermann GN, Chyou P, Ikuki K, Perez-Perez GI, Blaser MJ. *Helicobacter pylori* infection and gastric carcinoma among Japanese Americans in Hawaii. N Engl J Med. 1991;325:1132–6.
4. Forman D, Newell DG, Fullerton F *et al*. Association between infection with *Helicobacter pylori* and risk of gastric cancer: evidence from a prospective investigation. Br Med J. 1991;302:1302–5.
5. Parsonnet J, Friedman GD, Vandersteen DP *et al*. *Helicobacter pylori* infection and the risk of gastric carcinoma. N Engl J Med. 1991;325:1127–31.
6. Blaser MJ, Perez-Perez GI, Kleanthous H *et al*. Infection with *Helicobacter pylori* strains possessing cagA is associated with an increased risk of developing adenocarcinoma of the stomach. Cancer Res. 1995;55:2111–15.
7. Kuipers EJ, Uyterlinde AM, Pena AS *et al*. Long-term sequelae of *Helicobacter pylori* gastritis. Lancet. 1995;345:1525–8.
8. Correa P. Human gastric carcinogenesis: a multistep and multifactorial process. Cancer Res. 1992; 52:6735–40.
9. Correa P, Haenszel W, Cuello C, Tannenbaum S, Archer M. A model for gastric cancer epidemiology. Lancet. 1975;2:58–60.
10. Sipponen P, Kekki M, Haapakoski J, Ihamaki T, Siurala M. Gastric cancer risk in chronic atrophic gastritis: statistical calculations of cross-sectional data. Int J Cancer. 1985;35:173–7.
11. Fontham ETH, Ruiz B, Perez A, Hunter F, Correa P. Determinants of *Helicobacter pylori* infection and chronic gastritis. Am J Gastroenterol. 1995;90:1094–101.
12. Kuipers EJ, Perez-Perez GI, Meuwissen SGM, Blaser MJ. *Helicobacter pylori* and atrophic gastritis: importance of the cagA strain. J Natl Cancer Inst. 1995;87:1777–80.
13. Crabtree JE, Taylor JD, Wyatt JI *et al*. Mucosal IgA recognition of *Helicobacter pylori* 120kDa protein, peptic ulceration, and gastric pathology. Lancet. 1991;338:332–5.
14. Telford JL, Ghiara P, Dellorco M *et al*. Gene structure of the *Helicobacter pylori* cytotoxin and evidence of its key role in gastric disease. J Exp Med. 1994;179:1653–8.
15. Ihamaki T, Saukkonen M, Siurala M. Long-term observation of subjects with normal mucosa and with superficial gastritis: results of 23–27 years' follow-up examinations. Scand J Gastroenterol. 1978;13:771–4.
16. Correa P, Haenszel W, Cuello C *et al*. Gastric precancerous process in a high risk population: cohort follow-up. Cancer Res. 1990;50:4737–40.
17. Villako K, Kekki M, Maaroos HI *et al*. Chronic gastritis: progression of inflammation and atrophy in a six-year endoscopic follow-up of a random sample of 142 Estonian urban subjects. Scand J Gastroenterol. 1991;186(Suppl.):135–41.
18. Maaroos HI, Salupere V, Uibo R, Kekki M, Sipponen P. Seven-year follow-up study of chronic gastritis in gastric ulcer patients. Scand J Gastroenterol. 1985;20:198–204.
19. Jonsson KA, Strom M, Bodemar G, Norrby K. Histologic changes in the gastroduodenal mucosa after long-term medical treatment with cimetidine or parietal cell vagotomy in patients with juxtapyloric ulcer disease. Scand J Gastroenterol. 1988;23:433–41.
20. Solcia E, Fiocca R, Havu N, Dalvag A, Carlsson R. Gastric endocrine cells and gastritis in patients receiving long-term omeprazole treatment. Digestion. 1992;51(Suppl. 1):82–92.
21. Lamberts R, Creutzfeldt W, Struber HG, Brunner G, Solcia E. Long-term omeprazole therapy in peptic ulcer disease: gastrin, endocrine cell growth, and gastritis. Gastroenterology. 1993;104: 1356–70.

22. Klinkenberg-Knol EC, Festen HPM, Jansen JBMJ et al. Efficacy and safety of long-term treatment with omeprazole for refractory reflux esophagitis. Ann Intern Med. 1994;121:161–7.
23. Kuipers EJ, Lee A, Klinkenberg-Knol EL, Meuwissen SGM. The development of atrophic gastritis – Helicobacter pylori and the effects of acid suppressive therapy. Aliment Pharmacol Ther. 1995; 9:331–40.
24. Kuipers EJ, Lundell L, Klinkenberg-Knol EC et al. Atrophic gastritis and Helicobacter pylori infection in patients with reflux esophagitis treated with omeprazole or fundoplication. N Engl J Med. 1996;334:1018–22.
25. Logan RPH, Walker MM, Misiewicz JJ, Gummett PA, Karim QN, Baron JH. Changes in the intragastric distribution of Helicobacter pylori during treatment with omeprazole. Gut. 1995;36: 12–16.
26. Dunn BE, Phadnis SH, Henderson J. Induction of gastric dyspepsia by H. felis in p53-deficient mice. Gastroenterology. 1996;110:A99(abstract).
27. Lundegardh G, Ekbom A, McLaughlin JK, Nyren O. Gastric cancer risk after vagotomy. Gut. 1994;35:946–9.
28. Moller H, Nissen A, Mosbech J. Use of cimetidine and other peptic ulcer drugs in Denmark 1977–1990 with analysis of the risk of gastric cancer among cimetidine users. Gut. 1992;33: 1166–9.
29. Moller H, Toftgaard C. Gastric cancer occurrence in patients previously treated for peptic ulcer disease. Eur J Gastroenterol Hepatol. 1994;6:1104–10.
30. Colin Jones DG, Langman MJ, Lawson DH, Logan RF, Paterson KR, Vessey MP. Postmarketing surveillance of the safety of cimetidine: 10 year mortality report. Gut. 1992;33:1280–4.
31. La Vecchia C, Negri E, Franceschi S, D'Avanzo B. Histamine-2-receptor antagonists and gastric cancer: update and note on latency and covariates. Nutrition. 1992;8:177–82.
32. Langman MJS. Postmarketing surveillance and the examination of the long-term safety of anti-ulcer drugs. Bailliere's Clin Gastroenterol. 1993;7:183–90.
33. Aarimaa M, Soderstrom KO, Kalimo H, Inberg M. Morphology and function of the parietal cells after proximal selective vagotomy in duodenal ulcer patients. Scand J Gastroenterol. 1984;19: 787–97.
34. Cuesta Valentin MA, Doblas Dominguez M, Rodrigez Alonso M, Bengoechea Gonzalez E. Vagal regeneration after parietal cell vagotomy: an experimental study in dogs. World J Surg. 1987;11: 94–100.
35. Correa P, Miller MJS. Helicobacter pylori and gastric atrophy – cancer paradoxes. J Natl Cancer Inst. 1995;87:17–18.
36. Brones F, Ruiz B, Correa P et al. Helicobacter pylori causes hyperproliferation of the gastric epithelium: pre- and post-eradication indices of proliferating cell nuclear antigen. Am J Gastroenterol. 1993;88:1870–5.
37. Lynch DAF, Mapstone NP, Clark AMT et al. Cell proliferation in Helicobacter pylori associated gastritis and the effects of eradication therapy. Gut. 1995;36:346–50.
38. Bechi P, Brandi ML, Fabiani S, Benvenuti F, Cianchi R. Nitric oxide involvement in Helicobacter pylori infection. Gastroenterology. 1996;110:A63(abstract).
39. Crabtree JE, Wyatt JI, Trejdosiewicz LK et al. Interleukin-8 expression in Helicobacter pylori infected, normal and neoplastic gastroduodenal mucosa. J Clin Pathol. 1994;47:61–6.
40. Moss SF, Calam J, Agarwal B, Wang S, Holt PR. Induction of gastric epithelial apoptosis by Helicobacter pylori. Gut. 1996;38:498–501.
41. Jones NL, Yeger H, Cutz E, Gherman PM. Helicobacter pylori induces apoptosis of gastric antral epithelial cells in vivo. Gastroenterology. 1996;110:A933(abstract).
42. Peek RM, Moss SF, Tham KT et al. Infection with H. pylori CagA+ strains dissociates gastric epithelial proliferation from apoptosis. Gastroenterology. 1996;110:A575(abstract).
43. Bedi A, Pasricha PJ, Akhtar AJ et al. Inhibition of apoptosis during development of colorectal cancer. Cancer Res. 1995;55:1811–16.
44. Moss SF, Scholes J, Wang S, Holt PR. Progressively disordered apoptosis during the multistep process of colorectal carcinogenesis. Gastroenterology. 1995;107:A511(abstract).
45. Lauwers GY, Scott GV, Hendricks J. Immunohistochemical evidence of aberrant bcl-2 protein expression in gastric epithelial dysplasia. Cancer. 1994;73:2900–4.
46. Bravo LE, Mannick EE, Zhang XJ, Ruiz B, Correa P, Miller MJ. H. pylori infection is associated with inducible nitric oxide synthase expression, nitrotyrosine and DNA damage. Gastroenterology. 1995;108:A63(abstract).

47. Fukuda T, Arakawa T, Fujiwara Y, Nakagawa K, Uno H, Watanabe T. Nitric oxide induces apoptosis in gastric mucosal cells *in vitro*. Gastroenterology. 1996;110:A111(abstract).
48. Rieder G, Hatz RA, Stolte M, Enders G. INOS in *H. pylori*-associated gastritis: possible roles in carcinogenesis. Gastroenterology. 1996;110:A1002(abstract).
49. Stachura J, Konturek JW, Karczewska E, Domschke W. Inducible nitric oxide (NO) synthase in *Helicobacter pylori* associated gastritis in duodenal ulcer patients. Gastroenterology. 1996;110A:1010(abstract).

26
Essential co-factors in gastric carcinogenesis

D. FORMAN

INTRODUCTION

There is now a large body of evidence which supports the association between *Helicobacter pylori* infection and an increased risk of gastric cancer. This is reflected in the decision by the International Agency for Cancer Research to categorize *H. pylori* infection as a definite cause of human cancer[1]. It is, however, readily apparent that, whereas infection with *H. pylori* is an extremely common event, gastric cancer is a relatively rare outcome of such infection. For every 100 people infected, no more than five, and probably only one or two, are likely to develop a malignancy. This poses the problem of how to identify the small percentage of infected individuals who are at increased risk of cancer. Clearly unravelling the co-factors involved in the process may be of public health significance, and should help in improving the focus of screening programmes which have, as their objective, preventing the future occurrence of gastric cancer.

Before addressing this issue in detail it is worthwhile emphasizing two aspects of the problem. Firstly the hypothesis of a cause-and-effect relationship between *H. pylori* infection and gastric cancer is not weakened by the infrequency of the outcome. Most aetiological relationships in carcinogenesis involve the development of cancer in a small minority of exposed individuals. Even for such well-established causes of cancer as tobacco smoking and infection with the hepatitis B virus, only a fraction of those exposed (in the order of 10%) will develop cancers of the lung and liver respectively. The random occurrence of disease among an apparently homogeneously exposed population is, therefore, a common problem in cancer research. Secondly, although much insight will be gained by understanding the essential co-factors which result in cancer, it should not be automatically assumed that such knowledge will benefit the cost-effectiveness of cancer prevention programmes. Screening individuals for *H. pylori* infection and treating those who are positive is, in comparative terms, a relatively inexpensive health intervention. It may cost considerably more to screen for the additional presence of co-factors in a subset of the population than to treat the entire infected population.

There are three categories of co-factor which may have a bearing on this problem: co-factors associated with the bacterial strain, the genetic background of the host and other environmental exposures. Each of these will be considered in turn.

BACTERIAL STRAIN

Nearly all research on the risk of gastric cancer associated with specific strains of *H. pylori* has been concerned with the difference between strains which express the *cagA* gene product (CagA-positives) and those which do not (CagA-negatives). Although the first papers on the spectrum of diseases associated with CagA-positivity indicated a role in ulcerogenesis[2,3], it rapidly became clear that it was increased pathogenicity in general which characterized the difference in infection between CagA-positive and CagA-negative strains[4]. It is now known that it is not the *cagA* gene product *per se* which is the pathogenic determinant, but that of a closely linked gene[5]. Nevertheless, characterization of CagA-positive strains using an ELISA with the *cagA* gene product, or components of it, can be used to classify individuals in epidemiological studies and assess the disease-specific association with the so-called 'pathogenicity island' of which the *cagA* gene is one part (see Chapter 4).

One longitudinal study from Kuipers and colleagues[6], in which there had previously been demonstrated a strong association between *H. pylori* infection and progression to atrophic gastritis and/or intestinal metaplasia[7], has recently shown a quantitatively increased risk of such progression if infection was with CagA-positive strains of the bacteria. The relative risks for progression, in comparison with uninfected individuals, were 10.5 (95% CI, 2.5–44.3) and 6.0 (95% CI, 1.4–26.2) for those infected with CagA-positive and CagA-negative strains respectively. Thus, although there was an important difference in risk between the two strains, there was still a significant risk of development of precancerous lesions associated with infection by CagA-negative strains.

A few studies have directly investigated the association between gastric cancer and CagA strain type, and these are summarized in Table 1. The results show the additional risk associated with having a CagA-positive infection in comparison with a CagA-negative infection. In all of the studies, previous reports had shown a significant risk of cancer associated with *H. pylori* infection[8–10]. For intestinal

Table 1 Odds ratio for gastric cancer associated with CagA-positive *H. pylori* infection compared with CagA-negative infection by histological subtype

Gastric cancer histology	Odds ratio (95% CI)	Reference
Intestinal	2.3 (1.0–5.2)	Blaser *et al.*, 1995[11]
	3.7 (1.7–8.3)	Parsonnet *et al.*, 1996[12]
Diffuse	1.0 (0.1–7.1)	Blaser *et al.*, 1995[11]
	2.2 (0.8–6.4)	Parsonnet *et al.*, 1996[12]
	1.0 (0.5–1.9)	Kikuchi *et al.*, 1996[13]

type adenocarcinoma the two prospective studies of Blaser et al.[11] and Parsonnet et al.[12] showed increased additional risks with odds ratios of 2.3 and 3.7, albeit with borderline significance in the former[11]. For diffuse-type adenocarcinoma, however, neither study showed any additional risk, nor did a study from Japan with all cases under the age of 40 years[13].

There have to date been no studies reported looking at the prevalence of CagA-positive infection in patients with gastric lymphoma and matched controls. One small study in Germany[14] found that, although 89% of a group of 55 lymphoma patients had evidence of *H. pylori* infection, the prevalence of CagA-positive strains was 47%, no more than would be expected in the general population.

Whereas there is some evidence that gastric cancer is more strongly associated with a CagA-positive infection compared with a CagA-negative infection, this association currently appears to be confined to intestinal-type gastric adenocarcinoma. Further, individuals infected with Cag-A-negative strains still show progression of the *H. pylori*-associated gastritis to pathologies strongly associated with cancer. On available evidence, therefore, it would appear that eradicating the infection only in those with CagA-positive strains would not be fully effective as a means of gastric cancer prevention.

GENETIC BACKGROUND OF THE HOST

The concept that individuals differ in their response to an infection as a result of genetic variation is well established, and one would expect that the pathogenic effects of an organism as prevalent throughout the world as *H. pylori* would be modified by host factors. There has been very little direct human genetic research on this topic, although mouse model systems show striking strain variation in the development of atrophy subsequent to *H. felis* infection[15]. Such human research that has been reported relates to variation in HLA haplotypes. In a small study from the UK, Beales and colleagues[16] have shown a significantly higher prevalence of the DQ5 genotype in individuals with *H. pylori* infection and accompanying atrophic gastritis or intestinal metaplasia in comparison with infected individuals and accompanying superficial gastritis or with uninfected individuals. In Japan, Azuma and colleagues have extensively investigated the DAQ1 alleles[17,18] and found no association with atrophic gastritis[18] and a lower prevalence of DQA1*0102 among patients with gastric cancer and coexisting *H. pylori* infection. This work on HLA may be pointing in an interesting direction, but requires much larger studies, appropriately adjusted for the multiple comparisons being made, before any conclusions can be drawn.

A different insight into host factors is provided by the work of McColl and colleagues looking at the role of gastric acid production, basal and stimulated, associated with *H. pylori* infection. They have shown that, whereas most individuals show an increase in acid output in response to infection with a return to normal after eradication[19], a small group of subjects appear to show profound suppression of gastric acidity as a result of infection and, in these individuals, eradication of the infection increases acid output back to normal levels[20]. The latter group could be those destined to develop severe gastric atrophy, further hypoacidity and the precancerous lesions characteristic of gastric cancer.

Why there should be a divergent response in acid output after infection is unclear but, as Dixon has suggested[21], this could be related to the size of the parietal cell mass at the time of infection. Those with a large cell mass and high acid output have infection confined to the antrum, which does not disrupt acid-secreting cells in the gastric corpus. Acid output may then be further enhanced as a result of increased gastrin release. In those with a small parietal cell mass, acid production is insufficient to 'protect' the corpus from infection, and subsequent cellular degeneration compromises acid output still further. Size of the parietal cell mass may be under direct genetic influence and differ, for example, between different ethnic groups. Alternatively, infection at young age may be acquired when the parietal cell mass is immature, thus the corpus would be more sensitive to bacterial colonization at such a time.

Indirect evidence in support of the above hypothesis is provided by Blaser *et al.*[22] who showed, among Japanese Hawaiians, that gastric cancer (but not duodenal ulcer) risk was increased, within an *H. pylori*-positive population, in children who have a higher birth order within a family. Such children are, by definition, in families with an increased number of elder siblings and may therefore have a greater likelihood of acquiring an infection at a particularly young age.

ENVIRONMENTAL EXPOSURES

Several environmental exposures have been proposed as risk factors for gastric cancer. These include diet, smoking and a variety of occupational exposures[23]. Probably the best-established association, which has been consistently confirmed in studies from many countries, is that between risk and a diet deficient in fresh fruit and vegetables[24]. The evidence establishing this and other associations dates back to the pre-*H. pylori* era, and there are few studies which have looked simultaneously at the relative contributions to risk made by *H. pylori* infection and other exposures. Almost the only exception is the study, from Sweden, by Hansson and colleagues[25], results from which are shown in Table 2. This was a retrospective case–control study, a methodology which may produce an under-ascertainment of the risk conferred by *H. pylori* infection[26]. Nevertheless, the results show that infection, low fruit intake, smoking and high alcohol and coffee consumption all significantly increased the risk of gastric cancer after multivariate analysis (with

Table 2 Odds ratio for gastric cancer associated with multiple risk factors in Sweden (from ref. 25)

Risk factor	Odds ratio* (95% CI)
H. pylori	2.7 (1.3–5.8)
High vegetable intake	1.7 (0.8–3.4)
High fruit intake	0.2 (0.1–0.5)
Smoking	1.9 (0.9–3.4)
High alcohol intake	4.5 (1.4–14.0)
High coffee intake	10.5 (2.9–37.7)
Long-term refrigeration use	0.3 (0.1–1.3)
High social class	0.9 (0.4–2.0)

*Multivariate analysis

results of borderline significance for smoking). Of additional interest is the fact that social class was not a risk factor in this analysis, even though gastric cancer is usually observed to be strongly inversely related to socioeconomic status. This may be because the relationship with social class is fully accounted for after adjusting for *H. pylori* infection and the other environmental risk factors.

It is unwise to draw too many conclusions from a single epidemiological study, especially considering the inherent uncertainties involved in using questionnaires to measure dietary exposures. The results concerning coffee in the Swedish study have not been replicated elsewhere and should, therefore, be treated with particular caution. It is, however, important to repeat this type of study, especially using prospective designs, in order to define in quantitative terms the cancer risk associated with *H. pylori* in those with an adverse diet and lifestyle.

One other environmental exposure that has been subject to scrutiny in recent years, because of its suggested association with gastric cancer, is nitrate consumption. Considerable attention has been paid to nitrate levels in drinking water, as it has been believed that consumption of water with a high nitrate content may enhance the formation of carcinogenic *N*-nitroso compounds in the stomach[27]. Evidence relating to this specific hypothesis remains equivocal[28], although the nitrate and *N*-nitroso compound association is now of interest for other reasons. Several studies have shown that, under conditions of chronic infection (bacterial and parasitic), one level of host response is to synthesize nitric oxide as a result of inducing nitric oxide synthase activity[29]. Such induced nitric oxide can be oxidized to other nitrogen oxides and result in formation of nitrite and nitrate ions. In such circumstances endogenous production of nitrate might be substantively more important than exogenous exposure. There is now evidence that *H. pylori* infection can also induce nitric oxide synthase activity[30–32]. It is plausible, therefore, that nitrate exposure might be of relevance to gastric carcinogenesis, but by a mechanism that does not depend on direct environmental exposure. Infected individuals might be capable of nitrosating dietary amides and amines, giving rise to *N*-nitroso compounds, with greater efficiency than uninfected individuals.

SUMMARY

This chapter has attempted to review the different lines of research which help define the conditions that increase the risk of gastric cancer in those infected with *H. pylori*. Although none of the evidence is conclusive, it is apparent that there are likely to be bacterial strain, host and environmental factors of importance. It is tempting to construct a picture of a high-risk individual with a CagA-positive *H. pylori* infection, acquired at an early age, together with a poor diet and unfavourable HLA haplotype. Considerably more research is required, however, before such pictures can be drawn with any degree of certainty.

References

1. International Agency for Research on Cancer. IARC Monographs on the evaluation of carcinogenic risks to humans, Vol. 61: Schistosomes, liver flukes and *Helicobacter pylori*. Lyon: IARC; 1994.

2. Cover TL, Dooley CP, Blaser MJ. Characterisation of a human serologic response to proteins in *Helicobacter pylori* broth culture supernatants with vacuolizing cytotoxin activity. Infect Immun. 1990;58:603–10.

3. Crabtree JE, Taylor JD, Wyatt JI *et al.* Mucosal IgA recognition of *Helicobacter pylori* 120 kDa protein, peptic ulceration and gastric pathology. Lancet. 1991;338:332–5.

4. Crabtree JE, Wyatt JI, Sobala GM *et al.* Systemic and mucosal humoral responses to *Helicobacter pylori* in gastric cancer. Gut. 1993;34:1339–43.

5. Tummuru MKR, Cover TL, Blaser MJ. Mutation of the cytotoxin-associated cagA gene does not affect the vacuolating cytotoxin activity of *Helicobacter pylori*. Infect Immun. 1994;62:2609–13.

6. Kuipers EJ, Pérez-Pérez GI, Meuwissen SGM, Blaser MJ. *Helicobacter pylori* and atrophic gastritis: importance of the cagA status. J Natl Cancer Inst. 1995;87:1777–80.

7. Kuipers EJ, Uyterlinde AM, Peña AS *et al.* Longterm sequelae of *Helicobacter pylori* gastritis. Lancet. 1995;345:1525–8.

8. Nomura A, Stemmermann GN, Chyou PH *et al.* *Helicobacter pylori* and gastric carcinoma among Japanese Americans in Hawaii. N Engl J Med. 1991;325:1132–6.

9. Parsonnet J, Friedman GD, Vandersteen DP *et al.* *Helicobacter pylori* infection and the risk of gastric carcinoma. N Engl J Med. 1991;325:1127–31.

10. Kikuchi S, Wada O, Nakajima T *et al.* Serum anti-*Helicobacter pylori* antibody and gastric carcinoma among young adults. Cancer. 1995;75:2789–93.

11. Blaser MJ, Pérez-Pérez GI, Kleanthous H *et al.* Infection with *Helicobacter pylori* strains possessing cagA is associated with an increased risk of developing adenocarcinoma of the stomach. Cancer Res. 1995;55:2111–15.

12. Parsonnet J, Friedman GD, Orentreich N *et al.* Infection with the type 1 phenotype of *H. pylori* increases risk of gastric cancer independent of corpus atrophy. Gastroenterology. 1996;110:A221.

13. Kikuchi S, Forman D, Covacci A *et al.* Diffuse gastric cancer in young *H. pylori* positive Japanese patients: lack of association with CagA status. Gut. 1996 (abstract) (In press).

14. Foerster EC, Koch P, Koch O *et al.* Serum response to *Helicobacter pylori* in primary B-cell gastric lymphoma. Gut. 1995;37(Suppl. 1):A6.

15. Lee A. *Helicobacter* infections in laboratory animals: a model for gastric neoplasias? Ann Med. 1995;27:575–82.

16. Beales ILP, Davey NJ, Pusey CD *et al.* Long-term sequelae of *Helicobacter pylori* gastritis. Lancet. 1995;346:381–2 (letter).

17. Azuma T, Konishi J, Tanaka Y *et al.* Contribution of HLA-DQA gene to host's response against *Helicobacter pylori*. Lancet. 1994;343:542–3.

18. Azuma T, Ito Y, Miyaji H *et al.* Immunogenetic analysis of the human leukocyte antigen DQA1 locus in patients with duodenal ulcer or chronic atrophic gastritis harbouring *Helicobacter pylori*. Eur J Gastroenterol Hepatol. 1995;7(Suppl. 1):S71–3.

19. El-Omar E, Penman I, Dorrian CA *et al.* *Helicobacter pylori* infection lowers gastrin releasing peptide stimulated gastrin release in duodenal ulcer patients. Gut. 1993;34:1060–6.

20. McColl KEL, El-Omar E. *Helicobacter pylori* and disturbance of gastric function associated with duodenal ulcer disease and gastric cancer. Scand J Gastroenterol. 1996;31(Suppl. 215):32–7.

21. Dixon M. Acid, ulcers and *H. pylori*. Lancet. 1993;342:384–5.

22. Blaser MJ, Chyou PH, Nomura A. Age at establishment of *Helicobacter pylori* infection and gastric carcinoma, gastric ulcer, and duodenal ulcer risk. Cancer Res. 1995;55:562–5.

23. Fuchs CS, Mayer RJ. Gastric carcinoma. N Engl J Med. 1995;333:32–41.

24. Steinmetz KA, Potter JD. Vegetables, fruit, and cancer. I. Epidemiology. Cancer Causes Control. 1991;2:325–57.

25. Hansson LE, Engstrand L, Nyren O *et al.* *Helicobacter pylori* infection: independent risk indicator of gastric adenocarcinoma. Gastroenterology. 1993;105:1098–103.

26. Forman D. The prevalence of *Helicobacter pylori* infection in gastric cancer. Aliment Pharmacol Ther. 1995;9(Suppl. 2):77–84.

27. Forman D. Are nitrates a significant risk factor in human cancer? Cancer Surv. 1989;8:443–58.

28. Gangolli SD, van den Brandt PA, Feron VJ *et al.* Nitrate, nitrite and *N*-nitroso compounds. Eur J Pharmacol. 1994;292:1–38.

29. Iyengar R, Stuehr BJ, Marletta MA. Macrophage synthesis of nitrate and N-nitrosamines: precursors and the role of the respiratory burst. Proc Natl Acad Sci USA. 1987;84:6369–73.

30. Rachmilewitz D, Karmeli F, Eliakim R *et al.* Enhanced gastric nitric oxide synthase activity in duodenal ulcer patients. Gut. 1994;35:1394–7.

31. Bravo LE, Mannick EE, Zhang XJ *et al.* *Helicobacter pylori* infection is associated with inducible nitric oxide synthase expression, nitrotyrosine and DNA damage. Gastroenterology. 1995;108:A63 (abstract).
32. Rieder G, Hatz RA, Stolte M, Enders G. Inos in *H. pylori*-associated gastritis – possible role in carcinogenesis. Gastroenterology. 1996;110:A1002 (abstract).

27
Mechanisms of spread of *Helicobacter pylori* infection

S. M. KELLY

INTRODUCTION

Helicobacter pylori is the commonest bacterial infection in the world. The mode of transmission of *H. pylori* is of fundamental importance when considering strategies for its control. This is of increasing importance as the public health implications of infection become clear. However, despite much research the exact route of transmission of *H. pylori* remains controversial.

SOURCES OF *H. PYLORI*

Humans are generally believed to be the sole natural host of *H. pylori*. The organism is uniquely adapted to surviving in the hostile environment of the stomach. It possesses a potent urease to provide a buffering microclimate to protect it from gastric acid[1], active motility to enable it to move through gastric mucus[2] and the ability to adhere to the epithelium of gastric mucosal cells[3]. Organisms similar to *H. pylori* have been isolated from primates including rhesus monkeys[4] and pigtailed macaques[5]. Of more importance is the recent report of the isolation of *H. pylori* from a population of domestic cats[6]. Spiral organisms have long been observed in the gastric mucosa of cats and dogs, but have been largely ignored as they were believed to be commensals. It has previously proved very difficult to isolate the organism from any domestic animal. Experimental attempts to infect animals with *H. pylori* have also proved largely unsuccessful, with the exception of studies in gnotobiotic pigs[7] and athymic or germfree mice[8]. However, Fox and colleagues recently cultured *H. pylori* from a group of commercially reared cats. The organism was associated with an active gastritis in these cats and its identity was confirmed as *H. pylori* by 16S rRNA sequence analysis. This group have subsequently demonstrated that oral dosing with *H. pylori* can lead to persistent infection in cats treated with cimetidine[9]. The results of studies to determine the prevalence of the organism in pet cats outside of laboratory conditions are awaited with interest, and will help to determine the potential for the domestic cat to act as a reservoir of infection.

It is believed that the major route of transmission of *H. pylori* is by person-to-person spread. In support of this is the observation of clustering of infections in conditions of close proximity, such as institutions[10] and within families[11]. Although there is great variability in DNA and RNA profiles, studies of DNA or RNA finger-printing of *H. pylori* strains obtained from family members have given results which generally support spread of infection within the home[12], most likely by interpersonal spread. If transmission outside of interpersonal spread is important, then the organism must be able to survive in the environment. The finding of an association between infection with *H. pylori* and a municipal water supply in families of both high and low socioeconomic status in Peru is consistent with water acting as a vehicle of transmission[13]. The association between infection and consumption of vegetables produced on farms using irrigation water contaminated with sewage is also consistent with faecally contaminated water as a vehicle for transmission[14].

H. pylori can be cultured under laboratory conditions from water at 7°C 14 days after inoculation. However, it was not possible to culture the organism after 1–3 days at room temperature[15]. *H. pylori* labelled with [³H]thymidine have also been recovered from water and induced to proliferate[16]. These findings raise the possibility of the presence of viable, but largely non-culturable, forms of *H. pylori* in water supplies as a potential source of infection. This may well be of particular importance in spread of infection in the developing world.

EPIDEMIOLOGY

In the developed world the prevalence of infection with *H. pylori* increases with age. Rates of infection are low in childhood and progressively increase up to the age of around 50 years[17]. At present the incidence of infection in adults in the developed world is low at approximately 0.5% per year[18,19], so the pattern of infection within the developed world is likely to be due to a cohort effect. Earlier this century the rate of *H. pylori* infection would have been closer to that observed now in developing countries, and infection was acquired at an early age. However, with socioeconomic development and subsequent improvement in hygiene and living conditions, the rate of infection has declined, resulting in the lower rates of infection we see today. *H. pylori* serological studies have demonstrated an age-related pattern of infection consistent with this cohort phenomenon, with a break in the rate of infection curve at the age of 40[18]. At present it appears that childhood remains the most important time for acquiring infection, but that in the developed world rates of infection at this time are now lower, and some subjects may be infected at later ages[20].

In the developing world prevalence of infection is very high and infection occurs at a young age with rates of infection of around 75% by the age of 20[21-24]. A vital risk factor for infection is socioeconomic status. This is well documented by comparison of groups within the same country[25,26], and when comparing developed and developing countries[17,27]. There is a strong link between infection in adults and overcrowding in childhood, and also the absence of a fixed hot-water supply[28,29], both of which are associated with low socioeconomic status. In poorer developing countries with low socioeconomic status the prevalent living conditions are an ideal environment for spread of the organism. Overcrowding, the lack of adequate sewage disposal and the absence of a safe, secure water supply are all likely to be important factors facilitating spread of the organism.

In the developed world rates of *H. pylori* infection in childhood have declined, whereas the infection rates at this time remain very high in the developing world, and represent a considerable public health challenge.

ROUTES OF INFECTION

The faeco-oral route

Many bacterial infections of the gastrointestinal tract are transmitted by the faeco-oral route and the epidemiological evidence is in favour of the faeco-oral route of transmission of *H. pylori*[30]. Prevalence data on viruses which are known to be transmitted by this route, such as hepatitis A, parallel data on *H. pylori*[31,32], while viruses known to have oro-oral transmission, such as EBV and herpes simplex, do not[33]. As previously seen, the case controlled study in Peru was consistent with contaminated water acting as a vehicle for transmission[13]. Children in families using a municipal water supply had a high prevalence of infection, whereas the infection rate was much lower when families had their own private supply. This study is highly suggestive of faeco-oral transmission via contaminated water as a route of infection in developing countries, but its relevance to the spread of infection in the developed world remains unclear. One long-standing problem with the faeco-oral route has been the difficulty in actually isolating the organism from faeces. *H. pylori* has been detected in faeces by PCR[34] and has been detected on metaplastic tissue in a rectal biopsy[35], suggesting that the organism can pass through the gastrointestinal tract. *H. pylori* was first isolated in human faeces from a group of Gambian children[36] and it was postulated that the different intra-luminal environment of the gastrointestinal tract in this population facilitated passage of the bacterium into faeces, enabling it to be cultured. Consequently the relevance of this finding to mechanisms of *H. pylori* infection in other populations was questioned. However, isolation of *H. pylori* in faeces was subsequently conclusively demonstrated in adults with dyspepsia in the United Kingdom[37]. The colonies obtained on initial cultures were very small and difficult to spot on a plate of mixed faecal flora, and this fact certainly goes some way to explain the failure of other groups to repeat this work[38]. The organism isolated contained *ureA* and *cagA* genes, both of which are believed to be highly specific for the organism, confirming that the isolate was indeed *H. pylori*. This work confirmed that faeco-oral transmission is possible, and so removes one of the major stumbling blocks to this route of spread.

The oro-oral route

H. pylori may possibly be regurgitated into the buccal cavity during episodes of gastro-oesophageal reflux, and via this route infect dental plaque and saliva. Attempts at isolating the organism from saliva have failed[39], but there has been some success in isolating *H. pylori* from dental plaque[40]. In one study the same strain of *H. pylori* was shown in dental plaque as that in the stomach in one patient[41]. A further study demonstrated that *H. pylori* may persist in the dental plaque of patients following eradication of the organism from the stomach[42], although in that study detection was simply on the basis of a positive urease test of plaque without firm identification of *H. pylori*. However, this does raise the interesting possibility of dental plaque acting as a reservoir of infection.

Against oro-oral spread is that studies on dental workers have shown no evidence of an increased risk of infection, and therefore that exposure to dental plaque and saliva is not a risk factor for *H. pylori* infection[43]. The fact that EBV and HSV show a different pattern of infection also argues against oro-oral transmission[44]. It has been suggested that in developed countries an increasing proportion of the population are infected outside of childhood, and in particular in adolescence with oro-oral contact with the opposite sex. However if this were a significant factor one would expect much higher rates of infection in this group than are actually observed at present. Oro-oral spread certainly plays a major role in some populations, as for example in Western Africa where premastication of food by mothers for their children is practised, and is associated with high rates of infection[45].

Some support for oro-oral transmission against faeco-oral is from a study demonstrating transmission of *Helicobacter felis* from gnotobiotic Beagle puppies to uninfected animals in close contact. However, such transmission was not observed under similar conditions in rats, who are coprophagous, suggesting that *H. felis* is predominantly transmitted by the oral route[46].

The gastro-oral route

H. pylori infection has been documented after gastroscopy[47] and following experiments with reusable pH probes[48]. Staff working in gastroscopy units appear to be at a greater risk of infection[49] due to exposure to endoscopes and regurgitated gastric juice. Therefore it is possible that transmission may occur via gastric juice and possibly vomitus[50]. A recent anecdotal report in support of this was the infection of a member of medical staff following mouth-to-mouth resuscitation where the collapsed patient's mouth was initially full of vomitus[51].

H. pylori infection is predominantly acquired in childhood, and vomiting is relatively common at this age. Acute infection with *H. pylori* has been associated with pain and vomiting which will facilitate transmission via this route. Low socioeconomic status, with overcrowding and a lack of a fixed hot-water supply, will also facilitate transmission via this route. At present the organism has not been cultured from vomitus, and it is not known how long the organism can survive in gastric juice outside of the stomach. This recent hypothesis is an interesting development which deserves further scrutiny, but for which there is no direct evidence at present. It may well contribute to spread of infection, but it is doubtful that it is as important a factor as faeco-oral spread in similar environments.

Reinfection

Once *H. pylori* has been successfully eradicated rates of reinfection in the developed world are generally low. Reinfection has been documented in 6% of cases after just 12 months following eradication[52], but such episodes have been shown to occur with *H. pylori* strains displaying identical genotypes, and have been attributed to recrudescence of infection rather than true infection[53]. A long-term follow-up study has shown a cumulative reinfection rate of 8.6% at 7 years after eradication[54], suggesting that the early rates of reinfection are not maintained. Reinfection has been documented with a strain of *H. pylori* identical to that of the patient's spouse, raising the possibility of an intrafamilial route of reinfection, although a common environmental source would also fit with these data[55]. As previously stated, dental plaque may act as a reservoir of infection in some patients[42], and can lead to reinfection of the stomach. However, *H. pylori* has not been conclusively identified in plaque after successful eradication, as in this particular study it was identified on the basis of a urease test alone. Another possible route of reinfection is if *H. pylori* can survive in the colon. The organism has been cultured from faeces, and in a follow-up study was persistently isolated in faeces after eradication from the stomach[56]. The colon is a complex microbial ecosystem with many favourable conditions for the resident microflora. It is not surprising that *H. pylori* may be able to establish itself in such an environment, and may not be cleared from the colon by treatment which eradicates the organism from the stomach. Niches of persistent infection may help to explain episodes of early reinfection, and more work is needed in this interesting area. It is of interest to note that early rates of reinfection are higher than *de-novo* rates of infection outside of childhood, and auto-reinfection in a subgroup of patients could explain this, although equally a persisting source of infection within the home is also possible.

In developing countries rates of reinfection are much higher[57]. This is likely to represent sub-optimal hygiene associated with poor socioeconomic conditions and reacquisition of infection by intrafamilial spread, a common environmental source, or possibly auto-reinfection as stated above.

SUMMARY

H. pylori infection is predominantly acquired in childhood. Poor socioeconomic conditions with overcrowding facilitate spread of the organism, resulting in high rates of infection in the developing world. Rates of infection in the developed world continue to fall with improved living conditions. Faeco-oral spread appears to be the main route of infection, particularly in the developing world where water may act as a vehicle for transmission. Oro-oral and gastro-oral transmission may occur, but are not as important. Further work is needed to identify environmental sources of *H. pylori*, on isolation from faeces and dental plaque, particularly after treatment, and on the possibility of domestic pets as a source of infection.

References

1. Kelly SM, Crampton J, Hunter JO. *Helicobacter pylori* increases gastric antral juxtamucosal pH. Dig Dis Sci. 1993;38:129–31.
2. Eaton KA, Morgan DR, Krakowka S. *Campylobacter pylori* virulence factors in gnotobiotic piglets. Infect Immun. 1989;57:1119–25.

3. Brassens-Rabbe MP, Megraud F, Lessier R, Cassagne C. Study of *Helicobacter pylori* interaction with epithelial cell glycolipid receptors. Rev Esp Enf Dig. 1990;78(Suppl. 1):53 – 4.
4. Newell DG, Hudson MJ, Baskerville A. Isolation of a gastric *Campylobacter*-like organism from the stomach of four rhesus monkeys, and identification as *Campylobacter pylori*. J Med Microbiol. 1988;27:41 – 4.
5. Brondson MA, Schoenknecht FD. *Campylobacter pylori* isolated from the stomach of the monkey, *Macaca nemestrina*. J Clin Microbiol. 1988;26:1725 – 8.
6. Handt LK, Fox JG, Dewhirst FE *et al*. *Helicobacter pylori* isolated from the domestic cat: public health implications. Infect Immun. 1994;62:2367 – 74.
7. Krakowa S, Morgan DR, Kraft WG, Leunk RD. Establishment of gastric *Campylobacter pylori* infection in the neonatal gnotobiotic piglet. Infect Immun. 1987;55:2789 – 96.
8. Karita M, Kouchiyama T, Okita K, Nakazama T. New small animal model for human gastric *Helicobacter pylori* infection: success in both nude and athymic mice. Am J Gastroenterol. 1991; 86:1596 – 603.
9. Fox JG, Batchelder M, Marini R *et al*. *Helicobacter pylori*-induced gastritis in the domestic cat. Infect Immun. 1995;63:2674 – 81.
10. Lambert JR, Lin SK, Nicholson L *et al*. High prevalence of *Helicobacter pylori* antibodies in institutionalized adults. Gastroenterology. 1990;98:A69.
11. Graham DY, Malaty HM, Klein PD, Evans DG, Evans DJ, Adam E. *Helicobacter pylori* infection clusters in families. Rev Esp Enf Dig. 1990;78(Suppl. 1):26 – 7.
12. Bamford KB, Bicley J, Collins JSA *et al*. *Helicobacter pylori*: comparison of DNA fingerprints provides evidence for intrafamilial infection. Gut. 1993;34:1348 – 50.
13. Klein PD, Graham DY, Gaillour A, Opekun AR, O'Brian Smith E. Water source as a risk factor for *Helicobacter pylori* infection in Peruvian children. Lancet. 1991;337:1503 – 6.,
14. Hopkins RJ, Vial PA, Ferreccio C *et al*. Seroprevalence of *Helicobacter pylori* in Chile: vegetables may serve as one route of transmission. J Infect Dis. 1993;168:222 – 6.
15. West AP, Millar MR, Tompkins DS. Survival of *Helicobacter pylori* in water and saline. J Clin Pathol. 1990;43:609.
16. Shahamat M, Paszko-Kolva C, Yamamoto H, Mai U, Pearson AD, Colwell RR. Ecological studies of *Campylobacter pylori*. Klin Wochenschr. 1989;67(Suppl. 18):62 – 3.
17. Megraud F, Brassens-Rabbe MP, Denis F, Belbouri A, Hoa DQ. Seroepidemiology of *Campylobacter pylori* infection in various populations. J Clin Microbiol. 1989;27:1870 – 3.
18. Parsonnet J, Blaser MJ, Perez-Perez GI, Hargrett-Bean N, Tauxe RV. Symptoms and risk factors of infection in a cohort of epidemiologists. Gastroenterology. 1992;102:41 – 6.
19. Kuipers JE, Pena AS, van Kamp G. Seroconversion for *Helicobacter pylori*. Lancet. 1993;342: 328 – 31.
20. Mewndall MA, Northfield TC. Transmission of *Helicobacter pylori* infection. Gut. 1995;37:1 – 3.
21. Holcombe C, Tsimiri S, Eldridge J, Jones DM. Prevalence of antibody to *Helicobacter pylori* in children in Northern Nigeria. Rev Esp Enf Dig. 1990;78(Suppl. I):39.
22. Glupczynski Y, Bourdeaux L, Verhas M, Balegamire B, Devos D, Devrecker T. Epidemiology of *Campylobacter pylori* infection in Zaire. Klin Wochenschr. 1989;67(Suppl. 18):23 – 4.
23. Yang HT, Zohn DY. Seroepidemiology of *Campylobacter pylori* infection in China. Rev Esp Enf Dig. 1990;78(Suppl. 1):130.
24. Al-Moagel MA, Evans DG, Abdulghani ME *et al*. Prevalence of *Helicobacter pylori* infection in Saudi Arabia and comparison of those with and without gastrointestinal symptoms. Am J Gastroenterol. 1990;85:944 – 8.
25. Fiedorek SC, Evans DG, Evans DJ *et al*. *Helicobacter pylori* infection epidemiology in children: importance of socioeconomic status, age, gender and race. Gastroenterology. 1990;98:A44.
26. Webberley MJ, Webbeley JM, Lowe P, Melikian V, Newell D. Seroepidemiology of *Helicobacter pylori* infection in vegans and meat eaters. Rev Esp Enf Dig. 1990;78(Suppl. 1):39.
27. Dwyer B, Kaldor J, Wee Tee, Marakowski E, Raios K. Antibody response to *Campylobacter pylori* in diverse ethnic groups. Scand J Infect Dis. 1988;20:349 – 50.
28. Mendall MA, Goggin PM, Molineux N *et al*. Childhood living conditions and *Helicobacter pylori* seropositivity in adult life. Lancet. 1992;339:986 – 7.
29. Galpin OP, Whitaker CJ, Dubiel AJ. *Helicobacter pylori* infection and overcrowding in childhood. Lancet. 1992;339:619.
30. Graham DY, Malaty HM, Evans DG, Evans DJ, Klein PD, Adam E. Epidemiology of *Helicobacter pylori* in asymptomatic population in the United States. Effect of age, race and socio-economic status. Gastroenterology. 1991;100:1495 – 501.

31. Perez-Perez GI, Taylor DN, Bodhidatta I *et al.* Seroprevalence of *Helicobacter pylori* infections in Thailand. J Infect Dis. 1990;161:1237–41.
32. Gill HH, Desai HG, Majiudar P, Mehta PR, Prabhu SR. Epidemiology of *Helicobacter pylori*: the Indian scenario. Indian J Gastroenterol. 1993;12:9–11.
33. De Korwin JD, Hartemann P, Remot P, Riche I, De La Vergne A, Schmidt J. *Campylobacter pylori* infection: a possible person to person transmission. Klin Wochenschr. 1989;67(Suppl. 18):35–6.
34. Mapstone NP, Lynch DAF, Lewis FA *et al.* PCR identification of *H. pylori* in faeces of gastritis patients. Lancet. 1993;342:1419–20.
35. Dye KR, Marshall BJ, Frierson HF, Pambianco DJ, McCallum RW. *Campylobacter pylori* colonizing heterotopic gastric tissue in the rectum. Am J Clin Pathol J Med Microbiol. 1990; 93:144–7.
36. Thomas JE, Gibson GR, Darboe MK, Dale A, Wever LT. Isolation of *H. pylori* from human faeces. Lancet. 1992;340:1194–5.
37. Kelly SM, Pitcher MCL, Farmery SM, Gibson GR. Isolation of *H. pylori* from feces of patients with dyspepsia in the UK. Gastroenterology. 1994;107:1671–4.
38. Levenstein-van Hall MA, van der Ende A, van Milligan de Wit M, Tytgan GN, Dankaert J. Transmission of *H. pylori* via faeces. Lancet. 1993;342:1419–20 (letter).
39. Krajden S, Fuksa M, Anderson J *et al.* Examination of the human stomach biopsies, saliva and dental plaque for *Campylobacter pylori.* J Clin Microbiol. 1989;322:2849–50.
40. Song QS, Zheng ZT, Yu H. *Helicobacter pylori* in dental plaque. Chinese J Int Med. 1994;33: 59–61.
41. Cellini L, Allocati N, Piatelli A, Petrelli I, Fanci P, Dainelli B. Microbiological evidence of *Helicobacter pylori* from dental plaque in dyspeptic patients. Microbiologica. 1995;18:187–92.
42. Desai HG, Gill HH, Shankaran K, Mehta PR, Prabhu SR. Dental plaque: a permanent reservoir of *Helicobacter pylori*? Scand J Gastroenterol. 1991;26:1205–8.
43. Banatvala N, Abdi Y, Clements L *et al. Helicobacter pylori* infection in dentists – a case control study. Scand J Infect Dis. 1995;27:149–51.
44. Adams E. The transmission of EBV infections. In: Hoks JG, editor. Viral infections in oral medicine. New York: Elsevier: 1982:211–25.
45. Albenque M, Tall F, Dabis F, Megraud F. Epidemiological study of transmission from mother to child in Africa. Rev Esp Enferm Dig. 1990;78(Suppl. 1):48.
46. Lee A, Fox JG, Otto G, Dick EH, Krakowa S. Transmission of *Helicobacter* spp.: a challenge to the dogma of faecal–oral spread. Epidemiol Infect. 1991;107:99–109.
47. Langenberg W, Rauws EAJ, Oudbier JH, Tytgat GNJ. Patient to patient transmission of *Campylobacter pylori* infection by fibreoptic OGD and biopsy. J Infect Dis. 1990;161:507–11.
48. Ramsey EJ, Carey KV, Peterson WL *et al.* Epidemic gastritis with hypochlorhydria. Gastroenterology. 1979;76:1449–57.
49. Reiff A, Jacobs E, Kist M. Seroepidemiological study of the immune response to *Campylobacter pylori* in potential risk groups. Eur J Clin Microbiol Infect Dis. 1989;8:592–6.
50. Axon ATR. Is *Helicobacter pylori* transmitted by the gastro-oral route. Aliment Pharmacol Ther. 1995;9:585–8.
51. Figura N. Mouth to mouth resuscitation and *H. pylori* infection. Lancet. 1996;347:1342.
52. Borody T, Cole P, Noonan S *et al. Campylobacter pylori* recurrence post eradication. Gastroenterology. 1988;94:A43.
53. Langenberg ML, Rauws EA, Schipper ME, Widjojokoruo A, Tytgat GTN. The pathogenic role of *Campylobacter pyloridis* studied by attempts to eradicate these organisms. In: Pearson AD, Skirrow MB, Lior H, Rowe B, editors. *Campylobacter.* III. Proceedings of the Third International Workshop on *Campylobacter* infections. Ottawa: PHLS; 1985:162–3.
54. Forbes GM, Glaser ME, Cullen DJE, Warren JR, Christiansen KJ, Marshall BJ. Duodenal ulcer treated with *Helicobacter pylori* eradication: seven-year follow-up. Lancet. 1994;343:258–60.
55. Schutze K, Hentschel E, Dragosics B, Hirschl AM. *Helicobacter pylori* reinfection with identical organisms: transmission by the patients' spouses. Gut. 1995;36:831–3.
56. Kelly SM, Gibson GR. Persistent faecal excretion of *Helicobacter pylori* in faeces after gastric eradication. Gut. 1994;35:S2–3.
57. Coelho LGV, Passos MCF, Chausson Y *et al.* Duodenal ulceration and eradication of *H. pylori*: an eighteen-month follow-up study. Scand J Gastroenterol. 1992;27:362–6.

28
Whom, how and when to test for *Helicobacter pylori* infection

A. AXON, P. MOAYYEDI and P. SAHAY

INTRODUCTION

With the recognition that *H. pylori* is an important pathogen, and that curative treatment is now reasonably effective, simple and inexpensive there has been increased interest in testing for *H. pylori*. As these investigations have become more accurate and widely used a number of questions have emerged.

Who should be tested? From a clinical standpoint there is no purpose in testing patients for *H. pylori* unless there is an intention to act upon the findings. It follows that the decision whether or not to test goes back to the selection of individuals for treatment.

Secondly, which test should be used? The number of tests available has increased rapidly in recent years, and they vary in sensitivity and specificity, but this is not the only consideration; clinical convenience is also important. Tests can now be done in the surgery on whole blood, and can provide an answer within 15 minutes; on the other hand the urea breath test not only screens the patient, but can also be used to assess eradication success. The cost of these tests is also of relevance.

Testing for *H. pylori* at endoscopy is now widely used, and techniques in this area have not changed substantially in recent years. This chapter therefore will concentrate mainly on non-invasive techniques of testing, as it is in this area that the greatest interest and controversy exists at present.

TESTING FOR *H. PYLORI* AT ENDOSCOPY

Is it necessary to test for *Helicobacter* in all patients who undergo endoscopy? There are several reasons why this should always be done. Firstly, the absence of *H. pylori* reassures the clinician that if the rest of the endoscopy is normal there probably has never been an ulcer, and there is unlikely to be one in the future. Secondly, patients who have gastro-oesophageal reflux disease may require treatment at some time with an acid pump inhibitor that may be used for a long period.

In patients infected with *H. pylori* these drugs cause a migration of the organism from the antrum of the stomach to the corpus[1], giving rise to a pan-gastritis[2]. Over a period this may cause gastric atrophy[2,3], a known precursor of gastric cancer[4]. Under these circumstances a clinician may feel it desirable to eradicate *Helicobacter* before starting long-term acid pump inhibitor therapy. Thirdly, most patients in the developed world who undergo endoscopy are aware that *H. pylori* is a potential cause of upper gastrointestinal disease, and they often enquire of the clinician, after endoscopy, whether or not the organism was present. It can be embarrassing if the clinician has not tested for it at the time of endoscopy. Finally, to take biopsies prolongs the examination for only a short period, and if the rapid urease test is used the costs of this extra test are negligible compared with the cost of the procedure itself.

Some doctors suggest that if a duodenal ulcer is present it is unnecessary to test for *H. pylori* because there is a 95% probability that the patient will be infected. The reason for taking biopsies in this instance, however, is not to detect the organism, but to determine if the patient is *Helicobacter*-negative as, if so, it then becomes necessary to consider alternative aetiologies for the ulcer. This may be the patient's surreptitious intake of non-steroidal anti-inflammatory drugs, Zollinger-Ellison syndrome or rare conditions such as Crohn's disease.

The most accurate method for detecting *H. pylori* at endoscopy is to take two biopsies from the antrum and two from the corpus, for examination by an experienced histopathologist. Although polymerase chain reaction (PCR) techniques provide a greater sensitivity they are not generally available to most endoscopy services, and great care has to be taken to ensure that extraneous DNA is not introduced into the system. Failure to do this causes a drop in the specificity of the technique. Culture of gastric mucosa is relatively simple, and not as expensive as histopathology; however, although very specific, its sensitivity is variable depending upon the endoscopy room set-up and the arrangements made with the microbiology laboratory. Culture enables the bacterial sensitivity to antimicrobial agents to be determined. In practice, with the newer *Helicobacter* eradication regimens, which have a 90% success rate, antibiotic sensitivities are not particularly helpful. Culture may also enable the strain of *Helicobacter* to be studied.

These latter tests are relatively expensive compared with the rapid urease test. With this technique biopsies are placed immediately into a medium containing urea and phenol red. The urease present within *H. pylori* converts urea to ammonia and carbon dioxide, causing a rise in the pH, which changes the colour of the medium from yellow to red. Commercially available rapid urease test kits are available at a cost of around £2.50, but an even less expensive 'do-it-yourself' rapid urease test is simple to prepare and may give a quicker result[5]. A suitable method is as follows: 0.5 ml of 10% unbuffered[1] urea in distilled water is placed in a 0.7 ml Eppendorf tube, and one drop of 1% phenol red is added. We have compared the accuracy of this test with the CLO test after 24 hours, comparing each against a gold standard of histology (two antral, two body biopsies), culture (one antral biopsy) and carbon-13 urea breath test. A patient was defined as *H. pylori*-positive if two or more tests were positive, and negative if all tests were negative. The *H. pylori* status was indeterminate if only one test gave a positive result.

Table 1 Comparison of a do-it-yourself rapid urea test (RUT) compared with the commercially prepared test (CLO) 95% confidence intervals for the difference in sensitivities between the two tests -14% to $+1\%$

	RUT-positive	RUT-negative	CLO-positive	CLO-negative
Gold standard positive	57	5	61	1
Gold standard negative	0	39	0	39

One hundred and four patients were recruited; 62 were gold standard positive, 39 negative and three indeterminate. The do-it-yourself test had a sensitivity of 92% and a specificity of 100%, while the CLO test had a sensitivity of 98% and a specificity of 100% when compared with the gold standard. Although there was a tendency for the CLO test to be more sensitive than the do-it-yourself test the difference was not statistically significant in the sample size we tested (Table 1).

SEROLOGICAL TESTING FOR *H. PYLORI*

Greater interest has recently been expressed in non-invasive tests for *Helicobacter* infection. The simplest and least expensive from the patient's point of view is a blood test for serology. Considerable advances have been made in this area, and some of the newer laboratory-based methods have a sensitivity and specificity that rivals histology. Kits for 'near patient testing' enable the result to be obtained in the surgery within 15 minutes. *H. pylori* antibodies can also be detected in saliva, and although no sufficiently accurate salivary test is available to date, there is considerable potential in this area, particularly for epidemiological studies in children.

Antigen specificity and categories

The normal gastric mucosa contains virtually no T or B lymphocytes. Following infection with *H. pylori* B lymphocytes appear in the mucosa, and produce a local antibody response predominantly of the IgA and IgG classes[6] with IgG seroconversion usually $22-33$ days after initial infection[7]. The extent of response of these antibodies does not correlate with the degree of inflammation[8], nor does it eliminate infection or prevent re-establishment of infection after clearance[9]. The molecular basis of the host response is dependent upon epithelial damage, infiltration of immunocompetent cells and the efficiency of the antigen-presenting cell.

The antigens used for serodiagnosis of *H. pylori* infection are of three kinds: (a) whole cell antigens and their ultrasonicates, (b) partially purified antigens and (c) highly purified antigens[10]. Whole cell antigens and their sonicates have the theoretical advantage of presenting the maximum number of surface antigens, but they increase the risk of crossreaction with other organisms, particularly the *Campylobacter* species[11]. Among the partially purified antigens, the ultra-centrifuged cell sonicate and an acid glycine extract give excellent specificity, but reduced sensitivity. Crude urease preparations give a high false-positive result[12], while highly purified urease is very specific.

Forms of anti-*H. pylori* antibodies

H. pylori-positive patients produce antibodies that react against 61, 56 and 28 kDa polypeptides which are specific for *H. pylori* and are associated with urease[13]. Other antigens frequently detected in positive sera are 110–120 kDa protein and several series of high and low molecular weight proteins[8]. Some of these polypeptides are not specific for *H. pylori* and no single protein antigen has been detected that consistently reacts with all the positive sera investigated. As the same major antigens are detected in heterologous and homologous strains by individual sera this supports the view that variation in antibody specificity is host-mediated rather than reflecting antigenic differences between infecting strains of *H. pylori*[14].

Technique for serodiagnosis

The current technique of choice is an enzyme-linked immunosorbent assay (ELISA), as this is simple, quick, economical and reproducible. The test measures IgG antibodies, as *H. pylori* is a chronic infection. It involves the addition of patients' serum to a mixture of antigens, derived from *H. pylori*, dried on the ELISA plate[10]. After washing off the excess antigen the bound antigen–immunoglobulin complex is detected by adding a second antibody which is coupled either to a colour reagent or an enzyme which is capable of producing a coloured product that can be read off an ELISA plate reader, quantifying the amount of antibody present. The real problem is to decide upon the cut-off point between positive and negative results. Hence ELISA test kits require local validation[15].

Selection criteria for ELISA antigens

There should be a mixture of antigens which are common to all *H. pylori* strains (although including more strains in antigen preparation only marginally increases the sensitivity of the serological test[11]). The antigens should be easily prepared and purified, be stable on storage and should not crossreact with other organisms or bind non-specifically to immunoglobulins. ELISA tests with complex antigens detect 95% of infected patients with over 90% specificity. The highly purified antigens include the urease and 120–128 kDa product of the gene *cagA*. A major problem in producing purified antigens is organizing the large-scale growth of *H. pylori*. Chemostat culture techniques can produce up to 1 g of bacterial mass per day (M. Hudson and K. Lee, unpublished data). In spite of the fact that the 120 kDa protein is quite specific it is not expressed by all strains of *H. pylori*[12]. Urease, which is generally regarded as specific for *H. pylori*, is also found in *H. heilmannii*[16]. A 400–700 kDa protein reported to have urease activity in *H. pylori* has over 98% sensitivity and 100% specificity[17].

Detection of IgA as well as IgG antibodies increases the sensitivity[18]. However, it is the *H. pylori* IgG that is used in commercial serology kits now marketed. Preliminary evidence shows that IgG subclass detection may be important, with IgG-4 being an excellent indicator of *H. pylori* infection[16].

Clinical uses of serological tests

Screening young patients with dyspepsia

The demand for digestive endoscopy continues to spiral upwards. Dyspepsia accounts for 2–3% of all general practitioner consultations, and about 40% of outpatient referrals to the gastroenterology department[19]. This trend is continuing in spite of the fact that patients under the age of 45 years who are *H. pylori*-negative and not taking NSAIDs have a low incidence of peptic ulcer disease and gastric malignancy. Still, 0.5% of the population of the UK undergo gastroscopy each year, with the demand being at least double that[20]. Open-access endoscopy plays an important role, but there has been an increase in the workload[21], with younger patients perhaps being over-investigated[22].

Screening dyspepsia patients under age 45 years by *H. pylori* serology has been recommended as a way of reducing the endoscopy workload by 25–37%[23,24]. Using this strategy Sobala *et al.*[23], who studied 1153 patients, showed that this would reduce the endoscopy workload by 23.3% with a 97.4% sensitivity for detecting peptic ulcers. Tham *et al.*[25] concluded that 35% of endoscopies would have been saved without missing any patient with duodenal ulcer disease. Williams *et al.*[22] undertook a retrospective analysis over a 6-year period in Leicester, and found that only 1.8% of gastric cancers occurred in the under-45-year-olds and none of them had uncomplicated simple dyspepsia. They all had additional worrying features such as dysphagia, weight loss, postprandial vomiting or gastrointestinal bleeding which would, in any event, have selected them as high priority for gastroscopy. Serology as a complement to endoscopy in screening dyspepsia saves money, as one serology test costs about £10 as opposed to gastroscopy which costs around £200 in the UK National Health Service.

Epidemiological studies

Seroepidemiology is an important investigative tool used to characterize the prevalence of *H. pylori* infection, its reservoirs and its modes of transmission. Other non-invasive methods, such as the breath tests and study of saliva and urine, are being used increasingly, but serological methods are most commonly used for population-based epidemiological studies.

The performance of serological methods varies with the antigens chosen, age and ethnicity of the population from which the reference sera are drawn, and the homologous and heterologous infection rates in the population being studied. The major variables are the definitions of true positive and negative, replicability and comparability of the tests when used by different laboratories and the number of results near the cut-off value[26]. The sensitivity and specificity of a test is not affected by the prevalence of infection. However, as the prevalence of infection rises in the population, the positive predictive value (PPV) rises and the negative predictive value (NPV) falls. The accuracy measurements for the tests are therefore of limited value as they vary with changes in *H. pylori* prevalence. An alternative is to report likelihood ratios which indicate the probability of a person with a particular result being truly positive when compared with the probability of a person with the result being truly negative[26].

Diagnosis of gastroduodenal disease in children

Serology is useful in diagnosing *H. pylori*-related gastroduodenal diseases in children; however, the criteria for seropositivity need adjustment because standardization of epidemiological assays is done in adults while the antibody levels in childhood infections are lower.

Monitoring treatment

IgG levels decrease following eradication of *H. pylori*, but the fall is slow and takes about 6 months or more to reach normal values[27]. Reinfection leads to a rapid rise in titre[28]. Serology is therefore unsuitable for checking eradication as it is a slow indicator of effective treatment.

Commercial serology kits

Serology is quick, non-invasive, inexpensive, easy to perform and reproducible. Many kits are now commercially available and once validated locally they will provide useful results. There are a number of reasons why serology kits give different results. Kits themselves vary, bacterial antigenicity differs between local strains and the immune response between populations may be different. However, a number of workers have undertaken comparative studies of 18 different commercial kits[26,29,30]. The kits tested were manufactured by Biorad, Biowhitaker, Genesis, Kenstar, Launch, Orion EIA and dry latex test, Porton, Sigma, Biometra, Roche, Amrad, Biolab, Radim and Danish in House ELISA.

The positive and negative predictive values (PPV + NPV) of the serology test results depend on the prevalence of *H. pylori* infection in the study population. Lower prevalence is associated with lower PPV and higher NPV. Laboratories which provide reference services are unable to provide predictive values because of their heterogeneous patient population.

Two kits which performed extremely well when tested by workers in Addenbrookes Hospital, Cambridge were Pylori-ELISA II (Biowhitaker) and Premier (Launch)[29]. The Biowhitaker kit had 100% sensitivity and NPV with 96% specificity and 97% PPV. The Launch kit, which was initially qualitative, had 100% sensitivity, specificity, PPV and NPV. It has now been modified to give a quantitative result. False-positive results occur either as a result of cross-reacting antibodies or due to the presence of long-lived antibodies. About 12% of kits have equivocal results. As a result, some manufacturers recommend retesting sera giving equivocal results, but this makes the test more expensive and creates extra work. The most important thing is to evaluate a kit adequately in the population on which it is to be used. There is a difference in the results obtained in the under-20-year age group compared to the rest.

For epidemiological studies using serology the problem is defining the 'cut-off' value which separates the positives from the negatives. The higher the cut-off value the fewer the false-positives and the greater the number of false-negatives. The other difficulty with a cut-off value is the variation which takes place when these tests are used in children as opposed to adults[31,32]. There is therefore need for selection of antigens which are region-specific, with different cut-off values for children and adults. One of the important alternatives, as mentioned earlier, is to report the likelihood ratio (LR). Thus, there is the true positive (LR+) and true negative (LR−) together with a LR(grey) in a three-zone test. A receiver operating characteristic (ROC) curve is a useful way to describe the effect of varying the cut-off value. This also can compare the performance of two or more different tests. Test variability can also be highlighted using the calibration curve (EV), the log of EV value and the square root of the EV value. Both the log and square root of EV give equal weight to changes at both the high and lower titres.

The problem, however, with the use of a grey zone, which is incorporated into a number of tests, is that it leads to uncertainty in serological diagnosis. The correlation between *H. pylori* infection and seropositivity is greater in the under-45-year-olds[33], probably because of reduced immunological responses in the elderly[34]. No advantage has been recorded when a combination of IgG, IgA and IgM antibodies to *H. pylori* are measured together[35]. Separate measurement of IgA or IgM for the diagnosis of *H. pylori* is also unhelpful[36].

Clinic room tests

Test kits have now been produced enabling the clinician to ascertain the *H. pylori* status of the patient by using a fingerprick whole blood method. This provides an answer in 10 minutes. Cortecs Diagnostics have recently introduced the Helisal rapid whole blood test, which is the first near-patient test to be available commercially in the UK. This has been assessed recently for its sensitivity and specificity against a standard serology kit (Helico-G; Porton, Cambridge) and a 'gold standard' which consisted of histology, microbiology, CLO test and [^{13}C]urea breath test[37]. It was found to be as accurate as the laboratory-based commercial serology kit when compared to the 'gold standard'. Helisal was slightly more expensive (£15 per patient) than other serology kits. Its advantage, however, is the quick result, which makes it useful in the outpatient or primary-care setting. The proviso here, as with all serology kits, is its need for validation in the population to be studied. This is particularly important for Helisal, as it is a qualitative test rather than quantitative and hence cut-off points cannot be redefined to improve accuracy[38]. Smith Kline Diagnostics have developed a test called Flexsure™, which will soon be available in Europe, but requires serum. Boehringer Mannheim have introduced their BM test *Helicobacter pylori*™. These tests will be useful in clinical practice, and further development is inevitable. Another test kit which may soon be offered is measurement of antibodies to the 120–128 kDa product of the gene *cagA*, as this is present more often in patients with gastric pathology such as ulcers or cancer. Unfortunately, not all patients with these diseases will give a positive result; therefore the value of such a test in clinical practice may be limited[18].

UREA BREATH TESTS

The [^{13}C]urea breath test (^{13}C-UBT) was first described by Graham *et al.* in 1987[39], but interest was limited initially. The equipment required was expensive and protocols varied, making direct comparisons from different centres difficult. Over the past 5 years cheaper dedicated ^{13}C-UBT equipment has become available[40] and the protocol has been standardized[41] and simplified[42]. As a result the ^{13}C-UBT has gained widespread acceptance as a useful method of diagnosing *H. pylori* infection.

Principles of the ^{13}C-UBT

The ^{13}C-UBT relies on the powerful urease enzyme produced by *H. pylori*, which hydrolyses urea to CO_2. [^{13}C]urea is ingested, and if *H. pylori* is present $^{13}CO_2$ is produced. The $^{13}CO_2$ is absorbed into the blood stream and then excreted by the lungs, where it can be measured in breath samples. The ^{13}C-UBT is more accurate if a test meal is given with the [^{13}C]urea to delay gastric emptying, thereby increasing the exposure of the labelled substrate to *H. pylori*[43]. A false-negative ^{13}C-UBT can occur if administered within 1 month of a course of antibiotics[44], proton pump inhibitors[45] or bismuth salts[46], or after gastric surgery[45].

The European standard ^{13}C-UBT protocol

In the initial description of the ^{13}C-UBT 250 mg [^{13}C]urea was used, and breath samples were obtained every 10 min for 180 min in a collecting bag to obtain a $^{13}CO_2$ excretion curve[39]. Subsequently it has been shown that a baseline and subsequent 30 min breath sample give similar accuracy, and are simpler and quicker to collect[42]. Furthermore, 100 mg of [^{13}C]urea produced similar results, suggesting that less of this expensive substrate was required[43]. In an effort to standardize the ^{13}C-UBT a European protocol was recommended based on these findings[41]. Patients were starved for 4 h before being given a fatty test meal (50 ml Callogen® and 50 ml Ensure®). A baseline breath sample was obtained in an excutainer and the patient was given 100 mg [^{13}C]urea dissolved in 50 ml of water. The [^{13}C]urea was distributed throughout the stomach by turning the patient on each side for 2 min. A further breath sample was taken at 30 min and $^{13}CO_2$ excreted in the breath was measured by mass spectrometry.

Measurement of $^{13}CO_2$ for the ^{13}C-UBT

$^{13}CO_2$ is naturally present in expired air, and in patients with a positive breath this may increase by only 1 part per 1000. The methods used to measure $^{13}CO_2$ must, therefore, be extremely accurate, and as it is a non-radioactive isotope this presents a major problem. The most appropriate technique to measure $^{13}CO_2$ is by mass spectrometry, which can detect particles of a given molecular weight with extreme precision. Initial studies purified CO_2 from other breath gases with a cryogenic purification unit before measuring $^{13}CO_2$ using an isotope ratio mass spectrometer (IRMS). The process of purifying the breath was slow and expensive, and limited the availability of the ^{13}C-UBT. Recently, dedicated automated breath ^{13}C analysers (ABCA) have become available which are quicker and cheaper[40]. These use an in-built gas chromatograph that separates CO_2 from N_2 and O_2 in the breath before analysis by an IRMS. The ABCA systems can process samples within 2 min and consumable costs are low, but the machines are still relatively expensive. Improvements in technology and increased demand should reduce these costs substantially over the next few years.

Expression of results

Accurate measurement of $^{13}CO_2$ is meaningless unless results can be expressed in a form that is reproducible with different conditions, equipment and centres. The amount of $^{13}CO_2$ excreted in the breath varies according to the quantity of $^{12}CO_2$ expired. Situations of high $^{12}CO_2$ excretion are mirrored by higher $^{13}CO_2$ excretion. To control for this, results are expressed as a ratio of $^{13}C/^{12}C$. This ratio may vary between different mass spectrometers and so all instruments are calibrated to an international standard. The standard used in this case is PBD (*Belemnitella americana* extracted from the Pe Dee formation of South Carolina, USA[47]). The $^{13}C/^{12}C$ excreted by the patient is expressed relative to the $^{13}C/^{12}C$ found in PBD. In this way results obtained in different centres using different instruments can be compared directly. The isotopic composition (δ) of CO_2 detected in an individual breath sample is therefore calculated according to the following equation:

$$\delta\,^{13}CO_2 = \{[(^{13}C/^{12}C)\text{sample}/(^{13}C/^{12}C)\text{PBD}] - 1\} \times 10^3$$

The amount of $^{13}CO_2$ in the breath also varies according to diet. Individuals eating a ^{13}C-rich diet (contained in corn and maize products[48]) have a higher $^{13}CO_2$ excretion. It is therefore important to compare the breath sample taken at 30 min with the baseline $^{13}CO_2$ excretion. The final result is expressed as excess $\delta^{13}CO_2$ excretion per mil at 30 min compared with baseline calculated as follows:

$$\text{Excess } \delta^{13}CO_2 = \delta^{13}CO_2(30\,\text{min}) - \delta^{13}CO_2(\text{baseline})$$

The authors of the European standard ^{13}C-UBT defined an upper limit of normal for excess $\delta^{13}CO_2$ of 5 per mil. This was derived from 3 standard deviations above the mean exhaled excess $\delta^{13}CO_2$ in *H. pylori*-negative patients[41]. Using this cut-off the ^{13}C-UBT had a 98% sensitivity and 92% specificity compared to a gold standard derived from histology, microbiology and rapid urease test.

Modifications to the European standard ^{13}C-UBT

Standardization of the ^{13}C-UBT has allowed results from different centres to be compared, and has facilitated multicentre clinical trial protocols. Standards are set so that they can be improved upon, and the ^{13}C-UBT is no exception, with advances being made in patient preparation, test meals and analysis of results.

Non-fasting ^{13}C-UBT

A 4-h fast is recommended before a ^{13}C-UBT. This is uncomfortable for patients and results in the test being less applicable to population studies. We have evaluated the impact of a light diet on the ^{13}C-UBT in 222 patients[49]. Patients had a standard fasting ^{13}C-UBT followed by a repeat ^{13}C-UBT after eating two slices of toast with butter and honey/jam, together with a cup of tea or coffee. Gold standard used histology, CLO test and culture.

Two hundred and twenty-two patients were recruited; 123 gold standard positives and 94 gold standard negatives, with five patients of indeterminate status. The fasting and non-fasting ^{13}C-UBT had a similar accuracy when compared to the gold standard. The non-fasting breath test had a sensitivity of 98% and a specificity of 96% when compared against a gold standard. The fasting and non-fasting ^{13}C-UBT agreed in 217/222 (98%) patients. These results suggest that a light diet does not reduce the accuracy of the ^{13}C-UBT. However, we do ask patients to avoid eating corn or maize products, as these are rich in ^{13}C and may theoretically alter results[48].

Test meal

A fatty test meal consisting of Callogen 50 ml and Ensure 50 ml is commonly employed to delay gastric emptying. This meal is relatively expensive (£1.04) and cannot be given to patients who are allergic to peanuts. A much cheaper (£0.04) citric acid test meal has been suggested as an alternative and gives similar results[50]. Four grams of citric acid are dissolved in 200 ml of water. The patient drinks 150 ml of the solution and the final 50 ml are used to dissolve the 100 mg urea. We have assessed this test meal in the same patients in whom we evaluated the non-fasting breath test. The citric acid test meal ^{13}C-UBT had a 96% sensitivity and 97% specificity against a gold standard of histology, micro-biology and rapid urease test. We compared the excess $\delta^{13}CO_2$ values in patients who had previously had a Callogen/Ensure test meal. The 265 H. pylori-positive patients given a Callogen and Ensure test meal had significantly lower excess $\delta^{13}CO_2$ values than the 122 patients taking the citric acid test meal (26.4±15.9 vs. 43.8±28.4; $p < 0.0001$, Student's t-test) (Figure 1). The 243 H. pylori-negative patients given a Callogen and Ensure test meal had significantly higher excess $\delta^{13}CO_2$ values than the 98 patients given a citric acid test meal (1.01±0.82 vs. 0.67±0.68; $p < 0.0001$, Student's t-test) (Figure 2). Furthermore, only 4% (10/222) patients taking citric acid had borderline values (excess $\delta^{13}CO_2$ 2–10 per mil) compared with 9% (46/508) of the Callogen and Ensure patients ($p = 0.03$, λ^2 test). The citric acid test meal therefore increases the separation of excess $\delta^{13}CO_2$ values between H. pylori-positive and -negative patients, making the test more robust with fewer results subject to misclassification.

The reasons for this are unclear, but patients ingesting a fatty meal will have a higher intragastric pH than those taking citric acid. The H. pylori urease enzyme may be more active at the lower pH[51] obtained with citric acid, and this may explain the higher excess $\delta^{13}CO_2$ values seen in H. pylori-positive patients. Oral bacteria have a small amount of urease activity and this may result in a small amount of $^{13}CO_2$ excretion even in H. pylori-negative patients[52]. Citric acid will act as a mouthwash to reduce oral bacterial load, thereby decreasing oral urease activity. This might explain the lower excess $\delta^{13}CO_2$ values seen in H. pylori-negative patients taking the citric acid test meal.

The cut-off point defining H. pylori-positive patients is an excess $\delta^{13}CO_2$ of > 5 per mil using Callogen/Ensure test meal[41]. This was defined by the mean excess

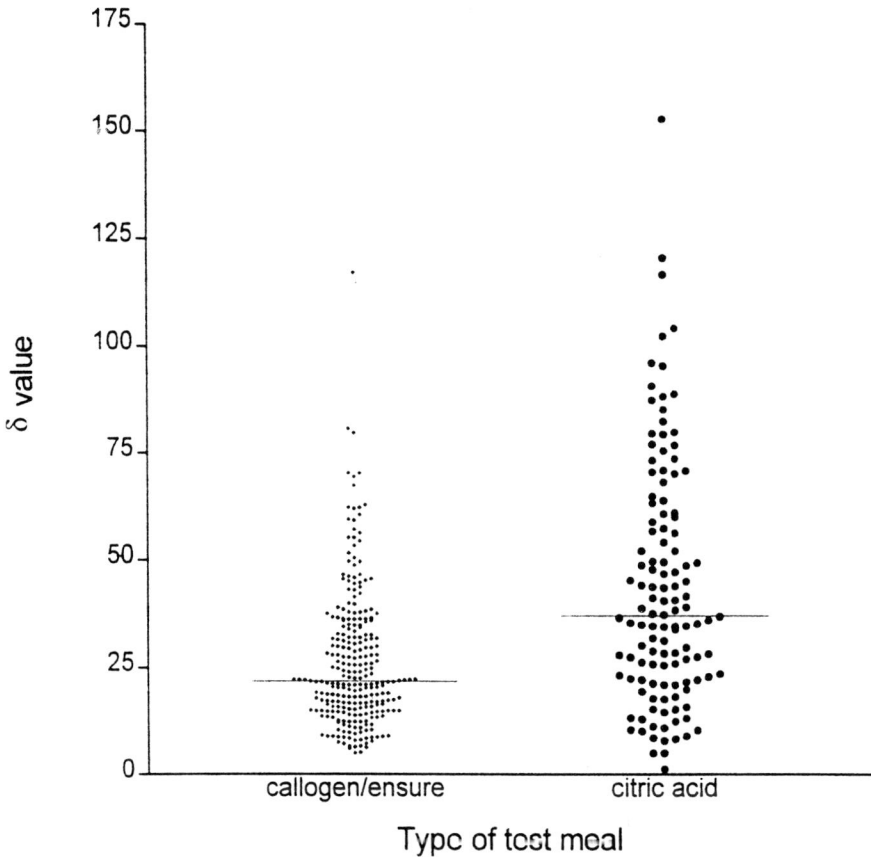

Figure 1 Comparison of test meals in *H. pylori*-positive patients

$\delta^{13}CO_2$ value + 3 standard deviations in *H. pylori*-negative patients. The cut-off point using the same definition for citric acid would be $0.67 + 3 \times 0.68 = 2.7$. In this series the accuracy of ^{13}C-UBT using a citric acid test meal would have improved if an excess $\delta^{13}CO_2$ excretion of 3 per mil was used as the approximate cut-off point. This would have resulted in the same number of false-positive results (specificity 97%) but 3/5 false-negative cases would have been correctly defined (Figure 2), increasing the sensitivity of the test from 96% to 98%. We suggest, therefore, that if the cheaper more robust citric acid test meal is used for the ^{13}C-UBT an excess of $\delta^{13}CO_2$ of 3 per mil should be used as the cut-off point.

Analysis of results

Despite the introduction of simpler, dedicated mass spectrometers these machines remain the most expensive component of the ^{13}C-UBT. Infrared technology has been developed in an attempt to produce cheaper and more compact spectrometers.

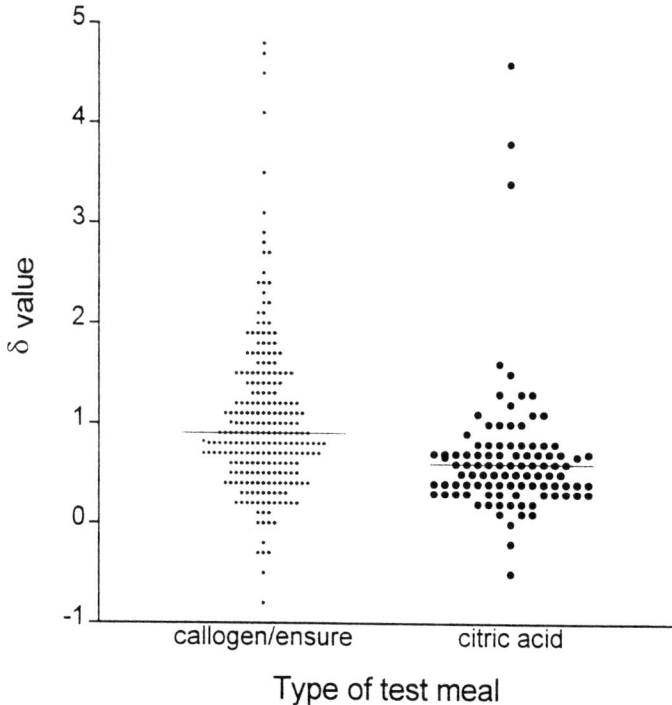

Figure 2 Comparison of test meals in *H. pylori*-negative patients

The principle of these machines is that they direct two infrared laser beams at the collected breath sample. One laser beam is set at a wavelength that will excite only $^{13}CO_2$, while the other beam interacts with $^{12}CO_2$. The amount of each respective laser beam that each isotope absorbs can be measured using a special optical detector (non-dispersive infrared spectrometry NDIR)[53,54]. Alternatively, the breath sample can be exposed to an electrical charge and after laser excitation this produces electrical signals that are characteristic of each isotope (laser-assisted ratio analyser LARA™ system)[55]. These analysers are reported to be as accurate as mass spectrometry, but do not require purification of the breath sample and so are substantially cheaper[56]. The disadvantage of the NDIR system is that it is temperature-dependent, and is prone to inaccuracy if the breath sample is heated by the laser beam. To avoid this a continuous flow of breath has to be passed through the spectrometer. This requires the patient to fill a 1500 ml collecting device, which may be impractical in some clinical settings[57]. The LARA™ system is not so temperature-dependent and can therefore analyse smaller breath samples. At present the manufacturers of this system are recommending breath samples taken over 60 min. This is more time-consuming than the requirements for mass spectrometer analysis. Neither of the infrared laser systems has been independently validated in large numbers of patients[57], so mass spectrometry remains the 'gold standard' analyser for the ^{13}C-UBT at present.

Alternative urea breath tests

Isotopes other than ^{13}C can be utilized in the urea breath test. Descriptions of a ^{14}C urea breath test followed soon after the ^{13}C-UBT[46,58], with similarly accurate results. The main advantage of the ^{14}C-UBT is that ^{14}C is a radioactive isotope and can be measured accurately and cheaply using a liquid scintillation counter. The radiation exposure to the patient is very low (bone marrow exposure is one-tenth that of a chest X-ray) but this limits the test to units that adhere to government guidelines on the use of radioactive isotopes[59]. This restricts the ^{14}C-UBT to hospital medical physics departments, whereas ideally a non-invasive test should be available in the community. Furthermore, there are ethical problems with using the ^{14}C-UBT for clinical trials, and it should be avoided in children and pregnant women. An ^{11}C urea breath test has also been described, but ^{11}C is also radioactive and subject to the same disadvantages as the ^{14}C-UBT[60]. The wider applicability and availability of the ^{13}C-UBT makes this the breath test of choice.

Comparison of serology and ^{13}C-UBT

The main non-invasive alternative to the ^{13}C-UBT is serology, but direct comparisons of the accuracy of these tests have been infrequent. One report suggested that 'in-house' ELISA serology can achieve similar results to the ^{13}C-UBT in dedicated centres[61]. The accuracy of the ^{13}C-UBT is similar in most centres, whereas the accuracy of serology varies in different populations[62]. This suggests that the ^{13}C-UBT is a more robust diagnostic test requiring less expertise to achieve accurate results. We have directly compared the accuracy of a commercial serology kit (Porton Cambridge Helico G kit), which performs well in our population, with the ^{13}C-UBT. *H. pylori* status was defined by a gold standard of histology, microbiology and rapid urease test. Patients were defined as *H. pylori*-positive if at least two of the gold standard tests were positive, and negative if all tests were negative. The *H. pylori* status was indeterminate if only one test gave a positive result. We recruited 122 patients with seven indeterminate cases. Sixty-one patients were gold standard *H. pylori*-positive and 54 were negative, with the ^{13}C-UBT giving one false-negative and one false-positive result (sensitivity and specificity = 98%). In the same population serology gave four false-negative and six false-positive results (sensitivity = 93%, specificity = 87%). The ^{13}C-UBT was significantly more accurate than serology (98% vs. 91%, $p = 0.04$ λ^2) with the 95% confidence intervals for the improvement in accuracy being 1–13%. These data suggest that the ^{13}C-UBT is desirable when accuracy is the most important criterion for choosing a test. In situations where cost and ease of use are more important (e.g. large epidemiological studies), serology may be more appropriate. Furthermore, as indicated earlier, serological testing is becoming more accurate.

NON-INVASIVE TESTS IN THE MANAGEMENT OF DYSPEPSIA

Although non-invasive tests are frequently used in epidemiological studies their major role is in screening dyspeptic patients prior to endoscopy, and in assessing the results of treatment.

The potential for screening dyspeptic patients has already been discussed. Either serology or the urea breath test is suitable for pre-endoscopy testing, and in younger patients a negative result implies that the likelihood of serious disease or peptic ulcer is unlikely unless the patient is taking non-steroidal anti-inflammatory drugs, or presents with alarm symptoms such as weight loss. One approach is that young patients, under 45 years of age, who are *H. pylori*-negative, should be reassured that there is no evidence of serious gastrointestinal disease and they should be counselled to make lifestyle changes or take simple antacids to avoid dyspepsia[63]. It is argued that young dyspeptic patients who are positive for *H. pylori* should be referred for endoscopy, as this group contains virtually all the significant pathology. An alternative policy would be to treat this group for *Helicobacter* infection without undertaking endoscopy in any patient under 45 years of age without alarm symptoms. This protocol would treat patients who had peptic ulcer in an appropriate way.

Some physicians consider this second scheme of management to be inappropriate, because it means that some individuals infected with *H. pylori*, but without ulcers, will have been treated unnecessarily. While this was a reasonable line of argument when effective treatments were not available, and when medication led to unacceptable side-effects, this is now a view that is more difficult to sustain. Although there is little evidence to suggest that *H. pylori* is responsible for non-ulcer dyspepsia it does, nevertheless, represent a risk factor not only for the future development of peptic ulceration, but also for gastric cancer. Furthermore, dyspeptic patients are often treated with acid suppression, and it is now recognized that long-term profound acid suppression causes a change in *Helicobacter*-associated gastritis such that it progresses to a pan-gastritis, with the potential for atrophy. For all of these reasons it appears more logical to treat patients who are *H. pylori*-positive and, if so, there seems little advantage to be gained in also performing an endoscopy. This pragmatic approach to the management of dyspepsia is one that is being used increasingly in primary care. If this policy is used it is desirable to check for eradication following medication, to ensure that treatment has been successful. In this way the patient can be reassured that there is no longer a risk of peptic ulcer disease.

CONCLUSION

The ability to test for *H. pylori* has made a considerable impact on the management of patients with dyspepsia. In particular, the non-invasive tests using serology and the [^{13}C]urea breath test enable patients to be screened for *H. pylori* infection without having to undergo endoscopy and, particularly in the younger age group, this is useful, as it enables appropriate treatment to be given to patients without them requiring an expensive, invasive and somewhat unpleasant examination.

Acknowledgement

We thank Miss Julie Mackintosh for her assistance in typing the manuscript.

References

1. Logan RPH, Walker MM, Misiewicz JJ, Gummett PA, Karim QN, Baron JH. Changes in the intragastric distribution of *Helicobacter pylori* during treatment with omeprazole. Gut. 1995; 36:12–16.
2. Kuipers EJ, Uyterlinde AM, Pena AS *et al.* Increase of *Helicobacter pylori*-associated corpus gastritis during acid suppressive therapy: implications for long-term safety. Am J Gastroenterol. 1995;90:1401–6.
3. Kuipers EJ, Lee A, Klinkenberg-Knol EC, Meuwissen SGM. Review article: the development of atrophic gastritis – *Helicobacter pylori* and the effects of acid suppressive therapy. Aliment Pharmacol Ther. 1995;9:331–40.
4. Sipponen P, Kekki M, Haapakoski J, Ihamaki T, Siurala M. Gastric cancer risk in chronic atrophic gastritis: statistical calculations of cross-sectional data. Int J Cancer. 1985;35:173–7.
5. Arvind AS, Cook RS, Tabaqchali S, Farthing MJG. One-minute endoscopy room test for *Campylobacter pylori*. Lancet. 1988;1:149.
6. Rathbone BJ, Wyatt JI, Worsley BW *et al.* Systemic and local antibody responses to gastric *Campylobacter pyloridis* in non-ulcer dyspepsia. Gut. 1986;27:642–7.
7. Morris A, Nicholson G. Ingestion of *Campylobacter pyloridis* causes gastritis and raised fasting pH. Am J Gastroenterol. 1987;82:192–9.
8. Von Wulffen H, Grote HJ, Gaterman S *et al.* Immuno-blot analysis of immune response to *Campylobacter pylori* and its clinical associations. J Clin Pathol. 1988;41:653–9.
9. Langenberg W, Rauws EAJ, Widjojokusumo A *et al.* Identification of *Campylobacter pyloridis* isolates by restriction endonuclease DNA analysis. J Clin Microbiol. 1986;24:414–17.
10. Hirschl AM, Rathbone BJ, Wyatt JI *et al.* Comparison of ELISA antigen preparations alone or in combination for serodiagnosing *Helicobacter pylori* infections. J Clin Pathol. 1990;43:511–13.
11. Newell DG. Identification of outer membrane proteins of *Campylobacter pyloridis* and antigenic cross reactivity between *Campylobacter pyloridis* and *Campylobacter jejuni*. J Clin Microbiol. 1987;133:163–70.
12. Newell DG, Stacey AR. Antigens for the serodiagnosis of *Campylobacter pylori* infection. Gastroenterol Clin Biol. 1989;13:37–41B.
13. Hawtin PR, Stacey AR, Newell DG. Investigation of the structure and localisation of the urease of *Helicobacter pylori* using monoclonal antibodies. J Gen Microbiol. 1990;136:1995–2000.
14. Newell DG. Human antibody responses to the surface protein antigens of *Campylobacter pyloridis*. Serodiagnosis Immunother. 1987;1:209–17.
15. Calam J. Diagnosis of infection. In: Calam J, editor. Clinician's guide to *Helicobacter pylori*, 1st edn. Cambridge: Chapman & Hall Medical; 1996:93–116.
16. Newell DG, Stacey AR. The serology of *Helicobacter pylori* infections. In: Rathbone BJ, Heatley RV, editors. *Helicobacter pylori* and gastroduodenal disease, 2nd edn. Oxford: Blackwell Scientific Publications; 1992:64–73.
17. Evans DJ, Evans DG, Graham DY, Klein PD. A sensitive and specific serologic test for detection of *Campylobacter pylori* infection. Gastroenterology. 1989;96:1004–8.
18. Von Wulffen H, Grote HJ. Enzyme linked immuno-sorbent assay for detection of immunoglobulin A and G antibodies to *Campylobacter pylori*. Eur J Clin Microbiol Infect Dis. 1988;77:559–65.
19. Knill-Jones RP. Geographical differences in the prevalence of dyspepsia. Scand J Gastroenterol. 1991;26(Suppl. 182):17–24.
20. Working Party of the Clinical Services Committee of the British Society of Gastroenterology. Provision of gastrointestinal endoscopy and related services for a district general hospital. Gut. 1991;32:95–105.
21. Gear MWL, Wilkinson SP. Open access upper alimentary endoscopy. Br J Hosp Med. 1989; 41:438–44.
22. Williams B, Luckas M, Ellingham JHM *et al.* Do young patients with dyspepsia need investigation? Lancet. 1988;2:1349–51.
23. Sobala GM, Crabtree JE, Pentith JA *et al.* Screening dyspepsia by serology to *Helicobacter pylori*. Lancet. 1991;338:94–6.
24. Patel P, Khulusi S, Mendall MA *et al.* Prospective screening of dyspeptic patients by *Helicobacter pylori* serology. Lancet. 1995;346:1315–18.
25. Tham TCK, McLaughlin N, Hughes DF *et al.* Possible role of *Helicobacter pylori* serology in reducing endoscopy workload. Postgrad Med J. 1994;70:809–12.

26. Feldman RA, Evans SJW. Accuracy of diagnostic methods used for epidemiological studies of *Helicobacter pylori*. Aliment Pharmacol Ther. 1995;9(Suppl. 2):21–31.
27. Newell DG, Bell GD, Weil J *et al.* The effect of treatment on circulating anti-*Helicobacter pylori* antibodies – a two year follow up study. In: Malfertheiner P, Ditschuneit H, editors. *Helicobacter pylori*, gastritis and peptic ulcer. Berlin: Springer-Verlag; 1990:172–5.
28. Langenberg W, Rauws EAJ, Houthoff HJ *et al.* Follow-up of individuals with untreated *Campylobacter pylori* associated gastritis and of non-infected persons with non-ulcer dyspepsia. J Infect Dis. 1988;157:1245–8.
29. Wilcox MH, Dent JHS, Hunter JO *et al.* Is serology sufficiently accurate for the diagnosis of *Helicobacter pylori* infection? – a comparison of eight kits. J Clin Pathol. (in press).
30. Jensen AKW, Andersen LP, Wachmann CH. Evaluation of eight commercial kits for *Helicobacter pylori* IgG antibody detection. APMIS. 1993;101:795–801.
31. Blecker V, Lanciers S, Hauser B *et al.* Diagnosis of *Helicobacter pylori* infection in adults and children by using the Malakit *Helicobacter pylori*, a commercially available enzyme-linked immuno-sorbent assay. J Clin Microbiol. 1993;31:1770–3.
32. Best LM, Veldhuyzen Van Zanten SJ, Sherman PM *et al.* Serological detection of *Helicobacter pylori* antibodies in children and their parents. J Clin Microbiol. 1994;32:1193–6.
33. Schembri MA, Lin SK, Lambert JR. Comparison of commercial diagnostic tests for *Helicobacter pylori* antibodies. J Clin Microbiol. 1993;31:2621–4.
34. Horan MA, Fox RA. Ageing and the immune response – a unifying hypothesis? Mech Ageing Dev. 1984;26:165–81.
35. Hoek FJ, Noach LA, Rauws EAJ, Tytgat GNJ. Evaluation of the performance of commercial test kits for detection of *Helicobacter pylori* antibodies in serum. J Clin Microbiol. 1992;30:1525–8.
36. Perez-Perez GI, Divorkin BM, Chodos JE, Blaser MJ. *Campylobacter pylori* antibodies in humans. Ann Intern Med. 1988;109:11–17.
37. Moayyedi P, Carter AM, Catto A *et al.* Validation of a rapid whole blood test for the diagnosis of *Helicobacter pylori* infection. Gut. 1996 (Submitted).
38. Moayyedi P, Tompkins DS, Axon ATR. Salivary antibodies to *Helicobacter pylori*: screening dyspeptic patients before endoscopy (letter). Lancet. 1994;344:1016–17.
39. Graham DY, Klein PD, Evans DJ *et al. Campylobacter pylori* detected non-invasively by the ^{13}C-urea breath test. Lancet. 1987;2:1174–7.
40. Bell GD, Powell K, Weil J, Harrison G, Brookes S, Prosser S. ^{13}C-urea breath test for *Helicobacter pylori* infection (letter). Gut. 1991;32:551–2.
41. Logan RPH, Dill S, Bauer FE *et al.* The European ^{13}C-urea breath test for the detection of *Helicobacter pylori*. Eur J Gastroenterol Hepatol. 1991;3:915–21.
42. Logan RPH, Polson RJ, Misiewicz JJ *et al.* Simplified single sample ^{13}carbon urea breath test for *Helicobacter pylori*: comparison with histology, culture and ELISA serology. Gut. 1991;32: 1461–4.
43. Logan RPH. Detection of *Helicobacter pylori* by the ^{13}C-urea breath test. In: Rathbone BJ, Heatley RV, editors. *Helicobacter pylori* and gastroduodenal disease, 2nd edn. Oxford: Blackwell Scientific Publications; 1992:88–106.
44. Marshall BT, Surveyor I. Carbon-14 urea breath test for the diagnosis of *Campylobacter pylori* associated gastritis. J Nucl Med. 1988;29:11–16.
45. Weil J, Bell GD. Detection of *Campylobacter pylori* by the ^{14}C-breath test. In: Rathbone BJ, Heatley RV, editors. *Campylobacter pylori* and gastroduodenal disease, 1st edn. Oxford: Blackwell Scientific Publications; 1989:83–93.
46. Bell GD, Weil J, Harrison G *et al.* ^{14}C-urea breath test analysis, a non-invasive test for *Campylobacter pylori* in the stomach. Lancet. 1987;1:1367.
47. Craig H. Isotopic standards for carbon and oxygen and correlation factors for mass spectrometric analysis of carbon dioxide. Geochim Cosmochim Acta. 1957;12:133–49.
48. Lerman JC, Troughton JH. Carbon isotope discrimination by photosynthesis: implications for the bio- and geosciences. Proceedings, Second International Conference on Stable Isotopes. Oak Brook, Illinois; 1975:630–44.
49. Moayyedi P, Axon ATR. Validation of a non-fasting ^{13}carbon urea breath test to diagnose *Helicobacter pylori* (*H. pylori*) infection. Gut. 1995;37(Suppl. 1):A12.
50. Braden B, Duan LP, Caspary WF, Lemboke B. More convenient ^{13}C-urea breath test modifications still meet the criteria for valid diagnosis of *Helicobacter pylori* infection. Gastroenterology. 1994;32:198–202.

51. Mobley HLT, Cortesia MJ, Rosenthal LE, Jones BD. Characterization of urease from *Campylobacter pylori*. J Clin Microbiol. 1988;26:5:831–6.
52. Eggers RH, Kulp A, Tegeler R *et al*. A methodological analysis of the ^{13}C-urea breath test for detection of *Helicobacter pylori* infections: high sensitivity and specificity within 30 min using 75mg of ^{13}C-urea. Eur J Gastroenterol Hepatol. 1990;2:437–44.
53. Haisch M, Hering P, Fuss W, Fabinski W. A sensitive isotope selective nondispersive infrared spectrometer for [13]CO_2 and [12]CO_2 concentration measurements in breath samples. Isotopenpraxis Environ Health Stud. 1994;30:247–51.
54. Braden B, Haisch M, Duan LP, Lemboke B, Baspary WF, Hering P. Clinically feasible stable isotope technique at a reasonable price: analysis of [13]CO_2/[12]CO_2 – abundance in breath samples with a new isotope selective nondispersive infrared spectrometer. Z Gastroenterol. 1994;32:675–8.
55. Murnick DE, Peer BJ. Laser-based analysis of carbon isotope ratios. Science. 1994;263:945–7.
56. Dagani R. Laser method measures carbon isotope ratios. Chem Eng News. 1994;72:6–7.
57. Koletzko S, Haisch M, Seeboth I *et al*. Isotope-selective non-dispersive infrared spectrometry for detection of *Helicobacter pylori* infection with ^{13}C-urea breath test. Lancet. 1995;345:961–2.
58. Rauws EAJ. Detecting *Campylobacter pylori* with the [13]C- and ^{14}C-urea breath test. Scand J Gastroenterol. 1989;24(Suppl. 160):25–56.
59. Catherton JC, Spiller RC. The urea breath test for *Helicobacter pylori*. Gut. 1994;35:723–5.
60. Hartman NG, Jay M, Hill DB, Bera RK, Nickl NJ, Ryo UY. Noninvasive detection of *Helicobacter pylori* colonization in stomach using (^{11}C] urea. Dig Dis Sci. 1992;37:618–21.
61. Cutler AF, Havstad S, Chen K, Blaser MJ, Perez-Perez GI, Schubert TT. Accuracy of invasive and noninvasive tests to diagnose *Helicobacter pylori* infection. Gastroenterology. 1995;109:136–41.
62. Glupczynski Y, Goossens H, Burette A, Deprez C, van Borre C, Butzler JP. Serology in *Helicobacter pylori* infection. Int J Med Microbiol Viro Parasitol Infect Dis. 1993;280:150–4.
63. Axon ATR, Bell GD, Jones RH, Quine MA, McCloy RF. Guidelines on appropriate indications for upper gastrointestinal endoscopy. Br Med J. 1995;310:853–6.

29
Helicobacter pylori infection in children

M. ROWLAND and B. DRUMM

INTRODUCTION

Helicobacter pylori infection occurs mainly in children. Studies on children are therefore vital if we are to answer many of the questions relating to this important global infection. The mode of transmission of *H. pylori*, and the risk of reinfection following treatment, can be evaluated adequately only in children. Epidemiological studies involving children depend on the validation of non-invasive methods for the diagnosis of *H. pylori*. Because relatively few children in developed countries are infected, they are an excellent population in which to evaluate whether or not specific symptoms are associated with *H. pylori* gastritis. The recent classification of *H. pylori* as a Group 1 carcinogen must stimulate us to evaluate the need to treat all children with this infection.

PATHOGENESIS

H. pylori is a Gram-negative spiral-shaped organism which is found within and beneath the mucous layer overlying the gastric epithelium. Colonization of the gastric mucosa by *H. pylori* is always associated with histological evidence of gastritis[1-5]. Infection of gastric epithelium has been reported not only in the stomach, but also in areas of gastric metaplasia in the duodenum[6], oesophagus[7] and ectopic gastric mucosa at other sites in the gastrointestinal tract, including Meckel's diverticulum[8] and the rectum[9].

Studies in children demonstrate that *H. pylori* is not an opportunistic colonizer of inflamed gastric tissue. Children with secondary gastritis due to Crohn's disease or eosinophilic gastritis are not colonized by *H. pylori*[4]. In contrast, the majority of children with primary gastritis are colonized by the organism[4,5,10-12].

The mucosal inflammatory infiltrate in children with *H. pylori* is very different from that in adults, but is identical to that which occurs in animal models of *Helicobacter* infection[13]. In children there is a lymphocyte and plasma cell infiltrate with a few neutrophils present[12].

Duodenal ulcer disease is associated with chronic gastritis, and *H. pylori* is present on the gastric mucosa of almost all individuals with duodenal ulcer disease[1,5,14,15]. Eradication of the organism from the gastric mucosa leads to long-term healing of the duodenal ulcer disease in adults[14–18]. Eradication of *H. pylori* also appears to lead to long-term healing of duodenal ulcer disease in children[10–12,19]. *H. pylori* will only colonize gastric epithelium; therefore its association with duodenal ulcer disease is difficult to understand. It has been hypothesized that *H. pylori* colonizes areas of gastric metaplasia in the duodenum with the subsequent development of duodenal inflammation and possibly ulceration[21]. In children *H. pylori* infection of the antral mucosa and gastric metaplasia in the duodenum are independent risk factors for duodenal ulceration and inflammation[22,23]. However, the presence of both *H. pylori* and gastric metaplasia results in a greatly increased risk of duodenal disease[23].

EPIDEMIOLOGY

The prevalence of *H. pylori* is about 10% in the first decade and increases to 60% by the age of 60 in developed countries[24]. This is unusual for an enteric infection and more recent studies indicate that *H. pylori* infection is acquired in childhood. The high prevalence seen in adults is due to a cohort effect, in that adults acquired the infection as children when socioeconomic conditions were much poorer[25]. The incidence of new infection in adults is estimated between 0.33%[26] and 0.49%[27] per person-year, based on serology studies. *H. pylori* infection appears to be lifelong in the absence of specific treatment. This persistence of infection occurs despite a marked serological and mucosal immune response to the infection[28,29]. Reinfection following eradication of *H. pylori* is uncommon in adults, ranging from 0.36%[30] to 1.2%[31] annually. However, as infection occurs mainly in children, this low reinfection rate in adults is not surprising. Reinfection of children who have been treated successfully is much more likely. Studies in children are necessary if we are to assess accurately the risk of reinfection following treatment. If reinfection does not occur in children it may indicate that the host immune response is capable of protecting against reinfection. This is important in relation to vaccine development.

H. pylori infection is much more prevalent among children in developing countries than in developed countries, and up to 70% of children may be infected by the age of ten[32]. The most significant risk factor for the development of *H. pylori* infection is poor socioeconomic conditions in childhood[33–36]. Over-crowding *per se*, rather than poor sanitary conditions, may be more important in the transmission of *H. pylori* infection[33]. In children under 16 years of age, increasing birth order and the number of children in the family are risk factors for the development of infection[36].

The mode of transmission of *H. pylori* infection has not been identified. *H. pylori* has not been repeatedly isolated from a site outside the gastrointestinal tract. There are a few reports of successful culture from dental plaque[37] and from faeces[38,39]. There is no known reservoir in the environment for this bacterium. A study of children and their families provides strong evidence supporting person-to-person transmission of this organism[5]. Clustering of *H. pylori* infection also has been identified within institutions for the mentally handicapped[40]. Strain identification using DNA digest patterns has shown the same strain infecting different members of the same family in European studies[41,42]. In Canada, young siblings were shown to be colonized by different strains[43]. Furthermore it appears that an individual can harbour more than one strain of the organism simultaneously. Recently it has been shown that cats can be naturally infected with *H. pylori*[44]. Naturally infected cats and experimentally infected cats both develop lesions which can mimic many of the features seen in *H. pylori*-infected children. Cats develop multifocal gastritis consisting of lymphoid aggregates plus multiple large lymphoid nodules which are most notable in the antral mucosa[45].

Gastric cancer

H. pylori has been classified as a Group 1 carcinogen by the World Health Organization[46], based primarily on serological studies from England[47], California[48] and Hawaii[49]. Infection of the gastric mucosa in childhood may be a particular risk factor for the development of gastric carcinoma in adult life[50,51]. Moreover, gastric carcinoma is associated with lower socioeconomic groups[52]. The incidence of gastric cancer has decreased rapidly over the past 30 years in developed countries, as has the prevalence of *H. pylori* gastritis[53]. While the current evidence for an association between *H. pylori* infection at a young age and the subsequent development of carcinoma of the stomach is strong, most individuals with *H. pylori* gastritis will not develop gastric cancer[54]. The suggestion that eradication of this infection in children may prevent a significant number of deaths from gastric cancer requires further careful study. The answer to this question will ultimately determine whether or not we need to screen children for this infection. It will also determine the likelihood of a successful vaccine being developed.

CLINICAL FINDINGS

There is no evidence that *H. pylori* gastritis is a cause of symptoms in children since *H. pylori* infection occurs in asymptomatic children[55,56]. The clustering of *H. pylori* infection within families, and the very high prevalence in underdeveloped countries, also suggest that the infection is not associated with specific symptoms[5,32].

Recurrent abdominal pain is not associated with an increased prevalence of *H. pylori*-associated gastritis[57]. Recent studies have shown that, prior to endoscopy, *H. pylori*-infected children cannot be differentiated from those who are not infected on the basis of their presenting symptoms[58]. Furthermore, *H. pylori* eradication was associated with an improvement in symptoms only in children who had duodenal ulcer disease, but not in those with gastritis alone[59]. This implies that the effect of *H. pylori* eradication on symptoms in these children relates to healing of duodenal ulcer disease rather than healing of gastritis.

DIAGNOSIS

Upper gastrointestinal endoscopy has, until recently, been the investigation of choice for the diagnosis of gastritis and peptic ulcer disease in children but the endoscopic appearance of the stomach often correlates poorly with the presence or absence of gastritis[4,12]. This is especially true in cases of *H. pylori*-associated gastritis, in which the stomach is often reported as macroscopically normal. More recently a nodularity of the antral mucosa has been described in association with *H. pylori* gastritis in children[11,60,61]. These nodules give the antrum a cobblestone appearance. This appearance is not usually seen in adults with *H. pylori* gastritis[62]. The reason for this appearance of the gastric mucosa in association with *H. pylori* in children is not known.

Colonization of the antrum by *H. pylori* can be identified by histological examination, rapid urease testing and culture[63]. Non-invasive methods to detect the presence of *H. pylori* in children are currently being evaluated, and approaches such as serology and the ^{13}C-urea breath test may lead to less invasive screening tests in the near future.

CULTURE

Culture of an antral biopsy is considered as the gold standard to confirm the presence of *H. pylori* on the gastric mucosa. However, a very small number of colonies may be present on plates when gastric biopsies from children are cultured. Biopsy specimens may be cultured on Columbia blood agar (GIBCO) plates containing 7% (vol/vol) defibrinated horse blood in an atmosphere of 5% O_2 and 10% CO_2. Organisms can then be identified as *H. pylori* on the basis of colony morphology, Gram stain, and the production of urease, oxidase and catalase.

UREASE TEST

As *H. pylori* produces high levels of the enzyme urease, this property can be used to screen for the presence of bacteria in antral biopsy specimens. In some children, because of the reduced number of bacteria, the colour reaction may take up to 24 hours and, on occasion, rapid urease tests have not been as sensitive as in adults[4,64]. When a full biopsy specimen is placed in the urea medium, as against a fragment of the biopsy, the sensitivity of this test increases and is close to 100%[63,65].

HISTOLOGY

A presumptive diagnosis of *H. pylori* infection can be made by identifying spiral-shaped organisms on gastric biopsy sections because of the characteristic appearance and unique location of *H. pylori* on the gastric mucosa. The Warthin Starry silver stain is 100% sensitive and specific[63]. A modified Giemsa stain is less expensive and easier to perform than the Warthin Starry silver stain, and is also very sensitive for identifying the presence of *H. pylori*[63].

SEROLOGY

The *H. pylori*-specific serum IgG response has been reported as highly specific (99%) and sensitive (96%) in detecting children with *H. pylori* colonization of the gastric antrum[5]. Sensitivity and specificity vary considerably, however, depending on the assay employed[66,67]. It is important that ELISA assays used to diagnose *H. pylori* colonization in children are standardized using children's sera. A positive serological response using an ELISA assay is generally defined as an optical density greater than 2 standard deviations above the mean value obtained for non-colonized individuals. This cut-off point is higher in adults than in children. If the assay is based on adult antibody levels, a significant number of children colonized with *H. pylori* will not be detected. Crabtree *et al.*[67] found that a *H. pylori*-specific serum IgG assay based on adult cut-off values was less than 50% sensitive in identifying infected children. Measurement of *H. pylori*-specific serum IgA antibodies in children is not a sensitive indicator of gastric colonization. Czinn *et al.* found that only 45% of children with *H. pylori* colonization of the gastric mucosa had increased *H. pylori*-specific serum IgA antibodies[66]. Moreover, *H. pylori*-specific serum IgM antibodies are not consistently elevated in children with *H. pylori*-associated gastritis.

^{13}C-UREA BREATH TEST

The ^{13}C-urea breath test (UBT) is a non-invasive test for the diagnosis of *H. pylori* infection. It is based on the fact that *H. pylori* produces large amounts of urease. When isotopically labelled urea is given to a patient who is infected with *H. pylori* the urease enzyme splits the urea into ammonia and labelled carbon dioxide, which can be measured in the expired breath. This test has been shown to be safe and highly sensitive and specific for the diagnosis of *H. pylori* infection in adults[68,69]. It is also accurate in determining the success of treatment in eradicating *H. pylori* infections[70]. The UBT has been shown recently to be 100% sensitive and 97.6% specific in the diagnosis of *H. pylori* infection in children[71].

TREATMENT IN CHILDREN

In children, standard therapy for the eradication of *H. pylori* infection has consisted of bismuth combined with one antibiotic often for periods up to 6 weeks. Compliance is probably reduced because of the long duration of treatment and the strong taste of ammonia which is associated with liquid bismuth. Israel has shown that compliance is a very important factor in achieving high eradication rates in children[11]. Combinations of bismuth and ampicillin or amoxycillin have eradicated *H. pylori* infection in approximately 70% of cases[10,11,19]. Oderda *et al.* eradicated *H. pylori* in 75% of children using tinidazole and bismuth[72], while more recently Gormally *et al.* have eradicated the organism in 84% using metronidazole and bismuth[59]. A more recent study indicated that a combination of furazolidone, amoxycillin and metronidazole administered for only 7 days eradicated *H. pylori* in 11/13 (85%) children[73]. Regimens which are of long duration and include liquid bismuth are unlikely to achieve a high compliance rate. In Europe colloidal bismuth subcitrate is the major bismuth preparation used to treat *H. pylori* infection, whereas in North America bismuth subsalicylate is used. While concern has been expressed about the use of bismuth salts in children none of the potential toxic side-effects have been so far reported.

A 1-week treatment regimen incorporating a proton pump inhibitor and two antibiotics, which has proven very successful in adults[74,75], should be examined in children to determine if eradication rates in excess of 90% can be achieved.

The NIH consensus statement recommends that adults with gastric or duodenal ulcer disease who are infected with *H. pylori* should receive antimicrobial treatment for this infection[76]. In children long-term remission of duodenal ulcer disease can also be achieved with antimicrobial regimens which eradicate *H. pylori* infection[11,20]. The necessity to treat *H. pylori* infection in the absence of duodenal ulcer disease is controversial[77] since *H. pylori* infection in the absence of duodenal ulcer does not appear to cause symptoms in children. In the past there has been no evidence to suggest that it is necessary to treat children who have *H. pylori* infection in the absence of ulcer disease. This situation will have to be reviewed as evidence supporting the association between *H. pylori* infection, gastric carcinoma and MALT lymphoma increases.

References

1. Warren JR, Marshall BJ. Unidentified curved bacilli on gastric epithelium in active chronic gastritis. Lancet. 1983;1:1273–5.
2. Goodwin CS, Armstrong JA, Marshall BJ. *Campylobacter pyloridis*, gastritis and peptic ulceration. J Clin Pathol. 1986;39:353–65.
3. Blaser MJ. Gastric *Campylobacter*-like organisms, gastritis and peptic ulcer disease. Gastroenterology. 1987;93:371–83.
4. Drumm B, Sherman P, Cutz E, Karmali M. Association of *Campylobacter pylori* on the gastric mucosa with antral gastritis in children. N Engl J Med. 1987;316:1557–61
5. Drumm B, Perez-Perez GI, Blaser MJ, Sherman PM. Intrafamilial clustering of *Helicobacter pylori* infection. N Engl J Med. 1990;322:359–63.
6. Wyatt JI, Rathbone BJ, Dixon MF, Heatley RV. *Campylobacter pyloridis* and acid-induced gastric metaplasia in the pathogenesis of duodenitis. J Clin Pathol. 1987;40:841–8.
7. Paull G, Yardley J. Gastric and oesophageal *Campylobacter pylori* in patients with Barett's oesophagus. Gastroenterology. 1988;95:216–18.
8. Morris A, Nicholson G, Zwi J, Vanderwee M. *Campylobacter pylori* infection in Meckel's diverticula containing gastric mucosa. Gut. 1989;30:1233–5.
9. Pambianco D, Dye K, Marshall B *et al*. Gastritis in the rectum: *Campylobacter*-like organisms in heterotrophic inflamed gastric mucosa. Gastroenterology. 1988;94:A340.
10. Yeung CK, Fu KH, Yuen KY *et al*. *Helicobacter pylori* and associated duodenal ulcer. Arch Dis Child. 1990;65:1212–16.
11. Israel D, Hassall E. Treatment and long term follow-up of *Helicobacter pylori* and associated duodenal ulcer. Arch Dis Child. 1990;123:53–8.
12. Hassall E, Dimmick JE. Unique features of *Helicobacter pylori* disease in children. Dig Dis Sci. 1991;36:417–23.
13. Bertram TA, Krakowka S, Morgan DR. Gastritis associated with infection by *Helicobacter pylori*: comparative pathology in humans and swine. Rev Infect Dis. 1991;13(Suppl. 8):S414–423.
14. Dooley CP, Cohen H. The clinical significance of *Campylobacter pylori*. Ann Intern Med. 1988;108:70–9.
15. Peterson WL. *Helicobacter pylori* and peptic ulcer disease. N Engl J Med. 1991;324:1043–8.
16. Marshall BJ, Goodwin CS, Warren JR *et al*. Prospective double-blind trial of duodenal ulcer relapse after eradication of *Campylobacter pylori*. Lancet. 1988;2:1437–42.

17. Coughlan JG, Gilligan D, Humphries H *et al. Campylobacter pylori* and recurrence of duodenal ulcers – a 12 month follow up study. Lancet. 1987;2:1109–11.
18. Hentschel E, Brandstatter G, Dragosics B *et al.* Effect of ranitidine and amoxicillin plus metronidazole on the eradication of *Helicobacter pylori* and the recurrence of duodenal ulcers. N Engl J Med. 1993;328:308–12.
19. Drumm B, Sherman P, Chiasson D, Karmali M, Cutz E. Treatment of *Campylobacter pylori*-associated antral gastritis in children with bismuth subsalicylate and ampicillin. J Pediatr. 1988; 113:908–12.
20. Goggin N, Rowland M, Clyne M, Drumm B. Effect of *Helicobacter pylori* eradication on the natural history of duodenal ulcer disease. Proc Br Paediatr Assoc. 1995;78:42.
21. Goodwin CS. Duodenal ulcer, *Campylobacter pylori* and the 'leaking roof' concept. Lancet. 1988;2:1467–9.
22. Shabib S, Cutz E, Drumm B, Sherman P. *Helicobacter pylori* infection is associated with gastric metaplasia in the duodenum. Am J Clin Pathol. 1994;102:188–91.
23. Gormally SM, Kierse B, Daly L, Bourke W, Durnin M, Drumm B. Gastric metaplasia and duodenal ulcer disease in children. Gut. 1996;38:513–17.
24. Megraud F, Brassens-Rabbe MP, Denis F, Belbouri A, Hoa DQ. Seroepidemiology of *Campylobacter pylori* infection in various populations. J Clin Microbiol. 1989;27:1870–3.
25. Banatvala N, Mayo K, Megraud F, Jennings R, Deeks JJ, Feldman RA. The cohort effect and *Helicobacter pylori.* J Infect Dis. 1993;168:219–21.
26. Cullen DJE, Collins BJ, Christiansen KJ *et al.* When is *Helicobacter pylori* infection acquired? Gut. 1993;34:1681–2.
27. Parsonnet J, Blaser MJ, Perez-Perez GI, Hargrett-Bean N, Tauxe RV. Symptoms and risk factors of *Helicobacter pylori* infection in a cohort of epidemiologists. Gastroenterology. 1992;102:41–6.
28. Dooley CP, Cohen H, Fitzgibbons PL *et al.* Prevalence of *Helicobacter pylori* infection and histologic gastritis in asymptomatic persons. N Engl J Med. 1989;321:1562–6.
29. Crabtree JE, Shallcross TM, Wyatt JI *et al.* Mucosal immune responses to *Helicobacter pylori* in patients with duodenitis. Dig Dis Sci. 1991;36:1266–73.
30. Borody T, Andrews P, Mancuso N, Jankiewicz E, Brandl S. *Helicobacter pylori* reinfection 4 years post eradication. Lancet. 1992;339–1295.
31. Forbes GM, Glaser ME, Cullen DJE *et al.* Duodenal ulcer treated with *Helicobacter pylori* eradication: seven year follow-up. Lancet. 1994;343:258–60.
32. Graham DY, Adam E, Reddy GT *et al.* Seroepidemiology of *Helicobacter pylori* infection in India. Dig Dis Sci. 1991;36:1084–8.
33. Fiedorek SC, Malaty HM, Evans DI *et al.* Factors influencing the epidemiology of *Helicobacter pylori* infection in children. Pediatrics. 1991;88:578–82.
34. Sitas F, Forman D, Yarnell JWG *et al. Helicobacter pylori* infection rates in relation to age and social class in a population of Welsh men. Gut. 1991;32:25–8.
35. Webb PM, Knight T, Greaves S *et al.* Relation between infection with *Helicobacter pylori* and living conditions in childhood: evidence for person to person transmission in early life. Br Med J. 1994;308:750–3.
36. Teh BH, Lin JT, Pan WH *et al.* Seroprevalence and associated risk factors of *Helicobacter pylori* infection in Taiwan. Anticancer Res. 1994;14:1389–92.
37. Shames B, Krajden S, Fuksa M, Babida C, Penner JL. Evidence of occurrence of the same strain of *Campylobacter pylori* in the stomach and dental plaque. J Clin Microbiol. 1989;27:2849–50.
38. Thomas JE, Gibson GR, Darboe MK, Dale A, Weaver LT. Isolation of *Helicobacter pylori* from human faeces. Lancet. 1992;340:1194–5.
39. Kelly SM, Pitcher MCL, Farmery SM, Gibson GR. Isolation of *Helicobacter pylori* from feces of patients with dyspepsia in the United Kingdom. Gastroenterology. 1994;107:1671–4.
40. Berkowicz J, Lee A. Person to person transmission of *Campylobacter pylori.* Lancet. 1987;2: 680–2.
41. Nwokolo CU, Bickley J, Attard AR, Owen RJ, Costas M, Fraser IA. Evidence of clonal variants of *Helicobacter pylori* in three generations of a peptic ulcer disease family. Gut. 1992;33:1323–7.
42. Bamford KB, Bickley J, Collins JSA *et al. Helicobacter pylori:* comparison of DNA fingerprints provides evidence for intrafamilial infection. Gut. 1993;34:1348–50.
43. Simor AE, Shames B, Drumm B, Sherman P, Low DE, Penner JL. Typing of *Campylobacter pylori* by bacterial DNA restriction endonuclease analysis and determination of plasmid profile. J Clin Microbiol. 1990;28:83–6.

44. Handt LK, Fox JG, Dewhirst FE *et al*. *Helicobacter pylori* isolated from the domestic cat: public health implications. Infect Immun. 1994;62:2367–74.

45. Fox JG, Batchwelder M, Marini R *et al*. *Helicobacter pylori*-induced gastritis in the domestic cat. Infect Immun. 1995;63:2674–81.

46. IARC monographs on the evaluation of carcinogenic risks to humans. Schistosomes, liver flukes and *Helicobacter pylori*. Lyon: IARC; 1994;61:177–240.

47. Forman D, Newell DG, Fullerton F *et al*. Association between infection with *Helicobacter pylori* and risk of gastric cancer: evidence from a prospective investigation. Br Med J. 1991;302: 1302–5.

48. Parsonnet J, Friedman GD, Vandersteen DP *et al*. *Helicobacter pylori* infection and risk for gastric cancer. N Engl J Med. 1991;324:1127–31.

49. Nomura A, Stemmermann GN, Chyou PH, Kato J, Perez-Perez GI, Blaser MJ. *Helicobacter pylori* infection and gastric carcinoma among Japanese Americans in Hawaii. N Engl J Med. 1991;325:1133–6.

50. Blaser MJ, Chyou PH, Nomura A. Age at establishment of *Helicobacter pylori* infection and gastric carcinoma, gastric ulcer, and duodenal ulcer risk. Cancer Res. 1995;55:562–5.

51. Blaser MJ, Parsonnet I. Parasitism by the 'slow' bacterium *Helicobacter pylori* leads to altered gastric homeostasis and neoplasia. J Clin Invest. 1994;94:4–8.

52. Howson CP, Hiyama T, Wynder EL. The decline in gastric cancer: epidemiology of an unplanned triumph. Epidemiol Rev. 1986;8:1–27.

53. Sipponen P. *Helicobacter pylori* infection – a common worldwide environmental risk factor for gastric cancer? Endoscopy. 1992;24:424–7.

54. Correa P. Is gastric carcinoma an infectious disease? N Engl J Med. 1991;325:1170–1.

55. Blecker U, Hauser B, Lanciers S, Peeters S, Suys B, Vandenplas Y. The prevalence of *Helicobacter pylori*-positive serology in asymptomatic children. J Pediatr Gastroenterol Nutr. 1993;16:252–6.

56. Fiedorek SC, Casteel HB, Pumphrey CL *et al*. The role of *Helicobacter pylori* in recurrent functional abdominal pain in children. Am J Gastroenterol. 1992;87:347–9.

57. van der Meer SB, Forget PP, Loffeld RJLF, Stobberingh E, Kuijten RH, Arends JW. The prevalence of *Helicobacter pylori* serum antibodies in children with recurrent abdominal pain. Eur J Pediatr. 1992;151:799–801.

58. Reifen R, Rasooly I, Drumm B, Millson ME, Murphy K, Sherman PM. Symptomatology and demographic features of *Helicobacter pylori* infection in children. Dig Dis Sci. 1994;39:1488–92.

59. Gormally SM, Prakash N, Durnin M *et al*. Symptoms in children before and after treatment of *Helicobacter pylori*. Gastroenterology. 1994;106:A83.

60. De Giacomo C, Fiocca R, Villani L *et al*. *Helicobacter pylori* infection and chronic gastritis: clinical, serological and histologic correlations in children treated with amoxicillin and colloidal bismuth subcitrate. J Pediatr Gastroenterol Nutr. 1990;11:310–16.

61. Mahony MJ, Wyatt JI, Littlewood JM. Management and response to treatment of *Helicobacter pylori* gastritis. Arch Dis Child. 1992;67:940–3.

62. Elta GH, Appleman HD, Behler EM, Wilson JA, Nostrant TJ. A study of the correlation between endoscopic and histological diagnoses in gastroduodenitis. Am J Gastroenterol. 1987;82:749–53.

63. Drumm B. *Helicobacter pylori* and the pediatric patient. Gastroenterol Clin N Am. 1993;22: 169–82.

64. McNulty CAM, Dent JC, Uff JS, Gear MW, Wilkinson SP. Detection of *Campylobacter pylori* by the biopsy urease test: an assessment in 1445 patients. Gut. 1989;30:1058–62.

65. Carvalho AST, Queiroz DMM, Mendes EN, Rocha GA, Penna FJ. Diagnosis and distribution of *Helicobacter pylori* in the gastric mucosa of symptomatic children. Braz J Med Biol Res. 1991; 24:163–6.

66. Czinn SJ, Carr HS, Speck WT. Diagnosis of gastritis caused by *Helicobacter pylori* in children by means of an ELISA. Rev Infect Dis. 1991;13:700–3.

67. Crabtree JE, Mahony MJ, Taylor JD, Heatley RV, Littlewood JM, Tompkins DS. Immune responses to *Helicobacter pylori* in children with recurrent abdominal pain. J Clin Pathol. 1991;44:768–71.

68. Graham DY, Evans Jr DJ, Alpert LC *et al*. *Campylobacter pylori* detected noninvasively by the ^{13}C-urea breath test. Lancet. 1987;1:1174–7.

69. Eggers RH, Kulp A, Tegeler R *et al*. A methodological analysis of the ^{13}C-urea breath test for detection of *Helicobacter pylori* infections: high sensitivity and specificity within 30 min using 75 mg of ^{13}C-urea. Eur J Gastroenterol Hepatol. 1990;2:437–44.

70. Slomianski A, Schubert T, Cutler AF. ^{13}C-urea breath test to confirm eradication of *Helicobacter pylori*. Am J Gastroenterol. 1995;90:224–6.

71. Rowland M, Lambert I, Gormally S *et al.* ^{13}C-urea breath test for the diagnosis of *Helicobacter pylori* infection in children. Proc BPA. 1996;68:46.
72. Oderda G, Dell'olio D, Morra I, Ansaldi N. *Campylobacter pylori* gastritis: long term results of treatment with amoxycillin. Arch Dis Child. 1989;64:326–9.
73. Queiroz DMM, Moura SB, Mendes EN, Rocha GA, Barbosa AJA, de Carvalho AST. Effect of *Helicobacter pylori* eradication on G-cell and D-cell density in children. Lancet. 1994;343: 1191–3.
74. Yousfi MM, El-Zimaity HMT, Al-Assi MT, Cole RA, Genta RM, Graham DY. Metronidazole, omeprazole and clarithromycin: an effective combination therapy for *Helicobacter pylori* infection. Aliment Pharmacol Ther. 1995;9:209–12.
75. Ozmen MM, Johnson CD. Is short-term triple therapy with lansoprazole, clarithromycin, and metronidazole a definitive answer for *Helicobacter pylori* eradication? Am J Gastroenterol. 1995;90:1542–3.
76. National Institutes of Health. *Helicobacter pylori* in peptic ulcer disease. NIH Consensus Statement. 1994;12:1–23.
77. Drumm B. *Helicobacter pylori.* Arch Dis Child. 1990;6:1278–82.

30
The problem ulcer: bleeding, perforation, *Helicobacter pylori*-negativity and intractability

M. BUCKLEY, J. LEE and C. O'MORAIN

INTRODUCTION

Since the discovery of *Helicobacter pylori* in 1982, this Gram-negative bacterium has been associated with a variety of clinical conditions. The bacterium was initially reported to be present in 80–100% of duodenal ulcer patients. In recent larger studies, with improved diagnostic techniques, the prevalence of *H. pylori* in uncomplicated duodenal ulcers is reported to be approximately 95%[1]. Duodenal ulcer disease is usually a chronic recurrent condition in untreated individuals. In excess of 50% of patients have dyspeptic symptoms for more than 2 years before presentation. In the pre-*H. pylori* era, of patients who were followed for 1 year after ulcer healing, 57% had one or two recurrences, 7% had more than three recurrences and 36% remained symptom-free[2]. Overall 50–80% of duodenal ulcer patients will have a recurrence during a 12-month follow-up after healing. Eradication of *H. pylori* alters the natural history of peptic ulcer disease and virtually abolishes ulcer relapse rates during 1 year follow-up[3].

There is also evidence that eradication of *H. pylori* may promote primary ulcer healing. Duodenal ulcers have been shown to heal when antibiotic monotherapy successfully eradicated the infection. In a recent study of 66 patients with active duodenal ulceration, healing rates at the end of a 2-week dual therapy eradication regime were 68% in patients in whom the bacterium had been eradicated and 73% in those with persistent infection. However, 4 weeks later, with no additional treatment, the healing rate had increased to 95.5% in patients who had been cleared of the infection but had reduced to 36.8% in those with persistent infection[4] (Figure 1). In the vast majority of patients, eradication of *H. pylori* may be regarded as an indirect indicator of ulcer healing; that is, eradication is a surrogate marker for ulcer healing[5].

Peptic ulcer is also associated with serious complications, such as bleeding, perforation and gastric outlet obstruction, leading to significant morbidity and mortality (Table 1). In a 15-year placebo-controlled follow-up study, 14% of ulcer

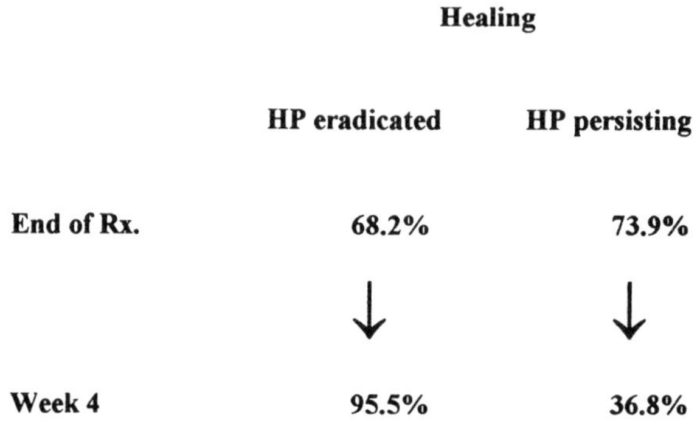

Healing

	HP eradicated	**HP persisting**
End of Rx.	68.2%	73.9%
	↓	↓
Week 4	95.5%	36.8%

Figure 1   Effect of *H. pylori* eradication on primary healing of duodenal ulcer (adapted from ref. 4)

Table 1   Complications of duodenal ulcer

Recurrence
Bleeding
Perforation
Pyloric outlet obstruction

patients developed haemorrhage and 8% developed perforation[6] and it is estimated that 1–3% of untreated duodenal ulcer patients will develop complications during the course of a year.

BLEEDING ULCER

Haemorrhage is a common complication of peptic ulcer disease, accounting for approximately 150 000 hospitalizations per year in the United States[7]. The incidence of peptic ulcer haemorrhage has not decreased over the past 20 years despite the decrease in hospitalization and surgery for uncomplicated ulcers[8].

The presence of *H. pylori* in patients who present with a bleeding peptic ulcer is higher than that of controls. There is some evidence that the prevalence of the infection is lower in patients with bleeding ulcers than in patients who have uncomplicated duodenal ulceration. In a study from Hong Kong, patients presenting with acute bleeding duodenal ulcer had a prevalence of *H. pylori* of 71% when compared to a prevalence of 91% in those presenting with recurrent pain from uncomplicated peptic ulcer[9]. Overall, the prevalence of *H. pylori* in patients with bleeding ulcers may be 15–20% lower than in patients with non-bleeding ulcer[10,11]. Non-steroidal anti-inflammatory drugs (NSAIDs) are also an important risk factor for bleeding ulcer disease[12]. Case–control cohort studies suggest that the risk of upper gastrointestinal haemorrhage is higher in those patients who ingest NSAIDs than those who do not. The risk of complications for NSAIDs appears to be more common during the first month of therapy, but may occur at any period during treatment[13,14]. In most studies to date the decreased prevalence of *H. pylori* in patients with bleeding ulcer may be partly accounted for by NSAID toxicity. However, there is some recent evidence that the sensitivity of

Table 2 Effect of *H. pylori* on peptic ulcer disease rebleeding

Authors	Reference	n	H. pylori eradicated (%)	H. pylori persistent (%)
Rokkas *et al.* (1995)	19	31	0	31.2
Labenz and Borsch (1994)	20	66	0	37.5
Graham *et al.* (1993)	21	31	0	28.5
Jaspersen *et al.* (1995)	22	33	3.5	50
Jaspersen *et al.* (1995)	23	51	0	27

the rapid urease test may be decreased when there is blood in the gastric lumen. In a study of patients with a bleeding ulcer who had a rapid urease and serological test, the rapid urease test was negative in 40.5% (30/74) of patients but serology was positive in 97% (29/30) of patients with a negative urease test[15]. In a recent study from our own unit the rapid urease test was positive in 54% of patients with bleeding duodenal ulcer compared to a *H. pylori*-positivity rate of 74% on histology. These results suggest that, in patients with upper gastrointestinal haemorrhage, false-negative rapid urease tests are more common than in patients with uncomplicated gastritis or peptic ulcer. This may be due to an indirect effect of acid-suppressing medication taken before or after admission to hospital, or a direct inhibitory effect of the blood on bacterial urease activity.

When a patient presents with a bleeding ulcer, the presence of *H. pylori* infection should be determined and the ingestion of NSAIDs should be excluded. Conventionally, patients with bleeding peptic ulcer disease are treated with maintenance therapy with H$_2$ receptor antagonists. Maintenance treatment decreases the rebleeding rate but does not abolish it. In recent studies fewer episodes of recurrent bleeding were reported among patients who received ranitidine 150 mg nocte (9%) than in those taking placebo (36%)[16–18].

There is now considerable evidence that eradication of *H. pylori* reduces rebleeding rates in patients who present with haemorrhage from a duodenal ulcer to virtually zero, while those continuing on H$_2$ receptor antagonists rebleed at a rate of about 12%[19–23] (Table 2). Long-term follow-up multi-centre studies are now needed to assess the need for medium- to long-term acid suppression in patients who present with a bleeding ulcer, and in whom *H. pylori* has been eradicated.

PERFORATED DUODENAL ULCER

Duodenal ulcers may extend through the serosa, resulting in acute visceral perforation or penetration into an adjacent organ. The site of perforation is usually the anterior wall of the first part of the duodenum, with less than 10% of perforations involving the posterior wall.

The prevalence of *H. pylori* infection is lower in patients who present with a perforated ulcer than in patients with chronic recurrent duodenal ulceration[24]. Approximately one-third of patients who present with an acute perforated duodenal ulcer do not have a history of dyspepsia or duodenal ulceration[25]. At surgery these patients seldom have any evidence of chronic ulcer disease. In one series the prevalence of *H. pylori* in 80 patients presenting with acute perforated

Table 3   Causes of *H. pylori*-negative duodenal ulcer (percentages)

Author	Reference	NSAID	Crohn's	Gastrosporillium hominis	Gastrinoma	Miscellaneous/ idiopathic
Borody *et al.* (1991)	31	44	11	11	–	34
Nensey *et al.* (1991)	32	75	–	–	–	25
McColl *et al.* (1993)	33	33	8	–	8	5

ulcer was only 49%, and was similar to the 50% prevalence in a control population[26]. In this study only 24% of patients had a previous history of peptic ulcer disease, and only one-third of these patients had ever received acid-suppressing medication. The lower prevalence of *H. pylori* in perforating duodenal ulcer compared to uncomplicated ulcer disease suggests that acute perforated duodenal ulcer has a different pathogenesis from chronic recurrent duodenal ulcer.

NSAIDs may play an important aetiological role in perforation. The prevalence of NSAID ingestion in patients who present with acute perforation ranges from 32% to 82%[27-29]. The use of NSAIDs was significantly more common in perforated duodenal ulcer patients (60%) than in a hospital control group (9.1%)[27].

It is likely that *H. pylori* infection is responsible for a proportion of ulcers that perforate. However, detailed pathophysiological studies are difficult to perform in this group of patients, because the majority present acutely and the natural physiology of gastric function is altered at surgery.

H. PYLORI-NEGATIVE ULCER

In addition to *H. pylori* infection, a number of other conditions are associated with duodenal ulcer (Table 3). Before these conditions are considered, the absence of *H. pylori* infection should be confirmed (Figure 2). False-negative testing for the infection may occur for a variety of reasons. When endoscopic biopsy-based techniques are used to diagnose the infection, sampling error may occur due to the patchy distribution of the infection. A sufficient number of biopsies, both from the antrum and the corpus, should be obtained. If a patient is receiving acid-suppressing medication at the time of endoscopy, migration of the infection to the corpus may occur, leading to false-negative results if antral biopsies only are obtained. Tests that depend on the biological activity of the bacterium, such as the rapid urease test and the urea breath test, may be negative if the patient is ingesting bacteriostatic medication (proton pump inhibitors and perhaps H_2 receptor antagonists and bismuth-based compounds). As mentioned earlier, there is preliminary evidence that blood in the gastric lumen may also inhibit the rapid urease test[15].

Crohn's disease may affect the stomach and upper small intestine, and in some circumstances isolated ulceration of the first part of the duodenum may occur. When *H. pylori* is not present, and there is no history of NSAID ingestion, a duodenal ulcer should be biopsied in an attempt to exclude Crohn's disease. A microscopic focal active gastritis may occur in patients with Crohn's disease. In a recent study of *H. pylori*-negative patients, gastritis was found in 59% of patients with Crohn's disease, compared with 36% of controls[30]. In this situation gastritis may be mistaken for an indirect marker of *H. pylori* infection.

Confirm absence of H.pylori

↓

YES

↓

Exclude NSAIDs

↓

YES

↓

↓   ↓   ↓   ↓

Serum Gastrin   **D2 biopsy**   **Ulcer biopsy**   **Abdo. ultrasound**
Serum Calcium
Renal/Liver function

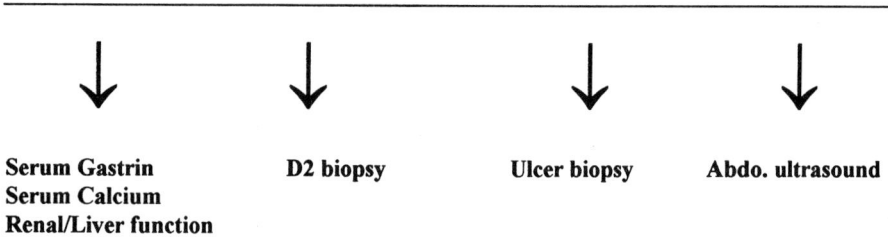

Figure 2 Management of *H. pylori* negative duodenal ulcer

Zollinger–Ellison syndrome

In 1955 Zollinger and Ellison described a syndrome of gastric hyperacidity, severe peptic ulcer disease and non-beta islet cell tumours of the pancreas. The true incidence of this condition is not known, but it is estimated to occur in between 0.1% and 1% of duodenal ulcer patients. It is slightly more common in males and the peak age of onset is between 30 and 50 years of age. Of patients with gastrinoma, 90–95% develop peptic ulceration during their illness, and approximately 70% of these ulcers are situated in the first part of the duodenum. Patients with this condition may develop atypical symptoms unrelated to ulceration, such as diarrhoea, steatorrhoea and vitamin B_{12} deficiency. The diagnosis can be made by measuring the serum gastrin in a fasting patient. Proton pump inhibitors (PPI) and gastric distension during endoscopy elevate the serum gastrin, and at the time of measurement of gastrin the patient should not be immediately post-endoscopy and should be off PPI treatment for several days.

Multiple ulcers in the small intestine are a rare but serious complication of coeliac disease. They occur most commonly in the jejunum, but are also found in the duodenum and colon. They may present as a worsening of the symptoms

299

Table 4   Causes of atypical duodenal ulceration

NSAIDs	Duodenal carcinoma
Aspirin	Penetrating pancreatic cancer
Zollinger–Ellison syndrome	Systemic mastocytosis
Crohn's disease	Amyloidosis Type IV
Coeliac disease	Renal failure
Ulcerative jejunitis	Stiff skin syndrome
Lymphoma	Pachydermoperiostosis
Hypercalcaemia	Cirrhosis
Gastrospirillium hominis	Polycythaemia rubra vera

Table 5   Pathophysiological mechanisms of *H. pylori*-negative ('idiopathic) duodenal ulcer (adapted from ref. 33)

Hypergastrinaemia
Increased acid secretion
Rapid gastric emptying
Absence of blood group A1 antigen gene

of malabsorption, abdominal pain, obstruction or perforation. The radiographic features on a small bowel series include diffuse ulceration, flocculation, segmentation, oedema and stricture formation. The presence of lymphoma should be excluded by biopsies, performed either at endoscopy or laparotomy. Strict exclusion of gluten from the diet may not have any beneficial effect, while corticosteroid therapy may help a minority of patients.

Other conditions that are associated with *H. pylori*-negative duodenal ulceration include lymphoma and carcinoma of the duodenum, penetrating pancreatic carcinoma, *Gastrospirilium hominis* infection, hypercalcaemia, chronic liver disease, and other rare conditions (Table 4)[31,32].

Idiopathic hypersecretors

The pathogenic mechanisms of true idiopathic *H. pylori*-negative duodenal ulceration have been assessed. Three abnormalities of gastric function were found in these patients: hypergastrinaemia, increased acid secretion and rapid emptying of both liquids and solids from the stomach (Table 5). The ABO blood group status of this patient group was also determined. The blood group antigen A1 was not found in any of six patients with 'idiopathic' ulceration, but was present in 38% of *H. pylori*-positive patients with duodenal ulceration and in 56% of controls. The absence of this gene may be consistent with a genetic basis for the altered gastric function found in these patients[33].

Intractable ulcer

The introduction of the H_2 receptor antagonists has revolutionized the treatment of peptic ulcer disease[34]. The vast majority of duodenal ulcers can be healed with a 4–8-week course of H_2 receptor antagonists or a 4-week course of PPI, and maintenance therapy with these drugs reduces ulcer relapse rates. However, ulcer recurrence during maintenance treatment may still occur in up to 20% of patients.

Eradication of *H. pylori* has been consistently shown to prevent ulcer recurrence and in a meta-analysis of patients with duodenal ulcer treated with anti-*H. pylori* therapy, eradication of the infection reduced the 1-year relapse rates from approximately 60% to 2.6%[35]. Moreover the ulcer recurrence rate at 5 years also is reduced significantly from 80% to approximately 9%[36].

The most common cause of duodenal ulcer relapse after attempted eradication is persistence of the infection. Effective regimes which consistently achieve over 90% eradication are now available. Several factors such as non-compliance, smoking and antimicrobial resistance may be responsible for treatment failure. In duodenal ulcer patients who have persistent infection after treatment the antimicrobial sensitivity of the bacterium should be assessed, and an appropriate second-line treatment prescribed. In compliant patients recurrent failure to eradicate the infection usually occurs when multi-drug resistance (usually to nitroimidazoles and clarithromycin) is present. When the bacterium has been eradicated ulcer recurrence is rare. The most common cause of *H. pylori*-negative ulcer relapse is NSAID ingestion[29]. NSAID consumption is often covert or inadvertent. In a recent study of NSAID ingestion in intractable peptic ulcer, nine of 60 patients with a refractory ulcer admitted to using daily NSAIDs. Platelet cyclooxygenase activity was positive in nine of 16 patients who denied any NSAID consumption, suggesting that surreptitious ingestion was responsible for ulcer relapse[37]. In this study it was found that 41% of refractory peptic ulcers were due to persistent *H. pylori* infection, 39% were due to NSAIDs or analgesic abuse, and in the remaining 20%, miscellaneous factors such as increased basal acid output or smoking were found. *H. pylori* infection and NSAIDs are independent risk factors for the development of peptic ulcer disease. It has not been established, however, whether there is an additive effect between these two agents[38].

When *H. pylori* has been eradicated successfully, and there is no evidence of NSAID ingestion, other causes of atypical duodenal ulceration should be considered.

CONCLUSION

H. pylori is present in the vast majority of patients who present with duodenal ulcer disease. When the infection is eradicated, the long-term recurrence rates are dramatically reduced. If a duodenal ulcer recurs after eradication NSAID ingestion should be excluded. If idiopathic ulceration or unexplained relapse occurs, other conditions associated with duodenal ulcer disease should be excluded. When a patient presents with a bleeding duodenal ulcer and the infection is present, eradication of *H. pylori* should be attempted and confirmed. The prevalence of *H. pylori* in complicated duodenal ulcer is lower than in recurrent uncomplicated ulcer, suggesting the importance of other risk factors in this subgroup of patients. NSAIDs, in particular, are associated with haemorrhage and perforation.

References

1. Kuipers EJ, Thijs JC, Festen HMP. The prevalence of *Helicobacter pylori* in peptic ulcer disease. Aliment Pharmacol Ther. 1995;9(Suppl. 2):59–69.

2. Malmros H, Hiertonn T. A post-investigation of 687 medically treated cases of peptic ulcer. Acta Med Scand. 1949;133:229.
3. Coghlan JD, Gilligan D, Humphries H et al. Campylobacter pylori and recurrence of duodenal ulcers. Lancet. 1987;2:1109–11.
4. Goh KL, Parasakthi N, Peh SC et al. Helicobacter pylori eradication with short-term therapy leads to duodenal ulcer healing without the need for continued acid suppressing therapy. Eur J Gastroenterol Hepatol. 1996;8:421–3.
5. Buckley M, O'Morain C. Helicobacter pylori eradication – a surrogate marker for duodenal ulcer healing. Eur J Gastroenterol Hepatol. 1996;8:415–16.
6. Fry J. Peptic ulcer: a profile. Br Med J. 1964;2:809.
7. Kurath JH, Corboy ED. Current peptic ulcer time trends: an epidemiological profile. J Clin Gastroenterol. 1988;10:259–68.
8. Makela J, Laitien S, Kairaluoma MI. Complications of peptic ulcer disease before and after the introduction of H2 receptor antagonist. Hepatogastroenterology. 1992;39:144–8.
9. Hoskings W, Young MY, Chung SC, Li AKC. Differing prevalence of Helicobacter pylori in bleeding and non bleeding peptic ulcers. Gastroenterology. 1992;102:A85.
10. Hodgkin SW, Ling TKW, Young MY et al. Randomised control trial of short term treatment eradicating Helicobacter pylori in patients with duodenal ulcer. Br Med J. 1992;305:502.
11. Jensen DM, You S, Pelayo E, Jensen ME. The prevalence of Helicobacter pylori and NSAID use in patients with severe UGI haemorrhage and their potential role in recurrence of ulcer bleeding. Gastroenterology. 1992;102:A85.
12. Kaufman DW, Kelly JP, Sheehan JE et al. Nonsteroidal anti-inflammatory drug use in relation to major upper gastrointestinal bleeding. Clin Pharmacol Ther. 1983;53:485–94.
13. Somerville K, Faulkner G, Langman M. Non-steroidal anti-inflammatory drugs and bleeding peptic ulcer. Lancet. 1986;1:462–4.
14. Hovoet J, Terriere L, van Hee W, Verbist L, Fierens E, Hauteteete ML. Relation of upper gastrointestinal bleeding to non-steroidal anti-inflammatory drugs and aspirin: a case control study. Gut. 1991;32:730–4.
15. Lai KC, Hui WM, Lam SK. Bleeding ulcers have high false negative rates for antral Helicobacter pylori when tested with urease test. Gastroenterology. 1996;110:A167.
16. Jensen DM, Cheng S, Kovacs TOG et al. A control study of ranitidine for the prevention of recurrent haemorrhage from duodenal ulcer. N Engl J Med. 1994;303:382–6.
17. Laine L, Peterson WL. Bleeding peptic ulcer. N Engl J Med. 1994;331:717–27.
18. Murray WR, Cooper G, Laferla G, Rogers P, Archibald M. Maintenance ranitidine treatment after haemorrhage from a duodenal ulcer: A 3 year study. Scand J Gastroenterol. 1988;23:183–7.
19. Rokkas T, Karameris A, Mavrogeorgis A, Rallis E. Eradication of Helicobacter pylori reduces the possibility of rebleeding in peptic ulcer disease. Gastrointest Endosc. 1995;41:1–4.
20. Labenz J, Borsch G. The role of Helicobacter pylori by eradication and the prevention of peptic ulcer bleeding relapse. Indigestion. 1994;55:19–23.
21. Graham DY, Hepps KS, Ramirez FC, Lew GM, Saeed ZA. Treatment of Helicobacter pylori reduces the rate of rebleeding in peptic ulcer disease. Scand J Gastroenterol. 1993;28:939–42.
22. Jaspersen D, Korner T, Schorr W, Brennensthul M, Raschka C, Hammar CH. Helicobacter pylori eradication reduces the rate of rebleeding of an ulcer haemorrhage. Gastrointest Endosc. 1995;41:5–7.
23. Jaspersen P, Korner T, Schorr W, Brennersthul M, Raschka C, Hammar CH. Omeprazole, amoxicillin therapy for eradication of Helicobacter pylori in duodenal ulcer bleeding: preliminary results of a pilot study. J Gastroenterol. 1995;30:319–21.
24. Debongnie JC, Legross G. Gastric perforation: an acute disease unrelated to H. pylori? Rev Esp Enferm Dig. 1990;78(Suppl. 1):71–2.
25. Turner FP. Acute perforations of the stomach, duodenum and jejunum. Surg Gynaecol Obstet. 1951;92:281.
26. Reinbach DH, Cruickshank G, McColl KEL. Acute perforated duodenal ulcer is not associated with Helicobacter pylori infection. Gut. 1993;34:1344–7.
27. Armstrong CP, Blower AL. Non-steroidal anti-inflammatory drugs in life threatening complications of peptic ulceration. Gut. 1987;28:527–32.
28. Horowitz J, Kukuora JS, Ritchie WP. All perforated ulcers are not alike. Ann Surg. 1989;209:693–7.
29. Collier D, Sant J, Pain JA. Non-steroidal anti-inflammatory drugs in peptic ulcer perforation. Gut. 1985;26:359–62.

30. Oberhuber G, Puspok A, Oesterreicher C *et al.* Crohn's disease of the stomach is histologically characterized by focal active gastritis. Gastroenterology. 1996;110:A982.
31. Borody TJ, George LL, Brandl S, Andrews P, Ostapowicz N, Hyland M, Devine M. *Helicobacter pylori* negative duodenal ulceration. Am J Gastroenterol. 1991;86:1154–7.
32. Nensey YW, Schubert TT, Bolonga SD, Ma CK. *Helicobacter pylori* negative duodenal ulceration. Am J Med. 1991;91:15–18.
33. McColl KEL, El-Nujumi AM, Chittajallu RS *et al.* A study of the pathogenesis of *Helicobacter pylori* negative chronic duodenal ulceration. Gut. 1993;34:762–8.
34. Black JW, Duncan WAM, Durant CJ, Ganellin CR, Parsons ME. Definition and antagonism of histamine H2 receptors. Nature. 1972;236:385.
35. Tytgat GNJ. Treatments that impact favourably upon the eradication of *Helicobacter pylori* and ulcer recurrence (review). Aliment Pharmacol Ther. 1994;8:359–68.
36. Miehlke S, Bayerdorrfer E, Lehn N *et al.* Recurrence of duodenal ulcers during five years of follow-up after cure of *Helicobacter pylori*. Eur J Gastroenterol. 1995;7:975–8.
37. Lanas AI, Remacha B, Esteva F, Sainz R. Risk factors associated with refractory peptic ulcers. Gastroenterology. 1995;109:1124–33.
38. Veldhuyzen van Zanten SOJ. *H. pylori* and NSAIDs: a meta-analysis on interactions of acute gastroduodenal injury, gastric and duodenal ulcers and upper gastrointestinal symptoms. In: Hunt RH, Tytgat GNJ, editors. *Helicobacter pylori*: basic mechanism to clinical cure. Dordrecht: Kluwer; 1994:449–57.

31
Role of *Helicobacter pylori* infection in gastro-oesophageal reflux disease

G. N. J. TYTGAT

INTRODUCTION

Long before *H. pylori* was discovered, it was already known that gastritis was common in patients with gastro-oesophageal reflux disease (GERD). In 1977 Volpicelli *et al.*[1] found that the symptom of heartburn was related to antral gastritis and duodenitis. In 1984 Fink and co-workers[2] published evidence that antral gastritis was common in patients with reflux disease. Moreover those patients with antral gastritis had evidence of delayed gastric emptying which was thought to contribute to reflux disease. We now know that *H. pylori* infection is the most common cause of gastric inflammation. The question therefore is whether this infection plays any role in the pathogenesis of GERD. This role, if any, turns out to be highly complex, which largely explains why the analysis of the literature appears confusing.

PREVALENCE OF *H. PYLORI* INFECTION IN GERD

Several studies have looked at the prevalence of *H. pylori* infection in GERD patients (summarized in Table 1). In general the prevalence of *H. pylori* in GERD is largely similar to that in the control population[3]. In those studies the rate of infection was similar across the grades of oesophagitis. Unfortunately information regarding the distribution of *H. pylori*-associated gastritis in the stomach in those reports is lacking. Whether the inflammation is mainly antrum-predominant, corpus-predominant or pangastritis, and whether the cardia is involved in the inflammatory process, is rarely mentioned. Genta *et al.*[4] stressed the importance of the cardia as a site of infection and inflammation, of an intensity comparable to the antrum. However, a systematic biopsy study of the cardia in GERD has not yet been carried out. In the study by O'Connor and Cunnane[3] almost half the patients with hiatal hernia had *H. pylori* infection of the herniated gastric mucosa; moreover infection of the hiatal hernia was especially common in patients with severe oesophagitis.

Table 1 Prevalence of *H. pylori* or gastritis in GERD

	GERD	
Reference	n GERD	Percentage H. pylori-*positive* or % gastritis
Fink et al.[2]	23	78
Marshall (Lancet 1984;1:1311)	34	41
Cheng (Ann Intern Med. 1989;149:1373)	27	52
Francoual (J. Infect Dis. 1990;162:1415)	21	52
Rosioru (Am J Gastroenterol. 1993;88:510)	457	28
Rintala (J Pediatr Surg. 1994;29:737)	Children	47
O'Connor and Cunnane[3]	93 of which 64 HH	54 of which 44 HH

HH = hiatus hernia

Table 2 Relationship of GERD with *H. pylori* infection

	n	Percentage H. pylori-*positive*	Percentage corpus gastritis
Dyspepsia	119	45	37
Reflux symptoms without oesophagitis	43	44	56
Reflux symptoms with oesophagitis	70	47	25

From ref. 5.

One important observation was made by De Koster and colleagues[5] in a large cohort of patients with *H. pylori* infection and GERD (Table 2). Patients with endoscopy-negative GERD more often had active corpus gastritis than did patients with endoscopy-positive GERD. The authors concluded from their study that GERD patients with active corpus gastritis may have an impairment of gastric acid secretion and therefore a limited acid load available for reflux, thereby lessening the risk of induction of mucosal damage. Similar findings were collected in Hiroshima (Haruma, personal communication). Patients with reflux oesophagitis had less active gastritis and less atrophy in the corpus mucosa compared to controls.

The prevalence of *H. pylori* infection was also examined in patients with columnar metaplasia in the oesophagus (Table 3). Overall the prevalence of *H. pylori* infection in columnar metaplasia or Barrett's oesophagus is comparable to that in the background population. Interestingly enough, when biopsies were taken first from the columnar metaplastic areas and then from the antrum, the prevalence of oesophageal infection appeared to be lower[6].

Moreover, in the study by Ectors et al.[7], 65% of the patients with ulcerated Barrett's mucosa were *H. pylori*-positive, whereas only 30% of those without ulcers were positive, indicating a probable role for infection in the pathogenesis of Barrett's ulcers.

PREVALENCE OF GERD IN PEPTIC ULCER DISEASE

It is well established that a variable proportion of patients with duodenal ulcer disease may present with reflux-like dyspepsia. This supports Earlam's hypothesis

Table 3 *H. pylori* in columnar metaplasia

Reference	n	Percentage H. pylori-positive
Paull (Gastroenterology. 1988;95:216)	26	15
Hazell (Gastroenterology. 1988;94:A178)	20	15
Talley (Mayo Clin Proc. 1988;63:1176)	23	52
Talley (Gastroenterology. 1988;94:A454)	47	15
Houck (A Pat Lab M. 1989;113:470)	34	0
Walker (Gut. 1989;30:1334)	7	29
Italian Task Force (Histopathology. 1991;18:568)	100	19
Cooper (Gullet. 1991;1:173)	40	18
Angholt et al.[6]	11	12
Loffeld (Am J Gastroenterol. 1992;87:1598)	71	62
Ectors et al.[7]	49	49 (+ ulcer 65) (− ulcer 30)
O'Connor and Cunnane[3]	8	12

that symptoms in duodenal ulcer are not always attributable to the ulcer itself, but commonly result from coexisting GERD[8,9]. Older studies have shown that recurrences of the original symptoms in duodenal ulcer patients commonly occur in the absence of recurrent ulcer[10]. Moreover, oesophageal acid infusion in duodenal ulcer disease can reproduce the usual epigastric symptoms experienced by the patient[8,11].

Especially in the older literature, the prevalence of the 'secondary reflux disease' in *duodenal ulcer* disease was high, but to a large extent this usually reflected selection bias in what were mainly surgical series[12]. About 40–70% of the patients in those surgical series had evidence of reflux oesophagitis. The prevalence of GERD may have been exaggerated by the inclusion of patients with pyloric stenosis or massive gastric acid hypersecretion. The presumed pathogenic sequence of events included: variable degrees of pyloric stenosis, delayed gastric emptying, antral ectasia, excessive gastrin release, excessive acid secretion and high-volume reflux. One can readily hypothesize that all those patients were indeed infected with *H. pylori*. Precise data on the prevalence of GERD in non-complicated *H. pylori*-associated duodenal ulcer disease are largely lacking. Recently Di Mario et al.[13] found reflux esophagitis in 15.5% of approximately 1000 patients with peptic ulcer disease.

PUTATIVE *H. PYLORI*-RELATED MECHANISMS INTERFERING WITH REFLUX DISEASE

At present only hypotheses can be formulated with respect to potential mechanisms whereby *H. pylori*-associated inflammation interferes in the regulation of lower oesophageal sphincter function and the pathogenesis of reflux disease.

Schematically one can distinguish mechanisms which may hypothetically *aggravate* reflux disease or mechanisms that might *be beneficial*.

Hypothetical aggravating or injurious mechanisms include the following:

1. Antral inflammation may interfere with adequate and orderly gastric emptying[2] and/or interfere with pyloric competence and the coordination of antro-

duodenal motility. Delayed gastric emptying is demonstrable in up to half the patients with GERD[14]. Patients with delayed emptying demonstrate greater oesophageal acid exposure than those without. Delayed emptying may provide a greater reservoir of gastric juice available for reflux and/or may prolong the distension stimulus leading to lower oesophageal sphincter relaxations. Interference with pyloric competence may in addition favour excessive duodenogastric reflux.

2. Especially in patients with antrum-predominant gastritis, subsequent hypergastrinaemia may drive the parietal cell mass to excessive acid production. This will augment the degree of acidity and the volume of gastric juice available for reflux.

3. The admixture of inflammatory mediators into the gastric content may potentially aggravate the injurious potential of the refluxate[15].

4. Extension of the inflammation in the upper part of the stomach may theoretically further jeopardize the barrier function of the gastro-oesophageal junction. It is now well established that transient lower oesophageal sphincter relaxations (TLOSR) represent the dominant mechanism that leads to reflux events[16]. It would appear that some of those TLOSR are triggered through distension of the upper part of the stomach. Hypothetically, mucosal inflammation in the gastric fundus may lower the threshold for triggering TLOSR and reflux episodes by intragastric stimuli[16] (altered sensitivity of vagal sensory receptors in the cardia?). Gastric distension is considered to be a major stimulus for TLOSR. This is the principal reason for the substantial increase in the rate of TLOSR and reflux episodes after meals[17,18]. Patients with GERD may have a high prevalence of fundic gastritis (R.H. Holloway, personal communication). Mucosal inflammation may alter the sensitivity of vagal sensory receptors[19], which in turn may alter the rate of triggering TLOSR. Although one could speculate that inflammation in the area of the cardia or in a hiatal hernia might have some effect on lower oesophageal sphincter pressure and competence[20], yet the overall significance remains unclear at present. The whole issue of upper intestinal inflammation has become more important by the discovery that powerful acid suppression with proton pump inhibitors (PPI) in *H. pylori*-infected individuals leads to worsening of the inflammation in the corpus area, and presumably also in the cardia, and this is accompanied by the accelerated development of atrophic changes[21,22]. Whether worsening of inflammation is somehow involved in explaining the often very rapid recurrence of reflux symptoms and oesophagitis after stopping PPI therapy, through aggravation of the underlying motor disorders, is entirely speculative, but deserves detailed study.

Putative mechanisms that are beneficial and might *counteract* those factors that aggravate reflux disease can be considered as follows:

1. Some components induced by *H. pylori* and/or generated in the inflammatory milieu can interfere with parietal cell function and might decrease acid secretion[15,23,24]. Especially in patients who appear to have inflammation in the corpus, acid secretion tends to be less during active inflammation[24].

2. It is still not entirely certain whether the permeability characteristics of an inflamed mucosa are changed to such an extent that there is excessive intra-

mural backflow of acid from the gastric lumen resulting in a lower intragastric acidity.

3. Ammonia production by *H. pylori* urease activity could provide a substantial buffering capacity, again decreasing the corrosive potential of the gastric juice available for reflux. The pK_a for the ammonia–ammonium buffer system is approximately 9.1. The low pH in the gastric contents favours diffusion of (lipid-soluble) ammonia into the gastric juice, where it is trapped as the positively charged ammonium. One of the arguments in this regard includes the recent studies showing that the acid inhibitory effect of PPI is substantially reduced after cure of the *H. pylori* infection[25,26]. This has been explained mainly by the absence of ammonia buffer with subsequent decreased acid neutralization after *H. pylori* eradication. A powerful buffer system composed of ammonia and volatile amines produced by *H. pylori* may disappear after cure of the infection[27,28]. Ammonia buffer is ineffective at low pH but highly effective at high pH.

It is impossible to predict what the ultimate balance will be in a given individual between the *aggravating* and the more or less *protective* mechanisms. This needs to be studied in much more detail in the future.

DISAPPEARANCE OF GERD OR REFLUX-LIKE DYSPEPSIA AFTER *H. PYLORI* CURE

There are anecdotal reports of patients with mild GERD who have had no further GERD symptoms after eradication of *H. pylori*. This could relate to regression of the *H. pylori*-associated hypergastrinaemic drive of the parietal cell mass, or perhaps to regression of the inflammatory changes in the (sub)cardiac area with lesser compromise of lower oesophageal sphincter function.

DEVELOPMENT OF REFLUX-LIKE DYSPEPTIC COMPLAINTS AND GERD AFTER *H. PYLORI* CURE

It is common experience that some patients, especially duodenal ulcer patients, do return with reflux-like dyspeptic complaints and GERD after successful cure of *H. pylori* infection. In some studies the proportion of patients may be up to 10%. Labenz *et al.*[29,30] followed 210 duodenal ulcer patients after *H. pylori* cure. Nineteen patients, corresponding to 4.8% per patient-year of follow-up, developed reflux oesophagitis. The most important factor predicting the occurrence of reflux oesophagitis was the severity of corpus gastritis before cure. The severity of gastritis in the corpus appeared related to the density of colonization by *H. pylori*[31]. Schütze *et al.*[32] discovered reflux oesophagitis in 10 out of 16 duodenal ulcer patients after successful cure of *H. pylori* infection.

Many mechanisms have been proposed to explain the development of reflux symptoms and occasionally oesophagitis:

1. Unmasking of latent disorders such as GERD after disappearance of the ulcer-related symptoms.

2. Liberalization of the eating habits and changes of lifestyle after cure of the infection. Patients may have changed to a more liberal diet as soon as gastro-intestinal symptoms resolved after *H. pylori* cure, especially by drinking more coffee or food containing xanthines (coffee, tea, chocolate etc.).
3. Weight gain.
4. Withdrawal of antisecretory drugs after cure of ulcer disease.
5. Perhaps increased basal and postprandial acid secretion. It is interesting to note from the study by Labenz *et al.*[30] that reflux symptoms or reflux-like dyspeptic symptoms developed especially in patients who had inflammation in the corpus prior to the eradication therapy. Presumably those patients have indeed higher acid secretion after cure of the infection. The overall effects of *H. pylori* cure on acid secretory potential are complex (see Chapter 12). As shown especially in McColl's group[33], many patients with prior hyperacidity develop lowering of acid production after cure of the infection. However, there is a subgroup in which acidity rises after cure of the infection, and this presumably comprises patients who, indeed, had corpus gastritis. Many patients with peptic ulcer disease have been treated in the past with potent antisecretory drugs. Treatment with PPI may be associated with more luxurious growth of *H. pylori* organisms in the corpus/fundus area[34]. The subsequent aggravation of the mucosal inflammation may interfere with the acid secretory capacity[23], further compounded by acceleration of the development of atrophy[22]. Subsequent healing of the mucosa after *H. pylori* cure may remove the suppressive effect of the inflammation with apparently increased basal and stimulated acid secretion.

In general, it would appear that the acid secretory outcome depends largely upon the distribution of the mucosal inflammation in the stomach prior to cure[24,25]. Inflammation of the oxyntic mucosa may interfere with acid secretion through various putative mechanisms. The organism produces an acid-inhibitory protein and unusual fatty acids which inhibit acid production and H^+, K^+, ATPase activity. In addition inflammation generates IL-1β, which is a potent inhibitor of acid secretion[23]. Although, usually, *H. pylori* eradication decreases the acid secretory responses to gastrin-releasing peptide (GRP) in most infected asymptomatic individuals, dyspeptics or ulcer patients, in some the eradication corrects a marked impairment of the oxyntic mucosa with subsequent increase in both basal and stimulated gastric acid secretory capacity[35–39].

CONCLUDING REMARKS

The relationship of *H. pylori* infection and GERD is complex. The epidemiologically rather crude observation that there does not appear to be an excess of patients with GERD who are *H. pylori*-infected when compared to the community prevalence would argue against any such relationship. Moreover, there is no evidence at present that eradication of *H. pylori* alone is of benefit in the management of GERD, again questioning the role of *H. pylori* in the causation of reflux disease. What really matters, however, relates to the way the *H. pylori* infection is impacting on the gastric mucosa. The topography of inflammation in the stomach may be relevant in determining whether oesophagitis develops, and may perhaps also play a role in altering the triggering of transient lower oesophageal sphincter relaxations, although this remains speculative at present.

Many factors promote the development of GERD after cure of *H. pylori*-associated (ulcer) disease. Patients at risk for GERD appear to have more severe corpus gastritis before cure, are often male and do gain weight. Healing of the corpus mucosa presumably increases acid secretion sufficiently to cause mucosal damage upon reflux.

References

1. Volpicelli NA, Yardley JH, Hendrix TR. The association of heartburn with gastritis. Am J Dig Dis. 1977;22:333–9.
2. Fink SM, Barwick KW, DeLuca V, Sanders FJ, Kandathil M, McCallum RW. The association of histologic gastritis with gastroesophageal reflux and delayed gastric emptying. J Clin Gastroenterol. 1984;6:301–9.
3. O'Connor HJ, Cunnane K. *Helicobacter pylori* and gastro-oesophageal reflux disease – a prospective study. IJMS. 1994;163:369–73.
4. Genta RM, Huberman RM, Graham DY. The gastric cardia in *Helicobacter pylori* infection. Hum Pathol. 1994;25:915–19.
5. De Koster E, Ferhat M, Deprez C, Deltenre M. *Helicobacter pylori*, gastric histology and gastro-oesophageal reflux disease. Gut. 1995;37(Suppl. 1):A36.
6. Agnholt J, Fallingborg J, Møller-Petersen J et al. The occurrence of *Helicobacter pylori* in the oesophagus. Eur J Gastroenterol Hepatol. 1991;3:685–8.
7. Ectors N, Geboes K, Janssens J, Ventrappen G. *Helicobacter pylori* and the oesophagus. In: Pajares JM et al., editors. *H. pylori* and gastroduodenal pathology. Berlin: Springer; 1993:142–50.
8. Earlam RJ. Production of epigastric pain by lower oesophageal acid perfusion. Br Med J. 1970;4:714–16.
9. Earlam RJ. Further experience with the epigastric pain reproduction test in duodenal ulceration. Br Med J. 1972;1:683–95.
10. McDonald AJ, Peden NR, Hayton R, Mallinson CN, Roberts D, Wormsley KG. Symptom relief and the placebo effect in the trial of an antipeptic drug. Gut. 1980;21:323–6.
11. Earlam RJ, Amerigo J, Kakvoulis T, Pollock DJ. Histological appearances of oesophagus, antrum and duodenum and their correlation with symptoms in patients with a duodenal ulcer. Gut. 1985;26:95–100.
12. Flook D, Stoddard CJ. Gastro-oesophageal reflux and oesophagitis before and after vagotomy for duodenal ulcer. Br J Surg. 1985;72:804–7.
13. Di Mario F, Leandro G, Battaglia G et al. Do concomitant diseases and therapies affect the persistence of ulcer symptoms in the elderly? Dig Dis Sci. 1996;41:17–21.
14. McCallum RW, Berkowitz OM, Lerner E. Gastric emptying in patients with gastroesophageal reflux. Gastroenterology. 1981;80:285–91.
15. Cover TL, Blaser MJ. *Helicobacter pylori* infection, a paradigm for chronic mucosal inflammation: pathogenesis and implications for eradication and prevention. Adv Intern Med. 1996;41:85–117.
16. Mittal RK, Holloway RH, Penagini R, Blackshaw LA, Dent J. Transient lower esophageal sphincter relaxation. Gastroenterology. 1995;109:601–10.
17. Holloway RH, Hongo M, Berger K, McCallum RW. Gastric distension: a mechanism for postprandial gastro-esophageal reflux. Gastroenterology. 1985;89:770–5.
18. Holloway RH, Dent J. Pathophysiology of gastroesophageal reflux disease. Lower esophageal sphincter dysfunction in gastroesophageal reflux disease. Gastroenterol Clin N Am. 1990;19:517–35.
19. Blackshaw LA, Grundy D. Effects of 5-hydroxytryptamine (5HT) on the discharge of vagal mucosal afferent fibres in the upper gastrointestinal tract of the anaesthetized ferret. J Autonom Nerv Syst. (In press).
20. Sloan S, Rademaker A, Kahrilas P. Determinants of gastroesophageal junction incompetence: hiatal hernia, lower esophageal sphincter, or both? Ann Intern Med. 1992;117:977–82.

21. Solcia E, Fiocca R, Villani L, Carlsson J, Rudbäck A, Zeijlon L. Effects of permanent eradication or transient clearance of *Helicobacter pylori* on histology of gastric mucosa using omeprazole with or without antibiotics. Scand J Gastroenterol. 1996;31(Suppl. 215):105–10.

22. Kuipers EJ, Lundell L, Klinkenberg-Knol EC *et al*. Atrophic gastritis and *Helicobacter pylori* infection in patients with reflux esophagitis treated with omeprazole or fundoplication. N Engl J Med. 1996;334:1018–22.

23. McGowan CC, Cover TL, Blaser MJ. *Helicobacter pylori* and gastric acid: biological and therapeutic implications. Gastroenterology. 1996;110:926–38.

24. Sipponen P, Kekki M, Seppälä K, Siurala M. The relationships between chronic gastritis and gastric acid secretion. Aliment Pharmacol Ther. 1996;10(Suppl. 1):103–18.

25. Verdú EF, Armstrong D, Idström J-P *et al*. Effect of curing *Helicobacter pylori* infection on intragastric pH during treatment with omeprazole. Gut. 1995;37:743–8.

26. Labenz J, Tillenburg B, Peitz U *et al*. *Helicobacter pylori* augments the pH-increasing effect of omeprazole in patients with duodenal cancer. Gastroenterology. 1996;110:725–32.

27. Goggin PM, Marrero JA, Ahmed H *et al*. Urea hydrolysis in *Helicobacter pylori* infection. Eur J Gastroenterol Hepatol. 1991;3:927–33.

28. Trindh LT, AlAssi MT, Graham DY, Lichtenberger LM. A comparison of gastric juice NH3 analysis by enzymatic kit (K) and electrode (E) in normal and *H. pylori* (HP) infected subjects. Am J Gastroenterol. 1994;89:1290–8.

29. Labenz J, Tillenburg B, Peitz U, Börsch G. Long-term consequences of *Helicobacter pylori* eradication: clinical aspects. Scand J Gastroenterol. 1996;31(Suppl. 215):111–15.

30. Labenz J, Blum AL, Stolte M, Börsch G. Curing *Helicobacter pylori* infection in duodenal ulcer patients may provoke reflux oesophagitis. (To be published).

31. Stolte M, Stadelmann O, Bethke B, Burkard G. Relationships between the degree of *Helicobacter pylori* colonisation and the degree and activity of gastritis, surface epithelial degeneration and mucus secretion. Z Gastroenterol. 1995;33:89–93.

32. Schütze K, Hentschel E, Dragosics B, Hirschl AM. *Helicobacter pylori* reinfection with identical organisms: transmission by the patients' spouses. Gut. 1995;36:831–3.

33. El-Omar EM, Penman ID, Ardill JES, Chittajallu RS, Howie C, McColl KEL. *Helicobacter pylori* infection and abnormalities of acid secretion in patients with duodenal ulcer disease. Gastroenterology. 1995;109:681–91.

34. Logan RPH, Walker MM, Misiewicz JJ, Gumnett PA, Karim QN, Baron JH. Changes in the intragastric distribution of *Helicobacter pylori* during treatment with omeprazole. Gut. 1995;36:12–16.

35. Chandrakumaran K, Vaira D, Hobsley M. Duodenal ulcer, *Helicobacter pylori* and gastric secretion. Gut. 1994;35:1033–6.

36. Yasumaga Y, Shinomura Y, Kanayama S *et al*. Improved fold width and increased acid secretion after eradication of the organism in *Helicobacter pylori* associated enlarged fold gastritis. Gut. 1994;35:1571–4.

37. Peterson WL. Gastrin and acid in relation to *Helicobacter pylori*. Aliment Pharmacol Ther. 1996;10(Suppl. 1):97–102.

38. Verhulst ML, Hopman WPM, Tangerman A, Jansen JBMJ. Eradication of *Helicobacter pylori* infection in patients with non-ulcer dyspepsia. Scand J Gastroenterol. 1995;30:968–73.

39. El-Omar EM, Penman ID, Ardill JE, Chittajallu RS, Howie C, McColl KE. *Helicobacter pylori* infection and abnormalities of acid secretion in patients with duodenal ulcer disease. Gastroenterology. 1995;109:681–91.

32
Are NSAIDs and *Helicobacter pylori* separate risk factors?

C. J. HAWKEY

INTRODUCTION

Now that *Helicobacter pylori* and NSAIDs have been shown to cause the vast majority of peptic ulcers it is natural to address the question of any interaction between them. Defining the precise interaction between *H. pylori* and NSAIDs is important for both theoretical and practical therapeutic reasons.

THEORETICAL ISSUES

One possibility is that NSAIDs and *H. pylori* induce quite separate processes resulting in lesions (ulcers) that appear similar, but are in fact different. If this were so, one would predict an additive effect on ulcer development. Alternatively, NSAIDs and *H. pylori* might each influence mechanisms otherwise capable of compensating for the harmful effects of them alone. Under these circumstances one would predict a greater than additive (synergistic) relationship. A relationship which is less than additive could arise in two main ways. Some individuals may be constitutionally incapable of developing ulceration so that there is in effect a ceiling for ulcer development. If NSAID consumption or *H. pylori* took the population close to this ceiling, addition of the other factor would have a minimal effect. Another way in which a less than additive relationship could arise is if the actions of one factor partially protected against the actions of the other whilst continuing to exert its own normal level of toxicity.

These theoretical issues can be addressed by considering the pathogenic mechanisms involved in damage caused by *H. pylori* and NSAIDs.

MECHANISMS OF DAMAGE

Figure 1 shows the effects of *H. pylori* and NSAIDs on potentially damaging and protective mechanisms[1,2]. As can be seen, some of these pathogenetic mechanisms are shared. For example both NSAIDs and *H. pylori* increase paracellular gastric

A: *Helicobacter pylori* ulcers		
Ulcer formation ↑		Ulcer healing ↓
↑ *Aggressive*	↓ *Defensive*	Competition + Growth factors
↑ Acid Back Diffusion	↓ Mucus* ↓ Bicarbonate*	Acid Destruction Growth Factors
↑ (Pepsin)	↓ Hydrophobicity*	
↑ Inflammation		
↑ Cytotoxin		
↑ Ammonia		
↑ Phospholipase		
	*Despite ↓ PGs	

B: NSAID ulcers		
Ulcer formation ↑		Ulcer healing ↓
↑ *Aggressive*	↓ *Defensive*	↓ Growth factor action
↑ (Acid)	↓ Mucus*	
↑ Acid Back Diffusion	↓ Bicarbonate*	
↑ Pepsin?	↓ Hydrophobicity*	
	Mucosal blood flow* ↓	
	Cell trapping	
	↓ Oxidative Phosphorylation	
	*Associated with ↓ PGs	

Figure 1 Pathogenesis of ulcers – a double balance, attack versus defence for ulcerogenesis, and ulcerogenesis vs healing

mucosal permeability and exposure of the mucosa to acid (and potential antigens). To this must be added, in the case of *H. pylori*, increased acid production secondary to stimulation of gastrin. Some studies, particularly those in animals, have also shown NSAIDs to increase gastric acid output, but others have not. Although the term 'peptic' is applied to ulcers caused by *H. pylori*, they can be healed by small changes in intragastric acidity which are insufficient to affect peptic activity. The description 'peptic' may, therefore, be misguided. Paradoxically, there is circumstantial evidence that pepsin may have more of a role in NSAID damage and oesophagitis in that both require an increase in 24-hour intragastric pH to 4 or more for effective healing or maintenance.

Conversely, NSAIDs and *H. pylori* each affect the mediators of mucosal defence in rather different ways. Prostaglandin synthesis, nitric oxide and enteric neuronal reflexes are recognized to synergize in mediating mucosal defence[3]. This redundancy means that there is not a simple relationship between an effect on the mediator and a defence mechanism. NSAIDs are known to inhibit prostaglandin synthesis whilst *H. pylori* increases it, probably by the induction of the inducible cyclooxygenase (COX-2) enzyme, even in the presence of NSAIDs[4,5]. Despite these opposite effects on prostaglandin synthesis, *H. pylori* is known to influence protective mechanisms normally regarded as prostaglandin-dependent, in the same direction as do NSAIDs – for example both reduce mucosal hydrophobicity, thickness of the mucus layer and bicarbonate secretion. Similarly, *H. pylori* induces expression of the inducible nitric oxide synthase (iNOS) enzyme. It is not clear, however, whether resulting increases in nitric oxide synthesis are protective or harmful.

PRACTICAL THERAPEUTIC ASPECTS

If *H. pylori* and NSAIDs interact synergistically or additively then eradication of *H. pylori* could assist in the management of NSAID users. If the interaction is less than additive it is even possible that eradication of *H. pylori* could be harmful – for example if, in an NSAID user, stimulation by *H. pylori* of defence mechanisms against NSAID damage (for example prostaglandin synthesis) outweighed the harmful effects of the infection itself. These considerations can in turn be broken down into a number of practical issues concerning the possible role of *H. pylori* eradication in NSAID users. Could *H. pylori* eradication:

1. be of itself sufficient to protect NSAID users against NSAID-associated problems;
2. increase rate of healing of NSAID-associated lesions, either spontaneously or under active treatment;
3. increase the effectiveness of maintenance treatment?

CANCER

One area where limited but fairly clear data suggest NSAIDs and *H. pylori* have opposite effects is in gastric cancer[6,7]. There appears to be a positive dose-dependence in terms of length of exposure to *H. pylori* and the development of gastric cancer, and a negative dose relationship with the amount of aspirin consumption (Figure 2). It will be important to define whether COX-2 is important in these relationships, as it may be in colon cancer.

INTERACTION BETWEEN NSAIDs AND *H. PYLORI* IN ULCER DISEASE

Possible sources of bias

Before examining the interaction between NSAIDs and *H. pylori* some sources of bias must be remembered.

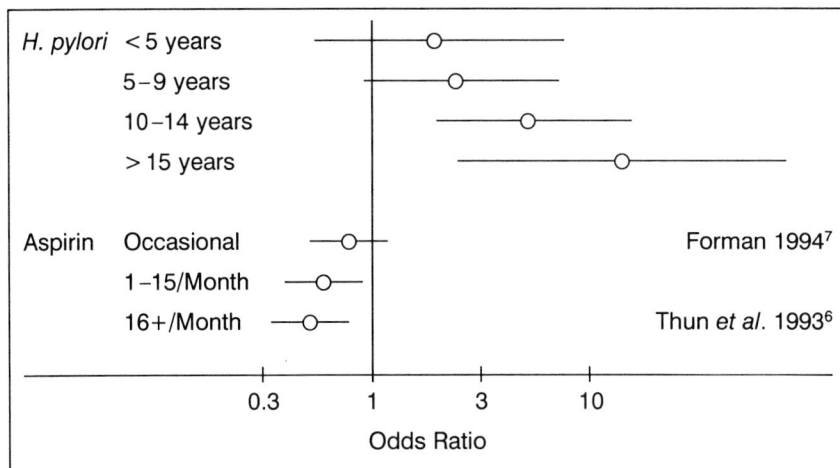

Figure 2 Opposite effects of *H. pylori* infection and NSAID consumption

Table 1 *H. pylori* prevalence in NSAID users

	H. pylori *prevalence (%)*		
	Patients	*Controls*	p *value*
Doube and Morris, 1988[11]	48	–	–
Upadhyay et al., 1988[12]	50	–	–
Iglehart et al., 1989[9]	32	69	<0.007
Caselli et al., 1989[8]	31	59	<0.001
Scherak et al., 1989[13]	56	67	n.s.
Maxton et al., 1990[14]	63	51	n.s.
Jones et al., 1991[15]	43	52	n.s.
Graham et al., 1991[16]	56	Not given	n.s.
Taha et al., 1993[10]	32	50	<0.02
Gubbins et al., 1991[17]	40	–	–

1. *NSAIDs could affect* H. pylori *colonization, viability or persistence. In vitro*, aspirin has been shown to be toxic to *H. pylori*[8], and some early studies showed a significant reduction in *H. pylori* prevalence compared to controls[8-10]. However, the majority of studies have selected patients thought to be at risk of ulcer, and their relevance to the unselected population of NSAID users is uncertain. The majority of studies have not found a difference in the prevalence of *H. pylori* in NSAID users[11-17] and if there is one it is likely to be relatively small (Table 1).

2. *Selective recruitment of NSAID users who are* H. pylori-*positive.* In clinical practice the knowledge that an NSAID user is positive for *H. pylori* may influence doctors to study that patient more readily. Equally, in supposedly unselected populations, those with low-grade dyspepsia may be more ready to volunteer for endoscopy than others.

We investigated this issue by asking patients to keep a 6-week diary before inviting them to undergo endoscopy as a prelude to a possible healing and maintenance

Table 2   Dyspeptic symptoms in NSAID users (percentages)

	H. pylori-*positive*	H. pylori-*negative*
Doube and Morris, 1988[11]	45	39
Upadhyay et al., 1988[12]	62	31*
Jones et al., 1991[15]	45	10*
Graham et al., 1991[16]	60	35
Loeb et al., 1992[20]	18	21
Gubbins et al., 1991[17]	54	44
Goggin et al., 1993[23]	72	33*
Hudson et al., 1992[24]	67	22*
Cullen et al., 1994[19]	81	63* (NUD)
Talley et al., 1995[21]		

*Significant difference

trial. Among this ostensibly asymptomatic population who had not consulted medically because of dyspepsia, 37.5% of those who recorded no dyspeptic symptoms whatsoever volunteered for endoscopy, compared to 67% of those who recorded some dyspeptic symptoms. Among these patients there was no difference in the prevalence of ulceration (20% for those not recording dyspepsia and 16% for those recording dyspepsia). When dyspepsia was related to *H. pylori* infection, 67% of those infected had recorded dyspepsia compared to 22% of those not infected ($p = 0.01$)[4,18]. This study, therefore, suggested that *H. pylori* enhanced NSAID-associated dyspepsia, and that this led to selective recruitment of infected patients. In this study some patients found to have ulcers were included. However, there did not appear to be an increased number of ulcers in the *H. pylori* group. In order to control for this possible confounding factor a further study of matched patients who did not have ulcers was conducted. In this study too, *H. pylori* infection was associated with higher levels of non-ulcer-associated dyspepsia[19]. In both studies *H. pylori* infection increased mucosal prostaglandin synthesis, probably by inducing COX-2 expression, even though the patients were taking NSAIDs. Since prostaglandins synergize with other irritants in pain perception, this increased prostaglandin synthesis may play a permissive role in the perception of non-ulcer dyspepsia.

H. PYLORI AND DYSPEPSIA IN NSAID USERS

Unfortunately, as shown in Table 2, other investigators have not found such clear-cut differences. In an early study, Upadhyay found an increased prevalence of dyspepsia among NSAID users who were *H. pylori*-positive compared with negative[12] and Jones *et al.* suggested such patients were particularly prone to multiple drug-related dyspepsia[15]. In Graham *et al.*'s study, a trend in favour of an association did not reach statistical significance[16], but other studies found no suggestion of an association[17,20–22].

   It is difficult to make sense of these discrepant data. One problem is that the endpoints in the studies were not the same. It is worth pointing out that none of the negative studies was specifically designed to investigate the relationship between *H. pylori* and dyspepsia. By contrast all five studies specifically designed to investigate this association as a primary endpoint did find a significant

Table 3 NSAIDs, *H. pylori* and peptic ulcer (percentages)

			Ulcer if	
	H. pylori	*Peptic ulcer*	H. pylori-*positive*	H. pylori-*negative*
Caselli *et al.*, 1989[8]	31*	8	12	7
Martin, 1989[23a]	52	35	41	15
Shallcross and Heatley, 1990[22]	61	31	38	20
Graham *et al.*, 1991[16]	73	18	21	10
Taha, 1993[10]	32	39	37	41
Safe, 1993[25]	49	34	38	32
Hudson *et al.*, 1993[4]	38	14	24	8
Overall			31	23

association[4,12,15,19,23]. It is probably also significant that all of these studies used a relatively simple definition of dyspepsia, although the definitions were not always stated and/or were not the same from study to study. The failure of Loeb, Gubbins and Talley[17,20,21] to find an association may reflect a broader definition of dyspepsia, while Talley's study[21] also was too small to have had substantial power.

Overall, it seems likely that there may be a true association between NSAID dyspepsia and infection with *H. pylori*. The relationship may in fact be stronger than suggested by the data reviewed. All of these studies were conducted in subjects who had been taking NAIDs for some time. One study has suggested a specific relationship between *H. pylori* infection and disabling multiple drug intolerance[15]. Such subjects would be forced to discontinue their NSAIDs, leading studies of chronic users to underestimate the influence of *H. pylori*. It also follows that if there is a true overall reduction of prevalence of *H. pylori* among NSAID users this may arise not because NSAIDs are toxic to *H. pylori* but simply by a process of attrition of infected patients stopping NSAID use because of dyspepsia.

Incidence and prevalence of NSAID-associated ulceration in NSAID users who are infected with *H. pylori*

As shown in Table 3, there is a reasonable consistency in the literature supporting the proposition that endoscopically detected ulceration is more common in NSAID users that are *H. pylori*-positive compared to those who are negative[4,8,16,24–29]. However, although the prevalence of *H. pylori* in patients with both gastric and duodenal ulcer is above that of matched or unmatched population controls, this prevalence, particularly for patients with duodenal ulcer, falls short of the values associated with ulceration in patients not taking NSAIDs. If the action of NSAIDs were simply to make ulceration more likely in *H. pylori*-infected individuals the rate of ulcer development would be high (as is known), but the percentage prevalence of *H. pylori* in this group would be the same as, or higher than, that seen in patients with ulcers not taking NSAIDs. The fact that this does not occur is strong circumstantial evidence in support of the idea that two types of ulcers occur in NSAID users – specifically NSAID-induced ulcers in patients who are *H. pylori*-negative and essentially *H. pylori*-related ulcers in the remainder.

Conversely, the relatively low prevalence of *H. pylori* in NSAID patients with duodenal ulcer is good circumstantial evidence that NSAIDs can cause duodenal ulcer and gastric ulcer *de novo*, as well as enhancing the development of those associated with *H. pylori*.

Overall, endoscopic studies of uncomplicated ulcer prevalence show that NSAID ulcers are more likely to be detected in patients infected with *H. pylori*. However, it is not known whether this arises simply because such patients are more likely to get dyspepsia and to be studied.

Ulcer complications

The possibility that *H. pylori*-induced dyspepsia leads to biased assessment of the prevalence of *H. pylori* in NSAID users developing ulcers needs to be borne in mind in interpreting apparently paradoxical data about the relationship between NSAIDs, *H. pylori* and ulcer complications. Four reasonably large studies have investigated the interaction between NSAIDs and *H. pylori* in patients presenting with ulcer bleeding (three studies) or perforation (one study[30–33]). In our own study cases were matched to controls prospectively, although there was an interval of approximately 2½ years on average between accession to the study and subsequent collection of serum to establish *H. pylori* status. This study showed that both NSAIDs and *H. pylori* were associated with an increased risk of bleeding peptic ulcer, and this risk appeared to be similar for both gastric and duodenal ulcer and for aspirin and non-aspirin usage (although confidence intervals for subgroups were wide[30]). While the upper confidence interval is compatible with the possibility of some synergy, it seems more likely that this is at the very most limited. Amongst NSAID users there was only a 1.16 (95% CI, 0.44–3.03) fold increase in the risk of bleeding peptic ulcer compared to NSAID users who were *H. pylori*-negative. Thus, in this study NSAID use appeared to be a greater influence than *H. pylori* status, there was little evidence of synergy and the relationship, if anything, appeared to be less than additive.

Such a conclusion is supported by the results of other studies which did not have formal controls. Thus, for ulcer bleeding, Jensen and his colleagues found a prevalence of *H. pylori* in patients presenting with duodenal ulcer bleeding of only 72%, not greatly different from the background population[31]. Similarly, when investigating ulcer perforation, Reinbach and colleagues reported a prevalence of *H. pylori* in those with perforated duodenal ulcer of only 44%, scarcely different from the prevalence of 50% in the background population[32]. In this study a substantial number of patients with perforation appeared to be neither infected with *H. pylori* nor to be taking NSAIDs, although it was retrospective and, since many NSAID users do not admit to taking the drugs, may have underestimated the influence of NSAID use.

Recently, a study using matched pairs as direct and contemporaneous controls reported relative risks for *H. pylori* of 3.4 (1.4–8.7), for NSAIDs 2.7 (1.0–7.6) and for both factors together of 2.4 (0.95–6.4[33]). This study is consistent with our own in showing no evidence of significant synergy, with no increase in the rate of NSAID ulcer bleeding in patients affected with *H. pylori*. It differs from our study and most other studies in the literature in showing a relatively low odds ratio for NSAIDs. Nevertheless, the question of whether, acting largely independently, *H. pylori* or NSAIDs represent the greater risk for ulcer complications remains undetermined.

DISCREPANCIES – POSSIBLE EXPLANATIONS

How can discrepancies between endoscopic studies showing an association between *H. pylori* and NSAID ulceration, but no such relationship for ulcer complications, be explained? Several possibilities exist:

1. The ulcer complication data represent the true relationship between NSAIDs and *H. pylori*. Patients present to endoscopic studies more readily if they are infected with *H. pylori* because they get more dyspepsia.
2. Endoscopic studies represent the true relationship between NSAIDs and *H. pylori*. NSAIDs specifically promote complications (e.g. by interfering with haemostasis) and do so particularly in those who are *H. pylori*-negative.
3. Endoscopic studies represent the true relationship between NSAIDs and *H. pylori*. *H. pylori* in some way protects against the development of ulcer complications, e.g. by promoting prostaglandin synthesis.
4. By developing dyspepsia, NSAID users who are infected with *H. pylori* are more likely to come to attention before they develop ulcer bleeding. Many bleeding peptic ulcers, particularly those associated with NSAID use, are relatively silent prior to presentation, and this may be because they represent the residue of patients without dyspepsia or dissociated *H. pylori* infection. By the same token, these may also be those with the most compromised defence mechanisms if prostaglandin levels are particularly low in this group.

If *H. pylori* does not synergize to enhance NSAID risk, it is difficult to explain the influence of past history – maybe this is a subgroup of *H. pylori*-infected patients with scars sufficient to have a high incidence of further bleeding but numerous enough to affect overall statistics.

Should *H. pylori* be eradicated in NSAID users?

The NIH Consensus meeting recommended eradication of *H. pylori* among patients who develop ulcers, regardless of NSAID status. There is a growing tendency to go beyond this advice in NSAID users and to eradicate *H. pylori* regardless of ulcer status on the basis that this approach can at best do no harm. Is such an approach evidence-based? If not is such an approach rational?

So far, two small studies have reported on the effect of *H. pylori* eradication on NSAID ulcer development. In one, no significant differences were found[34]. In a second study, patients were randomized to receive naproxen 750 mg daily with or without bismuth-based triple therapy[35]. After 2 months five of those randomized to naproxen alone (25%) developed ulcers compared to one (4.5%) of those also receiving triple therapy. While suggestive, this trial should not be taken as evidence in favour of the policy of *H. pylori* eradication, since the differences were not significant, the study was not blinded, the result is an interim one and the bismuth used in the eradication regimen is likely to have persisted in the mucosa and possibly had a mucosal protective effect.

Thus, at present, there is no evidence to support a policy of widespread *H. pylori* eradication in NSAID users. *H. pylori* eradication should not be attempted in this group until the results of a, now-complete, large prospective trial are known. *H. pylori* stimulates prostaglandin synthesis and could have a protective effect against NSAID ulceration, so the argument that eradication can at worse do no harm does not hold. Moreover, where active therapeutic agents are used, the influence of *H. pylori* is further paradoxical and appears beneficial rather than harmful.

Effect of *H. pylori* on NSAID ulcer healing or maintenance with active agents

These data arise from a recently analysed programme of studies comparing omeprazole with placebo, misoprostol or ranitidine for healing and maintenance of NSAID-associated ulcers (refs 36–38 and own unpublished data). All patients had their *H. pylori* status established by CLO test on entry to the study. During the healing phase of each study the primary endpoint was overall treatment success comprising healing of initial ulcer or multiple erosions, dyspeptic symptoms that were no more than mild and drug tolerability. Healing of gastric ulcer, duodenal ulcer and erosions were also assessed as in secondary analyses. During the maintenance phase overall therapeutic failure was recurrence of ulcer or erosions, development of moderate or severe dyspepsia or failure due to intolerance or adverse events.

In all phases of both studies, infection with *H. pylori* emerged as a good, rather than a bad, prognostic factor. This was not due to a selective association between *H. pylori* and duodenal ulceration. When analysed in terms of drug use, acid-suppressing drugs, particularly ranitidine, performed badly in patients not infected with *H. pylori*, while if anything the reverse was true for misoprostol. The reasons for these findings are not yet clear, but one can speculate that one of the following possibilities may apply.

1. Acid-suppression therapy may be particularly effective in the presence of *H. pylori*. Much evidence suggests that particularly profound acid suppression is needed to heal and protect against NSAID-associated ulcers.
2. Enhanced prostaglandin synthesis by *H. pylori* may contribute to ulcer healing and mucosal protection in patients receiving acid-suppressing drugs.
3. Ulcers occurring in NSAID users may be of two types: *H. pylori*-associated, particularly sensitive to acid suppression and *H. pylori*-independent, less influenced by acid suppression.

CONCLUSIONS

Much remains to be learnt about the relationship between NSAIDs and *H. pylori*. Many of the assumptions intuitively made in the absence of evidence are turning out to be wrong. Although much of the evidence in the literature is discrepant, the following conclusions are reasonable.

1. Patients infected with *H. pylori* are probably more likely to get dyspepsia when they take NSAIDs compared to those who are not infected.
2. The prevalence of *H. pylori* is higher among patients with endoscopically detected ulcers, but this may arise artefactually.
3. If anything, NSAIDs are the dominant influence on ulcer complications and there is little evidence that *H. pylori* modifies NSAID-associated risks.
4. Whether *H. pylori* eradication improves the prognosis for NSAID users not using prophylactic treatments is unknown.
5. *H. pylori* eradication has not been shown to be beneficial in NSAID users receiving acid-suppressing drugs, and could even be harmful.
6. NSAIDs and *H. pylori* probably have opposite effects upon the risk of developing gastric cancer.

These intriguing and paradoxical findings have many theoretical implications. The practical prescriber planning to eradicate *H. pylori* in NSAID users should pause to consider whether this is rational.

References

1. Hawkey CJ, Hudson N. Mucosal injury caused by drugs, chemicals and stress. In: Haubrich WS, Schaffner F, Berk JE, editors. Bockus gastroenterology, 5th edn, vol. 2. Philadelphia: WB Saunders; 1994:656–99.
2. Blaser MJ. Hypotheses on the pathogenesis and natural history of *Helicobacter pylori*-induced inflammation. Gastroenterology. 1992;102:20–7.
3. Hawkey CJ (Editorial). Future treatments for arthritis – new NSAIDs, NO-NSAIDs or no NSAIDs? Gastroenterology. 1995;109:614–16.
4. Hudson N, Balsitis M, Filipowicz B, Hawkey CJ. Effect of *Helicobacter pylori* colonisation on gastric mucosal eicosanoid synthesis in patients taking nonsteroidal antiinflammatory drugs. Gut. 1993;34:748–51.
5. Donnelly MC, Bishop AE, McLaughlan J, Polak J, Hawkey CJ. Elevated inducible cyclooxygenase in *H. pylori* infected gastric mucosa and gastric cancer. Gastroenterology. 1996;110:A897.
6. Thun MJ, Namboodiri MM, Calle E, Flanders WD, Heath CW. Aspirin use and risk of fatal cancer. Cancer Res. 1993;53:1322–7.
7. Forman D. *Helicobacter pylori* and gastric cancer. Scand J Gastroenterol. 1996;31(No. S215 S15):48–51.
8. Caselli M, Pazzi P, LaCorte R, Aleott A, Trevisani L, Stabellini G. *Campylobacter*-like organisms, non-steroidal anti-inflammatory drugs and gastric lesions in patients with rheumatoid arthritis. Digestion. 1989;44:101–4.
9. Iglehart IW 3rd, Edlow DW, Muills L Jr *et al.* The presence of *Campylobacter pylori* in non-steroidal anti-inflammatory drug associated gastritis. J Rheumatol. 1989;16:599–603.
10. Taha AS, Dahill S, Nakshabendi I, Lee FD, Sturrock RD, Russell RI. Duodenal histology, ulceration, and *Helicobacter pylori* in the presence or absence of non-steroidal anti-inflammatory drugs. Gut. 1993;34:1162–6.
11. Doube A, Morris A. Non steroidal anti-inflammatory drug-induced dyspepsia – is *Campylobacter pyloridis* implicated? Br J Rheumatol. 1988;27:110–12.
12. Upadhyay R, Howatson A, McKinlay A, Danesh BJZ, Sturrock RD, Russell RI. *Campylobacter pylori*-associated gastritis in patients with rheumatoid arthritis taking non steroidal anti-inflammatory drugs. Br J Rheumatol. 1988;27:113–16.
13. Scherak O, Hirschl AM, Nemec H, Amann B, Kolarz G, Thumb N. NSAID-associated gastritis and *Helicobacter pylori*. J Rheumatol. 1989;16:860–1.

14. Maxton DG, Srivastava ED, Whorwell PJ, Joner DM. Do non-steroidal anti-inflammatory drugs or smoking predispose to *Helicobacter pylori* infection? Postgrad Med J. 1990;66:717–19.
15. Jones STM, Clague RB, Eldridge J, Jones DM. Serological evidence of infection with *Helicobacter pylori* may predict gastrointestinal intolerance to nonsteroidal antiinflammatory drug (NSAID) treatment in rheumatoid arthritis. Br J Rheumatol. 1991;30:16–20.
16. Graham DY, Lidsky MD, Cox AM *et al*. Long-term non-steroidal anti-inflammatory drug use and *Helicobacter pylori* infection. Gastroenterology. 1991;100:1653–7.
17. Gubbins GP, Schubert TT, Artanasio F, Lubetsky M, Perez-Perez GI, Blaser M. Seroprevalence of *Helicobacter pylori* in rheumatoid arthritis patients. Gastroenterology. 1991;100:A405.
18. Hudson N, Everitt SJ, Taha AS, Russell RI, Sturrock RD, Hawkey CJ. Self-selection for endoscopic surveys in patients on NSAIDs. Gut. 1990;31:A1177.
19. Cullen DJE, Hull MA, Facer P, Bishop AE, Polak JM, Hawkey CJ. Substance P containing enteric neurones and prostaglandin E2 in non-steroidal, anti-inflammatory drug ulceration. Gastro-enterology. 1994;106:A66.
20. Loeb DS, Talley NI, Ahlquist DA *et al*. Long-term nonsteroidal antiinflammatory drug-use and gastroduodenal injury – the role of *Helicobacter pylori*. Gastroenterology. 1992;102:1899–905.
21. Talley NJ, Evans JM, Fleming KC, Harmsen WS, Zinsmeister AR, Melton LJ. Nonsteroidal antiinflammatory drugs and dyspepsia in the elderly. Dig Dis Sci. 1995;40:1345–50.
22. Shallcross TM, Heatley RV. Effect of non-steroidal anti-inflammatory drugs on dyspeptic symptoms. Br Med J. 1990;300:368–9.
23. Goggin PM, Collins DA, Jazrawi RP, Jackson PA, Corbishley CM, Bourke BE, Northfield TC. Prevalence of *Helicobacter-pylori* infection and its effect on symptoms and nonsteroidal anti-inflammatory drug-induced gastrointestinal damage in patients with rheumatoid arthritis. Gut. 1993;34:1677–80.
23a. Martin DF, Montgomery E, Dobek AS, Patrissi GA, Peura DA. *Campylobacter pylori*, NSAIDs, and smoking – risk factors for peptic ulcer disease. Am J Gastroenterol. 1989;84:1268–72.
24. Hudson N, Taha AS, Sturrock RD, Russell RI, Hawkey CJ. The influence of *Helicobacter pylori* colonisation of gastroduodenal ulceration in patients of non-steroidal anti-inflammatory drugs. Gut. 1992;33:T165.
25. Safe AF, Warren B, Corfield A, McNulty CA, Watson B, Mountford RA, Read A. *Helicobacter pylori* infection in elderly people – correlation between histology and serology. Age Ageing. 1993;22:215–20.
26. Publig W, Wustinger C, Zandle C. Nonsteroidal antiinflammatory drugs (NSAID) cause gastro-intestinal ulcers mainly in *Helicobacter pylori* carriers. Wiener Klin Wochenschr. 1994;106:276–9.
27. Schubert TT, Bologna SD, Nensey Y, Schubert AB, Mascha EJ, Ma CK. Ulcer risk factors – interactions between *Helicobacter pylori* infection, nonsteroidal use and age. Am J Med. 1993;94:413–18.
28. Kim JG, Graham DY, White DH *et al*. *Helicobacter pylori* infection and development of gastric or duodenal ulcer in arthritic patients receiving chronic NSAID therapy. Am J Gastroenterol. 1994;89:203–7.
29. Alassi MT, Genta RM, Karttunen TJ, Graham DY. Ulcer site and complications – relation to *Helicobacter pylori* infection and NSAID use. Endoscopy. 1996;28:229–33.
30. Cullen DJE, Hawkey GM, Humphries H *et al*. Role of non-steroidal, anti-inflammatory drugs and *Helicobacter pylori* in bleeding peptic ulcer. Gastroenterology. 1994;106:A66.
31. Jensen DM, You S, Pelayo E, Jensen ME, and the CURE Haemostasis Group. The prevalence of *Helicobacter pylori* and NSAID use in patients with severe UGI haemorrhage and their potential role in recurrence of ulcer bleeding. Gastroenterology. 1992;102:A90.
32. Reinbach DH, Cruickshank G, McColl KEL. Acute perforated duodenal-ulcer is not associated with *Helicobacter pylori* infection. Gut. 1993;34:1344–7.
33. Labenz J, Kohl H, Wolters S *et al*. *Helicobacter pylori*, NSAIDs and the risk of peptic ulcer bleeding – a prospective case–control study with matched pairs. Gastroenterology. 1996;110:A165.
34. Bianchi Porro G, Parente F, Imbesi V, Montrone F, Caruso I. Role of *H. pylori* infection in healing and recurrence of NSAID-associated peptic ulcers. Gastroenterology. 1996;110(4):A64.
35. Chan FKL, Sung JY, Leung VKS *et al*. Does eradication of *H. pylori* prevent NSAID-induced ulcers? A prospective randomised study. Gastroenterology. 1996;110:A79.
36. Hawkey CJ, Swannell AJ, Eriksson S *et al*. Benefits of omeprazole over misoprostol in healing NSAID-associated ulcers. Gastroenterology. 1996;110:A131.

37. Hawkey CJ, Swannell AJ, Eriksson S *et al.* Lower frequency of gastroduodenal ulcers and erosions and dyspeptic symptoms in NSAID users during maintenance with omeprazole compared to ranitidine. Gastroenterology. 1996;110:A131.
38. Yeomans ND, Swannell AJ, Eriksson S *et al.* Healing of NSAID-associated gastroduodenal ulcers and erosions: superiority of omeprazole over ranitidine. Gastroenterology. 1996;110:A303.

33
Helicobacter pylori and dyspepsia: a conceptual approach

D. ARMSTRONG and R. H. HUNT

INTRODUCTION

There is now overwhelming evidence that peptic ulcer disease is caused by *Helicobacter pylori* infection of the gastric mucosa, but numerous attempts to implicate *H. pylori* infection in the pathogenesis of dyspeptic symptoms have proved inconclusive. However, most studies have not defined critically the subgroups of dyspepsia, the extent of *H. pylori* gastritis or the strain of infecting organism. Moreover, clinical trial results have been largely equivocal for the same reasons. The absence of conclusive evidence does not, however, invalidate the concept that the inflammatory response to *H. pylori* infection might be associated with the pain syndromes of dyspepsia or disordered antro-pyloro-duodenal motility; the aim of this chapter is to review and present data which support the notion that gastrointestinal function and the perception of gastrointestinal stimuli may be modified by gastrointestinal inflammation produced by *H. pylori* and other gastrointestinal tract infections.

Dyspepsia has been defined, by an International Working Group, as 'persistent or recurrent abdominal pain or abdominal discomfort (a subjective, negative feeling) centred in (*mainly* localized to) the upper abdomen'[1]. Thus, dyspepsia is not a specific disease entity, and different symptom complexes compatible with the above definition may arise as a result of many different disease processes affecting the gastrointestinal tract and pancreaticobiliary system (Table 1). Furthermore, dyspepsia is common, with period prevalences ranging from 19% to 41% in different studies[2]; these differences reflect not only true geographical variations in disease prevalence, but also considerable variations in the definition of dyspepsia[1]. A thorough investigation of dyspepsia patients will reveal a probable cause for the symptoms in only about a half of the cases[3]; the remaining patients are considered to have functional, or non-ulcer dyspepsia. Consequently, an attempt has been made to differentiate dyspepsia into subcategories (Table 2) of ulcer-like, reflux-like and motility-like dyspepsia[4], and this offers some opportunity to study better both mechanisms and the results of therapeutic interventions. However, it should be emphasized that there is no clear explanation for the origin of symp-

Table 1 Dyspepsia – symptomatology

Upper abdominal pain	Vomiting
Upper abdominal discomfort	Upper abdominal bloating
Early satiety	Belching
Postprandial fullness	Anorexia
Nausea	Heartburn
Retching	Regurgitation

Table 2 Non-ulcer dyspepsia subgroups

Ulcer-like
Epigastric pain
    Nocturnal pain
    Relief by food/antacids
    Remitting/relapsing disease

Reflux-like
Heartburn
    Acid regurgitation

Motility-like
Nausea/vomiting
    Early satiety/anorexia
    Postprandial bloating/belching
    Upper abdominal discomfort

toms in patients with documented peptic ulceration; perfusion of an ulcer base with acid reproduces typical symptoms in less than half of the patients[5]; furthermore, recurrent ulcer symptoms do not invariably indicate recurrence of the ulcer[6]. Thus, 'ulcer dyspepsia' may, in some patients, be related to the underlying *H. pylori* infection rather than to the ulcer itself.

This chapter will review currently available data from studies which have examined whether there is direct evidence of a relationship between *H. pylori* and dyspepsia before examining, more generally, data supportive of a relationship between a chronic gastrointestinal infection, the consequent inflammatory response and the generation of gastrointestinal symptoms. Evidence concerning a possible aetiological role for *H. pylori* in dyspepsia has been sought by a number of approaches.

Symptomatology

It has been suggested that *H. pylori* infection is associated more with ulcer-like dyspepsia than with dysmotility-like dyspepsia[7,8] but, despite this, no individual dyspeptic symptom or symptom complex has been associated specifically with *H. pylori* infection[7], gastritis[9] or organic disease[10] and, even when identified, the putative *H. pylori*-related symptoms have differed greatly between study populations (Table 3). Failure to identify a symptom or symptom complex pathognomonic of *H. pylori* infection is further evidence that dyspepsia is not a discrete disease entity. However, it is also true that the symptoms experienced and described by a patient are modulated by many factors including expectations, prior life experiences, ethnic background and concurrent disease or medication; the difficulty

Table 3 Symptoms associated with *H. pylori*-positive functional dyspepsia

Reference	Functional dyspepsia (n)	H. pylori-positive (%)	H. pylori-associated symptom
Marshall and Warren, 1984[11]	65	58	'Burping'
Rokkas *et al.*, 1987[12]	55	45	Postprandial bloating
Andersen *et al.*, 1988[13]	33	39	Nil (symptom duration)
Deltenre *et al.*, 1989[14]	200	64	'Ulcer-like' symptoms
Tucci *et al.*, 1992[15]	45	60	Epigastric pain/burning
Börsch *et al.*, 1988[16]	69	52	Absence of flatulence
Sobala *et al.*, 1990[17]	186	41	Nil
Collins *et al.*, 1991[18]	18	50	Nil
Vaira *et al.*, 1990[19]	107	58	Postprandial bloating
Goh *et al.*, 1991[20]	71	56	Nil
Waldron *et al.*, 1991[21]	50	36	Nil
Strauss *et al.*, 1990[22]	37	60	Nil
Kemmer *et al.*, 1994[23]	149	51	Pain relief after food
Schubert *et al.*, 1992[9]	474	36	Nil
Hovelius *et al.*, 1994[7]	127	35	'Ulcer-like' symptoms

After Talley[111]

assessing subjective symptoms is compounded by the use of many different symptom assessment scales, few of which have been tested for validity[24].

Epidemiology

Epidemiological studies have done little to clarify the relationship between *H. pylori* infection and non-ulcer dyspepsia; in some studies there was no reported difference in *H. pylori* prevalence between dyspeptics and controls whereas, in others, *H. pylori* was more prevalent in asymptomatic controls[25–27]. However, analysis of pooled data from 18 studies[8,12,14,15,22,25–38] suggests that the prevalence of *H. pylori* is, indeed, greater in dyspeptic patients than in controls (Figure 1) with a rate difference of 23% (95% CI 13–32%) and an odds ratio of 2.3 (95% CI 1.9–2.7). This provides some support for the hypothesis that *H. pylori* plays a role in the pathogenesis of dyspepsia despite a number of methodological problems. In particular, the selection of control subjects in many studies did not account for variations in *H. pylori* prevalence related to the subjects' age[34,37,39,40], socioeconomic status[41,42] and ethnic background[43,44].

Interestingly, Parsonnet *et al.*, in a study of 341 epidemiologists who had submitted paired sera, nearly 9 years apart, found that the symptoms of gastritis or upper gastrointestinal pain were associated not with the presence or absence of *H. pylori* antibodies, but rather with positive seroconversion in the interval between the two blood samples[45]. This suggests that *H. pylori* may produce symptoms in the medium term as well as in the short term[11] without necessarily producing chronic dyspepsia.

Pathophysiology

Attempts to implicate specific pathophysiological processes as the cause of *H. pylori* dyspepsia have been few and they have, thus far, met with little success.

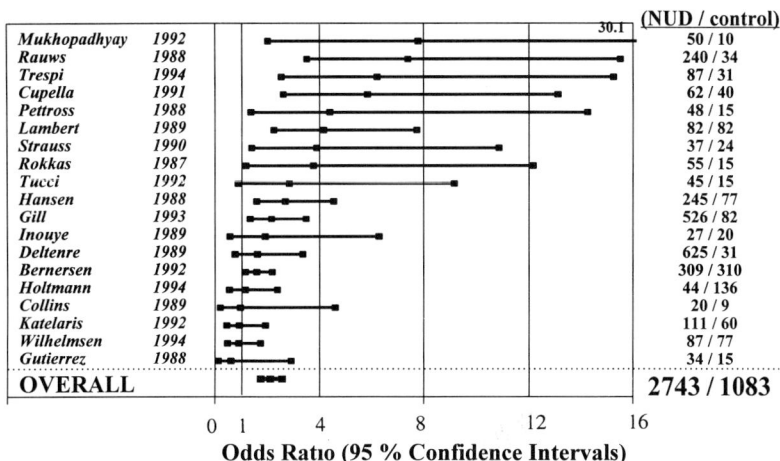

Figure 1 Meta-analysis of *H. pylori* prevalence rates in patients with non-ulcer dyspepsia (NUD) and asymptomatic controls. Overall odds ratios (95% confidence intervals) for the presence of *H. pylori* infection in dyspeptic patients are given along with the odds ratios and number of dyspeptic and control subjects in each study[8,12,14,15,23,25–38]

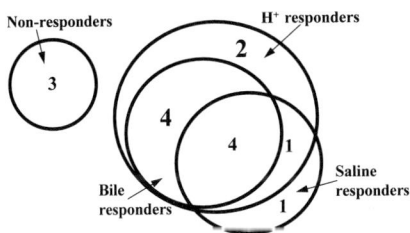

Figure 2 Venn diagram showing the number of *H. pylori*-positive dyspeptic patients who developed symptoms after the instillation of saline, autologous duodenal contents and acid[47]

The role of gastric acidity in the generation of dyspeptic symptoms remains controversial. Tucci *et al.*[15] reported that functional dyspepsia patients had acid outputs comparable to those of healthy controls, regardless of whether or not they had *H. pylori* gastritis, but more recent studies of GRP-stimulated gastric acid secretion[46] suggest that *H. pylori*-positive non-ulcer dyspepsia patients, like duodenal ulcer patients, have a higher acid secretion than *H. pylori*-uninfected subjects. There is, however, no clear indication that *H. pylori* infection renders dyspeptic patients more sensitive to the instillation of acid or autologous duodenal contents into the stomach (Figure 2)[47]. Thus, *H. pylori* infection has not been associated with increased gastric sensitivity to either gastric luminal chemical stimuli or distension[48]. *H. pylori* is, however, associated with failure of antral distension to inhibit pentagastrin-stimulated acid secretion, and cure of the infection produces a normalization of the distension-induced inhibition of acid secretion[49]. Thus, *H. pylori* can modify physiological responses to gastric stimuli, and it is

327

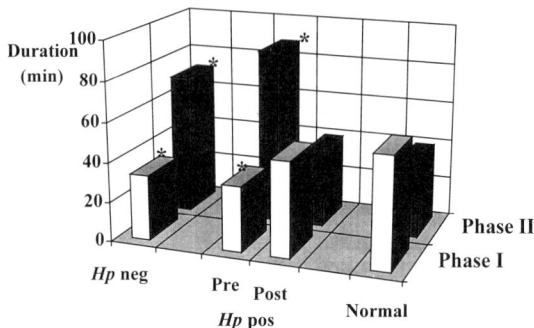

Figure 3 Mean duration of phases I and II of the antral migrating motor complex in six *H. pylori*-negative dyspeptics, 19 *H. pylori*-positive dyspeptics and 25 normal controls; phase I was shorter and phase II longer in both groups of dyspeptics than in controls, but cure of the *H. pylori* infection (*n* = 9) was associated with normalization of the phase durations[58]

conceivable that it may alter the perception of upper gastrointestinal stimuli. The relationship between infection and symptoms is not, however, likely to be simple and clear-cut; dyspeptic subjects are, for example, more sensitive to duodenal distension than are healthy controls, although *H. pylori* infection is not, in itself, associated with a change in duodenal sensitivity[50].

It has long been assumed that dyspepsia is associated, at least in a proportion of subjects, with altered gastrointestinal motility[21,51–53] but there is no clear evidence of any motor abnormality attributable specifically to *H. pylori* infection[15,54–57]. However, in a carefully conducted study, Qvist and colleagues reported that cure of *H. pylori* infection is associated with normalization of MMC activity in *H. pylori*-positive dyspeptic patients[58] (Figure 3). Thus, there may indeed be *H. pylori*-associated changes in upper gastrointestinal sensorimotor function; however, such changes may be obscured by inter-individual variability and they may become evident only if subjects are studied before and after cure of the *H. pylori* infection and resolution of the related inflammatory processes.

Treatment

Surprisingly, despite many trials over the past 10 years, there is still no consensus as to whether cure of *H. pylori* reduces dyspeptic symptoms. The limitations of published therapeutic studies in *H. pylori*-positive functional dyspepsia have been reviewed comprehensively by Talley in a paper which also provides detailed guidelines for the design and conduct of future studies[24]. It should also be noted that dyspeptic symptoms are probably the result of a number of different mechanisms; thus, cure of *H. pylori* would not be expected to render all patients completely symptom-free[24].

In many initial trials, anti-*H. pylori* therapy suppressed the infection without necessarily producing a definitive cure. It is possible that reduction of the bacterial load may have some beneficial effect, since trials which reported an improve-

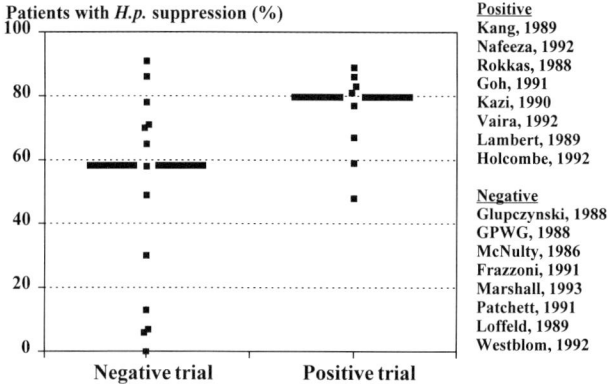

Figure 4 Percentage of dyspeptic patients with suppression of their *H. pylori* infection noted in studies which reported improvement (positive) and no change (negative) in treatment trials for non-ulcer dyspepsia; horizontal bars indicate median values[20,32,59–72]

ment in symptoms were, in general, associated with a greater degree of bacterial suppression than were the negative studies[20,32,59–72] (Figure 4). If, on the other hand, symptoms are due more to the associated gastritis, they may not improve after suboptimal therapy if there is persistent gastritis. Even if the infection is cured, it can take many months for the chronic gastritis to resolve[73], as demonstrated clearly by the persistence of gastric lymphoid follicles in gastric biopsies taken 12 months after cure of *H. pylori* infection[74]. Thus, it is conceivable that *H. pylori*-related symptoms may persist for many months, analogous to the prolonged persistence of symptoms in the post-infectious form of the irritable bowel syndrome[75].

Most therapeutic trials, to date, have evaluated symptom status within 1–2 months of completing treatment, and this may, therefore, have been too soon to assess outcome. A well-designed recent study, with follow-up of patients for 6 months after confirmed cure of *H. pylori* infection, also failed to show a significant effect of *H. pylori* cure compared with placebo[76]. However, the importance of extended follow-up is emphasized by the results of the study reported by Patchett *et al.*[70], in which cure of *H. pylori* was accompanied by decrease in gastritis severity after 4 weeks of therapy, but the improvement in symptoms was comparable, regardless of the change in *H. pylori* or gastritis status. The authors concluded initially that antral infection with *H. pylori* was not an important aetiological factor in non-ulcer dyspepsia. However, when the patients were re-evaluated 11 months later[77] (Figure 5), it was found that dyspepsia symptom scores had decreased further in the *H. pylori*-negative patients while they had risen again, almost to pre-treatment levels, in patients whose infection had not been cured[77]. However, since the patients in this study were not blinded to the outcome of treatment, it is important that double-blind treatment studies of comparable duration be conducted in the future; such studies must also account for the magnitude of the placebo response in dyspepsia[14,70,78] and spontaneous variations in symptom severity[79–81].

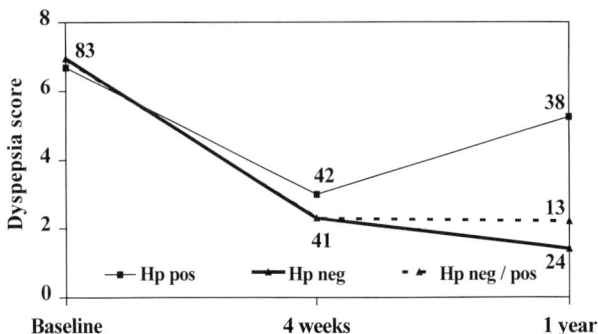

Figure 5 Dyspepsia symptom scores in 83 *H. pylori*-positive patients showing dyspepsia scores at 4 and 52 weeks after treatment for cure of *H. pylori*; scores are analysed based on the cure (thick solid line), persistence (thin solid line) and recurrence of infection (thick dotted line)[77]

CHRONIC GASTRIC INFLAMMATION AND LYMPHOID RESOLUTION

It is well known that *H. pylori* is associated with a chronic gastritis. Lymphoid follicles, which are not seen in the normal healthy stomach, develop during infection with *H. pylori*, and are seen more frequently in the gastric antrum than the corpus. They are also seen more commonly in ulcer patients[74]. Moreover, the number of lymphoid follicles correlates with the apparent density of infection[82]. Eradication of *H. pylori* infection is associated with a reduction in lymphoid follicles, but these do not resolve completely[74].

INFLAMMATION AND A HYPOTHESIS FOR DYSPEPSIA

H. pylori infection is characterized by a chronic active gastritis. This is predominantly a neutrophilic gastritis with a monocytic infiltrate and the development of a follicular lymphoid gastritis as described above. This inflammatory response to *H. pylori* colonization of the gastric epithelium is associated with the release of a repertoire of chemokines and cytokines[83]. Initially, gastric epithelial cells release IL-8 and the interstitial cell adhesion molecule, ICAM-1, which leads to the recruitment of neutrophils to the mucosa[84]. Moreover, the recruitment of neutrophils is *H. pylori* strain-dependent, with type I strains, which are *cagA* and *vacA* positive, producing a more prominent response. The neutrophils secrete further IL-8, responsible for the recruitment of further inflammatory cells which in turn secrete IL-1β, IL-6 and TNFα and there is a strong correlation between the production of IL-8 and IL-1β[83]. However, these authors found no difference in the expression of these cytokines and various *H. pylori*-associated clinical outcomes. IL-1 is also associated with the production of mucosal prostanoids and it is well recognized that PGE1 and PGI sensitize nociceptors. Furthermore, it has been shown that IL-1 increases pain reflexes in a rabbit ear model through an increase in PGE2 levels[85].

Gastric peptides are altered during infection with *H. pylori*. Gastrin levels are universally increased and return to normal after successful eradication of the infection[86]. The mechanism is thought to result from inhibition of the D cell or somatostatin-producing cell which reduces the secretion of somatostatin and hence the endocrine brake on the G cell, which results in uninhibited gastrin secretion[87]. Inhibition of the D cell is thought to be due to the action of TNFα, although this still remains to be proved. To date, few studies have looked at the role of gastric peptides in patients with dyspepsia. McColl and colleagues[46] have shown that patients with *H. pylori* infection, but no ulcer, have a higher gastrin response and also acid secretion than healthy volunteers, but their acid secretion is lower than those with ulcer. Kaneko and colleagues[88,89] studied 56 patients with non-ulcer dyspepsia, 34 of whom had ulcer-like dyspepsia and 22 dysmotility-like dyspepsia, who were compared with 51 controls and 30 peptic ulcer patients. Somatostatin levels were significantly higher in ulcer-like dyspepsia when compared to those with dysmotility-like dyspepsia, those with peptic ulcer disease or the controls. Substance P levels were also higher in the patients with ulcer-like dyspepsia compared to those with peptic ulcer disease, but no changes were seen in levels of calcitonin gene-related peptide.

MECHANISMS OF ALTERED SMOOTH MUSCLE FUNCTION

In a series of studies it has been shown that intestinal smooth muscle function may be deranged by two principal mechanisms; the first due to the inflammatory response and the second due to subsequent antigen stimulation.

INFLAMMATION AND SMOOTH MUSCLE FUNCTION

The inflammatory response in the intestine to infection with *Nippostrongylus brasiliensis* or *Trichinella spiralis* is associated with the expression of chemokines and cytokines[90]. IL-1β is increased in this inflammatory response and this, in turn, has been shown to stimulate further the secretion of IL-1 and also IL-6 and TNFα by intestinal smooth muscle cells, thus amplifying the inflammatory response by further secretion of these mediators of inflammation[91–95]. Further studies have confirmed that the intestinal smooth muscle cell responds to IL-1β, and that this leads to transcription of the IL-6 gene and the secretion of IL-6[95]. Moreover, in these studies the investigators showed that IL-1β stimulated substance P synthesis in myenteric nerves and that IL-1β and IL-6 synergism may result in the suppression of norepinephrine release[95]. Other studies, using the rat TNB colitis model, in which the inflammation is confined to the distal colon, have shown that tritiated nor-adrenaline release is significantly reduced, not only from the damaged area but also from the transverse colon and ileum (Figure 6), both of which were shown to be unaffected by the TNB injury[96].

ANTIGEN-STIMULATED SMOOTH MUSCLE FUNCTION

In a rat model of inflammation with *Trichinella spiralis* or *Nippostrongylus brasiliensis*, acute inflammatory changes are seen in the jejunal smooth muscle

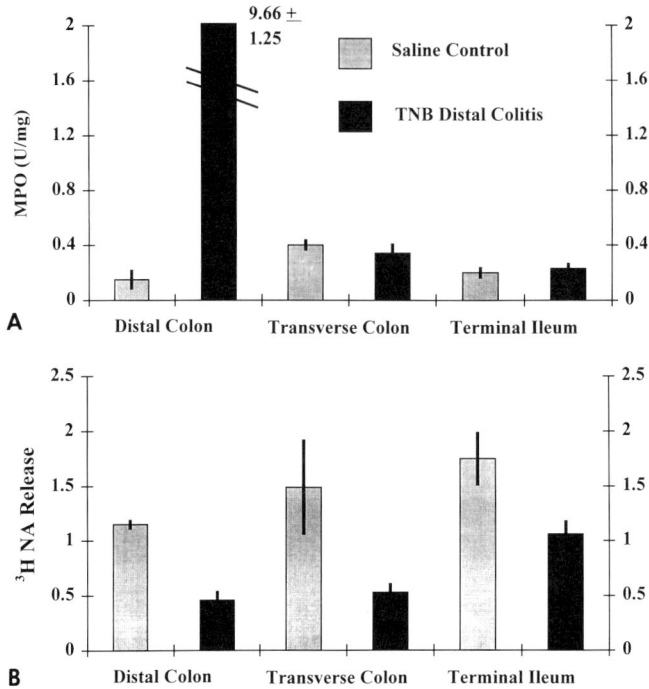

Figure 6 **A**: Myeloperoxidase activity in distal colon, transverse colon and terminal ileum of rats with TNB distal colitis compared with saline-treated control animals. **B**: Potassium chloride-stimulated [³H]nor-adrenaline release from distal colon, transverse colon and terminal ileum of rats with TNB distal colitis, compared with saline-treated controls, showing decreased nor-adrenaline release in areas unaffected directly by the inflammatory response[96]

and are accompanied by changes in muscle function as outlined above. When subjected to antigen-specific stimulation, 1–3 months after acute infection, an increase in mast cells was observed and a positive contractile response in jejunal muscle was reported[97]. Moreover, muscle contraction was inhibited by the mast cell stabilizer, cromoglycate.

Thus, there is evidence from models of intestinal infection that smooth muscle function is altered, and that smooth muscle cells may amplify the inflammatory response by the production of inflammatory mediators. In addition, these mediators may alter myenteric nerve function and this may occur at sites in the gastro-intestinal (GI) tract which are different from the site of initial inflammation. The evidence from studies of antigen stimulus is conceptually important, since it indicates that patients may become sensitized to luminal antigens in the GI tract, and this may be more likely if macromolecular permeability is increased[98,99].

Under normal circumstances the gastric mucosa presents a tight epithelium. This might be expected to be altered in the presence of *H. pylori* infection. One study has shown that *H. pylori* infection is associated with an apparently normal permeability to sucrose; however, permeability fell by about 50%, still within the normal range (Figure 7), when the infection was successfully eradicated[100]. Clearly, further studies are needed to examine this process in greater detail.

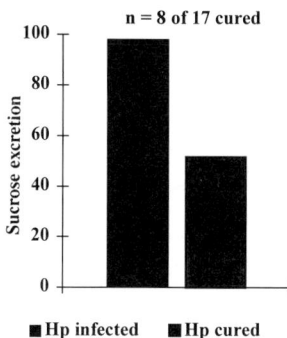

Figure 7 Urinary sucrose excretion after administration of oral sucrose in 17 subjects before cure of *H. pylori* infection; cure of the infection produced a significant fall in sucrose excretion indicative of decreased gastric permeability[100]

NEURAL AND CENTRAL NERVOUS SYSTEM MECHANISMS OF DYSPEPSIA

A number of possible mechanisms involving the enteric nervous system and the central nervous system may be disordered in patients with dyspepsia, and several of these may be associated with *H. pylori* infection.

Modification of afferent signalling might occur as a result of inflammation due to *H. pylori* infection. The stimulus–response curve to bladder distension is shifted by the presence of bladder inflammation, and there is evidence for the recruitment of new afferent fibres[101,102].

The release of cytokines due to mucosal inflammation in *H. pylori* infection can lead to the release of IL-1β, which has been shown to excite neurons, and increase pain perception by the release of mucosal prostanoids[85]. The alteration of nor-adrenaline release in models of intestinal inflammation may be due to alterations in cytokines in the mucosa[95]. The release of neuropeptides such as somatostatin and substance P may also lead to changes in myenteric nerve function. Lastly, there is evidence in *H. pylori* infection for remodelling of mucosal nerves as a consequence of the inflammatory process where there is a decrease in PGP 9.5 immunoreactive nerves[103].

As a consequence of altered afferent stimulation or perception, central perception may be altered and lead to altered efferent output, resulting in abnormal stimulation of the GI tract (Figure 8). Studies of the afferent and efferent gut–brain–gut connections are in their infancy, but sophisticated methods are becoming increasingly available[104–107].

It is also possible that conditioning may play an important role in patients with dyspepsia. In the study reported by Parsonnet *et al.*[45] of GI symptoms which were related to *H. pylori* seropositivity at two time-points on average 8.5 years apart, serological reactors (*H. pylori*-positive) were not significantly different from non-reactors (*H. pylori*-negative) with respect to gastritis symptoms or upper GI tract pain, but converters who were initially *H. pylori*-negative and subsequently became positive reported significantly more gastritis and upper GI tract pain (Figure 9). It is interesting to speculate that symptoms were more pronounced in

333

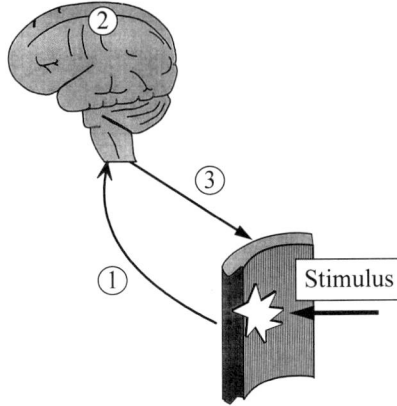

Figure 8 Neural mechanisms whereby the perception of a gastric stimulus may be modified: (1) recruitment of previously 'silent' C fibres which fire in response to mechanical stimulus[101,102]; (2) psychological status related to development of functional bowel disease[75]; (3) efferent autonomic neural abnormalities related to response to upper gastrointestinal stimuli[105]

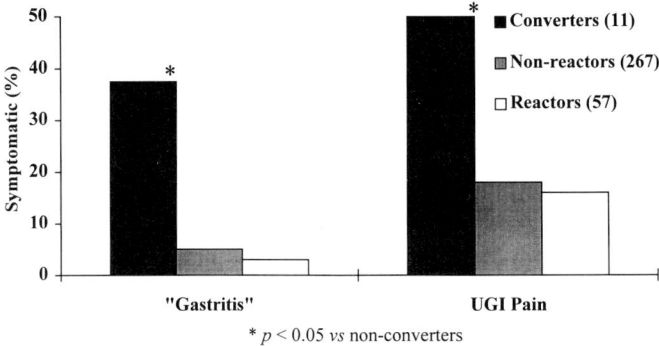

* *p* < 0.05 *vs* non-converters

Figure 9 Percentage of epidemiologists with dyspeptic symptoms: symptoms of 'gastritis' and 'upper gastrointestinal pain' were significantly more prevalent in subjects who had seroconverted from *H. pylori*-negative to *H. pylori*-positive ('Converters') than in subjects who were seronegative ('Non-reactors') or seropositive ('Reactors') on both test occasions[45]

those who acquired their infection subsequent to the maturation of their GI tract and that, perhaps, in those who became infected early in life, their upper GI tract circuitry adapted to the infection during development.

CONCLUSION

H. pylori infection is common in patients with dyspepsia. Currently published studies to determine a possible relationship between *H. pylori* and dyspepsia have serious limitations, and better design with careful stratification of patient subgroups is necessary for future studies. It is clear that inflammation of the GI tract is associated with myenteric nerve and smooth muscle dysfunction, which may occur at sites distant from the inflammation. Mechanistic studies are required to determine the possible relationship of the inflammatory process which occurs in *H. pylori* gastritis to alterations in the function of the antro-pyloro-duodenal segment. Our knowledge of the mechanisms underlying the generation of visceral symptoms is rudimentary. Dysmotility, defined by abnormal transit studies or manometric findings, does not seem to be a major factor, but there is good reason to suppose that a chronic inflammatory process affecting the gastric mucosa might alter enteric neuromuscular function[108] or afferent[109] and efferent signalling in response to normal stimuli[110] as a basis for the production of visceral symptoms. *H. pylori* is, for example, associated with an increased production of neuropeptides such as somatostatin and substance P, particularly in ulcer-like dyspepsia[89]. There is also increased production of the cytokines TNFα, IL-8 and IL-1β in both non-ulcer dyspepsia and ulcer disease[83]; IL-1β has been shown to increase enteric neural sensitivity[85].

Overall, epidemiological studies suggest that *H. pylori* is more prevalent in subjects with dyspepsia than in asymptomatic controls. Despite problems with the selection of control groups, these data cannot be dismissed lightly. As with therapeutic trials, it is important that future studies be meticulous in the choice of controls[111]. Furthermore, both types of study will need to account for differences in host response and *H. pylori* virulence.

References

1. Talley NJ, Colin-Jones D, Koch KL, Koch M, Nyrén O, Stanghellini V. Functional dyspepsia: a classification with guidelines for management. Gastroenterol Int. 1991;4:145–60.
2. Knill-Jones RP. Geographical difference in the prevalence of dyspepsia. Scand J Gastroenterol. 1991;26(Suppl. 182):17–24.
3. Thompson WG. Non-ulcer dyspepsia. Can Med Assoc J. 1984;130:565–9.
4. Colin-Jones DG. Management of dyspepsia: report of a Working Party. Lancet. 1988;1:576–9.
5. Kang JY, Jap I, Guan R, Tay HH. Acid perfusion of duodenal ulcer craters and ulcer pain: a controlled double-blind study. Gut. 1986;27:942–5.
6. Armstrong D, Arnold R, Classen M *et al.* and the RUDER Study Group. RUDER – a prospective, two-year multicentre study of risk factors for duodenal ulcer relapse during maintenance therapy with ranitidine. Dig Dis Sci. 1994;39:1425–33.
7. Hovelius B, Andersson SI, Hagander B *et al.* Dyspepsia in general practice: history and symptoms in relation to *Helicobacter pylori* serum antibodies. Scand J Gastroenterol. 1994;29: 506–10.
8. Trespi E, Broglia F, Villani L, Luinetti O, Fiocca R, Solcia E. Distinct profiles of gastritis in dyspepsia subgroups. Their different clinical responses to gastritis healing after *Helicobacter pylori* eradication. Scand J Gastroenterol. 1994;29:884–8.
9. Schubert TT, Schubert AB, Ma CK. Symptoms, gastritis, and *Helicobacter pylori* in patients referred for endoscopy. Gastrointest Endosc. 1992;38:357–60.
10. Talley NJ, Weaver AL, Tesmer DL, Zinsmeister AR. Lack of discriminant value of dyspepsia subgroups in patients referred for upper endoscopy. Gastroenterology. 1993;105:1378–86.
11. Marshall BJ, Warren JR. Unidentified curved bacilli in the stomach of patients with gastritis and peptic ulceration. Lancet. 1984;1:1311–15.
12. Rokkas T, Pursey C, Uzoechina E *et al.* *Campylobacter pylori* and non-ulcer dyspepsia. Am J Gastroenterol. 1987;82:1149–52.
13. Andersen LP, Elsborg L, Justesen T. *Campylobacter pylori* in peptic ulcer disease. III. Symptoms and paraclinical and epidemiological findings. Scand J Gastroenterol. 1988;23:344–50.
14. Deltenre M, Nyst J-F, Jonas C, Glupczynski Y, Deprez C, Burette A. Données cliniques, endoscopiques et histologiques chez 1100 patients dont 574 colonisés par *Campylobacter pylori*. Gastroenterol Clin Biol. 1989;13:89–95B.

15. Tucci A, Corinaldesi R, Stanghellini V *et al. Helicobacter pylori* infection and gastric function in patients with chronic idiopathic dyspepsia. Gastroenterology. 1992;103:768–74.
16. Börsch G, Schmidt G, Wegener M. *Campylobacter pylori:* prospective analysis of clinical and histological factors associated with colonization of the upper gastrointestinal tract. Eur J Clin Invest. 1988;133–8.
17. Sobala GM, Dixon MF, Axon ATR. Symptomatology of *Helicobacter-*associated dyspepsia. Eur J Gastroenterol Hepatol. 1990;2:445–9.
18. Collins JSA, Knill-Jones RP, Sloan JM. A comparison of symptoms between non-ulcer dyspepsia patients positive and negative for *Helicobacter pylori.* Ulster Med J. 1991;60:21–7.
19. Vaira D, Holton J, Osborn J. Endoscopy in dyspeptic patients: is gastric mucosal biopsy useful? Am J Gastroenterol. 1990;85:701–4.
20. Goh KL, Parasakthi N, Peh SC, Wong NW, Lo YL, Puthucheary SD. *Helicobacter pylori* infection and non-ulcer dyspepsia: the effect of treatment with colloidal bismuth subcitrate. Scand J Gastro-enterol. 1991;26:1123–31.
21. Waldron B, Cullen PT, Kumar R. Evidence for hypomotility in non-ulcer dyspepsia: a prospective multifactorial study. Gut. 1991;32:246–51.
22. Strauss RM, Wang TC, Kelsey PB *et al.* Association of *Helicobacter pylori* infection with dyspeptic symptoms in patients undergoing gastroduodenoscopy. Am J Med. 1990;89:464–9.
23. Kemmer TP, Domingo-Munoz JE, Klingel H, Zemmler T, Kuhn K, Malfertheiner P. The association between non-ulcer dyspepsia and *Helicobacter pylori* infection. Eur J Gastroenterol Hepatol. 1994;6:571–7.
24. Talley NJ. A critique of therapeutic trials in *Helicobacter pylori-*positive functional dyspepsia. Gastroenterology. 1994;106:1174–83.
25. Collins JSA, Hamilton PW, Watt PCH, Sloan JM, Love AHG. Superficial gastritis and *Campylobacter pylori* in dyspeptic patients – a quantitative study using computer-linked image analysis. J Pathol. 1989;158:303–10.
26. Gutiérrez D, Sierra F, Gomez MC, Camargo H. *Campylobacter pylori* in chronic environmental gastritis and duodenal ulcer patients. Gastroenterology. 1988;94:A163(abstract).
27. Wilhelmsen I, Tangen Haug T, Sipponen P, Berstad A. *Helicobacter pylori* in functional dyspepsia and normal controls. Scand J Gastroenterol. 1994;29:522–7.
28. Mukhopadhyay DK, Tandon RK, Dasarathy S, Mathur M, Wali JP. A study of *Helicobacter pylori* in North Indian subjects with non-ulcer dyspepsia. Indian J Gastroenterol. 1992;11:76–9.
29. Rauws EAJ, Langenberg W, Houthoff HJ, Zanen HC, Tytgat GNJ. *Campylobacter pyloridis-*associated chronic active antral gastritis. A prospective study of its prevalence and the effects of antibacterial and antiulcer treatment. Gastroenterology. 1988;94:33–40.
30. Cupella F, Alessio I, Intropido L, Pozzi V, Einaudi E, Possi U. Dispepsia ed infezione da *Helicobacter pylori.* Studio su una popolazione di lavatori. G Ital Med Lav. 1991;31:81–4.
31. Pettross CW, Appleman MD, Cohen H, Valenzuela JE, Chandrasoma P, Laine LA. Prevalence of *Campylobacter pylori* and association with antral mucosal histology in subjects with and without upper gastrointestinal symptoms. Dig Dis Sci. 1988;33:649–53.
32. Lambert JR, Dunn K, Borromeo M, Korman MG, Hansky J. *Campylobacter pylori* – a role in non-ulcer dyspepsia? Scand J Gastroenterol. 1989;24(Suppl. 160):7–13.
33. Hansen IM, Axelsson CK, Lundborg CJ. Distribution of *Campylobacter pylori* in dyspeptic and non-dyspeptic gastroenterologic patients. Dan Med Bull. 1988;35:282–5.
34. Gill HH, Desai HG, Majmudar P, Mehta PR, Prabhu SR. Epidemiology of *Helicobacter pylori:* the Indian scenario. Indian J Gastroenterol. 1993;12:9–11.
35. Inouye H, Yamamoto I, Tanida N. *Campylobacter pylori* in Japan: bacteriological features and prevalence in healthy subjects and patients with gastroduodenal disorders. Gastroenterol Jpn. 1989;24:494–504.
36. Bernersen B, Johnsen R, Bostad L, Straume B, Sommer A-I, Burhol PG. Is *Helicobacter pylori* the cause of dyspepsia? Br Med J. 1992;304:1276–9.
37. Holtmann G, Goebell H, Holtmann M, Talley NJ. Dyspepsia in healthy blood donors: pattern of symptoms and association with *Helicobacter pylori.* Dig Dis Sci. 1994;39:1090–8.
38. Katelaris PH, Tippett GHK, Norbu P, Lowe DG, Brennan R, Farthing MJG. Dyspepsia, *Helico-bacter pylori* and peptic ulcer in a randomly selected population in India. Gut. 1992;33:1462–6.
39. Greenberg RE, Bank S. The prevalence of *Helicobacter pylori* in nonulcer dyspepsia. Importance of stratification according to age. Arch Intern Med. 1990;150:2053–5.
40. Al-Moagel MA, Evans DG, Abdulghani ME *et al.* Prevalence of *Helicobacter* (formerly

Campylobacter) *pylori* infection in Saudi Arabia and comparison of those with and without upper gastrointestinal symptoms. Am J Gastroenterol. 1990;85:944–8.

41. Graham DY, Malaty HM, Evans DG, Evans DE, Klein PD, Adam E. Epidemiology of *Helicobacter pylori* in an asymptomatic population in the United States. Effect of age, race, and socioeconomic status. Gastroenterology. 1991;100:1495–501.

42. Mendall MA, Goggin PM, Molineaux N *et al.* Childhood living conditions and *Helicobacter* seropositivity in adult life. Lancet. 1992;339:896–7.

43. Uyub AM, Raj SM, Visvanathan R, Nazim M, Aiyar S, Anuar AK. *Helicobacter pylori* infection in north-eastern Peninsular Malaysia. Evidence for an unusually low prevalence. Scand J Gastroenterol. 1994;29:209–13.

44. Kang JY, Wee A, Math MV *et al.* *Helicobacter pylori* and gastritis in patients with peptic ulcer and non-ulcer dyspepsia: ethnic differences in Singapore. Gut. 1990;31:850–3.

45. Parsonnet J, Blaser MJ, Perez-Perez I, Hargrett-Bean N, Tauxe RV. Symptoms and risk factors of *Helicobacter pylori* infection in a cohort of epidemiologists. Gastroenterology. 1992;102:41–6.

46. El-Omar E, Penman ID, Ardill JES, McColl KEL. A substantial proportion of non-ulcer dyspepsia patients have the same abnormality of acid secretion as duodenal ulcer patients. Gut. 1995;36:534–8.

47. George AA, Tsuchiyose M, Dooley CP. Sensitivity of the gastric mucosa to acid and duodenal contents in patients with non-ulcer dyspepsia. Gastroenterology. 1991;101:3–6.

48. Mearin F, de Ribot X, Bartolomé R, Malagelada J-R. Does *Helicobacter pylori* gastritis increase perception of gastric accommodation in functional dyspepsia? Gastroenterology. 1993;104:A550.

49. Olbe L, Hamlet A, Dalenbäck J, Fändriks L. A mechanism by which *Helicobacter pylori* infection of the antrum contributes to the development of duodenal ulcer. Gastroenterology. 1996;110:1386–94.

50. Holtmann G, Goebell H, Hüber J, Talley NJ. *H. pylori* and sensory dysfunction in patients with functional dyspepsia and healthy controls. Gastroenterology. 1995;108:A615 (abstract).

51. Malagelada J-R, Stanghellini V. Manometric evaluation of functional upper gut symptoms. Gastroenterology. 1985;88:1223–31.

52. Camilleri M, Malagelada J-R, Kao PC *et al.* Gastric and autonomic responses to stress in functional dyspepsia. Dig Dis Sci. 1986;31:1169–77.

53. Kerlin P. Postprandial hypomotility in patients with idiopathic nausea and vomiting. Gut. 1989;30:54–9.

54. Scott AM, Kellow JE, Shuter B *et al.* Intragastric distribution and gastric emptying of solids and liquids in functional dyspepsia. Lack of influence of symptom subgroups and *H. pylori*-associated gastritis. Dig Dis Sci. 1993;38:2247–54.

55. Wegener M, Börsch G, Schaffstein J, Schulz-Flake C, Mai U, Leverkus F. Are dyspeptic symptoms in patients with *Campylobacter pylori*-associated Type B gastritis linked to delayed gastric emptying? Am J Gastroenterol. 1988;83:737–40.

56. Minocha A, Mokshagundam S, Gallo SH, Rahal PS. Alterations in upper gastrointestinal motility in *Helicobacter pylori*-positive nonulcer dyspepsia. Am J Gastroenterol. 1994;89:1797–800.

57. Pieramico O, Ditschuneit H, Malfertheiner P. Gastrointestinal motility in patients with non-ulcer dyspepsia: a role for *Helicobacter pylori* infection? Am J Gastroenterol. 1993;88:364–8.

58. Qvist N, Rasmussen L, Axelsson CK. *Helicobacter pylori*-associated gastritis and dyspepsia. The influence on migrating motor complexes. Scand J Gastroenterol. 1994;29:133–7.

59. Rokkas T, Pursey C, Uzoechina E *et al.* Non-ulcer dyspepsia and short-term De-Nol therapy: a placebo-controlled trial with particular reference to the role of *Campylobacter pylori*. Gut. 1988;29:1386–91.

60. Kang JY, Tay HH, Wee A, Guan R, Math MV, Yap I. Effect of colloidal bismuth subcitrate on symptoms and gastric histology in non-ulcer dyspepsia. A double blind placebo controlled study. Gut. 1990;31:476–80.

61. Nafeeza MI, Shahimi MM, Kudva MV *et al.* Evaluation of therapies in the treatment of *Helicobacter pylori* associated non-ulcer dyspepsia. Singapore Med J. 1992;33:570–4.

62. Kazi JI, Jafarey NA, Alam SM *et al.* A placebo-controlled trial of bismuth salicylate in *Helicobacter pylori* associated gastritis. JPMA. 1990;40:154–6.

63. Vaira D, Holton J, Ainley C *et al.* Double blind trial of colloidal bismuth subcitrate versus placebo in *Helicobacter pylori* positive patients with non-ulcer dyspepsia. Ital J Gastroenterol. 1992;24:400–4.

64. Holcombe C, Thom C, Galuba J, Lucas SB. *Helicobacter pylori* clearance in the treatment of non-ulcer dyspepsia. Aliment Pharmacol Ther. 1992;6:119–23.

65. Glupczynski Y, Burette A, Labbe M, Deprez A, De Reuck M, Deltenre M. *Campylobacter pylori*-associated gastritis: a double-blind placebo-controlled trial with amoxycillin. Am J Gastroenterol. 1988;83:365–72.

66. The Gastrointestinal Physiology Working Group of Cayetano Heredia and the Johns Hopkins University, Morgan D, Kraft W, Bender M, Pearson A. Nitrofurans in the treatment of gastritis associated with *Campylobacter pylori*. Gastroenterology. 1988;95:1178–84.

67. McNulty CMA, Gearty JC, Crump B *et al*. *Campylobacter pyloridis* and associated gastritis: investigator blind, placebo-controlled trial of bismuth salicylate and erythromycin ethylsuccinate. Br Med J. 1986;293:645–9.

68. Frazzoni M, Lonardo A, Grisendi A *et al*. Are routine duodenal and antral biopsies useful in the management of 'functional' dyspepsia? A diagnostic and therapeutic study. J Clin Gastroenterol. 1993;17:101–8.

69. Marshall BJ, Valenzuela JE, McCallum RW *et al*. Bismuth subsalicylate suppression of *Helicobacter pylori* in nonulcer dyspepsia: a double-blind placebo-controlled trial. Dig Dis Sci. 1993;38:1674–80.

70. Patchett S, Beattie S, Leen E, Keane C, O'Morain C. Eradicating *Helicobacter pylori* and symptoms of non-ulcer dyspepsia. Br Med J. 1991;303:1238–40.

71. Loffeld RJLF, Potters HVJP, Stobberingh E, Flendrig JA, van Spreeuwel JP, Arends JW. *Campylobacter*-associated gastritis in patients with non-ulcer dyspepsia: a double blind placebo controlled trial with colloidal bismuth subcitrate. Gut. 1989;30:1206–12.

72. Westblom TU, Madan E, Subik MA, Duriex DE, Midkiff BR. Double-blind randomized trial of bismuth subsalicylate and clindamycin for treatment of *Helicobacter pylori* infection. Scand J Gastroenterol. 1992;27:249–52.

73. Valle J, Seppala K, Sipponen O, Kosumen T. Disappearance of gastritis after eradication of *Helicobacter pylori*: a morphometric study. Scand J Gastroenterol. 1991;26:1057–65.

74. Genta RM, Hamner HW, Graham DY. Gastric lymphoid follicles in *Helicobacter pylori* infection: frequency, distribution, and response to triple therapy. Human Pathol. 1993;24:577–83.

75. Gwee KA, Graham JC, McKendrick MW *et al*. Psychometric scores and persistence of irritable bowel after infectious diarrhoea. Lancet. 1996;347:150–3.

76. Veldhuyzen van Zanten S, Malatjalian D, Tanton R *et al*. The effect of eradication of *Helicobacter pylori* on symptoms of non-ulcer dyspepsia: a randomized, double-blind, placebo-controlled trial. Gastroenterology. 1995;108:A250.

77. McCarthy C, Patchett S, Collins RM, Beattie S, Keane C, O'Morain C. Long-term prospective study of *Helicobacter pylori* in nonulcer dyspepsia. Dig Dis Sci. 1995;40:114–19.

78. Elta GH, Murphy R, Behler EM *et al*. *Campylobacter pylori* in patients with dyspeptic symptoms and endoscopic evidence of erosions. Am J Gastroenterol. 1989;84:643–6.

79. Jones RH, Lydeard SE, Hobbs FDR *et al*. Dyspepsia in England and Scotland. Gut. 1990;31;401–5.

80. Talley NJ, McNeil D, Hayden A, Colreavy C, Piper DW. Prognosis of chronic unexplained dyspepsia. A prospective study of potential predictor variables in patients with endoscopically diagnosed nonulcer dyspepsia. Gastroenterology. 1987;92:1060–6.

81. Talley NJ, Weaver AL, Zinsmeister AR, Melton LJ III. Onset and disappearance of gastrointestinal symptoms and functional gastrointestinal disorders. Am J Epidemiol. 1992;136:165–77.

82. Eidt S, Stolte M. Prevalence of lymphoid follicles and aggregates in *Helicobacter pylori* gastritis in antral and body mucosa. J Clin Pathol. 1993;46:832–5.

83. Noach LA, Bosma NM, Jansen J, Hoek FJ, van Deventer SJH, Tytgat GNJ. Mucosal tumour necrosis factor-a, interleukin-1b, and interleukin-8 production in patients with *Helicobacter pylori* infection. Scand J Gastroenterol. 1994;29:425–9.

84. Crowe SE, Alvarez L, Dytoc M *et al*. Expression of interleukin 8 and CD54 by human gastric epithelium after *Helicobacter pylori* infection *in vitro*. Gastroenterology. 1995;108:65–74.

85. Schweizer A, Feige U, Fontana A, Muller K, Dinarello CA. Interleukin-1 enhances pain reflexes. Mediation through increased prostaglandin E2 levels. Agents Actions. 1988;25:246–51.

86. Levi S, Beardshall K, Swift I *et al*. Antral *Helicobacter pylori*, hypergastrinaemia and duodenal ulcers: effect of eradicating the organism. Br Med J. 1989;299:1504–5.

87. Moss SF, Legon S, Bishop AE, Polak JM, Calam J. Effect of *Helicobacter pylori* on gastric somatostatin in duodenal ulcer disease. Lancet. 1992;340:930–3.

88. Kaneko H, Mitsuma T, Fujii S, Uchida K, Kotera H, Furusawa A, Morise K. Immunoreactive-somatostatin concentrations of the human stomach and mood state in patients with functional dyspepsia: a preliminary case–control study. J Gastroenterol Hepatol. 1993;8:322–7.
89. Kaneko H, Mitsuma T, Uchida K, Furusawa A, Morise K. Immunoreactive-somatostatin, substance P, and calcitonin gene-related peptide concentrations of the human gastric mucosa in patients with nonulcer dyspepsia and peptic ulcer disease. Am J Gastroenterol. 1993;88: 898–904.
90. Collins SM, Hurst SM, Main C *et al.* Effect of inflammation of enteric nerves. Cytokine-induced changes in neurotransmitter content and release. [Review]. Ann NY Acad Sci. 1992; 664:415–24.
91. Hurst SM, Stanisz AM, Sharkey KA, Collins SM. Interleukin 1 beta-induced increase in substance P in rat myenteric plexus. Gastroenterology. 1993;105:1754–60.
92. Hurst SM, Collins SM. Interleukin-1 beta modulation of norepinephrine release from rat myenteric nerves. Am J Physiol. 1993;264:G30–5.
93. Hurst SM, Collins SM. Mechanism underlying tumor necrosis factor-alpha suppression of norepinephrine release from rat myenteric plexus. Am J Physiol. 1994;266:G1123–9.
94. Khan I, Collins SM. Expression of cytokines in the longitudinal muscle myenteric plexus of the inflamed intestine of rat. Gastroenterology. 1994;107:691–700.
95. Khan I, Blennerhassett MG, Kataeva GV, Collins SM. Interleukin 1 beta induces the expression of interleukin 6 in rat intestinal smooth muscle cells. Gastroenterology. 1995;107:1720–8.
96. Jacobson K, McHugh K, Collins SM. Experimental colitis alters myenteric nerve function at inflamed and noninflamed sites in the rat. Gastroenterology. 1995;109:718–22.
97. Vermillion DL, Ernst PB, Scicchitano R, Collins SM. Antigen-induced contraction of jejunal smooth muscle in the sensitized rat. Am J Physiol. 1988;255:G701–8.
98. Perdue MH, Kosecka U, Crowe S. Antigen-mediated effects on epithelial function. [Review]. Ann NY Acad Sci. 1992;664:325–34.
99. Crowe SE, Soda K, Stanisz AM, Perdue MH. Intestinal permeability in allergic rats: nerve involvement in antigen-induced changes. Am J Physiol. 1993;264:G617–23.
100. Graham DY, Malaty HM, Goodgame R, Ou CN. Effect of cure of *H. pylori* infection on the gastric mucosal permeability. Gastroenterology. 1996;110:A122.
101. McMahon SB, Koltzenburg M. The changing role of primary afferent neurons in pain. Pain. 1990;43:269–72.
102. McMahon SB, Koltzenburg M. Changes in the afferent innervation of the inflamed urinary bladder. In: Mayer EA, Raybould HE, editors. Basic and clinical aspects of chronic abdominal pain. Amsterdam: Elsevier; 1993:155–72.
103. Stead RH, Hewlett BR, Lhotak S, Colley ECC, Frendo M, Dixon MF, Do gastric mucosal nerves remodel in *H. pylori* gastritis? In: Hunt RH, Tytgat GNJ, editors. *Helicobacter pylori*: basic mechanisms to clinical cure. Dordrecht: Kluwer; 1994:281–91.
104. Tougas G, Hudoba P, Fitzpatrick D, Hunt RH, Upton AR. Cerebral-evoked potential responses following direct vagal and esophageal electrical stimulation in humans. Am J Physiol. 1993; 264:G486–91.
105. Spaziani RM, Djuric V, Kamath MV *et al.* A low resting vagal tone predicts response to acid perfusion in patients with esophageal symptoms. Gastroenterology. 1996;110:A762.
106. Hollerbach S, Kamath MV, Chen Y, Fitzpatrick D, Upton ARM, Tougas G. The amplitude of the cerebral evoked response to electrical stimulation of the esophagus is intensity-dependent. A dose–response study. Gastroenterology. 1996;110:A679.
107. Armstrong D, Spaziani RM, Fallen EL, Kamath MV, Collins SM, Tougas G. Barostat-controlled esophageal balloon distension produces a pressure-dependent heart rate decrease in healthy subjects. Gastroenterology. 1996;110:A624.
108. Collins SM. Gastritis and altered motility: the ability of a mucosal inflammatory reaction to alter enteric nerve and smooth muscle in the gut. In: Malfertheiner P, Ditschuneit H, editors. *Helicobacter pylori*, gastritis and peptic ulcer. Berlin: Springer Verlag; 1990:370–4.
109. Mearin F, Cucala M, Azpiroz F, Malagelada J-R. The origin of symptoms on the brain–gut axis in functional dyspepsia. Gastroenterology. 1991;101:999–1006.
110. Mayer EA. The sensitive and reactive gut. Eur J Gastroenterol Hepatol. 1994;6:470–7.
111. Talley NJ. Functional dyspepsia and *H. pylori*: a controversial link. In: Hunt RH, Tytgat GNJ, editors. *Helicobacter pylori*: basic mechanisms to clinical cure. Dordrecht: Kluwer; 1994: 437–48.

34
Aspects of anti-*Helicobacter pylori* eradication therapy

G. N. J. TYTGAT

INTRODUCTION

The flood of data related to *H. pylori* eradication continues to appear, and further fuels the level of confusion about the choice of treatment, not only in the primary-care setting but also in referral centres. Many studies contribute to confusion because they lack power, because they fail to register primary or secondary resistance; because they fail to provide data 'per protocol' or 'intention to treat' or 'all patients treated' analysis; because they fail to monitor side-effect profiles but above all because they lack state-of-the-art monitoring of antimicrobial efficacy.

The purpose of this overview is to attempt to simplify the issue and to provide guidelines for therapy. Simplification is possible if one accepts the following presumptions: anti-*H. pylori* therapy should last no longer than 7 days, should be universally acceptable and guarantee a cure rate of around or above 90%, should induce a minimal incidence of antimicrobial resistance and a frequency of severe side-effects of less than 5%. In addition to antimicrobial recommendations, several aspects of current treatment modalities will be discussed, thereby hoping to improve the level of knowledge of the practising physician.

THE KEY ANTIMICROBIAL AGENTS CURRENTLY USED

The list of the key antimicrobial agents in current use has not changed recently and has been covered extensively in prior publications[1-4]. The list includes: bismuth salts (BIS) (colloidal bismuth subcitrate, bismuth subsalicylate), tetracycline (TET), metronidazole/tinidazole (MET), amoxycillin (AMO), clarithromycin (CLA) and proton pump inhibitors (PPI). Newer antimicrobials include ranitidine bismuth citrate (RBC) and azithromycin (AZI)[5].

Azithromycin (AZI) is a new acid-stable macrolide that achieves 10- to 40-fold higher tissue levels than erythromycin after oral dosing. The MIC_{90} for *H. pylori* is less than 1 mg/L. AZI has a long half-life in tissue. After a single 500 mg dose, AZI remains detectable at >2 mg/g gastric tissue for at least 5 days[6].

Table 1 *H. pylori*: possible mode of action of PPI therapy

Competition from overgrowing microorganisms
Autotoxicity from unbuffered ammonia
Direct antimicrobial effect
Synergy with other antimicrobials
Increased topical concentration of antimicrobials; lower gastric juice viscosity
Optimizing antimicrobial efficacy through enhanced pH
Prolonged topical contact through delayed gastric emptying
Enhanced bioavailability of CLA
Strong anti-urease effect
Effect on bacterial metabolism ($\downarrow$ urease production?) ($\downarrow$ ATP-ase activity?)
Effect on host immunity ($\downarrow$ Ig breakdown. improved PMN function)
Combinations of the above

MECHANISMS OF ACTION OF PPI

It is still unknown whether PPI only act *in vivo* through acid inhibition or whether there is a direct additive or synergistic antimicrobial effect (Table 1). PPI (omeprazole, lansoprazole, pantoprazole) potently decrease acid secretory capacity by inhibiting the H^+,K^+-ATPase of gastric parietal cells. *In vitro*, PPI also inhibit *H. pylori* survival at a neutral pH[7,8] and attenuate the ability of survival at acid pH[9]. The MIC values of lansoprazole are lower than for omeprazole; in addition, PPI may inhibit the urease activity of the organism[8].

The precise mode of action of PPI against *H. pylori in vivo* remains obscure.

1. It is not known whether PPI achieve significant levels within the gastric mucus layer to exert a direct antimicrobial effect. If a sufficient concentration can be reached, then PPI might have an intrinsic antimicrobial activity.
2. More important is the fact that the effectiveness of many antibiotics is enhanced at or near neutral pH. PPI are potent antisecretory drugs. A more neutral milieu in the stomach decreases the MIC_{90} of AMO, presumably prolongs intragastric stability and results in a higher concentration because of a reduced gastric volume[1]. Also for CLA the MIC falls from 10 mg/L at pH 5.5 to 0.3 at pH 6.5[10]. The efficacy of MET and TET is largely independent of pH[11]. Whether high pH favours penetration of BIS in the foveolae is speculative.

PPI may influence the bioavailability of antibiotics, especially CLA and TET, but not AMO[12,13]. Combining PPI with CLA leads to prolonged half-lives of both components, and higher CLA concentrations in antral mucosa and gastric mucus[14]. PPI may decrease the viscosity of gastric juice by a pH-dependent mechanism, perhaps facilitating the delivery of antimicrobials to the site of *H. pylori* organisms[15]. PPI (like H_2RA) tend to delay gastric emptying, perhaps perpetuating the exposure of the organisms to the antimicrobials in the gastric content[16].

OVERALL EFFICACY OF CURRENT EFFICACIOUS REGIMENS

A survey of current therapeutic possibilities is summarized in Table 2[2]. Obviously the best eradication rates are obtained with quadruple therapy [PPI–BIS–TET–MET] but the results obtained with other regimens are almost comparable.

Treiber (1996)[5] recently carried out a meta-analysis of various *H. pylori* eradication trials. He found [PPI–BIS–TET–MET] most effective but [PPI–CLA–

Table 2 *H. pylori*: amalgamated eradication rates with ±90% successful 1-week therapies

	No. of studies	No. of patients	Eradication mean	95% confidence interval
[BIS–TET–MET]	13	826	85	79–91
[PPI–CLA–MET]	24	1123	85	80–89
[PPI–CLA–AMO]	13	441	88	84–92
[PPI–AMO–MET]	14	521	77	68–87
[PPI–BIS–TET–MET]	9	461	96	93–99

MET] provided the best cost–benefit ratio. Based upon such very high cure rates, despite the inclusion of a variable percentage of patients with MET-resistant strains, the PPI–BIS–TET–MET quadruple regimen has been advocated as the current 'gold standard' to which other therapies should be compared[17].

FREQUENCY OF METRONIDAZOLE AND CLARITHROMYCIN RESISTANCE

Although precise data are lacking one may readily conclude that the incidence of metronidazole resistance is rising. In many major European cities MET resistance is above 50% of the population. In Hong Kong a dramatic and rapidly rising MET resistance has been recorded over the past few years, now amounting to 70–80%[18]. In the developing world MET resistance may be almost universal.

MET sensitivity testing is now usually carried out with the Epsilometer test (E-test). Strains are considered susceptible when the MIC is less than 8 mg/L. Recently, however, patients infected with strains with intermediate resistance to MET ($4 \leq MIC < 8$ mg/L) were shown to manifest a poor response to MET-containing triple therapy as seen in resistant strains, thus questioning the 8 mg/L cut-off value of the E-test[19]. In general the E-test has been found to be quite accurate and easy to use in assessing MIC values[20].

The mechanisms leading to MET resistance have not been fully elucidated. Most of what is known about MET mode of action was obtained under strict anaerobic conditions. To reduce the nitro group a very low redox potential must be generated. Smoking may interfere with reaching this low redox potential and thereby induce apparent resistance[21]. Furthermore, some MET-resistant strains may regain susceptibility after strict anaerobic incubation[22,23]. Because of such observations, a second mode of action for MET has been proposed. In that model the reduced nitroimidazole radical, in the presence of a sufficient oxygen tension, reverts into the native MET with production of oxygen radicals, ultimately leading to the toxic hydroxyl radical. This is the so-called 'futile cycling'. Apparent resistance along this pathway is explained by adequate microbial defence against the toxic oxygen radical attack through production of catalase and superoxide dismutase[22,24]. The futile cycling theory has been seriously challenged recently, when high and low oxygen tensions were found not to have any effect on MET activity[25]. Moreover, resistance was not correlated with levels of superoxide dismutase or catalase.

Expert testing for MET resistance is challenging. Not uncommonly a few colonies of *H. pylori* are visible within the zone of inhibited growth with the

E-test, the clinical significance of which is uncertain[26]. In the Amsterdam study, involving 156 patients[26], 33% were found to be infected with *H. pylori* populations, heterogeneous for their susceptibility to MET. Reassessment of MIC values in those patients revealed genuine MET resistance in 18% of them. Ten per cent of the isolates heterogeneous in MET susceptibility were heterogeneous at the genome level. This study clearly shows the limitations and the risks of possible misinterpretations when only a single colony is analysed for MET susceptibility. Moreover, there is the possibility to overcome *in-vitro* MET resistance *in vivo* as resistant organisms may be successfully eradicated using a MET-containing regimen[27,28].

Accurate data regarding CLA resistance (MIC > 0.5 mg/L) are limited[29,30]. In France and also in Brussels CLA resistance is high (> 10%). In London CLA resistance is roughly 9% (see Chapter by Dr Mégraud).

HOW TO OVERCOME MET RESISTANCE *IN VIVO*

Many studies have shown in the past that the eradication efficacy of [BIS – MET – TET] or [BIS – MET – AMO] substantially drops in cases of primary MET resistance. Adding PPI to regimens containing MET appears to overcome, in part, the deleterious influence of MET resistance upon final outcome. From the available literature, it would appear that the magnitude by which the deleterious effect of MET resistance can be overcome is somewhat larger with quadruple therapy com-pared to PPI-triple regimens.

The mechanisms involved in this phenomenon are not clear; only speculation can be offered for the time being. PPI may influence the metabolism of *H. pylori* through an interaction with disulphide bridges present in many enzyme systems of the organism. Is it possible that this may alter the oxidative chain metabolism and perhaps weaken the organism's defence against oxidative attack?

SELECTION OF THE PROTON PUMP INHIBITOR

Most studies with PPI so far reported have been carried out with OME. After initiating treatment with an OME-containing regimen it may take a few days before maximal acid suppression is achieved[31,32]. This may be somewhat disadvantageous in short-lasting eradicating regimens. The acid-suppressive effect of LAN appears superior to OME in the first few days of therapy, perhaps because of superior bioavailability[33,34]. Furthermore LAN manifests a 4–10 times stronger intrinsic anti-*H. pylori* activity *in vitro*[7,8,35,36]. Whether earlier acid suppression and lower MIC values *in vitro* translate into superior eradication efficacy *in vivo* is unclear at the present time. According to Takimoto *et al.*[37] *H. pylori* suppression by LAN monotherapy was superior to OME. De Boer achieved 95% cure with 7 days [LAN – BIS – MET – TET][38].

Since both OME and LAN quadruple regimens achieve very high cure rates (> 95% per protocol analysis) it will be impossible to demonstrate any clinically relevant difference between them for 7-day treatment schedules. Whether differences may become obvious for shorter therapy durations needs to be studied.

Table 3 *H. pylori* – impact of metronidazole resistance; amalgamation of world literature: therapy duration 1–2 weeks

	MET–SENS	MET–RES	Δ%
BIS–TET–MET	667/761 (92%)	208/306 (68%)	24
PPI–CLA–MET	140/161 (93%)	95/128 (74%)	19
PPI–AMO–MET	194/204 (95%)	105/151 (70%)	25
PPI–BIS–TET–MET	283/291 (97%)	93/98 (95%)	2

Table 4 *H. pylori* – impact of clarithromycin resistance; amalgamation of the world literature: therapy duration 1–2 weeks

	CLA–SENS	CLA–RES	Δ%
PPI–CLA–MET	101/118 (86%)	3/9 (33%)	53
PPI–CLA–AMO	45/45 (100%)	0/3 (0%)	100

IMPACT OF METRONIDAZOLE AND CLARITHROMYCIN RESISTANCE

Most intriguing is the impact of MET and CLA resistance in the various eradication schemes. As shown in Table 3, MET resistance is of critical importance in the overall efficacy of BIS-triple regimens [BIS–MET–TET] or [BIS–MET–AMO]. Also, in MET-containing PPI-triple regimens, the efficacy in MET-resistant patients is somewhat reduced. The efficacy of PPI–BIS-quadruple regimens [PPI–BIS–MET–TET] appears largely independent of MET resistance. Data on the impact of CLA resistance in CLA-containing PPI-triple regimens [PPI–CLA–MET] [PPI–CLA–AMO] are very limited, as summarized in Table 4.

COMPLIANCE WITH THERAPY

Compliance with therapy is, in all probability, a factor of decisive importance in antimicrobial efficacy. Yet proof of this statement with more recent studies employing efficacious eradication regimens is hard to come by. In general, the more potent the antimicrobial regimen, the less the impact of poor compliance. The reduction of therapy duration to 1 week certainly has contributed to overall patient compliance and acceptability.

TRIPLE OR QUADRUPLE THERAPY

The current treatment of choice should be based on high efficacy, overall patient acceptability and good compliance. Based upon currently available evidence it is to some extent possible to predict cure rates above 90%, provided the resistance patterns in the background population to be treated are known. The outcome of such a calculation is summarized in Table 5. Comparison between triple and quadruple therapies is given in Table 6.

In the absence of a high prevalence of MET or CLA resistance, both the [BIS-triple] and [PPI-triple] as well as [PPI–BIS-quadruple] regimens guarantee high

Table 5 *H. pylori* therapy: 1996 recommendations

Absent or low (<10%) MET resistance
BIS-triple   [BIS–TET–MET]
PPI-triples   [PPI–CLA–MET/PPI–CLA–AMO/PPI–AMO–MET]
PPI–BIS-quadruple   [PPI–BIS–TET–MET]
High MET resistance (>10%)
No regimens with MET except [PPI–BIS–TET–MET]
[PPI–CLA–AMO]
High CLA resistance (>5?)
No regimen with CLA
[BIS–TET–MET]
[PPI–AMO–MET]
[PPI–BIS–TET–MET]
High MET and CLA resistances
Only PPI–BIS-quadruple [[PPI–BIS–TET–MET]

Table 6 *H. pylori* therapy: 1996 standards–1 week

BIS–TET–MET	PPI–CLA–MET PPI–CLA–AMO PPI–AMO–MET	PPI–BIS–MET–TET
q.i.d. or b.i.d. dosing	b.i.d. dosing	q.i.d. dosing
Up to 11–15 pills/day	Up to 6 pills/day	Up to 13 pills/day
High failure rate in MET resistance	Failure in MET resistance; failure in CLA-resistance	No failure in MET resistance
Cheap	Expensive	Expensive
Severe side-effects <5%	Severe side-effects <5%	Severe side-effects <5%

Table 7 *H. pylori* – therapeutic recommendations in case of failure

[BIS–TET–MET] failure	→	[PPI–CLA–AMO] [PPI–BIS–TET–MET] ([PPI–AMO/or/CLA])
[PPI–CLA–MET] failure [PPI–CLA–AMO]	→	[PPI–BIS–TET–MET] [BIS–TET–MET]? [PPI–AMO]?
[PPI–AMO–MET] failure	→	[PPI–BIS–MET–TET] [PPI–CLA–AMO]
[PPI–BIS–TET–MET] failure	→	[PPI–CLA–AMO]? [PPI–AMO/or/CLA]?

eradication rates. How these regimens compare to each other is summarized in Table 6. Many experts suggest [PPI-triple] as first-line therapy because of the complexity of quadruple regimens, and because of the low frequency of severe side-effects and of better overall patient acceptability[39,40]. However, the side-effect profiles of all three treatment classes are more or less comparable. Compliance with [BIS-triple] or [PPI–BIS-quadruple] also seems adequate, provided meticulous instruction, motivation and warning of the patients has been carried out. Indeed, studies with a quadruple regimen have shown acceptable patient tolerability and a drop-out rate of <5%, comparable to that seen in PPI-triple regimens[41].

THERAPEUTIC RECOMMENDATIONS AFTER INITIAL FAILURE OF *H. PYLORI* ERADICATION

No generally accepted recommendations are available in the case of initial failure of *H. pylori* eradication when faulty compliance is excluded. From the limited data that are available in the literature, it would appear that retreatment with the same regimen cannot be recommended[42]. The choice of a CLA-containing regimen after failure of a CLA-containing scheme is also to be discouraged because of the high chance of secondary CLA resistance. Provisional recommendations for retreatment in the case of eradication failure are given in Table 7.

References

1. Tytgat GNJ. Treatments that impact favourably upon the eradication of *Helicobacter pylori* and ulcer recurrence. Aliment Pharmacol Ther. 1994;8:359–68.
2. Axon ATR. Eradication of *Helicobacter pylori*. Scand J Gastroenterol. 1996;31(Suppl. 214): 47–53.
3. Tytgat GNJ. Current indications for *Helicobacter pylori* eradication therapy. Scand J Gastroenterol. 1996;31(Suppl. 215):70–3.
4. van der Hulst RWM, Keller JJ, Rauws EAJ, Tytgat GNJ. Treatment of *Helicobacter pylori* infection: a review of the world literature. Helicobacter. 1966;1:6–19.
5. Treiber G. The influence of drug dosage on *Helicobacter pylori* eradication: a cost-effectiveness analysis. Am J Gastroenterol. 1996;91:246–52.
6. Al-Assi MT, Genta RM, Karttunen TJ, Cole RA, Graham DY. Azithromycin triple therapy for *Helicobacter pylori* infection: azithromycin, tetracycline and bismuth. Am J Gastroenterol. 1995; 90:403–4.
7. Iwahi T, Satoh H, Nakao M, Iwasaki T, Kubo K, Tamura T, Imada A. Lansoprazole, a novel benzimidazole proton pump inhibitor, and its related compounds have selective activity against *Helicobacter pylori*. Antimicrob Agents Chemother. 1991;35:490–6.
8. Nagata K, Satoh H, Iwahi T, Shimoyama T, Tamura T. Potent inhibitory action of the gastric proton pump inhibitor lansoprazole against urease activity of *Helicobacter pylori*: unique action selective for *H. pylori* cells. Antimicrob Agents Chemother. 1991;35:490–6.
9. McGowan CC, Cover TL, Blaser MJ. The proton pump inhibitor omeprazole inhibits acid survival of *Helicobacter pylori* by a urease-independent mechanism. Gastroenterology. 1994;107:1573–8.
10. Darmaillac V, Bouchand S, Lamouliatte H, Mégraud F. Macrolides and *Helicobacter pylori* determination of MICs and effect of pH. Gut. 1995;37(Suppl. 1):361:A91.
11. Grayson ML, Eliopoulos GM, Ferraro MJ, Moellering RC. Effect of varying pH on the susceptibility of *Campylobacter pylori* to antimicrobial agents. Eur J Clin Microbial Infect Dis. 1989;8: 888–9.
12. Paulsen O, Höglund P, Walder M. No effect of omeprazole-induced hypoacidity on the bioavailability of amoxillin or bacampicillin. Scand J Infect Dis. 1989;21:219–23.
13. Pommerien W, Braun M, Idström JP, Wrangsstadh M, Londong W. No interaction between omeprazole and amoxillin during combination therapy in *Helicobacter pylori*-positive subjects. Gastroenterology. 1995;108:A194.
14. Gustavson LE, Kaiser JF, Mukherjee DX, De Bartolo M, Schneck DW. Evaluation of pharmacokinetic drug interactions between clarithromycin and omeprazole. Am J Gastroenterol. 1994;89: 1373 (abstract).
15. Goddard AF, Spiller RC. The effect of omeprazole on gastric juice viscosity, pH and bacterial counts. Aliment Pharmacol Ther. 1996;10:105–9.
16. Benini L, Castellani G, Bardelli E *et al*. Omeprazole causes delay in gastric emptying of digestible meals. Dig Dis Sci. 1996;41:469–74.

17. de Boer WA, Tytgat GNJ. Ninety percent cure: which anti-*Helicobacter pylori* therapy can achieve this treatment goal? Am J Gastroenterol. 1995;90:1381–2 (editorial).

18. Ling TKW, Cheng AFB, Sung JJY, Yiu PYL, Chung SSC. An increase in *Helicobacter pylori* strains resistant to metronidazole: a five-year study. Helicobacter. 1996;2:57–61.

19. Xia HA, Keane CT, Beattie S, O'Morain CA. Standardization of disk diffusion test and its clinical significance for susceptibility testing of metronidazole against *Helicobacter pylori*. Antimicrob Agents Chemother. 1994;38:2357–61.

20. Hirschl AM, Hirschl MM, Rotter ML. Comparison of three methods of the sensitivity of *Helicobacter pylori* to metronidazole. J Antimicrob Chemother. 1993;32:45–9.

21. Witteman EM, Hopman WPM, Becx MCJ *et al*. Smoking habits and the acquisition of metronidazole resistance in patients with *Helicobacter pylori*-related gastritis. Aliment Pharmacol Ther. 1993;7:683–7.

22. Cederbrant G, Kahlmeter G, Ljungh A. Proposed mechanism for metronidazole resistance in *Helicobacter pylori*. J Antimicrob Chemother. 1992;29:115–20.

23. VanZwet AA, Thijs JC, de Graaf B. Explanations for high rates of eradication with triple therapy using metronidazole-resistant *Helicobacter pylori* strains. Antimicrob Agents Chemother. 1992; 36:163–6.

24. Xia JA, Keane CT, Beattic S, O'Morain CA. Culture of *Helicobacter pylori* under aerobic conditions on solid media. Eur J Clin Microb Infect Dis. 1994;13:406–9.

25. Smith MA, Edwards DI. Redox potential and oxygen concentration as factors in susceptibility of *Helicobacter pylori* to nitroheterocyclic drugs. J Antimicrob Chemother. 1995;35:751–64.

26. Weel JFL, van der Hulst RWM, Gerrits Y, Tytgat GNJ, van der Ende A, Dankert J. Heterogeneity in susceptibility to metronidazole among *Helicobacter pylori* isolates from patients with gastritis or peptic ulcer disease. J Clin Microbiol. 1996;34:(in press).

27. Rautelin H, Seppälä K, Renkonen OV, Vainio U, Kosunen TU. Role of metronidazole resistance in therapy of *Helicobacter pylori* infections. Antimicrob Agents Chemother. 1992;36:163–6.

28. Noach LA, Langenberg WL, Bertola MA, Dankert J, Tytgat GN. Impact of metronidazole resistance on the eradication of *Helicobacter pylori*. Scand J Infect Dis. 1994;26:321–7.

29. Al-Assi, Genta RM, Kartrunen TJ, Graham DY. Clarithromycin–amoxycillin therapy for *Helicobacter pylori* infection. Aliment Pharmacol Ther. 1994;8:453–6.

30. Cayla R, Lamouliatte HC, Brugman M, Mégraud F. Pre-treatment resistances of *Helicobacter pylori* to metronidazole and macrolides. Acta Gastroenterol Belg. 56(Suppl.):65.

31. Cederberg C, Ekenved G, Lind T, Olbe L. Acid inhibitory characteristics of omeprazole in man. Scand J Gastroenterol. 1985;20(Suppl. 108):105–12.

32. Cederberg C, Thomson ABR, Mahachai V *et al*. Effect of intravenous and oral omeprazole on 24 hour intragastric acidity in duodenal ulcer patients. Gastroenterology. 1992;103:913–18.

33. Damman HG, Richter G, Wolf N, Burkhardt F. Influence of lansoprazole 15 and 30 mg and omeprazole 20 and 40 mg on meal-stimulated gastric acid secretion. Gut. 1995;37(Suppl. 2): A45–6.

34. Ripke H, Fuder H, Kleistl P *et al*. Intragastric pH under various dosage regimens of lansoprazole as compared to a reference treatment with omeprazole. Gut. 1995;37(Suppl. 2):A23.

35. Mégraud F, Boyanova L, Lamouliatte H. Activity of lansoprazole against *Helicobacter pylori*. Lancet. 1993;337:1486 (letter).

36. Nagata K, Tagaki E, Tsuda M *et al*. Inhibitory action of lansoprazole and its analogs against *Helicobacter pylori*: inhibition of growth is not related to inhibition of urease. Antimicrob Agents Chemother. 1995;39:567–70.

37. Takimoto T, Ido K, Taniguchi Y *et al*. Efficacy of lansoprazole in eradication of *Helicobacter pylori*. J Clin Gastroenterol. 1995;20(Suppl. 2):S121–4.

38. de Boer WA, van Etten RJXM, Lai J, Schneeberger P, v.d. Wouw BAM, Driessen WMM. Effectiveness of 7-day quadruple therapy using lansoprazole, instead of omeprazole, in curing *Helicobacter pylori* infection Helicobacter. 1996;1:(in press).

39. Axon ATR. The role of acid inhibition in the treatment of *Helicobacter pylori* infection. Scand J Gastroenterol. 1994;29(Suppl. 201):16–23.

40. Harris A, Misiewicz JJ. Hitting *H. pylori* for four. Lancet. 1995;345:806–7 (editorial).

41. de Boer WA. How to achieve a near 100% cure rate for *H. pylori* infection in peptic ulcer patients. J Clin Gastroenterol. 1996 (in press).

42. v.d. Hulst RWM, Weel JFL, Verheul SB *et al*. Treatment of *H. pylori* infection with low or high dose omeprazole combined with amoxicillin and the effect of early treatment: a prospective randomized double blind study. Aliment Pharmacol Ther. 1996;10:165–71.

35
What is the relevance of resistance of *Helicobacter pylori* to antimicrobial agents?

F. MÉGRAUD

INTRODUCTION

The need to treat a *Helicobacter pylori* infection when associated with diseases such as peptic ulcer is now universally recognized.

The first regimen proposed to eradicate *H. pylori*, in 1990, was a triple therapy including a bismuth salt, tetracycline or amoxycillin and a nitroimidazole compound. The outcome of the treatment was shown to be dependent on the susceptibility of *H. pylori* to nitroimidazoles. More recently, triple therapies using two antibiotics and a proton pump inhibitor have been proposed. These regimens include clarithromycin and/or a nitroimidazole compound. The success of eradication of these regimens also has been claimed to be dependent on the susceptibility of *H. pylori* to these agents. In this chapter the relevance of resistance of *H. pylori* to these antimicrobial agents will be reviewed.

RESISTANCE OF *H. PYLORI* TO ANTIMICROBIAL AGENTS: WHAT DOES IT MEAN?

Resistance of an organism to an agent should be defined according to the concentration of drug which is able to reach the niche where the organism is present, in relation to the concentration of drug which is necessary to inhibit the growth of the organism. It is usually accepted that, to be efficacious, the drug concentration in the niche must be at least 4 times higher than the minimal inhibitory concentration (MIC)[1]. However, because it is too complicated to have specific breakpoint values for each tissue, the level of antibiotics present in the blood is usually considered, rather than within the specific niche colonized by the bacterium.

Furthermore, with regard to *H. pylori*, it is difficult to know the concentration of drugs in the gastric mucosa because it is not possible to do an endoscopy on a given subject at many different time-points. Furthermore, the concentration of an antimicrobial agent may vary at different sites in the stomach and at different levels of the mucosa. Another very important point is that the MIC values for some drugs are very dependent on the pH. It is possible to get some insight into this problem by performing studies on gastric juice[2], on resected gastric tissue[3] and by determining the MIC at a pH lower than 7 but usually not lower than 5.5, for technical reasons[4].

So how can a breakpoint value for resistance to antimicrobial agents be defined under such circumstances? A clue should come from clinicobacteriological correlations, i.e. the correlation between the MIC values determined using a reference method and the clinical efficacy in terms of eradication of the organism and cure of the infection. Such data are not currently available because in most trials, and especially those performed with the new short-term triple therapies, *H. pylori* strains have not been isolated for antimicrobial testing before treating the patients[5], and when strains have been isolated, a reference technique to determine MIC was not used. This is the reason for the controversy, because it has been stated that strains are resistant without giving the breakpoint used; indeed it may well be that the strains were falsely categorized as resistant. This is especially true for nitroimidazole compounds.

In this respect one must also keep in mind that, when a triple therapy with two antibiotics is used, even if one antibiotic is ineffective, the effect of the second antibiotic can still be expected. If the second antibiotic is amoxycillin, an eradication rate of 30–60% is possible to be achieved[6], i.e. the baseline for eradication will not be 0% but 30–60%. It is also possible that, in the future, a different breakpoint value will have to be used for metronidazole using different triple therapy regimens.

WHICH METHOD SHOULD BE USED TO TEST *H. PYLORI* ANTIMICROBIAL SUSCEPTIBILITY?

No reference method has yet been agreed upon to test the antimicrobial susceptibility of *H. pylori*. However, for other bacteria, especially fastidious species, the agar dilution method is recommended. From our experience the best results are obtained with this agar dilution method. Different groups of bacteriologists are presently working on the standardization of this method, including the NCCLS and a European group. The major points to consider are the agar, the blood supplement, the inoculum and the incubation atmosphere.

When this method is standardized and proved to be reproducible and reliable, the next step will be to compare it to the other methods such as broth dilution, disc diffusion and the E-test. It is clear that these latter methods will be better adapted to routine testing, but they should not be used to define susceptibility and resistance, especially in clinical trials, before being assessed against a reference technique.

RELEVANCE OF *H. PYLORI* RESISTANCE TO MACROLIDES

Macrolides constitute an exception to the argument above. The mode of testing is not as important because there is clearly a bimodal population of bacterial

**Cumulative %
of inhibition**

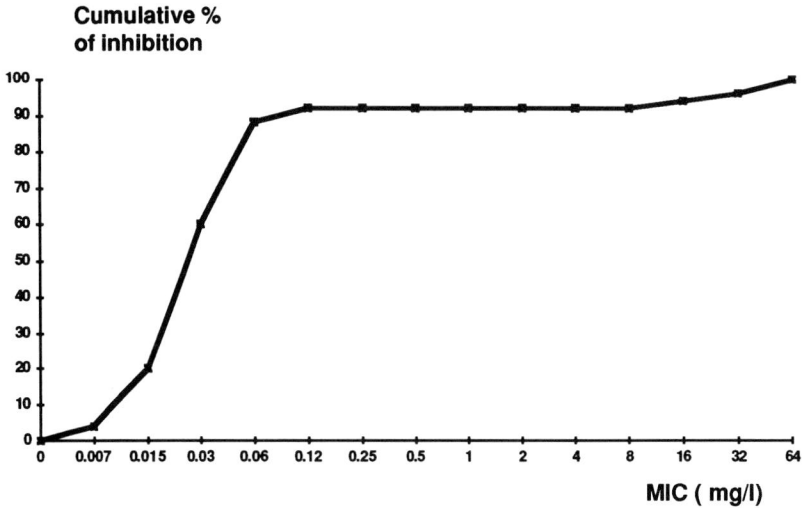

Figure 1   Distribution of MICs to clarithromycin in 50 *H. pylori* strains isolated in the southwest of France (agar dilution method). Ninety per cent have an MIC <0.12 mg/L and 10% >8 mg/L

strains, with most being highly susceptible and some being highly resistant (Figure 1). Because of the big gap existing between the first group (<0.125 mg/L) and the second (>16 mg/L), all techniques seem to be relevant, including disc diffusion. A small number of *H. pylori* strains nevertheless have a slightly higher MIC than the other susceptible strains, so it is not clear today what the clinical relevance of these last results is; in other words, breakpoints have not yet been definitely established[7].

It must be pointed out that a bacterial strain resistant to one macrolide is always resistant to others, therefore there is no benefit in changing to another macrolide. The mechanism for this, now clearly defined, is a lack of binding to ribosomes where macrolides normally interfere with protein synthesis. This is also the case for *H. pylori* resistant strains. We found that there was a decrease in binding to the ribosomes of a resistant strain, in comparison to a parent wild-type strain[8].

The molecular mechanism was first studied by Versalovic *et al.*[9], who found an association between resistance to macrolides and a point mutation in position 2058 or 2059 (A→G) in part of the gene coding for the V domain of the 23S rRNA, i.e. the peptidyl transferase. This first study, based on strains from the USA, has been confirmed, and similar mutations have also been found in European strains[8]. The frequency was the same between both positions of the mutation. A point mutation A→C has been documented in one case. This resistance can therefore be detected by amplification of the relevant gene and subsequent sequencing. There has been some controversy about the stability of macrolide resistance. It was claimed that some strains could revert to the wild-type when they were no longer in contact with the antibiotic[10]. Our results, based on resistant strains subcultured 25 times and then tested as well as resistant strains subsequently isolated from the same patient after a 1–18-month period, do not support this hypothesis[11].

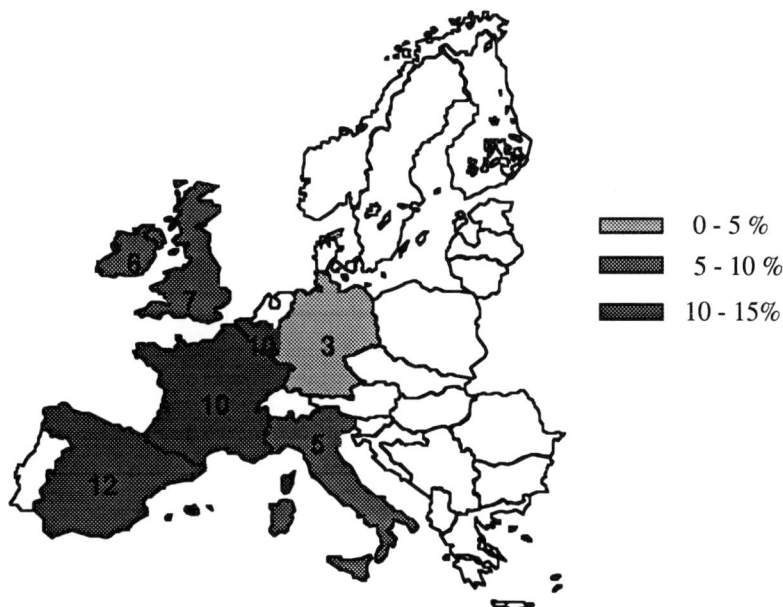

Figure 2 Distribution of macrolide resistant strains in some countries of Western Europe

Extent of resistance

Resistance of *H. pylori* to macrolides is low in general. Three patterns can be distinguished: (a) countries which have had a high consumption of macrolides for a long period of time (e.g. France); (b) countries which are using essentially the so-called 'new macrolides' (e.g. Spain); (c) countries for which macrolide use has always been low (e.g. Germany).

The resistance level in group (a) is in the range of 10% and was already in this range in 1985, i.e. 2–3 years after the introduction of macrolides for respiratory tract infection. Despite a long-standing consumption independent of *H. pylori* infection, the resistance has remained quite stable and is consistent, in Bordeaux, in the southwest of France and throughout France[12]. In group (b), countries such as Spain and Belgium, the resistance was virtually nil 10 years ago. It has progressively increased to about 10% during recent years, following the introduction of the new macrolides. In group (c), with such a low consumption of macrolides, no significant resistance is seen. An overview based on 1995 data in Europe is presented in Figure 2.

Clinical outcome

Very few studies are available which detail the clinical outcome, and resistance being uncommon (≤10%), few cases are documented in each study. Some studies concern clarithromycin in dual therapy. When the *H. pylori* strain is susceptible

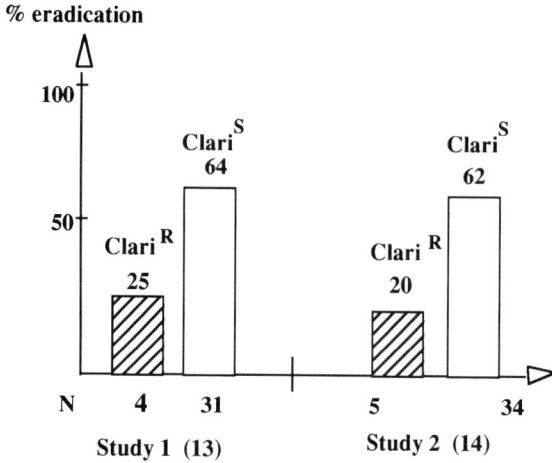

Figure 3 Correlation between resistance to clarithromycin and *H. pylori* eradication using dual therapy regimens: antisecretory + clarithromycin (14 days)

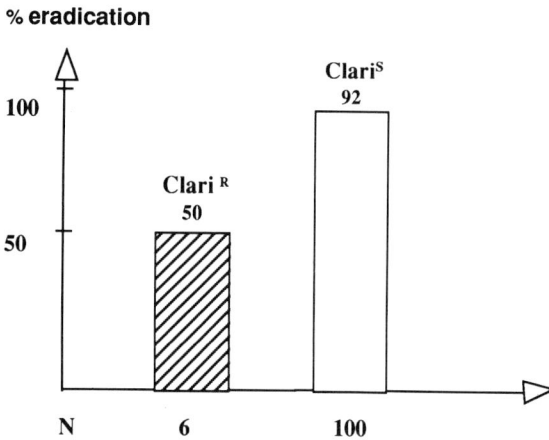

Figure 4 Correlation between resistance to clarithromycin and *H. pylori* eradication using a triple therapy regimen: omeprazole–clarithromycin–amoxycillin for 10 days[15]

to clarithromycin an eradication rate of 60% can be expected, and when the strain is resistant the eradication rate is about 20% (Figure 3). Furthermore, resistance occurs in about two-thirds of treatment failures, which jeopardizes the chance of subsequent success with the same treatment and highlights the need for culture when the first treatment fails[13,14].

Using triple therapy (omeprazole 20 mg, amoxicillin 1 g b.i.d., clarithromycin 500 mg b.i.d., for 10 days in patients with duodenal ulcer, the cure rate was 92% in those with susceptible strains versus 50% in those with resistant strains (Figure 4) and again most of the susceptible strains which were not eradicated became resistant[15].

**Cumulative %
of inhibition**

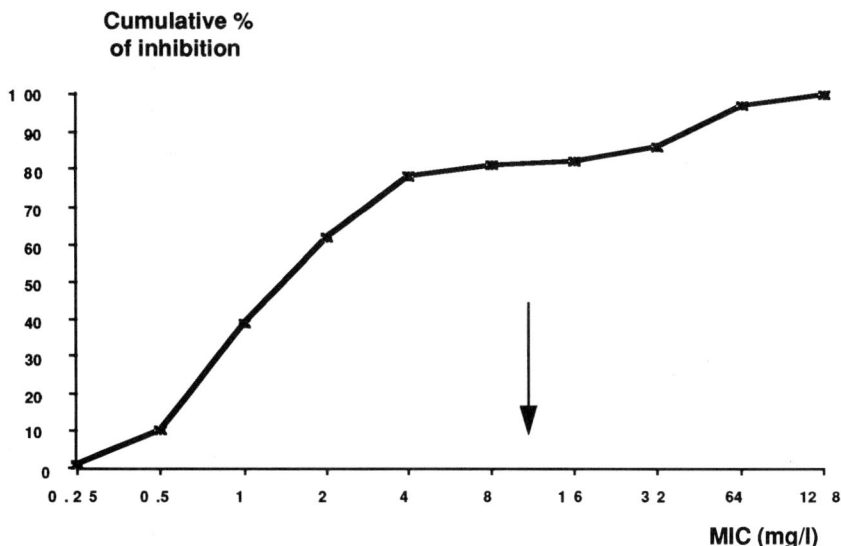

Figure 5 Distribution of MICs for metronidazole determined by an agar dilution method in 95 *H. pylori* strains isolated in France

This difference is highly significant and testifies to the clinical relevance of *H. pylori* resistance to macrolides.

RELEVANCE OF *H. PYLORI* RESISTANCE TO NITROIMIDAZOLE COMPOUNDS

As described with macrolides, there is also a cross-resistance between the different nitroimidazole compounds (metronidazole, tinidazole, and ornidazole). When MICs are performed on successive *H. pylori* strains, in contrast to what is seen for macrolides, a continuum of MIC is observed, indicating that there is not a bimodal population of bacterial strains (Figure 5). This result highlights the importance of the breakpoint value to define a resistant strain. The breakpoint value had been fixed at > 8 mg/L when the standard triple therapy with bismuth was used. It remains to be proven if the same value can be used for other triple therapies.

Another important factor is the method of testing. We were not able to confirm reports that metronidazole susceptibility determined by E-test gives the same value as the agar dilution method[16,17]. There has been a striking increase in resistance levels noted since the E-test has become popular. There is speculation that resistance to nitroimidazoles is overestimated when using the E-test. This may explain why the relevance of metronidazole resistance can be questioned.

The mechanism of action and of resistance to nitroimidazoles is also not clearly understood. Normally the NO_2 function of metronidazole is reduced and the compound breaks down bacterial DNA. One possible mechanism of resistance is linked to the failure in reducing the concentration of nitroimidazole administered. It has been proposed to lower the redox potential of the bacterial cell by a transitory

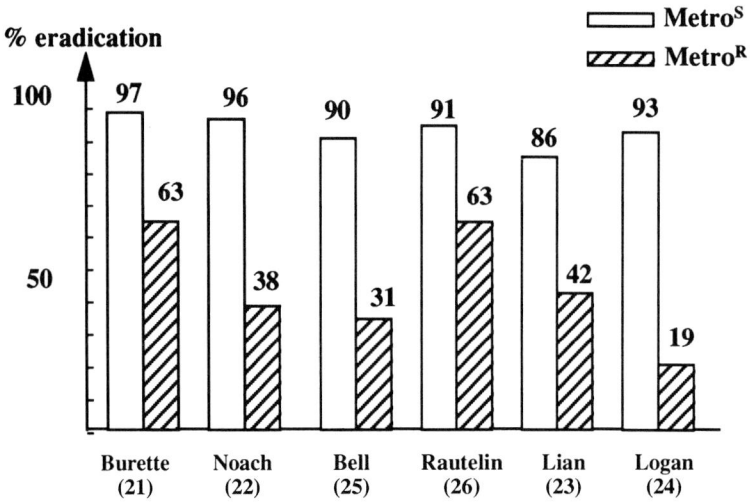

Figure 6 Comparative efficacy of the standard triple therapy (> 7 days) according to *H. pylori* suscep-tibility status for metronidazole in different studies

anaerobic incubation[18–20], under which circumstances the efficacy of the com-pound is maintained in a proportion of the strains. However, it is probable that another mechanism of resistance also exists, since metronidazole resistance has been shown to be transferable and a gene conferring metronidazole resistance has also been recently cloned.

These uncertainties with regard to the breakpoints used to define resistance, the method of testing, and the mechanism of action of the antimicrobial drug may be the cause of great variations in the level of resistance reported worldwide, a rate higher than 50% being reported in some countries.

CLINICAL OUTCOME

The relevance of metronidazole resistance has already been questioned by some authors when the standard bismuth triple therapy has been used. However, when the eradication rates obtained in different studies were broken down according to strain status, a statistically significant difference was observed between susceptible and resistant strains (Figure 6).

Bazzoli and others, surprisingly, obtained an eradication rate higher than 90% using a low-dose, short-term, triple therapy including a nitroimidazole compound. In the first trial, culture was not performed. In another trial, Moayyedi *et al.* per-formed disc diffusion studies and found that the resistant strains were eradicated[27]. This result was later confirmed by Bazzoli. Buckley *et al.* were not as successful, and their eradication rate among metronidazole-resistant strains was only 55%[28].

How can these divergent results be explained? The answer lies possibly in the methodology, with *H. pylori* strains being classified as resistant when they are not.

We have recently correlated the MICs of *H. pylori* strains to the treatment outcome using a triple therapy combination given for 10 days (lansoprazole 30 mg, amoxycillin 1 g b.i.d., metronidazole 500 mg b.i.d.) and found a clear difference between strains with MIC ≥ 16 mg/L versus those < 16 mg/L. In a study by Misiewicz *et al.* the odds of failure when harbouring a resistant strain of *H. pylori* were 5 times higher using a lansoprazole – amoxycillin – metronidazole combination, and 10 times higher using a lansoprazole – clarithromycin – metronidazole combination when compared to the wild-type[29]. Therefore, it is possible that the breakpoints used to define resistance should also be different, depending on the combination used.

CONCLUSION

It is clear that, as for any other bacteria, *H. pylori* resistance to antimicrobial agents is a major predictor of failure to cure the infection. The clinical relevance is not questioned for resistance to macrolides (except for some strains with a borderline MIC) because there is a bimodal population of strains and the mechanism of resistance is well understood.

The clinical relevance is questioned for metronidazole because the situation is more complex with regard to the mechanism of resistance and the mode of testing. However, when an agar dilution method is used, and results are expressed according to the MIC, a correlation with clinical outcome is found. More data are needed, and it is important that, in clinical trials, culture be performed and MIC values determined by a reference technique.

References

1. Davis DB. Chemotherapy. In: Davis DB, Dulbecco R, Eisen HN *et al.*, editors. Microbiology, 4th edn. Philadelphia: Lippincott; 1990;201–8.
2. Veldhuyzen Van Zanten SJ, Goldie J, Holligsworth J *et al.* Secretion of intravenously administered antibiotics in gastric juice: implication for management of *Helicobacter pylori*. J Clin Pathol. 1992;45:225–7.
3. Harrison JD, Jones JA, Morris DC. Azithromycin levels in plasma and gastric tissue, juice and mucus. Eur J Clin Microbiol Infect Dis. 1991;10:862–4.
4. Darmaillac V, Bouchard S, Lamouliatte H, Mégraud F. Macrolides and *Helicobacter pylori* – determination of MICs and effect of pH. Gastroenterology. 1995;108:A78.
5. Mégraud F, Malfertheiner P. Treatment of *Helicobacter pylori* infection: summary of a meeting at the fourth United European Gastroenterology Week. Helicobacter. 1996;1:118–21.
6. Labenz J, Gyenes E, Rühl GH, Borsch G. Omeprazole plus amoxicillin: efficacy of various treatment regimens to eradicate *Helicobacter pylori*. Am J Gastroenterol. 1993;88:491–5.
7. Butzler JP, Mégraud F. *Campylobacter* and *Helicobacter pylori*. In: Zinner S, Young L, Acar J, editors. New macrolides, azalides and streptogramins in clinical practice. New York: Marcel Dekker; 1996 (In press).
8. Occhialini A, Urdaci M, Doucet-Populaire F, Lamouliatte H, Bébéar CM, Mégraud F. *Helicobacter pylori* resistance to macrolides – confirmation of point mutation and detection by PCR-RFLP. Gut. 1996 (In press).
9. Versalovic J, Shortridge D, Kibler K *et al.* Mutations in 23S rRNA are associated with clarithromycin resistance in *Helicobacter pylori*. Antimicrob Agents Chemother. 1996;40: 477–80.
10. Xia HX, Buckley M, Keane CT, O'Morain CA. Clarithromycin resistance in *Helicobacter pylori*: prevalence in untreated dyspeptic patients and stability *in vitro*. J Antimicrob Chemother. 1996; 37:473–81.

11. Mégraud F, Camou-Juncas C, Occhialini A, Birac C. *Helicobacter pylori* resistance levels to clarithromycin remain stable. Gastroenterology. 1996;100:A192.
12. Camou C, Ancelle J, Lamouliatte H, Mégraud F. Evolution of the resistance of *Helicobacter pylori* to macrolides. ICMAS 96, Lisbon.
13. Cayla R, Zerbib F, Talbi P, Mégraud F, Lamouliatte H. Pre and post treatment clarithromycin resistance of *Helicobacter pylori* strains: a key factor of treatment failure. Gut. 1995;37(Suppl. 1):A55.
14. Shültze K, Hentschel E, Hirschl AM. Clarithromycin or amoxicillin plus high dose ranitidine in the treatment of *Helicobacter pylori* positive functional dyspepsia. Eur J Gastroenterol Hepatol. 1996;8:41–6.
15. Wurzer H, Rodrigo L, Archambault A *et al.* Short course therapy with amoxicillin–clarithroymcin triple for 10 days (ACT 10) eradicates *H. pylori* and heals duodenal ulcer. Gut. 1996 (In press).
16. Glupczynski Y, Labbé M, Hansen W *et al.* Evaluation of the E test for quantitative antimicrobial susceptibility testing of *Helicobacter pylori*. J Clin Microbiol. 1991;29:2072–5.
17. Hirschl AM, Hirschl MM, Rotter ML. Comparison of three methods for the determination of the sensitivity of *Helicobacter pylori* to metronidazole. J Antimicrob Chemother. 1993;32:45.
18. Cederbrant G, Kahlmeter G, Ljungh A. Proposed mechanism for metronidazole resistance in *Helicobacter pylori*. J Antimicrob Chemother. 1992;29:115–20.
19. Van Zwet AA, Thijs JC, de Graaf B. Explanation for high rates of eradication with triple therapy using metronidazole in patients harboring metronidazole-resistant *Helicobacter pylori* strains. Antimicrobiol Agents Chemother. 1995;39:250–2.
20. Smith MA, Edwards DI. Redox potential and oxygen concentration as factors in the susceptibility of *Helicobacter pylori* to nitroheterocyclic drugs. J Antimicrobiol Chemother. 1995;35:751–64.
21. Burette A, Glupczynski Y, Deprez C *et al.* Omeprazole alone or in combination with clarithromycin for eradication of *Helicobacter pylori*: results of a randomized double-blind controlled study. Gastroenterology. 1993;104:49.
22. Noach LA, Bosma NB, Tytgat GNJ. Clarithromycin resistance and *Helicobacter pylori* infection. European United Gastroenterology Week, Barcelona 1993;A103.
23. Lian JX, Carrick J, Daskalopoulos G. Metronidazole resistance significantly affects eradication of *Helicobacter pylori* infection. Gastroenterology. 1993;104:133.
24. Logan RPH, Gummett PA, Misiewicz JJ *et al.* One week eradication regimen for *Helicobacter pylori*. Lancet. 1991;338:1249–52.
25. Bell GD, Powell K, Burridge SM *et al.* Experience with triple anti-*Helicobacter pylori* eradication therapy: side effects and the importance of testing the pre-treatment bacterial isolate for metronidazole resistance. Aliment Pharmacol Ther. 1992;6:427–35.
26. Rautelin H, Kosunen TU, Seppala K. Eradicating *Helicobacter pylori*. Lancet. 1992;339:55.
27. Moayyedi P, Sahay P, Tompkins DS, Axon ATR. Efficacy and optimum dose of omeprazole in a new 1-week triple regimen to eradicate *Helicobacter pylori*. Eur J Gastroenterol Hepatol. 1996;7:835–40.
28. Buckley M, Xia HX, Hyde D, O'Morain C. Cost effective, European approach to *Helicobacter pylori* eradication. Gut. 1995;37(Suppl. 2):A175.
29. Misiewicz JJ, Harris AW, Bardhan KD, Levis S, Langworthy H. One week low-dose triple therapy for eradication of *H. pylori*: a large multi centre randomised trial. Gastroenterology. 1996;110:A198.

36
Treatment of patients with failed eradication – a personal view

T. J. BORODY and N. P. SHORTIS

INTRODUCTION

When we reflect upon the success or failure of *Helicobacter pylori* eradication therapies it is instructive to compare *H. pylori* infection with other well-known clinical infections, for it can help us gain an insight into the character of this infective agent. *H. pylori* infection is unlike a bacterial meningitis, a urinary tract infection or a bacterial pneumonia. These infections may be severe or even overwhelming; their severity is generally proportional to the number or load of infecting bacteria, and even their description relates to the clinical illness or condition they cause. *H. pylori* does not cause a state of 'overwhelming infection', and although it invariably causes gastritis we are generally called upon to treat its complications, particularly duodenal or gastric ulcers. *H. pylori* resembles in some respects slow-growing infections such as some fungal skin infections, tuberculosis or leprosy, in which therapy has to be very effective, either using multiple agents simultaneously or single agents for prolonged periods, otherwise the therapy will fail, suppression will result and frequently resistant strains of the organism will emerge.

Although *H. pylori* infection has certain features in common with the above infections we have learnt from clinical experience that it does have unique characteristics which set it apart from other infections. For example:

1. *H. pylori* is capable of surviving in an environment which is hostile to most other infecting agents, yet *in vitro* it is sensitive to a broad range of antimicrobials.
2. Single antimicrobial agents merely suppress and generally fail to eradicate *H. pylori*, which requires a combination of agents to achieve eradication rates of >90%.
3. The greater the combined number of appropriate antimicrobial agents the higher the eradication success rate and the shorter the length of therapy.
4. Unlike pneumonia, or a urinary tract infection, following successful eradication of *H. pylori* reinfection is rare.

This chapter will focus on the specific questions of why and in what setting we encounter eradication failure, and what can be done therapeutically for patients who have ongoing *H. pylori* infection after completing a course of therapy.

WHAT IS ERADICATION FAILURE?

Now that we understand better the character of *H. pylori*, it would be unfair to say that eradication failure occurred if a patient took a course of penicillin for an infected tooth, even though *H. pylori* is known to be sensitive to this antibiotic and some transient suppression of the infection might have occurred in the gastric mucosa during the treatment. In fact, it is difficult to categorically define eradication failure since we do not have a set of strictly accepted eradication protocols. However, we can define eradication failure generally as ongoing infection following an adequate course of anti-*H. pylori* combination therapy. Clearly eradication failure will occur more commonly after less efficacious than highly efficacious therapies.

WHY DOES ERADICATION FAILURE OCCUR?

Therapeutic protocols for the eradication of *H. pylori* which can achieve almost 100% are beginning to be described, and these will reduce the problem of eradication failure in the hands of experienced physicians who know how to use such protocols. The occasional user of eradication treatments will continue to create a pool of eradication failure patients. With the availability of simplified *H. pylori* detection methods many physicians with little experience in *H. pylori* eradication have been diagnosing the presence of this infection, and have commenced therapy using out-of-date dual therapies, or have lacked experience in adequately explaining and administering 'triple' therapies, thus leading to eradication failures. For example, in the past 8 months 56 patients have been referred to the Sydney Centre for Digestive Diseases for treatment of eradication failure. On review of the original therapy for *H. pylori* infection 35/56 (63%) had been treated with a protocol that has not been recommended in the literature and often constituted a 'cut-down' or personalized version of an accepted protocol. More worrying was the finding that 48/56 of these patients had been commenced on the ineffective therapy by a 'board-certified' specialist physician, and 8/56 by a general practitioner.

With the availability of serological testing *H. pylori*-positive patients are more frequently being detected in general practice, and are commenced on various therapies, but in the absence of an easily-available confirmatory post-therapy test, such as ^{13}C or ^{14}C-urea breath test, the physician does not realize that the eradication rate may be quite low. In fact, the level of understanding of *H. pylori* infection can be so poor that patients are sometimes retested with a serological test soon after therapy and declared *H. pylori*-positive.

Yet another reason why we are likely to continue to see many patients with eradication failure is the ongoing publication and subsequent promotion, by interested pharmaceutical sponsors, of suboptimal therapies. The gastroenterology literature abounds in eradication trials which report on 'promising' combination therapies with an efficacy of 85%, for example. Clearly such a protocol would produce an eradication failure rate of 15%. Since we now have available reliable protocols which in large trials result in >90% efficacy[1], it would be irresponsible to recommend any therapy which does not achieve eradication rates of 90–95%. In fact trials which demonstrate eradication rates of <90% should probably be reported to document an ineffective treatment.

THE IMPORTANCE OF ERADICATION FAILURE

If patients who failed initial *H. pylori* therapy could be reliably cured of their infection on a second-round treatment, this chapter would not have any relevance. However, with *H. pylori* infection 'life wasn't meant to be easy'. Not only do we not have a reliable cure for eradication failures, but we are beginning to see second-round, third-round, and ultimately 'incurable' patients[2]. These patients not only continue to suffer with their symptoms, and therefore require long term symptomatic therapy, but they may now be carrying unusual, perhaps resistant bacteria, which could conceivably be passed on to others, thus spreading potentially incurable *H. pylori* bacteria.

CLINICAL TYPES OF ERADICATION FAILURE PATIENTS

Patients who are eradication failures fall into two groups. They are either salvageable or 'incurable':

1. Generally salvageable eradication failure patients: this group usually constitutes patients who 'failed' a single course of *H. pylori* therapy. They are referred because of ongoing symptoms of dyspepsia poorly controlled by H_2-receptor antagonists, or because they know they harbour a carcinogen. More complex combination treatment protocols can cure >90% of these patients.
2. Generally unsalvageable eradication failure patients: this is fortunately a smaller but nevertheless a growing group of patients who have taken one or more forms of combination therapy a number of times[2]. These patients appear to be genuine therapy failures and yet are very particular about their compliance to therapy, still failing to be cured. Even very complex combinations of anti-*H. pylori* antibiotics may prove futile.

WHAT ARE THE MECHANISMS OF ERADICATION FAILURE?

It is likely that a number of mechanisms discussed below could be responsible for eradication failure. However, in any individual patient it is likely that one cause was of paramount importance while secondary causes may have contributed, e.g. non-compliance together with a partially-effective therapy taken for too short a period. In other words eradication failure is likely to be multifactorial, with a predominating mechanism carrying the brunt of the blame for eradication failure.

The factors which contribute to the development of eradication failure may include the following five factors:

Ineffective therapy

No matter how good patient compliance, monotherapy has been amply shown to suffer from poor efficacy, reaching almost 100% eradication failure with single agents such as doxycycline or tinidazole[3]. Provided appropriate antimicrobial agents are used, dual therapy improves eradication rates and so reduces eradication failure to around 50%[3]. It is only when we use the more successful triple therapies that eradication rates reach over 90%[3,4] to what is now considered clinically acceptable levels[1], while with the latest quadruple therapies eradication failure can fall to as low as 2–3%[5,6]. It is clear that improvement in eradication rates from 0% to 98% increases with the simultaneous increase in the number of appropriate antimicrobial agents. Stated in another way, eradication failures fall from 100% to 2% by using effective combination therapies. Eradication failure therefore appears to have most to do with our inability to damage irreparably the internal functioning of the *H. pylori* bacterial cell. We prevent eradication failures most successfully by exposing *H. pylori* to a range of noxious agents simultaneously.

Non-compliance

It is obvious that if a patient ingests no medications (zero compliance) of an efficacious therapy the result will be a zero eradication rate. On the other hand 100% compliance will result in no more than the maximal eradication possible for that particular treatment protocol. Graham *et al.*[7] quantified this expected phenomenon and found that, using a triple therapy, 96% of patients who took >60% of the prescribed medication achieved cure of the infection. From such figures it is clear that, given adequate patient explanation and training in taking a relatively short course of medications, high compliance is virtually always possible. From clinical experience with well over 12 000 patients treated at the Sydney Centre for Digestive Diseases for *H. pylori* infection, and a resultant large database, some 97.5% of our patients take >75% of their medications in often complex five-times-a-day triple therapies[8]. Similar rates of high compliance have been reported by others using complex protocols[5,9]. Overall, then, although non-compliance has the potential to cause eradication failure, in practice it is rather the use of ineffective therapy which constitutes the major problem.

Resistance to antibiotics

Acquisition of bacterial resistance to antimicrobials, especially to metronidazole, has always been an attractive explanation for eradication failure, especially since antimicrobial resistance is known to develop, and it can explain failure of cure in other infections such as tuberculosis. However, upon re-examination of various eradication failure data on *H. pylori*, invoking existing or acquired resistance does not explain the phenomena we observe clinically. For example, the pattern of 'resistance' does not follow that seen in a typical urinary tract infection, otherwise a simple switch of antibiotics would suffice to effect a cure of *H. pylori* eradication failures. Hence, for the following reasons the situation appears to be somewhat more complex:

1. If metronidazole resistance was an important cause of eradication failures the use of antimicrobial agents with little or no evidence of *H. pylori* resistance should prove effective. For example, bismuth salts, amoxicillin or tetracyline should have emerged as front-line monotherapy drugs. Yet bismuth subcitrate eradicates *H. pylori* in <20% of cases, amoxicillin in 5–35% and tetracycline in only 0–1%[10].

2. A non-metronidazole 'triple therapy' would, perhaps, be the answer. Indeed, such a combination of tetracycline, amoxicillin and bismuth was studied, but this resulted in an eradication rate of around 44%[11]. Clearly factors other than bacterial resistance were operating to cause such a profound eradication failure of 56%.

3. 'Metronidazole resistance' as measured *in vitro* in the laboratory can demonstrate unusual behaviour. It can develop without metronidazole exposure[12], it can develop after antibiotic use or disappear following a further eradication failure[2], and previously 'resistant' strains can regain susceptibility upon anaerobic incubation[13].

4. Eradication failure mechanisms other than bacterial resistance can be demonstrated when studying an individual case. Beji *et al.*[14] described a patient with several strains of *H. pylori* followed with serial cultures during failed antimicrobial polytherapy. MIC determinations on each endoscopic culture revealed that the differences between isolates were not related to the emergence of an antibiotic-resistant strain, but rather to the presence of multiple strains infecting the mucosa. Perhaps on occasions the presence of multiple strains in the mucosa may require an array of antibiotics to ensure collective eradication in a single course of treatment. The presence of multiple strains may therefore play a role in eradication failure in a small proportion of patients[15,16].

5. Studies of metronidazole resistance in therapeutic trials need specifically to differentiate between patients with *de-novo* and post-therapy metronidazole resistance[17], as the inclusion of previously treated patients in eradication trials biases against their eradication success, and metronidazole resistance is blamed for eradication failure. Indeed, when compliant patient populations with and without *de-novo* metronidazole-resistant bacteria are compared (but excluding previously treated patients), *H. pylori* eradication with triple and quadruple therapies results in virtually equivalent eradication in both groups[6,18]. Hence, metronidazole resistance *de novo* becomes clinically irrelevant, precluding the need to do sensitivity studies, as was shown by Hosking *et al.*[19], who achieved 98% eradication using quadruple therapy despite 48% metronidazole resistance.

Sanctuary sites and dormant forms

There are reasons to believe that sanctuary sites can exist in the gastric mucosa for *H. pylori*, and such sites might be induced by antimicrobial therapy. Boixeda *et al.*[20] found that in 20 patients with eradication failure eradication was site-specific in that 'eradication' was achieved in 62.5% of patients in the antrum while in the body in only 46.9%, suggesting unevenness of eradication, or possible 'sanctuary sites'. Site recrudescence was studied more recently by Atherton *et al.*[21], who showed, using polymerase chain reaction techniques, that after unsuccessful amoxycillin treatment it was again the antrum which was preferentially 'cleared' of *H. pylori* while the fundus and the body of the stomach remained infected significantly more frequently. If weak anti-*H. pylori* therapy can induce sanctuary sites then perhaps the subsequent therapy might find it more difficult to effect successful eradication. Indeed, Labenz *et al.*[22] showed evidence of a 50% reduction in eradication efficacy of amoxycillin/omeprazole in patients pretreated for 1 week with 40 mg omeprazole – a weak antimicrobial agent. Our own review of recurrent eradication failure patients showed that 14/21 had a history of recent antibiotic pretreatment in the form of either monotherapy for unrelated conditions (e.g. amoxycillin for respiratory infection), or partial or inappropriate *H. pylori* therapies[2].

Although *H. pylori* is not normally thought to be an invasive microorganism, electron microscopic (EM) studies of infected gastric mucosa have shown these bacteria can reside in the cytoplasm of gastric epithelial cells, and more so in metaplastic gastric cells of subjects with active duodenal ulceration[23–25], with a frequency reaching 10% of those with duodenal ulcers. Others have demonstrated *H. pylori* in the parietal cell canaliculi[26–28], quantified recently by Taniguchi *et al.*[29] to occur in 2.2% of parietal cell canaliculi. Recently *in-vitro* evidence has been presented showing that *H. pylori* is capable of invading mammalian cells[30]. It is therefore possible that there are intracellular sanctuary sites where *H. pylori* might avoid antimicrobial agents.

A separate potential sanctuary site is the apparent intracellular survival of *H. pylori* within polymorphonuclear leucocytes and within monocytes, as demonstrated using *in-vitro* studies[31].

Dormant or coccoid forms of *H. pylori* may also play a role in eradication failure. *H. pylori* is known to possess a bacillary and a coccoid morphological form. Little is known concerning the coccoid form as it is rarely seen *in vivo*, and is generally unculturable using standard techniques. Conversion of the bacillary to the coccoid form can be achieved by incubation with subinhibitory concentrations of some antibiotics such as roxithromycin and omeprazole[32]. In one study, coccoid forms have been observed in 3/14 eradication failure patients, suggesting that they are resistant to treatment. Such a finding has not been the general experience in the broad histological publications; indeed coccoid forms may be, with exceptions, an *in-vitro* phenomenon.

Unexplained factors

This section is included because we need to acknowledge that the ultimate cause of eradication failure is not necessarily known at the present time. Simply stating that a combination of factors causes eradication failure in every case is probably incorrect. The evidence for such a view comes from our observations of patients with recurrent eradication failure where up to seven different often complex therapies have been used in the most interested and compliant patients[2]. From culture sensitivities, histology, and EM studies we know that these patients do not appear to have any detectable, distinct features such as, for example, coccoid forms – which we could readily use to explain their plight. Hence, for the moment, we need to conclude that yet another factor is operating in eradication failure, which to date remains obscure. It may yet prove to be the most important factor.

HOW SHOULD WE PREVENT ERADICATION FAILURE?

The use of the most effective available therapies with proven eradication rates of over 95% will, by definition, result in the lowest eradication failure rates. Currently, the only combination therapy with published results in several hundred patients on three continents giving reproducible 95–98% eradication rates, is 'quadruple therapy'[5,6,9,19], and this is described as the 'gold standard' for other therapies in a recent editorial[1]. Although complex, this protocol achieves the highest eradication rates and, in our experience, with excellent compliance and acceptably low levels of side-effects. It is also the cheapest, more effective protocol. Although a four-times-a-day version is described[5,9,19], our preference is for the more frequent five-times-a-day regimen[6], which in our hands results in rare side-effects:

1. Omeprazole 20 mg, twice a day (7 am and 7 pm).
2. Bismuth subcitrate 108 mg, five times a day (7 am, 11 am, 3 pm, 7 pm, 11 pm).
3. Tetracycline HCl 250 mg, five times a day (7 am, 11 am, 3 pm, 7 pm, 11 pm).
4. Metronidazole 200 mg, five times a day (7 am, 11 am, 3 pm, 7 pm, 11 pm).

All to be taken over 7 days. (Bismuth subcitrate can be replaced by bismuth sub-salicylate.)

The alternative, simpler, perhaps only slightly less efficacious triple therapy protocol, albeit more expensive, uses clarithromycin:

1. Omeprazole 20 mg, twice a day (7 am and 7 pm).
2. Clarithromycin 250 mg, twice a day (7 am and 7 pm).
3. Metronidazole 400 mg or tinidazole 500 mg, twice a day (7 am and 7 pm).

All to be taken over 7 days.

HOW SHOULD WE TREAT PATIENTS WITH FAILED ERADICATION?

There are currently sporadic abstract reports on this topic, and certainly no consensus available based on any published data. Based on the fact that the more antimicrobial agents (currently up to four) given together will result in the highest eradication rates, we have previously reported a salvage therapy[33] which is a form of the quadruple treatment now being advocated as primary treatment. This therapy achieved an overall eradication in all eradication failure patients entered of 78%. A similar approach was taken by Barry Marshall, obtaining an overall 71% eradication in metronidazole-resistant patients[34]. With further optimization of the therapy for eradication failure patients we now use a 12-day course of five-times-daily quadruple therapy which achieves a 93% eradication in first-time eradication failure patients and approximately 70% in recurrent eradication failure patients. It consists of:

1. Omeprazole 20 mg, five times a day (7 am, 11 am, 3 pm, 7 pm, 11 pm).
2. Bismuth subcitrate 108 mg, five times a day (7 am, 11 am, 3 pm, 7 pm, 11 pm).
3. Amoxycillin 500 mg, five times a day (7 am, 11 am, 3 pm, 7 pm, 11 pm).
4. Clarithromycin 250 mg, three times a day (7 am, 3 pm, 11 pm).

By initially using a highly efficient eradication therapy we save patients from failing their therapy. Nevertheless, about 5% may return with ongoing *H. pylori* infection. A second-round protocol can be applied in these patients so that, overall, fewer than 0.5% of the original cohort will remain infected. In those with recurrent eradication failure no standard therapy is available and maintenance with H_2 receptor antagonists may suffice for the present until better *H. pylori* eradication treatments or novel medications emerge. Others will benefit from long-term bismuth therapy by suppression of the bacteria and associated inflammation. The potential carcinogenicity of *H. pylori* needs to be remembered, and monitoring mucosal biopsies considered in those with gastric atrophy or developing intestinal metaplasia.

References

1. de Boer WA, Tytgat GNJ. 90% cure: which anti-*Helicobacter pylori* therapy can achieve this treatment goal? Am J Gastroenterol. 1995;90:1381–2 (editorial).
2. Borody TJ, Andrews P, Shortis NP. Features of patients who fail all attempts at *Helicobacter pylori* (HP) eradication. Am J Gastroenterol. 1994;89:1365.
3. Chiba N, Rao BV, Rademaker JW, Hunt RH. Meta-analysis of the efficacy of antibiotic therapy in eradicating *Helicobacter pylori*. Am J Gastroenterol. 1992;87:1716–27.
4. Moayyedi P, Axon ATR. Efficacy of a new one week triple therapy regime in eradicating *Helicobacter pylori*. Gut. 1994;35(Suppl. 1):F248.
5. de Boer W, Driessen W, Jansz A, Tytgat G. Concomitant acid suppression increases the efficacy of traditional anti-*Helicobacter* triple therapy. Lancet. 1995;345:817–20.
6. Borody TJ, Andrews P, Fracchia G, Brandl S, Shortis NP, Bae H. Omeprazole enhances efficacy of triple therapy in eradicating *Helicobacter pylori*. Gut. 1995;37:477–81.
7. Graham DY, Lew GM, Malaty HM *et al*. Factors influencing the eradication of *Helicobacter pylori* with triple therapy. Gastroenterology. 1992;102:439–96.
8. Borody TJ, Brandl S, Andrews P, Ferch N, Jankiewicz E, Hyland L. Use of high efficacy, lower dose triple therapy to reduce side effects of eradicating *Helicobacter pylori*. Am J Gastroenterol. 1994;89:33–8.
9. de Bower WA, Driessen WMM, Jansz AR, Tytgat GNJ. Quadruple therapy compared with dual therapy for eradication of *Helicobacter pylori* in ulcer patients: results of a randomised prospective single-centre study. Eur J Gastroenterol Hepatol. 1995;7:1189–94.
10. Axon ATR. *Helicobacter pylori* therapy: effect on peptic ulcer disease. J Gastroenterol Hepatol. 1991;6:131–7.
11. Graham DY Lew GM, Ramirez FC *et al*. Short report: a non-metronidazole triple therapy for eradication of *Helicobacter pylori* infection – tetracycline, amoxicillin, bismuth. Aliment Pharmacol Ther. 1993;7:111–13.
12. Daskalopoulos G, Carrick J, Lian RX, Lee A. The silent minority – eradication of *Helicobacter pylori* where standard triple therapy has failed. In: *H. pylori*. Basic mechanisms to clinical cure. Interfalk Conference proceedings: Ritz-Carlton Hotel, Amelia Is, FL, 3–6 November 1993:36.
13. Cederbrant G, Kahlmeter G, Ljungh A. Proposed mechanism for metronidazole resistance in *Helicobacter pylori*. J Antimicrob Chemother. 1992;29:115–20.
14. Beji A, Vincent P, Dachis I, Husson MO, Cortol A, Leclerc H. Evidence of gastritis with several *Helicobacter pylori* strains. Lancet. 1989;2:1402–3.

15. Lelwala-Guruge J, Akopyanz N, Ljumgh A, Wadstrom T, Berg DE. Multiple *Helicobacter pylori* strains can colonize an individual patient. Acta Gastro-Enterol Belg. 1993;50(Suppl.):90.
16. Prewett E, Bickely J, Owen RJ, Pounder RE. DNA patterns of *Helicobacter pylori* isolated from gastric antrum, body and duodenum. Gastroenterology. 1992;102:829–33.
17. Burette A, Glupczynski Y, De Prex C. Evaluation of various multi-drug eradication regimens for *Helicobacter pylori*. Eur J Gastroenterol Hepatol. 1992;4:817–23.
18. Borody T, Andrews P, Brandl S, Devine M. Relevance of *in-vitro* metronidazole resistance to *H. pylori* (HP) eradication and eradication failure. Gastroenterology. 1993;104:A44.
19. Hosking SW, Ling TKW, Chung SCS *et al*. Duodenal ulcer healing by eradication of *Helicobacter pylori* without anti-acid treatment: randomised controlled trial. Lancet. 1994;343:508–10.
20. Boixeda D, De Rafael L, Martin De Argila C *et al*. Importance of biopsy sampling at the gastric body for follow-up of therapeutic trials directed against *Helicobacter pylori*. Ital J Gastroenterol. 1991;23(Suppl. 2):84–5.
21. Atherton JC, Cockayne A, Balsitis M, Hawkey CJ, Spiller RC. Polymerase chain reaction detects the sites at which *Helicobacter pylori* evades treatment with amoxycillin and cimetidine. Gut. 1993;34(Suppl. 1):S36.
22. Labenz J, Gyenes GH, Ruhl G, Borsch G. Pretreatment with omeprazole endangers the efficacy of amoxycillin/omeprazole treatment to eradicate *Helicobacter pylori*. Irish J Med Sci. 1992;161 (Suppl. 10):15.
23. Bode G, Malfertheiner P, Ditschuneit H. Pathogenic implications of ultrastructural findings in *Campylobacter pylori*-related gastroduodenal disease. Scand J Gastroenterol. 1988;23(Suppl. 142):25–39.
24. Meyrick-Tomas J, Poynter D, Goodling C *et al*. Gastric spiral bacteria. Lancet. 1984;2:100.
25. Lee WK, Gourley WK, Buck GE, Subramanyam K. A light and electron microscopic study of a *Campylobacter*-like bacteria inhabiting the human stomach. Gastroenterology. 1985;88:1470.
26. Chen XY, Correa P, Offerhaus J *et al*. Ultrastructure of the gastric mucosa harboring *Campylobacter*-like organisms. Am J Clin Pathol. 1986;86:575–82.
27. Rollason TP, Stone J, Rhodes JM. Spiral organisms in endoscopic biopsies of the human stomach. J Clin Pathol. 1984;37:23–6.
28. Jiang SJ, Liu WZ, Zhang DZ *et al*. *Campylobacter*-like organisms in chronic gastritis, peptic ulcer, and gastric carcinoma. Scand J Gastroenterol. 1987;22:553–8.
29. Taniguchi Y, Kimura K, Satoh K *et al*. *Helicobacter pylori* detected deep in gastric glands: an ultrastructural qualitative study. J Clin Gastroenterol. 1995;21(Suppl. 1):S169–73.
30. Evans DG, Evans DJ, Graham DY. Adherence and internalization of *Helicobacter pylori* by HEp-2 cells. Gastroenterology. 1992;102:1557–67.
31. Andersen LP, Blom J, Nielsen H. Survival and ultrastructural changes of *Helicobacter pylori* after phagocytosis by human polymorphonuclear leucocytes and monocytes. APMIS. 1993;100:61–72.
32. Cellini L, Allocati N, Di Campali E, Massuli M, Dainelli B. Morphological forms in *Helicobacter pylori*. Acta Gastro-Enterol Belg. 1993;53(Suppl.):108.
33. Borody TJ, Brandl S, Andrews P, Jankiewicz E, Ostapowicz N. *H. pylori* eradication failure (EF) – further treatment possibilities. Gastroenterology. 1992;102:A43.
34. Marshall BJ, Guerrant RL, Hoffman SR, Barrett L, McCallum RW. Eradication of metronidazole resistant *H. pylori*. Am J Gastroenterol. 1991;86:1315.

37
What is the role of the primary care physician in the treatment of *Helicobacter pylori* infection?

P. MALFERTHEINER and T. BREUER

INTRODUCTION

Progress in our knowledge of *H. pylori* infection has moved on at a relentless pace in basic as well as clinical science. Since *H. pylori* infection is now known to be the most common cause of chronic gastritis, overwhelming evidence has implicated it as an aetiological factor in a spectrum of gastrointestinal diseases including peptic ulcer, gastric carcinoma and gastric lymphoma[1-11]. More recently, other non-gastrointestinal diseases, such as coronary heart disease, skin rashes (urticaria) and growth retardation have also been linked with *H. pylori* infection[12]. However, these latter associations are still strongly disputed.

Since almost all discoveries related to *H. pylori* are recent, yet largely confirmed, the question is whether, and to what depth, this extensive knowledge should be transferred to the general community of practising physicians. General practitioners (GPs) are the primary-care providers who stand first in line, and treat the majority of patients. Therefore, they need preselected information on scientific progress ready for clinical application.

We have examined the extent to which knowledge about *H. pylori* has influenced GPs' diagnostic and therapeutic practices, and this helps us to define the role which the primary-care physician can fulfil in the management of *H. pylori*-associated diseases at present. Thorough education of physicians, in terms of the new knowledge in the area of gastrointestinal diseases, is extremely important because inadequate treatment of peptic ulcer disease is linked to therapy failures with high recurrence rates of ulcer disease, the emergence of resistant strains and, overall, to higher costs of health care.

Several issues need to be addressed in the definition of the role of GPs in handling *H. pylori*-associated diseases:

1. understanding of disease entities related to *H. pylori* infection;
2. clinical conditions necessitating *H. pylori* testing and strategy thereafter;

3. reliability of the many therapy regimens proposed;
4. follow-up protocols after treatment.

DISEASE ENTITIES RELATED TO *H. PYLORI* INFECTION

The first step for consideration in educating physicians is to clarify what knowledge is now appropriate for transfer to primary-care physicians for clinical application, and what knowledge is still in the experimental state. The reasons for this are obvious, as penetration of uncontrolled data would create, and unfortunately (in the case of *H. pylori*) have created, confusion among physicians.

Treatment studies have clearly shown that this bacterium has a primary role in the occurrence and recurrence of peptic ulcer disease. This knowledge has dramatically changed the possibilities for treating this condition. In the past recurrent peptic ulcers were treated with acid-suppressive therapy (pharmacological or surgical); current approaches use antimicrobial therapy for *H. pylori*-positive cases of peptic ulcer disease in order to cure patients of the causal infection[13]. According to the 1994 NIH Consensus Conference[14], ulcer patients with *H. pylori* infection require treatment with antimicrobial agents, whether on first presentation or on recurrence.

Epidemiological studies have demonstrated a relationship between *H. pylori* gastritis and gastric cancer, and have also estimated the relative risk for cancer development[2,4,11,15]. Because of sufficient epidemiological evidence of carcinogenic effects in humans, *H. pylori* infection has been classified as a Group I carcinogen by the International Agency for Research on Cancer (IARC)[16]. More evidence can be expected from large intervention studies in which *H. pylori*-infected population groups are randomly assigned to antibiotic therapy for *H. pylori* infection or placebo therapy, and are followed up to compare the rates of gastric cancer. Such studies are under way, but results cannot be expected in the near future.

Consequently, from the clinical point of view, guidelines regarding prophylactic treatment of *H. pylori* infection in order to prevent gastric cancer have not been established.

H. pylori seems to play a major role in the pathogenesis of low-grade mucosa-associated lymphoid tissue lymphoma (MALT lymphoma). The therapeutic approach in treating this kind of lymphoma with antibiotics in order to cure the *H. pylori* infection, despite successful short-term results, is still under study, and should preferably be undertaken within clinical trials.

The relationship between non-ulcer dyspepsia and *H. pylori* is less clear-cut, and continues to be an issue of major controversy. Therefore, therapeutic guidelines have not been established here either.

A recent study[17] revealed the possibility that patients with reflux oesophagitis and *H. pylori* infection who are treated with omeprazole on a long-term basis are at increased risk of atrophic gastritis, and that antimicrobial therapy for *H. pylori* infection should be considered. Despite strongly suggestive evidence, it may well need further and more controlled data in different populations before becoming mandatory to search for and treat *H. pylori* in these patients.

KNOWLEDGE BACKGROUND OF *H. PYLORI* INFECTION IN PHYSICIANS

Data on physicians' knowledge of the aetiological role of *H. pylori* in peptic ulcer disease are scarce[18-24], most only being available in abstract form. In a study conducted in 1992[18], *H. pylori* was recognized as the main cause of duodenal ulcer disease by 47–84% of physicians, depending on the country of investigation. The same study revealed that *H. pylori* treatment in duodenal ulcer disease was undertaken by 60–93% of the physicians who responded. Triple therapy using a bismuth salt, metronidazole and either amoxycillin or tetracycline was most frequently used (57%) at that time.

Another study conducted in 1993 investigating attitudes and practices of gastro-enterologists in the United Kingdom[20] revealed different results: 87% agreed that *H. pylori* was a cause of antral gastritis; whereas for gastric ulcer, duodenal ulcer, non-ulcer dyspepsia and gastric cancer, comparable figures were 47%, 73%, 25% and 17%, respectively. For the treatment of duodenal ulcer at initial presentation, 25% stated they would use *H. pylori* eradication therapy, in comparison with 38% for a duodenal ulcer at first recurrence and 80% for a chronic recurrent ulcer. The study further revealed that there was a general belief that therapy for *H. pylori* infection causes more side-effects and problems of compliance compared with acid-suppression therapy. This study was performed before the better-tolerated therapeutic regimens had been introduced.

A retrospective study published in 1996 conducted in five general practices in different parts of Scotland investigated the proportion of patients appropriately selected for *H. pylori* eradication therapy[21]. Eighty per cent received therapy for peptic ulcer disease, the remaining 20% for non-ulcer dyspepsia or gastro-oesophageal reflux diseases. Fifty-six different regimens were used, most commonly omeprazole plus amoxycillin. *H. pylori* status was known in only one-third of the patients before treatment.

More recent data are available from a German study conducted by the authors in September 1995[22-24] comparing two groups of physicians (gastroenterologists and GPs). The survey revealed that responding GPs treat almost 50% of their patients without ordering further diagnostic tests for the initial presentation of *suspected ulcer disease*. Both of the physician groups rarely recommended treatment for *H. pylori* infection for suspected ulcer disease. Nearly all of the responding physicians use antibiotics to treat recurrent *H. pylori*-positive gastroduodenal ulcer disease. More than 25% of the GPs, and 14% of the gastroenterologists, did not treat diagnosed *H. pylori* infection in the first presentation of duodenal ulcer disease. Around half of both physician groups used dual therapy containing amoxycillin and omeprazole. Twenty-two per cent of responding GPs treated the first presentation of *H. pylori*-positive ulcer disease with ineffective regimens as defined by the available literature[25]. Standard bismuth triple therapy does not play a role in the therapy of *H. pylori* infection in Germany.

In comparison, GPs from the United States often use bismuth-based triple therapy regimens. The use of ineffective regimens is comparable to the German data (Breuer T, Graham DY *et al.*, unpublished data).

To conclude, although *H. pylori* infection as the main cause of ulcer disease becomes increasingly accepted by the primary-care physician, treatment choices seem to differ extensively depending on the country of investigation.

CLINICAL CONDITIONS NECESSITATING *H. PYLORI* TESTING AND STRATEGY THEREAFTER

Peptic ulcer disease

There is no way around a firm recommendation to test all patients with suspected gastric or duodenal ulcer and/or with a history of peptic ulcer disease. Some clinicians object to the opinion that, due to the high prevalence of over 90% of *H. pylori* infection in patients with endoscopically proven duodenal ulcer, there is no need for *H. pylori* testing in these patients, especially as there is no single test with 100% accuracy. This argument has been overcome since the use of a combination of tests, in the rare circumstances when an individual test fails, offers the only reliable way to identify the *H. pylori*-negative duodenal ulcer patient. This would encourage the search for rare aetiologies of duodenal ulcer. The straightforward diagnostic approach is to refer the patient for endoscopy and biopsy. This diagnostic scheme is still the most pragmatic, as it can differentiate between a gastric ulcer and gastric malignancy. If duodenal ulcer has been proven recently by endoscopy, and no *H. pylori* testing has been performed, then the GP can rely on non-invasive tests such as serology or the ^{13}C urea breath test.

Non-ulcer dyspepsia

Controversy surrounds the question as to how extensive the diagnostic procedures should be in patients presenting with dyspeptic symptoms. The strategies vary in different countries as well as among doctors; however, the most frequent strategy adopted is to start an empirical therapy directed towards the leading symptom and then switch to more specific diagnostic investigations in the case of treatment failure or further relapses.

Now *H. pylori* testing by non-invasive means may be considered either in the subgroup of patients with ulcer-like symptoms or in all dyspeptics. Stratifying patients who are currently not on NSAIDs and suffer from ulcer-like symptoms in age groups above and below 45 years for further management seems to be economically advantageous. A study conducted in England was able to show savings of 37% in endoscopies by selecting patients on the basis of *H. pylori* serology, sinister symptoms and on the basis of a history of NSAID use[26]. Possible strategies derived from this approach could accordingly either screen patients for endoscopy based on *H. pylori* serology, or treat those younger than 45 years of age and not on NSAIDs, with *H. pylori* eradication therapy, and perform endoscopy only in those above age 45 years as more than 90% of gastric malignancies are to be expected in this age group (Figures 1 and 2).

The major objection by GPs to testing all dyspeptic patients for *H. pylori*, either by the ^{13}C urea breath test or by serology, derives from the fact that only one centre was able to provide convincing evidence of a major benefit for those with dyspeptic symptoms from the eradication of *H. pylori*[27]. A randomized controlled study that set the endpoint earlier than 1 year failed to show any benefit from this approach[28].

What should one recommend as a general rule to the primary-care physician? Should such physicians select patients on the basis of their *H. pylori* status and symptoms for referral to the gastroenterologist, or should they ignore *H. pylori*?

```
┌─────────────────────────────────────────────────────────┐
│                  Dyspepsia; Age < 45                      │
│              No alarm symptoms; no NSAIDs                 │
└─────────────────────────────────────────────────────────┘
        │                      │                     │
        ▼                      ▼                     ▼
┌──────────────┐      ┌──────────────┐      ┌──────────────┐
│  "Ulcer-like"│      │  "GERD-like" │      │"Motility-like"│
└──────────────┘      └──────────────┘      └──────────────┘
        │                      │                     │
        ▼                      └──────┐      ┌───────┘
┌─────────────────────────────┐   ┌─────────────────────────┐
│ Review history for alcohol, │   │  Appropriate empiric     │
│     smoking, NSAIDs         │   │      treatment           │
├─────────────────────────────┤   └─────────────────────────┘
│ Serologic test for H. pylori│              ▲
└─────────────────────────────┘              │
      │             │                         │
  POSITIVE      NEGATIVE─────────────────────┘
      │
      ▼
┌─────────────────────────────┐
│ Investigate or treat infection│
└─────────────────────────────┘
```

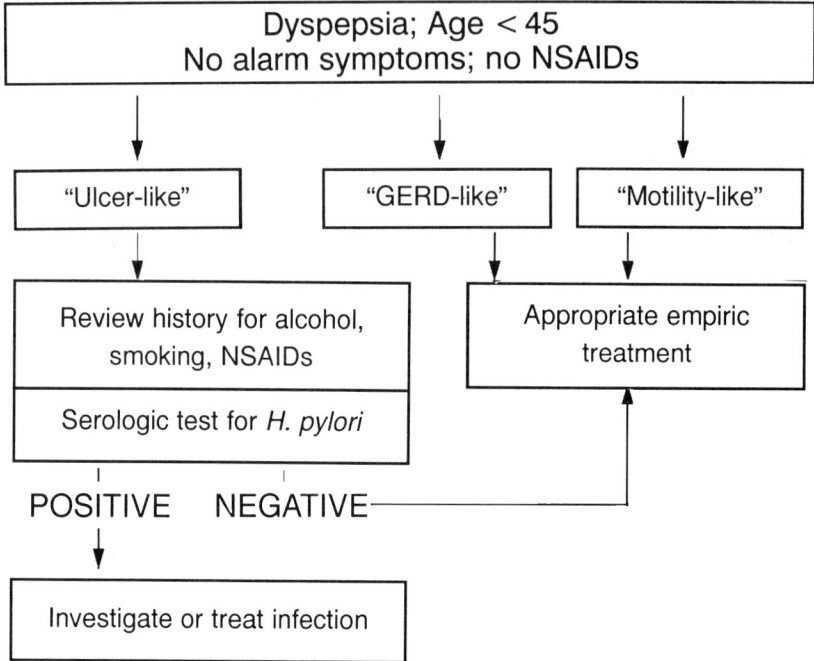

Figure 1   Flow sheet on diagnostic steps in new onset of dyspepsia (age < 45)

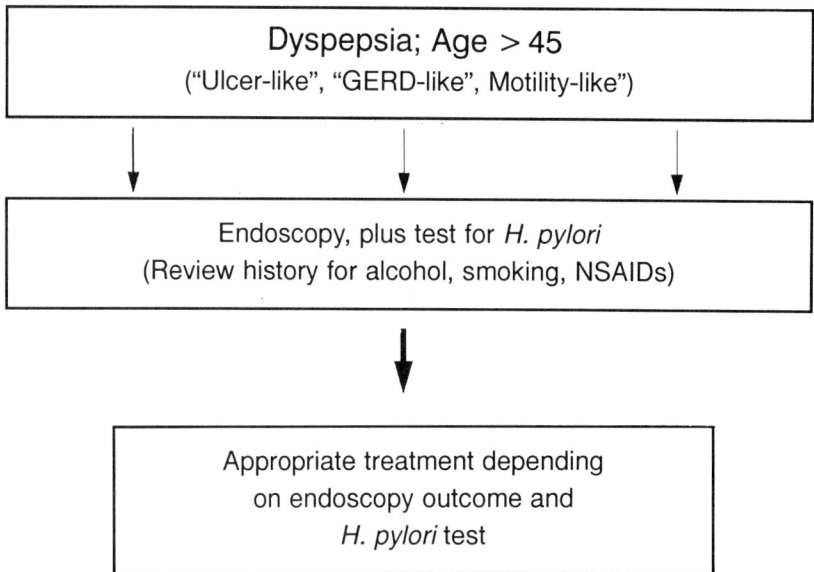

```
┌─────────────────────────────────────────────────────────┐
│                  Dyspepsia; Age > 45                      │
│        ("Ulcer-like", "GERD-like", Motility-like")        │
└─────────────────────────────────────────────────────────┘
        │                      │                     │
        ▼                      ▼                     ▼
┌─────────────────────────────────────────────────────────┐
│           Endoscopy, plus test for H. pylori              │
│    (Review history for alcohol, smoking, NSAIDs)          │
└─────────────────────────────────────────────────────────┘
                            │
                            ▼
┌─────────────────────────────────────────────────────────┐
│           Appropriate treatment depending                 │
│              on endoscopy outcome and                     │
│                  H. pylori test                           │
└─────────────────────────────────────────────────────────┘
```

Figure 2   Flow sheet on diagnostic steps in new onset of dyspepsia (age > 45)

Firm recommendations cannot be given, as yet, but testing of the 'ulcer-like' dyspeptic patients for *H. pylori* by the GPs based on non-invasive tests (serology, ^{13}C urea breath test) seems a reasonable approach in the industrialized, high-technology countries which have an approximate 30% prevalence of *H. pylori* infection in those aged below 45. This approach would not be appropriate in developing countries, where much higher prevalence rates for *H. pylori* are usually found. The future management could then consist of treating *H. pylori* infection without further investigations for those found to be infected with *H. pylori* who are below 45 years old and not on NSAIDs, and reserving endoscopy for those older than 45, since this group of patients is more likely to have more serious disease. Again, this point has to be taken into serious consideration and may not be rare in regions of the world with a higher incidence of gastric malignancy occurring at a younger age. For *H. pylori*-positive patients above 45 years of age, the GPs and their patients would be on the safe side if they have an endoscopic assessment before treatment. *H. pylori*-negative dyspepsia in the young dyspeptic not on NSAIDs may need only symptomatic treatment, while the older patient not on NSAIDs, and with a recent onset of symptoms, will need endoscopy.

WHAT THERAPEUTIC REGIMEN SHOULD BE USED BY THE GP?

Although *H. pylori* infection is susceptible to many different antimicrobial agents, curing the infection remains a major challenge. The ideal drug should be simple, effective, inexpensive, free of side-effects and successful in eradicating *H. pylori* infection in close to 100% of cases. Unfortunately, such a drug, or a combination of different drugs, has still not been found. To date, therapy of *H. pylori* infection is always a compromise between the above-mentioned criteria.

Major progress has been achieved with the 7-day regimens consisting of a proton pump inhibitor and clarithromycin plus either metronidazole or amoxycillin. All these regimens have cure rates of around 90%, which is comparable to standard 14-day triple therapy with bismuth, metronidazole and tetracycline, but the former regimens are superior in terms of patient compliance and reduced side-effects.

The major point in applying these therapies to patients is that different populations do not necessarily produce the same cure rates. This has been proven with different regimens and can be explained partly by different compliance rates in different populations, which is relevant especially with bismuth triple therapy, and also by the bacterial resistance to antibiotics used in the various regimens.

To summarize, physicians should use therapies with a high cure rate, preferably above 90%, and should rely on regimens which have been proven in the population with which they are working.

FOLLOW-UP AFTER TREATMENT OF THE *H. PYLORI* INFECTION

The follow-up protocol of patients treated for *H. pylori* infection is still an issue of controversy among clinical researchers. The only general agreement is the definite need to test the effects of treatment in patients with complicated ulcer disease such as those with bleeding ulcer. Patients with *H. pylori*-positive, non-complicated duodenal ulcer may be followed only by assessing of symptoms, as proposed in a recent study[29]. The study investigated the correlation between *H. pylori* status, confirmed by the ^{13}C-urea breath test, and dyspeptic symptoms 1 and 6 months after the completion of treatment. Of the breath test-negative patients 87.5% were free of all dyspeptic symptoms after 1 month (97.5% after 6 months). The reported specificity was 56.3% versus 90.6%, respectively. Figures for sensitivity were even better when only the absence of epigastric discomfort was used for assessment, 88.8% and 100%, respectively. This may be an option only for patients with duodenal ulcer and not gastric ulcer, since they are not at risk for gastric malignancies.

Our personal conviction is that the outcome in dyspeptic patients with *H. pylori* infection also should be checked for by non-invasive means (^{13}C-urea breath test) as it reassures the patient and indicates the efficacy of the treatment regimen.

CONCLUSION

In suspected ulcer only endoscopy can differentiate between duodenal ulcer, gastric ulcer and gastric malignancies. For ulcer treatment physicians should use *H. pylori* eradication treatments with a high cure rate, which are preferably above 90%, and should rely on regimens which have been proven in the population for which they are responsible.

Firm recommendations for treating non-ulcer dyspepsia cannot be given as yet, but testing 'ulcer-like' dyspeptic patients who are aged less than 45 years for *H. pylori* infection by the GPs using non-invasive tests seems a reasonable approach in industrialized countries with a low prevalence of *H. pylori* infection. For this subgroup of patients *H. pylori* treatment without further investigation appears a good option.

The follow-up of patients treated for *H. pylori* infection is still an important but controversial issue among clinical researchers. The only general agreement is the definite need to test the effects of treatment in patients with complicated ulcer disease. Since with the ^{13}C urea breath test a non-invasive control test for *H. pylori* eradication is possible, it should be used in all patients.

References

1. Correa P, Ruiz B, Hunter F. Clinical trials as etiologic research tools in *Helicobacter*-associated gastritis. Scand J Gastroenterol Suppl. 1991;181:15–19.
2. Parsonnet J, Friedman GD, Vandersteen DP *et al. Helicobacter pylori* infection and the risk of gastric carcinoma. N Engl J Med. 1991;325:1127–31.
3. Parsonnet J, Hansen S, Rodriguez L *et al. Helicobacter pylori* infection and gastric lymphoma. N Engl J Med. 1994;330:1267–71.
4. Nomura A, Stemmermann GN, Chyou PH, Kato I, Perez-Perez GI, Blaser MJ. *Helicobacter pylori* infection and gastric carcinoma among Japanese Americans in Hawaii. N Engl J Med. 1991;325:1132–6.
5. Fukao A, Komatsu S, Tsubono Y *et al. Helicobacter pylori* infection and chronic atrophic gastritis among Japanese blood donors: a cross-sectional study. Cancer Causes Control. 1993;4:307–12.

6. Craanen ME, Dekker W, Blok P, Ferwerda J, Tytgat GN. Intestinal metaplasia and *Helicobacter pylori*: an endoscopic bioptic study of the gastric antrum. Gut. 1992;33:16–20.

7. Graham DY, Lew GM, Klein PD *et al.* Effect of treatment of *Helicobacter pylori* infection on the long-term recurrence of gastric or duodenal ulcer. A randomized, controlled study. Ann Intern Med. 1992;116:705–8.

8. Graham DY, Hepps KS, Ramirez FC, Lew GM, Saeed ZA. Treatment of *Helicobacter pylori* reduces the rate of rebleeding in peptic ulcer disease. Scand J Gastroenterol. 1993;28:939–42.

9. Bayerdorffer E, Neubauer A, Rudolph B *et al.* Regression of primary gastric lymphoma of mucosa-associated lymphoid tissue type after cure of *Helicobacter pylori* infection. MALT Lymphoma Study Group. Lancet. 1995;345:1591–4.

10. Stolte M. *Helicobacter pylori* gastritis and gastric MALT-lymphoma. Lancet. 1992;339:745–6.

11. Forman D, Newell DG, Fullerton F *et al.* Association between infection with *Helicobacter pylori* and risk of gastric cancer: evidence from a prospective investigation. Br Med J. 1991;302:1302–5.

12. Mendall MA, Goggin PM, Molineaux N *et al.* Relation of *Helicobacter pylori* infection and coronary heart disease. Br Heart J. 1994;71:437–9.

13. Graham DY. Benefits from elimination of *Helicobacter pylori* infection include major reduction in the incidence of peptic ulcer disease, gastric cancer, and primary gastric lymphoma. Prev Med. 1994;23:712–16.

14. *Helicobacter pylori* in peptic ulcer disease. NIH Consensus Statement. 1994;12:1–23.

15. Forman D, Webb P, Parsonnet J. *H. pylori* and gastric cancer. Lancet. 1994;343:243–4.

16. IARC Working Group on the Evaluation of Carcinogenic Risks to Humans. Schistosomes, liver flukes and *Helicobacter pylori*. Lyon, 7–14 June 1994. IARC Monogr Eval Carcinog Risks Hum. 1994;61:1–241.

17. Kuipers EJ, Lundell L, Klinkenberg Knol EC *et al.* Atrophic gastritis and *Helicobacter pylori* infection in patients with reflux oesophagitis treated with omeprazole or fundoplication. N Engl J Med. 1996;334:1018–22.

18. Christensen AH, Logan RP, Noach LA, Gjorup T. Do clinicians accept the role of *Helicobacter pylori* in duodenal ulcer disease: a survey of European gastroenterologists and general practitioners. J Intern Med. 1994;236:501–5.

19. Babbs C. *H. pylori*-associated gastroduodenal disease: survey of British physicians' views. Gut. 1995;37(Suppl. 1):347 (abstract).

20. Forman D, Milne R, Logan R *et al.* Attitudes and practices of gastroenterologists in the UK towards *Helicobacter pylori* disease: results from a large survey. Am J Gastroenterol. 1994;89:398 (abstract).

21. Peniston JG, Mistry KR. Eradication of *Helicobacter pylori* in general practice. Aliment Pharmacol Ther. 1996;10:139–45.

22. Breuer T, Sudhop T, Goodman K *et al.* Does disease presentation influence treatment of *H. pylori* infection? A comparison of gastroenterologists and family practitioners. Gastroenterology. 1996;110(Suppl. 4):A69 (abstract).

23. Breuer T, Sudhop T, Goodman K *et al.* Treatment regimens used in *Helicobacter pylori* positive ulcer disease: a comparison of gastroenterologists and family practitioners (abstract). Gastroenterology. 1996;110(Suppl. 4):A69.

24. Breuer T, Sudhop T, Goodman K *et al.* Treatment of suspected gastroduodenal ulcer: is the German experience important for health policy decisions in the US? Gastroenterology. 1996;110(Suppl. 4):A42 (abstract).

25. van der Hulst RW, Keller IJ, Rauws EAJ, Tytgat GNJ. Treatment of *Helicobacter pylori* infection: a review of the world literature. Helicobacter. 1996;1:6–20.

26. Patel P, Mendall MA, Lloyd MA, Jazrawi R, Maxwell JD, Northfield TC. Prospective screening of dyspeptic patients by *Helicobacter pylori* serology. Lancet. 1995;346:1315–18.

27. McCarthy C, Patchett S, Collins RM, Beattie S, Keane C, O'Morain C. Long-term prospective study of *Helicobacter pylori* in nonulcer dyspepsia. Dig Dis Sci. 1995;40:114–19.

28. Veldhuyzen van Zanten SJ, Malatjalian DA, Tanton R *et al.* The effect of eradication of *Helicobacter pylori* (Hp) on symptoms of non-ulcer dyspepsia (NUD): a randomized double-blind placebo controlled trial. Gastroenterology. 1995;108:A250 (abstract).

29. Phull PS, Halliday D, Price AB, Jacyna MR. Absence of dyspeptic symptoms as a test for *Helicobacter pylori* eradication. Br Med J. 1996;312:349–50.

38
Novel therapies for *Helicobacter pylori* infection

J. LAMBERT and P. MIDOLO

INTRODUCTION

Helicobacter pylori colonizes the gastric mucosa. After surviving the acid environment of the gastric lumen it enters into gastric mucus aided by its motility. The organism adheres to gastric mucus and surface epithelial cells predominantly at the intercellular junctions. A local immune response is initiated, as well as the development of inflammation with associated attraction of inflammatory cells with chemokine and cytokine production. A systemic immune response is initiated as a consequence of the colonization.

Regimens to eradicate *H. pylori* have developed over the past 12 years, initially starting with monotherapy and then dual therapy. Currently, regimens consist of triple or quadruple therapy, but all these latter regimens have the problem that they are not universally successful in all patients[1,2]. Due to the numbers of tablets taken, these regimens are costly, with poor patient compliance and potential adverse effects. Moreover, as with other infectious diseases the natural drug resistance of *H. pylori* is increasing, with many isolated strains now resistant to nitroimidazoles, macrolides, tetracyclines and other antibiotics[3,4]. This chapter reviews some of the potentially novel therapies for *H. pylori* infection. The chapter initially will review the gastric microenvironment and then discuss new and alternative antimicrobial agents. Newer methods of drug delivery and formulation, agents modifying gastric mucus and anti-adherence strategies will be reviewed. Modulators of the immune and inflammatory response are now available and their role will be discussed.

GASTRIC ENVIRONMENT

Gastric mucus consists of a thin layer covering the surface epithelial cells. Composition is mainly water (90%) and mucin (10%). Gastric mucins largely consist of glycoproteins arranged in polymeric form consisting of four subunits with disulphide bridges. *H. pylori* are situated under and within gastric and duodenal mucus on the surface of gastric epithelial cells, in the intercellular spaces as well as in gastric glands. *H. pylori* may also be found in gastric juice, saliva, and stools[5]. Drugs may be delivered via the gastric lumen with local uptake (including bismuth compounds, amoxycillin and tetracycline), as well as via systemic absorption and distribution into the gastric environment[6]. Secretion of a number of antibiotics, including nitroimidazoles, macrolides, and clindamycin, does occur[6–8].

NEW ANTIMICROBIALS AGAINST *HELICOBACTER*

A number of agents with *in-vitro* activity against *H. pylori* are now becoming available for clinical use. Many of these agents have theoretical advantages in their tissue distribution, specific site of intragastric activity, safety, and local action via the gastric lumen.

New macrolide antibiotics with low minimal inhibitory concentrations against *H. pylori in vitro* include roxithromycin (MIC 0.2 mg/L) and azithromycin (MIC 0.25 mg/L)[9]. Human gastric tissue levels of azithromycin have been shown to be up to 10 times greater than those seen in gastric mucus following a 500 mg oral dose, and these levels persist over a 5-day period[10]. This may offer a significant advantage over clarithromycin with respect to dosing schedules. Cross-resistance between macrolides occurs against *H. pylori*, and their long-term efficacy may be questionable if macrolide resistance continues to increase.

The spectinomycin analogue trospectomycin has shown good *in-vitro* activity, a long tissue half-life and additive/synergistic activity with colloidal bismuth subcitrate, but there are few data on its activity *in vivo*[11].

The novel rifamycin antibiotic rifaximin has also shown good *in-vitro* activity against *H. pylori* and has the possible advantage of being non-absorbable in the stomach[12]. The disadvantage of this antibiotic is the development of resistance with exposure to subinhibitory concentrations, but its role in combination therapies *in vivo* warrants further investigation[13].

A number of new proton pump inhibitors are now available, and most show *in-vitro* and *in-vivo* activity against *H. pylori*. These include lansoprazole and its metabolites[14], pantoprazole[15] and E3810[16].

Several bismuth compounds are now available with both *in-vitro* and *in-vivo* activity against *H. pylori*. Those in most common use include colloidal bismuth subcitrate (Yamanouchi – De Nol) and bismuth subsalicylate (Procter & Gamble – Pepto-Bismol). Newer bismuth agents include ranitidine bismuth citrate (Glaxo – Pylorid®)[17], bismuth sucralfate[18], and a group of organic bismuths (CDTB, BTBT, TTCB), the latter of which have different activities against *H. pylori* as well as different ulcer healing properties[19].

A number of other agents are known to have *in-vitro* activity against *H. pylori*, with some of these agents now having undergone pilot studies and showing *in-vivo* effect. These include a zinc compound (Z103) which has been shown to have *in-vivo* activity along with other antibiotics[20]. A number of heavy metals including gold, copper, and silver are active *in vitro*[21]. No evidence exists, however, that these metals have activity against *H. pylori in vivo*. A lower prevalence of *H. pylori* does not occur in patients with rheumatoid arthritis taking oral-gold

Table 1 Potential alternative agents against *Helicobacter*

1. *Non-ionic surfactants and emulsifiers*
   Polysorbates, PEG ethers[29]

2. *Dietary compounds*
   Polyunsaturated fatty acids[30,31]
   Free fatty acids and monoglycerol esters[32]
   Manuka honey[33]

3. *Milk/milk products*
   Lactoferrin[34]
   Protein moiety[35]

4. *Probiotics – lactic acid bacteria*
   Organic acids[37]
   Supernatant *Lactobacillus acidophilus*[38]
   Bacteriocins – nisin+EDTA or citrate[39]

therapy. Moreover in a small pilot study oral gold was not effective in *H. pylori* eradication.

Other agents that have been evaluated include plaunotol, ecabet sodium, ebrotidine, and sulglycotide. Plaunotol is a 15 amino acid peptide which inhibits *H. pylori in vitro* at high doses (100 µg/ml). It also decreases adherence of *H. pylori* to cell culture *in vitro* and decreases *H. pylori*-induced IL-8 secretion[22]. In a randomized study plaunotol in combination with lansoprazole and clarithromycin was 100% effective in healing gastric ulcers, with a 69% *H. pylori* eradication rate[23]. Ecabet sodium, which has ulcer healing and mucosal protective properties, also inhibits *H. pylori* urease activity. The combination of ecabet sodium with lansoprazole and amoxycillin achieves eradication of *H. pylori* in 89% of infected subjects[24]. Ebrotidine is an H_2 receptor antagonist which is shown to inhibit *H. pylori* urease activity and to enhance the antibacterial actions of other antibiotics *in vitro* against *H. pylori*[25]. Sulglycotide is a mucin extract which again has been shown to enhance the action of other antibiotics against *H. pylori in vitro*[26].

Sucralfate, an aluminium octasulphate of sucrose, inhibits *H. pylori* haemagglutinin, protease and lipase, and as a single agent decreases *H. pylori* colonization and gastritis. In clinical studies sucralfate, tetracycline and metronidazole triple therapy is comparable in its eradication rate to bismuth triple therapy[27,28].

Agents may also kill *H. pylori* via an effect on cell wall and intermediary metabolism. Drugs may block metal transport (nickel, iron) or enzymes; however, it is unlikely that these could be delivered safely to the site of *H. pylori* without a significant adverse host effect.

ALTERNATIVE AGENTS AGAINST *HELICOBACTER*

A number of newer agents with local intragastric activity are now being considered (Table 1). These agents include non-ionic surfactants and emulsifiers, dietary compounds including fatty acids, milk products, as well as products of lactic acid bacteria. A number of non-ionic surfactants and emulsifiers have been shown to have anti-*Helicobacter* effects *in vitro*, including polysorbates and polyethylene glycol ethers[29].

Previous investigators have suggested possible links between dietary factors and peptic ulcer disease. Polyunsaturated fatty acids (PFA) have been implicated in the pathogenesis of peptic ulcer since decreased intake, as well as reduced subcutaneous concentrations of linolenic acid (a W-6 PFA), have been related to an increased incidence of the disease.

PFA, particularly linolenic acid (W-3 PFA) have been shown to exert *in vitro* activity against *H. pylori*[30]. In an open study of eight infected subjects, supplementation with PFA for 2 months (2 g per day; W6/W3 = 0.82), resulted in *H. pylori* suppression in six[31]. Confirmation by a double-blind placebo-controlled trial is required to support this observation. Free fatty acids (FFA) and their corresponding monoglyceryl esters (MG) are also known to have bactericidal properties. The medium chain MG and FFA C_8 and C_{12} have *in-vitro* killing activity against both *H. pylori* and *H. felis*. Infected mice given C_{10} monoglyceride (5 mg/ml) in a liquid diet showed clearance of infection suggesting *in-vivo* efficacy[32]. It has also been shown that Manuka honey from New Zealand has *in-vitro* properties against *H. pylori*[33].

Other milk products have also been found to possess anti-*Helicobacter* activity. Lactoferrin, a glycoprotein found in mammalian milk, possesses antibacterial activity against a variety of Gram-negative bacteria. Intact bovine lactoferrin has been shown to inhibit the growth of *H. pylori*, whereas a peptic digest was relatively inactive[34]. Within milk a component of the protein exerts *in-vitro* activity against *H. pylori*[35].

Lactic acid bacteria found within the human gastrointestinal tract produce bacteriocins (antibiotic-like substances) and organic acids including lactic acid and acetic acid. These bacteria have potential in the management of gastrointestinal problems[36]. Organic acids, particularly lactic acid, in a concentration-dependent manner, are inhibitory to the growth of *H. pylori*, and certain lactobacilli have been shown to exert anti-*Helicobacter* activity both from the organisms and culture supernatant[37]. In addition a supernatant of *Lactobacillus acidophilus* (strain LA1) has been shown, in infected humans, to cause suppression of the ^{13}C-urea breath test after 2 weeks of treatment[38].

Bacteriocins are peptides produced by a number of bacteria, including lactic acid bacteria, and are known to inhibit the growth of other organisms[39]. The food preservative nisin is a bacteriocin, and has *in-vitro* activity against *H. pylori* if chelated with either EDTA or citrate[40]. In animal studies using nisin in the treatment of *H. felis* infection in the mouse model, nisin, in a dose ranging from 0.3 to 3 mg per day, was found to eradicate the infection similarly to rates found with antibiotic monotherapy in the same model (Blackburn P, 1996, unpublished data). Human clinical trials are currently being undertaken.

DRUG DELIVERY SYSTEMS

Delivery of antimicrobial agents to the site of infection occurs via the topical or systemic route. Topical therapy has been incorporated by using the Jichi method, whereby subjects are pretreated with lansoprazole and pronase for a 2-day period[41]. A nasogastric tube is then inserted and a combination of amoxycillin, bismuth subnitrate, metronidazole, and pronase is placed intragastrically for a 2-h period.

The liquid is then removed and eradication rates of 88–94% have been reported[41]. This method has the advantages of a short-duration therapy as well as minimal side-effects from the agents administered. Moreover, this method confirms the importance of the local mucosal action of intragastric agents.

Modification of uptake of antibiotics into the gastric mucosa can occur by coadministration of other agents. Omeprazole has been found to increase the uptake of clarithromycin into gastric mucus and mucosa[42]. No such change in the uptake of amoxycillin into the gastric mucosa has been observed with coadministration of omeprazole[43]. Ranitidine has been shown to decrease the uptake of amoxycillin[44] and enhance that of clindamycin into the gastric mucosa[45].

Agents which disrupt the gastric mucus, including pronase, N-acetyl cysteine and non-steroidal anti-inflammatory drugs, may enhance the activity of antimicrobial agents against H. pylori. Pronase has been used in combination with antibiotics during topical therapy, as previously reported[41]. N-acetyl cysteine, a sulphydryl compound with potent mucolytic activity, induces a reduction of the gastric barrier mucus thickness of about 75% and reduces mucus viscoelasticity. A combination of omeprazole and amoxycillin, along with N-acetyl cysteine at a dose of 1200 mg b.i.d. for 10 days, was found to enhance the bacterial eradication rate[46]. Non-steroidal anti-inflammatory drugs which are known to affect the gastric mucosa have been shown in combination with ranitidine bismuth citrate, in an animal model, to increase the uptake of bismuth into the gastric mucus[47]. The levels of bismuth within the gastric mucus were maintained at a higher concentration in the indomethacin-treated animals[47].

BACTERIAL ADHERENCE, MODIFIERS

H. pylori adhere to gastric mucus as well as to surface epithelial cells, and at the intercellular junctions. A number of binding receptors have been proposed, and include binding to mucin, an extracellular matrix including laminin; collagen, type IV; heparin sulphate and fibronectin[48]. In addition a number of epithelial cell membrane constituents including carbohydrates (fucose and sialic acid), glycerolipids, gangliosides and cholesterol have been proposed. In a number of in-vitro studies receptor inhibition to the erythrocyte carbohydrate membrane constituents have been shown to inhibit the binding of H. pylori. These include competitive inhibitors such as fetuin, oromucoide, and sialoproteins[48,49]. Degradation of the carbohydrate moieties may occur with neuroaminidase, fucosidase and metaperiodate, the latter of which cleaves sialic acid residues[50,51]. Monoclonal antibodies directed against fucosylated blood group antigens may impair the binding of H. pylori to surface epithelium in vitro[51]. Thus, these agents have theoretical activity against binding of the bacteria to the gastric mucosa. As only up to 15% of the Helicobacter are bound it is unlikely that these agents will be of any clinical benefit. Moreover, delivery of these agents, even if they are safe, to the site of H. pylori is improbable.

Binding of Helicobacter also may be impaired with sucralfate preparations via competitive inhibition.

Table 2 *Helicobacter pylori* infection: immune/inflammatory modulation

Response to infection	Potential agents to treat
Immune response	Therapeutic immunization[55]
IgA	Bovine colostrum with *H. pylori*
IgG	antibodies[56]
Lymphocytes	Breast milk anti-*H. pylori* IgA[57]
Inflammatory response	Strategies:
Polymorphs	(A) Enhance inflammation
Monocytes	IL-2
Mast cells	IL-4
Cytokines	IL-10 antibody
IL1–8	(B) Immune deviation/suppress inflammation
TNFα	Th1 → Th2 lymphocytes
IFNγ	Anti-TNFα antibody/TNFα binding protein
	IL-10, IL-11
	IL-1 receptor antagonist
	Macrophage inhibitor (CNI-1493)

MODULATION OF THE IMMUNE AND INFLAMMATORY PROCESSES

In conjunction with *H. pylori*-induced inflammation, a local and systemic immune response occurs with production of IgA and IgG antibodies, the former found in gastric juice and from salivary secretions. In the inflammatory response that occurs in the gastric mucosa a number of polymorphonuclear leucocytes, monocytes and mast cells are attracted into the mucosa. Production of cytokines including interleukins, interferon gamma (IFNγ) and tumour necrosis factor alpha (TNFα) maintains the inflammatory response. Interleukins 10 and 11 have been shown to decrease inflammation as well as the levels of TNFα. Regulatory T cells including helper T cells (Th) are important in controlling the host response to infection. Th1 cells produce cytokines selecting for cell-mediated immunity, whereas Th2 cells secrete cytokines favouring induction of antibody responses including intestinal IgA. An imbalance may exist, with *H. pylori* infection persisting, due to the continued presence of Th1 cells resulting in inflammation and epithelial damage[52].

With the development of animal models of *Helicobacter* infection oral immunization strategies to prevent infection have been developed[53,54]. Immunization appears to enhance the Th2-driven responses in these models, favouring IgA responses and protective immunity.

Modification of the immune response has also been shown potentially to eradicate *H. pylori* infection (Table 2). Therapeutic immunization in animal models has been shown to abolish infection, again by enhancing the Th2 lymphocyte responses[55]. Cows immunized with *H. pylori* subsequently show, in both serum and colostrum, anti-*H. pylori* activity due to antibody production. Thus, post-colostral milk from immunized cows kills *H. pylori in vitro*[56]. In experimental mice infected with *H. felis*, administration of specific immune colostrum from cows immunized with *H. felis* strain CST, results in a decrease in colonization of the gastric antrum (Manila *et al.*, unpublished observations). No significant reduction in the degree of inflammation was noted, however.

It has been suggested by Thomas and colleagues that elevated breast milk anti-*H. pylori* IgA may help to prevent *H. pylori* infection in Gambian infants[57].

Enhancement of the inflammatory response in humans may thus theoretically increase the ability to eradicate *Helicobacter* from the mucosa. Proinflammatory cytokines (IL-1, IL-2, IL-4) may enhance immune responses, whereas other cytokines (IL-10, IL-11) suppress immune-mediated events. The use of human recombinant IL-2 and IL-4, as well as the use of antibodies against IL-10, may enhance the inflammatory response. Immune deviation using these above strategies will modify the stem cell development from Th2 to Th1 lymphocytes, resulting in increased inflammatory activity. These responses have been outlined in Chapter 15.

Suppression of inflammation in subjects with inflammatory bowel disease has resulted in a significant improvement in symptoms and remission of disease[58]. In *H. pylori* infection suppression of inflammation is unlikely to result in a decrease in bacterial colonization unless immune modulation in the direction of Th2 lymphocytes can be achieved. Immunosuppressive agents include lymphocyte activation inhibitors (e.g. rapamycin), monoclonal antibodies (e.g. anti-CD3, anti-CD4), cytokine-based therapies, and antiproliferative agents (e.g. brequinar sodium). Inflammatory suppression may occur via a number of agents including human recombinant IL-10 and IL-11[59]. In addition anti-TNFα antibodies and binding proteins will suppress the proinflammatory activity of TNFα. IL-1 receptor antagonists are currently available as are inhibitors of macrophage function (CNI-1493)[59]. *In-vitro* studies and animal models are necessary to provide further insights into the role of inflammation and its modification on regulating the immune response and achieving bacterial eradication.

SUMMARY

A number of novel agents, both alone and in combination with currently used antibiotics, may offer advantages over traditional multi-drug regimens. Further *in-vitro* studies are required to confirm the activity against *H. pylori*, as well as to understand the mechanisms of action. Studies in *H. pylori* and *H. felis* animal models should be undertaken to assess the optimal dose, duration of therapy, and modes of administration prior to human studies. Modification of the immune and inflammatory responses potentially offers the greatest promise in the eradication of *H. pylori*. Pilot studies which are well conducted, using pure substances, are necessary to support or refute the activity of some of these novel compounds. Publication of pilot studies also is essential to establish the potential role of these agents in treatment.

References

1. Van der Hulst RWM, Keller JJ, Rauws EAJ, Tytgat GNJ. Treatment of *H. pylori* infection: a review of the world literature. Helicobacter. 1996;1:6–19.
2. Holtmann G, Layer P, Goebell H. Proton pump inhibitors or H$_2$ receptor antagonists for *H. pylori* eradication: a meta-analysis. Lancet. 1996;345:817–20.
3. Megraud F. *H. pylori* resistance to antibiotics. In: Hunt RG, Tytgat GNJ, editors. *H. pylori*: basic mechanisms to clinical cure. Lancaster: Kluwer; 1994:540–83.

4. Midolo P, Korman MG, Turnidge JD, Lambert JR. *H. pylori* resistance to tetracycline. Lancet. 1996;347:1994–5.
5. Namavar F, Roosendaal R, Kuipers EJ *et al.* Presence of *H. pylori* in the oral cavity, oesophagus, stomach and faeces of patients with gastritis. Eur J Clin Microbiol Infect Dis. 1995;14:234–7.
6. Lambert JR, Arena G. Mucosal antibiotic levels. In: Hunt RG, Tytgat GNJ, editors. *H. pylori*: basic mechanisms to clinical cure. Lancaster: Kluwer; 1994:538–49.
7. Veldhuyzen van Zanten SJO, Goldie J, Hollingsworth J, Silletti C, Richardson H, Hunt RH. Secretion of intravenously administered antibiotics in gastric juice. Implications for management of *H. pylori*. J Clin Pathol. 1992;45:225–7.
8. Hextall A, Radley S. Andrews JM *et al.* Mucosal concentration and excretion of clindamycin by the human stomach. J Antimicrob Chemother. 1994;33:595–602.
9. Burette A, Glupczynski Y. *H. pylori*: the place of the new macrolides in the eradication of the bacteria in peptic ulcer disease. Infection. 1995(Suppl. 1);23:544–52.
10. Vogt K, Radloff AC, Hahn H. Combined activity of trospectomycin and colloidal bismuth subcitrate against *H. pylori in vitro*. Infection. 1991;19:138–9.
11. Debets-Ossekopp YJ, Namavar F, MacLaren DM. Effect of an acidic environment on the susceptibility of *H. pylori* to trospectomycin and other antimicrobial agents. Eur J Clin Microbiol Infect Dis. 1995;14:353–5.
12. Holton J, Vaina D, Menegatti M, Barbara L. The susceptibility of *H. pylori* to the rifamycin, rifaximin. J Antimicrob Chemother. 1995;35:545–9.
13. Megraud F, Bouffant F, Camoujuncas C. *In vitro* activity of rifaximin against *H. pylori*. Eur J Clin Microbiol Infect Dis. 1994;13:184–6.
14. Iwahi T, Satoh H, Hakao M. Lansoprazole: a novel benzimidozole proton pump inhibitor and its related compounds have selective activity against *H. pylori*. Antimicrob Agents Chemother. 1991;35:490–6.
15. Adamek RJ. Pantoprazole, clarithromycin and metronidazole vs pantoprazole and clarithromycin for cure of *H. pylori* infection in duodenal ulcer patients. Gastroenterology. 1996;110:A48.
16. Hirai M, Azuma T, Ito S, Kato T, Kohli Y, Kuriyama M. A proton pump inhibitor, E3810, has an antibacterial activity through binding to *H. pylori*. Gastroenterology. 1995;108:A114.
17. Pounder RE, Bailey R, Louw JA *et al.* GR122311X (ranitidine bismuth citrate) with clarithromycin for the eradication of *H. pylori*. Gut. 1995;37(Suppl. 1):A42.
18. Reijers MH, Noch LA, Tytgat GN. Evaluation of *H. pylori* eradication with bismuth sucralfate. Aliment Pharmacol Ther. 1994;8:351–2.
19. Le Blanc R, Van Zanten S, Bunford N, Agoc L, Leddin DJ. The efficacy of novel bismuth compounds in healing gastric ulceration in the rate varies with chemical structure implications for *H. pylori* treatment. Gastroenterology. 1995;108:A860.
20. Kuwayama H. Zinc compound is a novel, highly effective triple therapy for eradication of *H. pylori*. Gastroenterology. 1995;108:A139.
21. Vicari F, Foliguet B, Conroy MC *et al.* Comparative in vitro activity of 8 metal salts, lansoprazole and cefotiam against clinical isolates of *H. pylori*. Gastroenterology. 1995;108:A936.
22. Takagi A, Ohta U, Aiba Y *et al.* Suppression of *H. pylori*-induced IL-8 secretion by an anti-ulcer agent. Paunotol in vitro. Gastroenterology. 1995;110:A269.
23. Fukuda Y, Yamamoto I, Okui M, Tonokatsu Y, Tamura K, Shimoyama T. Combination therapy with mucosal protective agent for the eradication of *H. pylori*. Eur J Gastroenterol Hepatol. 1995;Suppl. 1:S45–7.
24. Matsukua N, Onda M, Shirakawa T *et al.* High eradication rate of *H. pylori* with lansoprazole and amoxicillin and ecabet sodium: new triple therapy with novel mucosal protective agent for the treatment of peptic ulcer. Gastroenterology. 1996;110:A190.
25. Slomiany BL, Piotrowski J, Majka J, Czaikowski A, Slomiany A, Gabryelewicz A. Enhancement in the protective qualities of gastric mucus by ebrotidine during duodenal ulcer healing. Gen Pharmacol. 1995;26:1039–44.
26. Slomiany BL, Murty VL, Piotrowski J, Slomiany A. Gastroprotective agents in mucosal defence against *Helicobacter pylori*. Gen Pharmacol. 1994;25:833–41.
27. Sung JJ, Leung VK, Chung SC *et al.* Triple therapy with sucralfate, tetracycline, and metronidazole for *H. pylori* associated duodenal ulcers. Am J Gastroenterol. 1995;90:1424–7.
28. Lam SK, Hu WH, Ching CK. Sucralfate in *H. pylori* eradication strategies. Scand J Gastroenterol. 1995;210:89–91.
29. Kane AV, Plaut AG. Unique susceptibility of *H. pylori* to simethicone emulsifiers in alimentary therapeutic agents. Antimicrob Agents Chemother. 1996;40:500–2.

30. Thompson L, Cockayne A, Spillar RC. Inhibitory effect of polyunsaturated fatty acids on the growth of *H. pylori*: a possible explanation of the effect of diet on peptic ulceration. Gut. 1994; 35:1557–61.

31. Frieri G, Marcheggiano A, Pimpo M *et al.* Polyunsaturated fatty acids (PFA) and *Helicobacter pylori* (*H. pylori*). An open study. Gastroenterology. 1995;108:A96.

32. Petschow BW, Batema RP, Ford LL. Susceptibility of *H. pylori* to bactericidal properties of medium-chain monoglycerides and free fatty acids. Antimicrob Agents Chemother. 1996;40: 302–6.

33. Al Somal N, Coley KE, Molan PC, Hancock BM. Susceptibility of *H. pylori* to the antimicrobial activity of manuka honey. J Roy Soc Med. 1994;87:9–12.

34. Dial EJ, Serna JH, Lichtenberger LM. Lactoferrin inhibits the growth of *H. pylori in vitro.* Gastroenterology. 1995;108:A82.

35. Luo F, Hull RR, Lambert JR. Milk derived substances inhibitory to *H. pylori in vitro.* Am J Gastroenterol. 1994;89:1395.

36. Lambert JR, Hull R. Upper gastrointestinal tract disease and probiotics. Asia Pacific J Clin Nutr. 1996;5:31–5.

37. Midolo PD, Lambert JR, Hull R, Luo F, Grayson ML. *In vitro* inhibition of *H. pylori* NCTC 11637 by organic acids and lactic acid bacteria. J Appl Bacteriol. 1995;79:475–9.

38. Michetti P, Dorta G, Brassard D *et al. L. acidophilus* supernatant as an adjunct in the therapy of *H. pylori* in humans. Gastroenterology. 1995;108:A166.

39. Mishra C, Lambert JR. Production of anti-microbial substances by probiotics. Asian Pacific J Clin Nutr. 1996;5:20–4.

40. Projan SJ, Blackburn P. The bacteriocin nisin activated by chelating agents is bactericidal for *H. pylori* in vitro. Gastroenterology. 1993;104:A173.

41. Kimura K, Ido K, Kihira K, Saifuko K, Tanigushi Y, Sato K. A 1-h topical therapy for the treatment of *Helicobacter pylori* infection. Am J Gastroenterol. 1995;90:60–3.

42. Gustavason LE, Kaiser JF, Edmonds AL, Locke CS, De Bartolo ML, Schmeck DW. Effect of omeprazole on concentrations of clarithromycin in plasma and gastric tissue at steady state. Antimicrob Agents Chemother. 1995;39:2078–83.

43. Cardaci G, Lambert JR, Aranda-Michel J, Underwood B. Omeprazole has no effect on the gastric mucosal bioavailability of amoxycillin. Gut. 1995;37(Suppl. 1):A90.

44. Cardaci G, Lambert JR, King RG, Onishi N, Midolo P. Reduced amoxycillin uptake into human gastric mucosa when gastric juice pH is high. Antimicrob Agents Chemother. 1995;39:2084–7.

45. Hextall A, Radley S, Andrews JM *et al.* Mucosal concentration and excretion of clindamycin by the human stomach. Antimicrob Chemother. 1994;33:595–602.

46. Zala G, Flury R, Wust J, Meyenberger C, Ammann R, Wirth HP. Omeprazole/amoxycillin: improved eradication of *H. pylori* in smokers because of *N*-acetylcysteine. J Swisse Med. 1994; 124:1391–7.

47. Tanaka S, Kaunitz JD. Indomethacin increases mucous bismuth concentration in ranitidine bismuth citrate treated rats. Gastroenterology. 1995;106:A234.

48. Sherman PM. Adherence and internalization of *H. pylori* by epithelial cells. In: Hunt RG, Tytgat GNT, editors. *Helicobacter pylori*: basic mechanisms to clinical cure. Lancaster: Kluwer; 1994: 148–62.

49. Armstrong JA, Cooper M, Goodwin CS *et al.* Influence of soluble haemagglutinins on adherence of *H. pylori* to Hep-2 cells. J Med Microbiol. 1991;34:181–7.

50. Lelwala-Guruge J, Ascencio F, Kreger AS, Ljungh A, Wadstrom T. Isolation of a sialic acid-specific surface haemagglutinin of *H. pylori* strain NCTC 11637. Zbl Bakt. 1993;280:93–106.

51. Falk P, Roth KA, Boren T, Westblom TU, Gordon JI, Normark S. An *in vitro* adherence assay reveals that *H. pylori* exhibits cell lineage-specific tropism in the human gastric epithelium. Proc Natl Acad Sci USA. 1993;90:2035–9.

52. Ernst PB, Crowe SE, Reyes VE. The immuno pathogenesis of duodenal disease associated with *Helicobacter pylori* infection. Curr Opin Gastroenterol. 1995;11:512–18.

53. Chen M, Lee A, Hazell S. Immunisation against gastric *Helicobacter* infection in a mouse/ *Helicobacter felis* model. Lancet. 1992;339:1120–1.

54. Chiara P, Michetti P. Development of a vaccine. Curr Opin Gastroenterol. 1995;11(Suppl. 1): 52–6.

55. Cvenca R, Blanchard T, Lee C *et al.* Therapeutic immunisation against *Helicobacter mustelae* infection in naturally infected ferrets. Gastroenterology. 1995;107:A78.

56. Korhonen H, Syvaoja EL, Ahola-Luttile H *et al*. Bactericidal effect of bovine normal and immune serum colostrum and milk against *H. pylori*. J Appl Bacteriol. 1995;78:655–62.
57. Thomas JE, Austin S, Dale A *et al*. Protection by human milk IgA against *Helicobacter pylori* infection in infancy. Lancet. 1993;342:121.
58. Fiocchi C, Podolsky DK. Cytokines and growth factors in inflammatory bowel disease. In: Kirsner JB, Shortner RG, editors. Inflammatory bowel disease, 4th edn. Philadelphia: Lea & Febiger; 1995:252–80.
59. Stevens AC, Shah SA, Bousvaros A. Immunosuppressive agents in gastrointestinal disease. Curr Opin Gastroenterol. 1995;11:554–61.

39
Economic evaluation of *Helicobacter pylori* eradication in the management of duodenal ulcer

B. O'BRIEN, R. GOEREE, R. HUNT, J. WILKINSON, M. LEVINE and
A. WILLAN

INTRODUCTION

The association between gastric *H. pylori* infection and peptic ulcer disease (PUD) is well established[1], and many studies have shown that eradication of *H. pylori* infection with various antimicrobial agents reduces ulcer recurrence[2,3]. This has important implications for the long-term clinical management of PUD where traditional emphasis has been on acid-suppressing drug therapy such as H_2-receptor antagonists (e.g. ranitidine) and, more recently, proton pump inhibitors (PPI) such as omperazole. A recent consensus conference of the US National Institutes of Health noted that 'nearly all patients with duodenal ulcer have *H. pylori*' and that the association with gastric ulcer is 'only slightly less strong'. The NIH consensus panel recommended treatment with antimicrobial agents for PUD patients with *H. pylori* in addition to antisecretory drugs, whether on first presentation with the illness or on recurrence[4]. Despite concerns about the cost implications of acid-suppressing drug therapy in a chronic recurrent disease such as PUD[5], the economic implications of *H. pylori* eradication compared to an alternative drug therapy such as omeprazole have received little research attention.

Growing pressure on limited drug budgets forces formularies to face difficult decisions about formulary listing of new, more effective but higher-priced drugs. The techniques of economic evaluation offer one way of synthesizing the available data on costs and outcomes associated with alternative treatment strategies, so that formulary decision-making can be based on the best evidence regarding value for money.

In this chapter we summarize a project commissioned by the Canadian Coordinating Office of Health Technology Assessment, investigating the economics of drug treatment for both peptic ulcer disease and reflux disease. Details of our methods and results are available elsewhere[6].

A BRIEF LITERATURE REVIEW

One of the earliest applications of economic appraisal to ulcer therapy was by Culyer and Maynard[7], who demonstrated the cost advantages of using cimetidine compared to surgery in duodenal ulcer. Much of the contemporary work has focused on comparisons between intermittent or maintenance therapy with histamine-2 receptor (H_2RA) antagonists and omeprazole; more recently these comparisons have also included combination antibiotic regimens to eradicate *H. pylori*. For example, Jonsson *et al.*[8] compared strategies of intermittent ranitidine and omeprazole in the UK, including both direct and indirect costs (i.e. value of time lost from work) and found omeprazole to be dominant, with fewer symptom days and lower cost over either a 1-year or 5-year period under most model assumptions. Sintonen and Alander[9] reached a similar conclusion for Finland with fewer days of symptoms and lower overall cost for an intermittent omeprazole regimen compared to ranitidine. The same general dominance conclusion for intermittent acid suppression with omeprazole over H_2RA was found in Sweden, using only direct health-care costs, by Walan and Eriksson[10].

Following the NIH Consensus Conference on *H. pylori*[4] a number of studies have examined the costs and outcomes of antibiotic therapy to eradicate *H. pylori* as an alternative to either intermittent or maintenance acid suppression with an H_2RA or PPI. For example, Sonnenberg[11] used a Markov model over 15 years to demonstrate that a combined strategy of healing ulcer with an H_2RA and eradicating *H. pylori* with antibiotics is dominant (lower cost and less time with ulcer symptoms) compared to maintenance or intermittent acid suppression with an H_2RA or surgery by vagotomy. Similarly, using a decision analytic model, Imperiale *et al.*[12] conclude that treatment with an H_2RA and bismuth triple therapy is less costly and more effective than treatment with an H_2RA alone. Unge *et al.*[13], in a modelling analysis from Sweden over a 5-year period, compared treatment of duodenal ulcer with either omeprazole or an *H. pylori* eradication regimen of omeprazole plus amoxycillin, and concluded that, despite higher initial costs, the eradication strategy is less costly and more effective than acid suppression alone.

Our own previous work[14] structured the economic problem as a comparison between three global treatment strategies for non-NSAID-related duodenal ulcer: intermittent acid suppression (H_2RA or PPI), maintenance acid suppression (H_2RA) or *H. pylori* eradication with either H_2RA and bismuth triple therapy or omeprazole plus amoxycillin. We concluded that the eradication strategies were less costly and more effective (fewer symptomatic recurrences) than the other two strategies; however, we had no good evidence to conclude *which* of the *H. pylori* regimens offered best value for money.

In 1995 we were commissioned by the Canadian Coordinating Office of Health Technology Assessment (CCOHTA) – a Federal-Provincial government agency – to develop further our model to evaluate a number of different *H. pylori* strategies. This chapter summarizes our findings.

STUDY OBJECTIVES AND COMPARATORS

We decided to compare three global therapeutic strategies for the management of uncomplicated duodenal ulcer, and within each strategy is nested a number of thera-

Table 1 Therapeutic strategies for patients with uncomplicated duodenal ulcer

'A' strategies *Heal ulcer and* *wait for recurrence*		*'B' strategies* *Heal ulcer and start* *maintenance H$_2$RA*		*'C' Strategies* *Heal ulcer and* *eradicate* H. pylori	
A$_1$	Heal with ranitidine (150 mg b.i.d., 8 weeks). No further treatment until ulcer recurrence then heal with ranitidine (150 mg b.i.d., 8 weeks)	B$_1$	Heal ulcer with ranitidine (150 mg b.i.d., 8 weeks) followed by continuous maintenance therapy with half-dose (150 mg o.d.) ranitidine. Recurrences treated with full-dose ranitidine (150 mg b.i.d., 8 weeks)	C$_1$	H. *pylori* eradication with omeprazole and amoxycillin (O + A)
A$_2$	Heal ulcer with omeprazole (20 mg o.d., 28 days). No further treatment until ulcer recurrence, then heal with omeprazole (20 mg o.d., 28 days)			C$_2$	H. *pylori* eradication with omeprazole and clarithromycin (O + C)
				C$_3$	H. *pylori* eradication with omeprazole and metronidazole and amoxycillin (O + A + M)
				C$_4$	H. *pylori* eradication with omeprazole and amoxycillin and clarithromycin (O + A + C)
				C$_5$	H. *pylori* eradication with omeprazole and clarithromycin and metronidazole (O + C + M)
				C$_6$	H. *pylori* eradication with ranitidine and triple therapy (BMT)

peutic permutations for comparison. Details of drug doses and duration of treatment for each strategy are contained in Tables 1 and 2.

Strategy A: Heal and wait for recurrence

A$_1$ Heal the ulcer with an H$_2$RA then follow up with intermittent H$_2$RA treatment conditional upon ulcer recurrence.

A$_2$ Heal the ulcer with omeprazole, then follow up with intermittent treatment with omeprazole conditional upon ulcer recurrence.

Strategy B: Maintenance H$_2$RA

B$_1$ Heal the ulcer with an H$_2$RA, followed by continuous half-dose maintenance treatment with an H$_2$RA.

Table 2 *H. pylori* eradication regimens in 'C' strategies

Regimen		Drugs	Dose	Days of therapy (from–to)
C_1	O+A	Omeprazole	20 mg b.i.d.	1–14
		Amoxycillin	1 g b.i.d.	1–14
		Omeprazole	20 mg o.d.	14–28
C_2	O+C	Omeprazole	20 mg b.i.d.	1–14
		Clarithromycin	500 mg t.i.d.	1–14
		Omeprazole	20 mg o.d.	14–28
C_3	O+A+M	Omeprazole	20 mg b.i.d.	1–14
		Metronidazole	500 mg b.i.d.	1–7
		Amoxycillin	1 g b.i.d.	1–7
		Omeprazole	20 mg o.d.	14–28
C_4	O+A+C	Omeprazole	20 mg b.i.d.	1–14
		Amoxycillin	1 g b.i.d.	1–7
		Clarithromycin	500 mg b.i.d.	1–7
		Omeprazole	20 mg o.d.	14–28
C_5	O+C+M	Omeprazole	20 mg b.i.d.	1–14
		Clarithromycin	500 mg b.i.d.	1–7
		Metronidazole	500 mg b.i.d.	1–7
		Omeprazole	20 mg o.d.	14–28
C_6	Ran-BMT	Ranitidine	150 mg b.i.d.	1–56
		Bismuth subsalicylate	151 mg q.i.d.	42–56
		Metronidazole	250 mg q.i.d.	42–56
		Tetracycline	500 mg q.i.d.	42–56

Strategy C: Heal ulcer and eradicate *H. pylori*

We examined six possible *H. pylori* eradication regimens:

C_1 omeprazole and amoxycillin (O+A)
C_2 omeprazole and clarithromycin (O+C)
C_3 omeprazole, metronidazole, and amoxycillin (O+A+M)
C_4 omeprazole, amoxycillin, and clarithromycin (O+A+C)
C_5 omeprazole, clarithromycin, and metronidazole (O+C+M)
C_6 H$_2$RA and bismuth triple therapy (Ran-BMT)

Our chosen set of comparators enable us to compare broad treatment strategies such as intermittent versus maintenance acid suppression and *H. pylori* eradication, but will also permit comparison of costs and outcomes among various *H. pylori* eradication regimens.

METHODS

Overview of analytical approach

There are three key components to understanding our analytical approach. The first is the structuring of the therapeutic decision problem in terms of the principles of clinical decision analysis. This is a conventional approach to clinical economic modelling[15] structuring relevant strategies, clinical events and costs using a decision tree. For calculation of expected costs and outcomes we determine the probabilities of relevant clinical events (i.e. ulcer healing rates, ulcer recurrence rates, *H. pylori* eradication rates) using principles of quantitative literature review or meta-analysis. We identify search criteria for retrieval of relevant published studies and then estimate pooled rates of events over these studies for inclusion in our model. Finally, we use principles of cost-effectiveness analysis for comparing treatment strategies in terms of weak and strong dominance and incremental cost-effectiveness, and use sensitivity analysis to explore key areas of uncertainty.

The viewpoint of this study is that of a governmental third-party payer for health care (i.e. Provincial Ministry of Health) in Canada. Much of our cost information comes from sources in the Province of Ontario. Costs are reported in 1995 Canadian dollars.

Decision analysis model

Details of our treatment alternatives are given in Tables 1 and 2, and presented as a decision tree in Figure 1. We consider a patient who has been diagnosed by endoscopy with uncomplicated duodenal ulcer and simplify the spectrum of treatment options facing a family doctor into our three global strategies: (a) heal the ulcer with either ranitidine or omeprazole and manage any subsequent recurrence(s) with either intermittent ranitidine, A_1, or omeprazole, A_2; (B) heal the ulcer and then initiate continuous maintenance therapy with half-dose ranitidine; (C) attempt to both heal the ulcer and eradicate *H. pylori* using one of six different regimens ranging from bismuth triple therapy to omeprazole plus one or two antibiotics.

The simplifying assumption of the patient(s) entering the model having confirmed and uncomplicated duodenal ulcer (DU) was necessary for two reasons: (a) the clinical data on the efficacy of the alternative treatments for long-term management of DU are from populations with diagnosed DU; (b) since the presence of DU on endoscopy is a highly sensitive and specific indicator of *H. pylori* infection[2], our model does not involve additional diagnostic testing for presence of *H. pylori*, or testing to confirm eradication. Therefore, our model addresses the question: *given* that a patient has DU, what is the cost-effectiveness of alternative clinical strategies?

Expected costs and outcomes per patient are calculated for each therapeutic strategy, where expected means a sum of items weighted by their probability of occurrence. Hence, on the cost side, we wish to capture both the 'up-front' costs of initial drug therapy (but excluding the confirmatory endoscopy which is common to all strategies) and any 'downstream' costs due to management of ulcer recurrence in the 12-month interval. Our model structure is simple in that it is recursive in two 6-month periods; hence probabilities of recurrence in the period to 12 months are conditional upon recurrence or non-recurrence in the period 0–6 months.

Outcome measures

Our primary outcome is time free from ulcer during the 12-month period of the model. For each regimen we pooled data from ulcer-healing trials to estimate

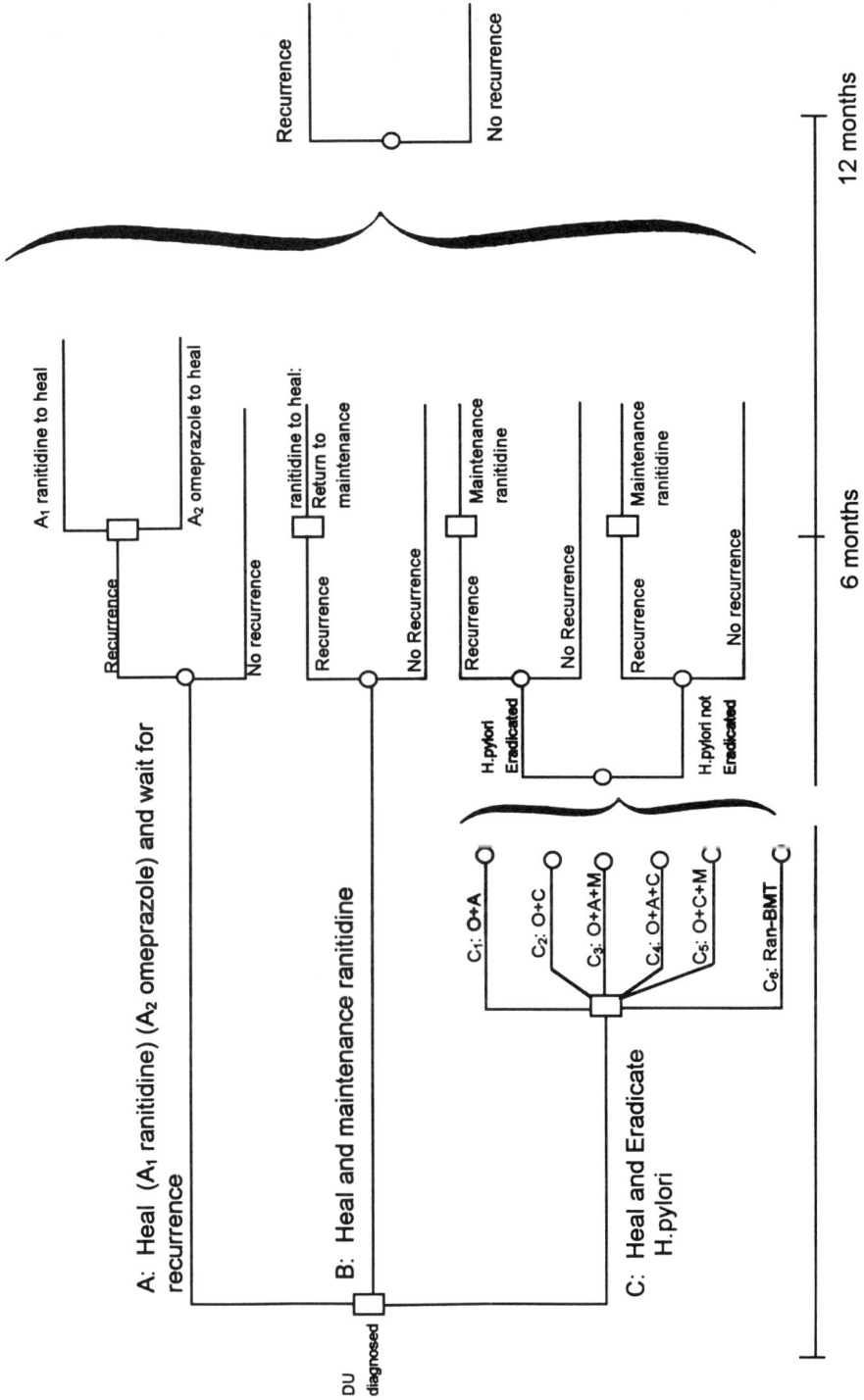

Figure 1 Decision tree for management of persons with confirmed duodenal ulcer (DU)

Table 3 Unit prices for pharmaceuticals, excluding dispensing fee

Drug	Dose (mg)	Cost per dose ($)
Ranitidine (generic)	150	0.45*
Ranitidine (Zantac)	150	1.20†
Cimetidine (generic)	400	0.15*
Cimetidine (Tagamet)	400	0.64†
Omeprazole (Losec)	20	2.57†
Bismuth (Pepto-Bismol)	151	0.21†
Amoxycillin (generic)	500	0.21*
Amoxycillin (Amoxil)	500	0.41†
Clarithromycin (Biaxin)	500	3.57†
Metronidazole (generic)	250	0.03*
Metronidazole (Flagyl)	250	0.05†
Tetracycline (generic)	250	0.02*
Tetracycline (Achromycin)	250	0.05†

Sources: *Ontario Drug Benefit Plan, plus 10% pharmacy up-charge.
†Survey of local pharmacies.

healing time curves. We searched by MEDLINE and other sources to find randomized controlled trials in adults where DU (>5 mm) healing was determined by endoscopy at set intervals (e.g. 4 weeks, 8 weeks). Estimation of the area under the healing curve yields information on expected time without (and with) ulcer during the acute healing treatment period. To determine total expected ulcer time over the period of the model, each acute healing ulcer duration is further weighted by the probabilities of ulcer recurrence (and retreatment) over the 12-month period, which will vary between regimens.

Costs

Our primary source of drug price information is Best Available Price from the Ontario Drug Benefit Plan with a 10% pharmacy up-charge. For drugs such as omeprazole that are a non-formulary benefit, and do not have the best available price on ODB, we conducted a small survey of local pharmacies to determine cost. These unit prices are presented in Table 3, and in Table 4 we estimate costs for the regimens that we analyse in our model. For example, an 8-week course of ranitidine, 150 mg, twice daily is $50.4 and a 4-week supply of omeprazole, 20 mg o.d. is $71.96. We also present drug costs for *H. pylori* eradication strategies. These range from ranitidine plus bismuth triple therapy at $66.08 up to omeprazole plus clarithromycin for 2 weeks at $257.88.

To estimate the costs associated with the management of patients with symptoms of ulcer recurrence, we required information on clinical practice patterns and resource utilization (e.g. diagnostic test ordering) and the prices of these resources. No published data were available on how physicians manage ulcer recurrence in Canada. We therefore used data from our previous study based on convening an expert physician panel (four gastroenterologists, two family doctors) and used a modified Delphi technique[18] to derive estimates and ranges on the percentage likelihood and volume of various services used when patients present with symptoms of ulcer recurrence. The panel was first mailed a questionnaire on resource

Table 4 Costs of drug regimens used in the model, excluding dispensing fee

Regimen	Cost ($)
Maintenance and intermittent acid suppression	
ranitidine (150 mg o.d.)	0.45 per day
ranitidine (150 mg b.i.d.×8 weeks)	50.40
omeprazole (20 mg o.d.×28 days)	71.96
Drug costs for eradication by strategy	
omeprazole+amoxycillin (20 mg omeprazole b.i.d.×14 days; 1 g amoxycillin b.i.d.×14 days)+20 mg omeprazole o.d.×14 days	119.70
omeprazole+clarithromycin (20 mg omeprazole b.i.d.×14 days; 500 mg clarithromycin t.i.d.×14 days)+20 mg omeprazole o.d.×14 days	257.88
omeprazole+amoxycillin+metronidazole (20 mg omeprazole b.i.d.×14 days; 1 g amoxycillin b.i.d. (500×2)×7 days; 500 mg metronidazole b.i.d. (250 mg×2)×7 days)+20 mg omeprazole o.d.×14 days	114.66
omeprazole+clarithromycin+metronidazole (20 mg omeprazole b.i.d.×14 days; 500 mg clarithromycin b.i.d.×7 days; 500 mg metronidazole b.i.d. (250 mg×2)×7 days)+20 mg omeprazole o.d.×14 days	158.76
omeprazole+amoxycillin+clarithromycin (20 mg omeprazole b.i.d.×14 days; 1 g amoxycillin (500×2 b.i.d.)×7 days; 500 mg clarithromycin b.i.d.×7 days)+20 mg omeprazole o.d.×14 days	163.80
H_2RA triple therapy (150 mg ranitidine b.i.d.×56 days; 151 mg bismuth q.i.d.×14 days; 250 mg metronidazole q.i.d.×14 days; 500 mg tetracycline q.i.d. (250×2)×14 days)	66.08

use based on a written scenario of DU recurrence, and then brought together in committee to discuss their estimates. The main focus was on the likelihood of expensive investigations being used such as urea breath test, upper gastro-intestinal series or endoscopy.

In Ontario, hospitals receive global budgets, and physician services are reimbursed by the government health insurance plan on a fee-per-item-of-service basis. Prices (combined hospital and physician service cost) for procedures such as upper gastrointestinal endoscopy were estimated from two sources: (a) a corporate cost model for Chedoke–McMaster hospitals in Hamilton, Ontario[17], which relates workload units assigned to procedures for managerial purposes[18–20] to hospital expenditures; (b) the physician fee schedule for Ontario[21] which itemizes allowable physician reimbursement by procedure under the provincial health insurance plan.

RESULTS

Ulcer healing probabilities

We found 26 ranitidine trials, either 150 mg b.i.d or 300 mg o.d., with 2641 patients, of whom 1895 (72%) were healed at 4 weeks and 2278 (86%) by 8 weeks. We found 24 omeprazole trials, 20 mg o.d., reporting on 2633 patients of whom 1688 (64%) were healed at 2 weeks, and 2286 (87%) were healed at 4 weeks. To illustrate the distribution of healing time curves for regimens we

omeprazole 20 mg   ranitidine 300 mg

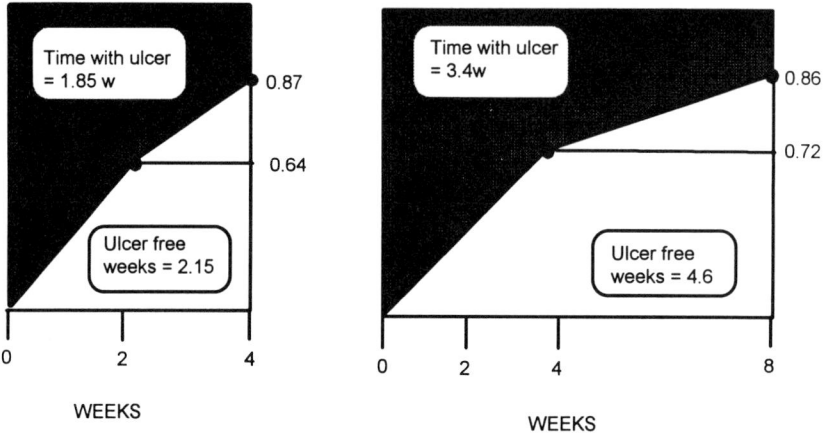

Figure 2   Ulcer healing curves and time with ulcer (shaded area) for 8-week ranitidine regimen and 4-week omeprazole

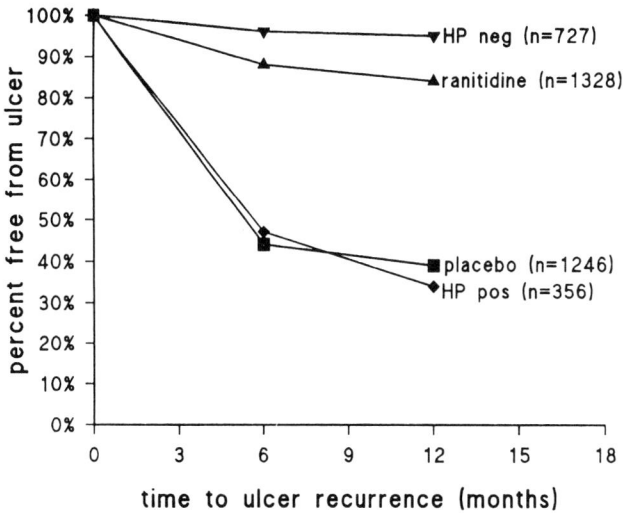

Figure 3   Time to ulcer recurrence

present the study curves and calculated expected time with and without ulcer in Figure 2.

Ulcer recurrence probabilities

Using similar techniques for the quantitative summary of the literature reviewed, we estimated rates of ulcer recurrence at 6 and 12 months for our model. Our ulcer recurrence probabilities are illustrated as a life table in Figure 3. These data

Table 5   *H. pylori* eradication rates

Regimen		Eradication rate (%)	Range for sensitivity analysis*	Source references
C_1	O+A	61	57–66	22
C_2	O+C	71	66–76	22
C_3	O+A+M	84	79–90	22
C_4	O+A+C	85	75–96	22
C_5	O+C+M	91	88–94	22
C_6	Ran+BMT	86	80–92	23–25

*Range is 95% CI for C_1 to C_5, from Chiba[22].

suggest a 56% recurrence of ulcer at 6 months in the placebo group, compared to a 12% rate of recurrence in patients receiving continuous maintenance ranitidine. Patients from trials who are *H. pylori*-positive have a recurrence rate of 53%, similar to that of placebo. For use in our model we adjusted endoscopically determined recurrence data based on information from the literature of the proportion of recurrences that are symptomatic to asymptomatic. Accordingly we used an adjustment factor of 0.75 based on the information that around 75% of ulcer recurrence is by endoscopy or symptomatic (for details see ref. 6).

Time with ulcer per healing episode

In Figure 2 we present the area-under-the-curve analysis for ranitidine and omeprazole required to estimate time with and without ulcer per healing regimen. Hence, of 4 weeks treatment with omeprazole (20 mg), 2.15 will be ulcer-free weeks. For ranitidine (300 mg) 8 weeks therapy yields 4–6 weeks free from ulcer.

H. pylori eradication probabilities

We based our eradication rates on a recent meta-analysis by Chiba *et al.*[22]. This meta-analysis was based on a MEDLINE search for papers and abstracts reporting *H. pylori* eradication rates for a number of the omeprazole combination regimens in our study. The study reports that it is a per-protocol analysis of the number eradicated per number treated when assessed at 4 weeks post-eradication therapy. Data from the study are presented in Table 5, indicating an eradication rate for O+A of 61%, O+C of 71%, O+A+M of 84%, O+A+C of 85%, and O+C+M of 91%. For bismuth triple therapy estimates vary between 90%[23], 84%[24] and 89%[25], and we assume a rate of 86% for our base case.

Cost-effectiveness

In Table 6 we present our base case estimates from the model, and for each of the nine strategies we present expected 1-year cost per patient, symptomatic ulcer recurrences per 100 patients, and the expected weeks per patient with ulcer in 1 year. These data indicate that both intermittent ranitidine and intermittent omeprazole have higher rates of symptomatic ulcer recurrence (69 per 100 patients)

Table 6   Expected cost, ulcer recurrences and weeks with ulcer: base case

Strategy		Expected 1-year cost per patient ($)	Symptomatic ulcer recurrences per 100 patients	Expected weeks per patient with ulcer in 1year
A	Heal and wait, treat duodenal ulcer with			
	A_1 ranitidine	306	69	5.7
	A_2 omeprazole	343	69	3.1
B	Heal and continuous maintenance ranitidine	353	18	4.0
C	Heal and *H. pylori* eradication			
	C_1 O+A	387	28	2.4
	C_2 O+C	482	22	2.3
	C_3 O+A+M	292	14	2.1
	C_4 O+A+C	337	13	2.1
	C_5 O+C+M	306	10	2.0
	C_6 Ran–BMT	228	12	3.8

than other strategies. However, because the speed of healing is greater with omeprazole, the expected weeks per patient with ulcer in the 1-year period is lower with intermittent omeprazole (3.1 weeks) than with intermittent ranitidine (5.7 weeks). Similarly, although continuous maintenance ranitidine has a lower rate of symptomatic ulcer recurrence (18 per 100 patients), it is associated with 4 weeks of ulcer per patient in a 1-year period because the lower rate of recurrence is partially offset by a slower speed of healing in the calculation of expected duration with ulcer. All of the omeprazole-based *H. pylori* eradication strategies are associated with approximately 2 weeks of ulcer per patient in a 1-year period. In contrast the time with ulcer is greater for ranitidine plus bismuth triple therapy as an *H. pylori* regimen because of the greater duration of this regimen and the slower speed of healing associated with ranitidine.

In considering the costs of alternative regimens, the six *H. pylori* eradication strategies contain both the least costly strategy of ranitidine bismuth triple therapy ($228), and also the most costly regimen C_2 of omeprazole plus clarithromycin ($482). The relatively high cost of the O+C regimen is largely explained by the need to use brand-name clarithromycin (Biaxin) three times daily.

In considering costs and outcomes together, it is apparent that strategies C_3 (O+A+M) and C_5 (O+C+M) are dominant over both intermittent strategies (A_1 and A_2) and continuous maintenance ranitidine, having both lower costs and greater outcomes with fewer weeks of ulcer in a 1-year period. For other *H. pylori* regimens such as O+A or O+C, there is a trade-off to be determined because, relative to regimens such as intermittent or continuous maintenance ranitidine, these strategies offer better outcomes but at a higher cost.

To better understand the cost and outcome relationships between the alternatives, it is instructive to organize this information in a graphical way. In Figure 4 we present the data on costs and expected weeks with ulcer per year using continuous maintenance ranitidine (strategy B_1) as our reference point or origin. In other words, every other point is presented as a difference relative to strategy B_1.

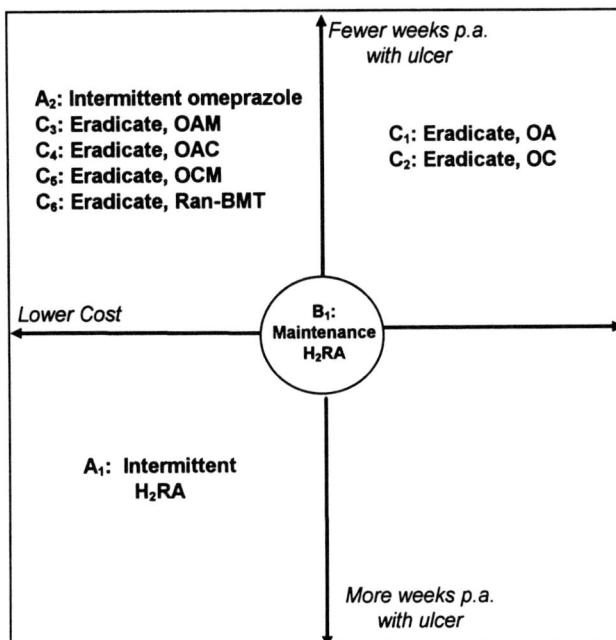

Figure 4 Dominance and trade-offs for all strategies relative to continuous maintenance ranitidine (B₁)

From this presentation it is clear that points lying above and to the left of B_1 at the origin are dominant, in that they offer increased effectiveness at reduced cost. These dominating strategies are intermittent omeprazole (A_2), O+A+C (C_4), O+C+M (C_5), O+A+M (C_3), and bismuth triple therapy (C_6). All of these strategies offer an unequivocal improvement over maintenance ranitidine because they offer better outcome at a lower cost.

DISCUSSION

We found that, relative to continuous maintenance therapy with ranitidine, intermittent omeprazole (A_2) and four of the *H. pylori* eradication strategies (O+A+M, O+A+C, O+C+M, Ran-BMT) were all dominant, having lower expected 1-year costs with fewer weeks of ulcer in the 1-year period. We also found that intermittent ranitidine had a lower cost, but was associated with more weeks of ulcer in the year than continuous maintenance ranitidine. Finally, relative to our reference strategy B_1, we found that two of the *H. pylori* eradication strategies (O+A, O+C) offered a better outcome, but at a higher cost. Therefore, our first general conclusion is that all of the *H. pylori* eradication regimens offer better outcomes than either intermittent or maintenance ranitidine. However, there is differentiation between the eradication regimens on grounds of cost with the combination of omeprazole with either amoxicillin or clarithromycin being the more costly of the eradication regimens.

In comparing among the *H. pylori* eradication strategies we calculated incremental cost-effectiveness relative to the reference of ranitidine bismuth triple therapy. This analysis revealed that the O + A + M and O + C + M strategies offer the best value for money among the eradication strategies, with an incremental cost-effectiveness of around $40 per ulcer-free week. We found that our analysis was generally robust to alternative assumptions explored in sensitivity analysis. However, one-way sensitivity analyses on each of the eradication strategies by its assumed eradication rate does suggest that the analysis is sensitive to these data. For example, if the base-case eradication rate of 86% for bismuth triple therapy is dropped to 50%, then the strategy goes from being the least costly to the second most costly eradication strategy.

If we assume that many physicians are currently treating duodenal ulcer with either intermittent or maintenance H_2RA then one general conclusion from our analysis is that a move towards treatment targeted at the eradication of *H. pylori* would both save money and improve health outcomes. Although bismuth triple therapy is the least costly of the eradication strategies, better outcomes for a modest increase in cost can be achieved with omeprazole plus two antibiotics given in a 7-day regimen, particularly O + A + M or O + C + M.

References

1. Peterson WL. Current concepts: *Helicobacter pylori* and peptic ulcer disease. N Engl J Med. 1991;324:1043–8.
2. Tytgat GNJ, Noach LA, Rauws EAJ. *Helicobacter pylori* infection and duodenal ulcer disease. Gastrointest Clin N Am. 1993;22:127–39.
3. Chiba N, Rao BV, Rademaker JW, Hunt RH. Meta-analysis of the efficacy of antibiotic therapy in eradicating *Helicobacter pylori*. Am J Gastroenterol. 1992;87:1716–27.
4. NIH Consensus Development Panel. *Helicobacter pylori* in peptic ulcer disease. J Am Med Assoc. 1994;272:65–9.
5. McIsaac W, Naylor CD, Anderson GM, O'Brien BJ. Reflections on a month in the life of the Ontario Drug Benefit Plan. CMAJ. 1994;150:473–7.
6. O'Brien BJ, Goeree RA, Hunt R, Wilkinson J, Levine M, Willan A. Economic evaluation of alternative therapies in the long term management of peptic ulcer disease and gastroesophageal reflux disease. Ottawa, Canadian Coordinating Office for Health Technology Assessment (CCOHTA); 1996:1.
7. Culyer AJ, Maynard AK. Cost-effectiveness of duodenal ulcer treatment. Soc Sco Med. 1981; 15C:3–11.
8. Jonsson B, Drummond MF, Stalhammar N-O. Cost-effectiveness of omeprazole and ranitidine in the treatment of duodenal ulcer. PharmacoEconomics. 1994;5:44–55.
9. Sintonen H, Alander V. Comparing the cost-effectiveness of drug regimens in the treatment of duodenal ulcers. J Health Econ. 1990;9:85–101.
10. Walan A, Eriksson S. Long-term consequences with regard to clinical outcome and cost-effectiveness episode treatment omeprazole or ranitidine for healing of duodenal ulcer. Scand J Gastroenterol. 1994;29:91–7.
11. Sonnenberg A, Townsend WF. Costs of duodenal ulcer therapy with antibiotics. Arch Intern Med. 1995;155:922–8.
12. Imperiale TF, Speroff T, Cebul RD, McCullough AJ. A cost analysis of alternative treatments for duodenal ulcer. Ann Intern Med. 1995;123:665–72.
13. Unge P, Jonsson B, Stalhammar N-O. The cost effectiveness of *Helicobacter pylori* eradication versus maintenance and episodic treatment in duodenal ulcer patients in Sweden. Pharmaco-Economics. 1995;8:410–27.
14. O'Brien BJ, Goeree RA, Mohamed H, Hunt R. Cost-effectiveness of *Helicobacter pylori* eradi-

cation for the long-term management of duodenal ulcer in Canada. Arch Intern Med. 1995; 155:1958–64.

15. Weinstein MC, Fineberg HV. Clinical decision analysis. Philadelphia: WB Saunders; 1980.
16. Park RE, Fink A, Brook RH *et al*. Physician ratings of appropriate indications for six medical and surgical procedures. Am J Publ Health. 1986;76:766–72.
17. Chedoke–McMaster Hospitals. Chedoke–McMaster Corporate hospital cost database. 1993 (abstract).
18. Health and Welfare Canada. Nuclear medicine workload measurement system. 1989 (abstract).
19. Health and Welfare Canada. Diagnostic radiology workload measurement system. 1988 (abstract).
20. Health and Welfare Canada. Laboratory workload measurement system. 1989 (abstract).
21. Ontario Ministry of Health. Schedule of benefits physician services under the health insurance act. 1 April 1991. 1992 (abstract).
22. Chiba N, Wilkinson JM, Hunt RH. Clarithromycin (C) or amoxicillin (A) dual and triple therapies in *H. pylori* (Hp) eradication: a meta-analysis. Gut. 1995;37:A31.
23. Graham DY, Lem GM, Malaty HM *et al*. Factors influencing the eradication of *Helicobacter pylori* with triple therapy. Gastroenterology. 1992;102:493–6.
24. Pentson JG. *Helicobacter pylori* eradication – understandable caution but no excuse for inertia. Aliment Pharmacol Ther. 1994;8:369–89.
25. Tytgat GNJ. Treatments that impact favourably upon the eradication of *Helicobacter pylori* and ulcer recurrence. Aliment Pharmacol Ther. 1994;8:359–68.

40
Model of *Helicobacter pylori* treatment and disease outcome: a threshold analysis

A. SONNENBERG

INTRODUCTION

An infection with *Helicobacter pylori* and the ensuing gastroduodenitis are considered the most important pathophysiological mechanisms in the development of common peptic ulcer disease that is not secondary to intake of non-steroidal anti-inflammatory drugs (NSAIDs)[1,2]. Several decision analyses have shown antibiotic eradication of *H. pylori* to be more cost-effective than other previous treatment modalities of peptic ulcer disease[3–5]. There is little doubt among gastroenterologists that all ulcers caused by *H. pylori* should be treated with antibiotics. Occasionally, other factors may contribute to the development of peptic ulceration, and the correct mode of ulcer management becomes questionable.

For instance, aspirin and other NSAIDs carry a high risk of causing ulcerations of the gastrointestinal tract[6–8]. Because a large fraction of the population is infected with *H. pylori*, it is not uncommon to confirm an infection with *H. pylori* in a patient who is also on NSAIDs[9–15]. This concordance is found all the more, because both infection with *H. pylori* and all diseases which require treatment with NSAIDs cluster in the elderly population. Zollinger–Ellison syndrome is found in about 1 out of 1000 duodenal ulcers. In a fraction of ulcer patients other mechanisms besides an infection by *H. pylori* seem to be responsible for the development of acute ulceration. It has been suggested that especially ulcers accompanied by haemorrhage and perforation are characterized by low levels of *H. pylori* infection[16]. In many instances the precise aetiology of a particular ulcer may remain unknown, because no gastric biopsies or serology for *H. pylori* are available.

In case of an NSAID-induced ulcer, the first lines of therapy would be to discontinue the NSAIDs whenever possible, reduce the dose, or change the type of medication. If none of these options is feasible the patient might be treated with a histamine-2 receptor antagonist (H$_2$RA) or a prostaglandin analogue, as both have been shown to be effective in NSAID-induced ulcers[17,18]. However, if

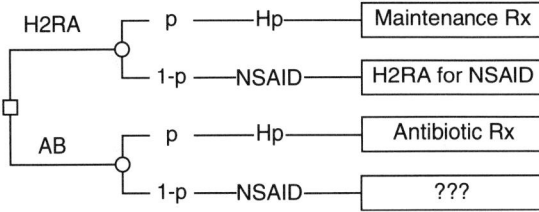

Figure 1 Decision tree for management of peptic ulcer in a patient on non-steroidal anti-inflammatory drugs (NSAIDs), p or $1-p$ representing the probabilities for an ulcer induced by NSAIDs or *Helicobacter pylori* (Hp), respectively. The boxes on the right represent the four outcomes of the initial decision, that is, maintenance therapy with histamine-2 receptor antagonists (H_2RA) for an *H. pylori*-induced ulcer, maintenance therapy with H_2RA for an NSAID-induced ulcer, antibiotic therapy for an *H. pylori*-induced ulcer, and the yet unknown (???) antibiotic therapy for an NSAID-induced ulcer

the ulcer resulted from an infection with *H. pylori*, antimicrobial therapy to eradicate the underlying infection would constitute the therapy of choice. Similarly, ulcers secondary to gastric hypersecretion or mechanisms other than *H. pylori* infection would require antisecretory treatment with H_2RA or proton-pump inhibitors. The physician is faced with the dilemma of whether a benign peptic ulcer associated with bleeding or diagnosed in a patient on NSAIDs stems from an infection with *H. pylori*, or from other mechanisms. Should the physician prescribe antibiotic therapy only in patients with proven *H. pylori* infection? How should the physician decide to treat a patient with *H. pylori* who also consumes NSAIDs? A decision tree and a threshold analysis were modelled to answer these questions.

DECISION MODEL

A decision tree is modelled to calculate the threshold probability of when to treat for *H. pylori* or for other causes of gastroduodenal ulceration. Since similar considerations apply to NSAIDs as to other causes of peptic ulcer besides *H. pylori*, the model is developed based on the example of an *H. pylori*-positive ulcer patient who is also on NSAIDs. In the sensitivity analysis the model is then expanded to include other clinical situations besides NSAID-induced ulcers.

For the purpose of the present analysis it is assumed that the patient cannot be taken off his/her NSAID medication, and that the physician has to decide between maintenance therapy with H_2RA or antibiotic therapy. Figure 1 shows the corresponding decision tree. After the initial decision to treat with H_2RA or antibiotics (AB), each branch has two potential daughter branches. Each daughter branch is governed by the probability p or $1-p$ for an *H. pylori*- or NSAID-induced ulcer, respectively. The boxes on the right represent the four outcomes of the decision, that is, maintenance therapy with H_2RA for an *H. pylori*-induced ulcer, maintenance therapy with H_2RA for an NSAID-induced ulcer, antibiotic therapy for an *H. pylori*-induced ulcer, and antibiotic therapy for an NSAID-induced ulcer. The costs to be expected over a time period of 15 years during an H_2-maintenance or an antibiotic therapy for an *H. pylori*-induced ulcer have been calculated in a

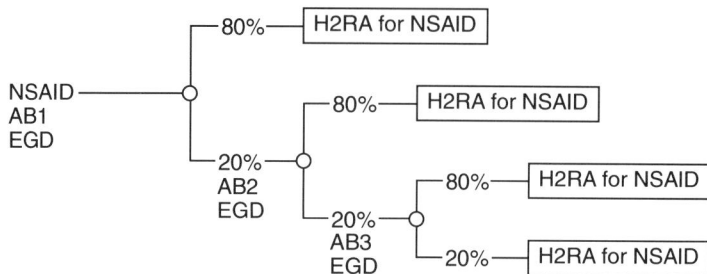

$(AB+EGD) \times (1+0.2+0.04) + H_2RA$ for NSAID

Figure 2 The expanded fourth branch from the decision tree of Figure 1, depicting the outcome of antibiotic therapy for an NSAID-induced ulcer. The outcome is shown in the formula below the tree, where AB = short-term treatment courses with antibiotics, EGD = oesophagogastroduodenoscopy

previous cost analysis[3]. The costs of H_2-maintenance therapy for an NSAID-induced ulcer and, especially, the costs of an 'erroneous' therapy of an NSAID-induced ulcer with antibiotics are presently unknown.

The last option is shown in greater detail in the second tree of Figure 2. It is assumed that persistent ulcer or ulcer recurrence, as well as persistence of *H. pylori* infection, require at least one oesophagogastroduodenoscopy (OGD) for their diagnosis. All types of antibiotic regimens are estimated to yield an 80% eradication rate of *H. pylori*. After the first treatment session with antibiotics (AB1), *H. pylori* will be eradicated in 80% of the patients. One additional OGD will be needed to confirm the successful *H. pylori* eradication associated with a persistent or recurrent NSAID-induced ulceration, before the 'correct' maintenance therapy is initiated. In 20% of the patients, however, the OGD reveals that *H. pylori* was not eradicated, and the persistent ulcer problems can still be ascribed 'erroneously' to an ongoing infection with *H. pylori*. In these patients a second antibiotic regimen (AB2) and a second OGD are needed, before the 80% eradication of *H. pylori* in a new subfraction of the patient population finally results in a 'correct' therapy with H_2RA maintenance. The remaining 20% with persistent infection may undergo yet another cycle of antibiotic therapy (AB3) and OGD. Eventually, everyone who was started initially on antibiotics for his/her NSAID-induced ulcer will end up with a 'correct' maintenance therapy. However, an additional one or more (mean: 1.24) treatment courses with antimicrobials, and as many upper gastrointestinal endoscopies, were required before antibiotic therapy became recognized as the 'erroneous' treatment approach. A similar argument would apply, if intermittent therapy with H_2RA or maintenance therapy with prostaglandin analogues are used instead of maintenance therapy with H_2RA.

The overall outcome of the tree from Figure 2 reduces to maintenance therapy with H_2RA for an NSAID-induced ulcer plus a mean of 1.24 treatment courses with antimicrobials and as many upper gastrointestinal endoscopies. This result has been added as fourth outcome to the upper decision tree of Figure 3. For both

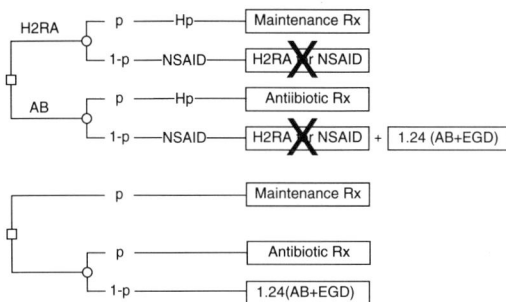

$$p \times \text{Maintenance} = p \times \text{Antimicrobials} + (1\text{-}p) \times 1.24 \text{ (AB+EGD)}$$

Figure 3 Updates of the decision tree from Figure 1, using the outcome from Figure 2 to complete the outcome of the fourth branch. Since both the second and fourth branch on the right, result in the outcome 'maintenance therapy with H_2RA for an NSAID-induced ulcer' multiplied with the identical probability $(1-p)$, they cancel out, leading to the reduced tree shown at the foot. This lower tree was used to calculate the threshold value for the probability p, when both decisions represented by the initial fork provide an equal outcome

initial decisions, ulcer treatment with H_2RA or antibiotics, to be equally feasible, the expected outcomes of both decisions need to be equal. Since maintenance therapy with H_2RA for an NSAID-induced ulcer appears in both decisions, multiplied by $(1-p)$, it cancels out, and the upper tree reduces to the lower decision tree of Figure 3. The equality of both decisions can be expressed as follows:

$$p \times \text{Maintenance Rx} = p \times \text{Antibiotic Rx} + (1-p) \times 1.24 \times (\text{AB} + \text{EGD}) \quad (1)$$

In this equation the term 'Maintenance Rx' refers to the overall expected costs of peptic ulcer disease managed by H_2RA over a time period of 15 years. Similarly, the term 'Antibiotic Rx' refers to the expected costs of peptic ulcer managed by antibiotic therapy over 15 years. It must not be confused with the term 'AB', i.e. antibiotics, also appearing in the equation, which refers to a single treatment course plus office visit. The equation (1) can be solved for p to yield a threshold probability when both treatment options are equally feasible[19].

$$p = \frac{1.24 \times (\text{AB} + \text{EGD})}{\text{Maintenance Rx} - \text{Antibiotic Rx} + 1.24 \times (\text{AB} + \text{EGD})} \quad (2)$$

COST ESTIMATES

Direct costs consist of medical expenditures for surgical operations, endoscopy, and medications, while indirect costs consist of income losses secondary to absenteeism from work, disability, or death. Total costs represent the sum of direct and indirect costs. Drug costs are estimated from their average wholesale prices plus $5.00 per prescription in 1993[20]. The initiation of any drug therapy is associated with one office visit. Ranitidine 150 mg b.i.d. and 150 mg q.h.s. are considered appropriate treatments for the active ulcer attack and maintenance therapy, respectively. Antibiotic therapy consists of bismuth subsalicylate 262 mg

Table 1 Threshold analysis for antibiotic therapy of peptic ulcer in patients on NSAIDs

Name	Cost item	Direct costs		Total costs	
		Allowed charges	Submitted charges	Allowed charges	Submitted charges
Antibiotic Rx	Long-term management with antibiotics for 15 years	$659	$784	$870	$995
Maintenance Rx	Long-term maintenance therapy with H₂RA for 15 years	$8517	$8855	$10849	$11186
Intermittent Rx	Long-term intermittent therapy with H₂RA for 15 years	$2395	$3086	$9660	$10350
EGD	Upper gastrointestinal endoscopy plus biopsy for *H. pylori*	$1169	$1428	$1169	$1428
AB	Office visit plus quadruple therapy of *H. pylori* for 2 weeks*	$151	$161	$151	$161
p	Threshold probability for antibiotic therapy				
	assuming maintenance Rx with H₂RA	18%	20%	14%	17%
	assuming intermittent Rx with H₂RA	54%	51%	16%	18%

Drug costs were estimated from average wholesale prices plus $5.00 per prescription. Other costs were estimated from the average charges allowed by and submitted to the HCFA in 1992. Estimates of long-term costs for management of peptic ulcer over 15 years were taken from ref. 3.
*For 2 weeks: bismuth subsalicylate two tablets q.i.d. + metronidazole 250 mg + tetracycline 500 mg q.i.d. + for 4 weeks: ranitidine 150 mg b.i.d.
NSAIDs: non-steroidal anti-inflammatory drugs, H₂RA: histamine-2 receptor antagonists.

tablets, two tablets q.i.d.; metronidazole 250 mg t.i.d.; tetracycline 500 mg q.i.d. Antimicrobials are given for 2 weeks. The cost for this particular regimen is similar to other 1-week regimens using, for instance, metronidazole, omeprazole, and clarithromycin. Other direct costs besides drugs are estimated from the US average of charges allowed by and submitted to the Health Care Financing Administration (HCFA) in 1992 (Table 1). Average annual income is used to estimate indirect costs[21]. In a previous study a Markov chain was used to accumulate the direct and total costs of various treatment strategies for peptic ulcer over a time period of 15 years[3]. Table 1 shows the cumulative costs that can be expected in an ulcer patient who is managed over 15 years, using intermittent or maintenance therapy with H₂RA or antibiotic therapy to eradicate *H. pylori*.

RESULTS AND SENSITIVITY ANALYSIS

If maintenance therapy with H₂RA is considered the appropriate long-term management option for an NSAID-induced ulcer in a patient who cannot be taken off his/her anti-inflammatory medication, the threshold probability for antibiotic therapy is less than 20%. Unless the physician is more than 80% certain that NSAIDs are the only responsible factor for the ulceration, the patient should be treated with antibiotics first. In other words, even as small a probability as 20% for an *H. pylori*-induced ulcer should represent a sufficient indication to start a patient on antibiotics before considering any other long-term management strategy. Basically, this low threshold probability is given in any ulcer patient in whom serology, CLO test, or biopsy establish an infection with *H. pylori*, irrespective of whether other potential causes of peptic ulceration are considered. The unequivocal outcome in favour of *H. pylori* eradication even in patients on NSAIDs is a reflection of the low expected costs associated with antibiotic therapy as compared with any other form of ulcer management.

The differences between allowed and submitted charges or direct and indirect costs do not affect the low threshold. However, the threshold probability rises to about 50%, if the antibiotic strategy and long-term management using intermittent H_2RA are compared with respect to their direct costs. Intermittent therapy with H_2RA during an acute ulcer attack and discontinuation of the H_2RA after the ulcer has healed is a very cheap treatment option with respect to the direct costs. Its few direct costs stem from expenses for drugs and a few emergencies of gastric surgery necessitated by severe ulcer complications. The perspective of medical costs alone, however, ignores the additional expenses to the patient secondary to painful ulcer recurrences, that are likely to keep him/her partly incapacitated or could result in life-threatening complications. Therefore, this treatment strategy has fallen into disfavour with most physicians treating peptic ulcer on a long-term basis, and it is unlikely that it would be considered a valid option to manage large fractions of patients, for instance, with recurrent NSAID-induced ulceration. It has been included in the present analysis primarily to delineate the extreme range of the threshold probability that one might expect. As most management options for recurrent NSAID-induced ulcers would be much more expensive than the direct costs of intermittent therapy, the threshold probability for *H. pylori* eradication would fall well below 50%. These options also include maintenance or intermittent therapy with prostaglandin analogues.

The threshold probability of equation (2) reflects primarily the ratio of the expenses for pursuing a wrong strategy over the difference between H_2RA maintenance and antibiotic therapy. The expenses for the mistake of adhering to antibiotic therapy, when other modes of therapy would be more appropriate, amounts to $1.24 \times (AB + EGD) = 1.24 \times (\$161 + \$1428) = \$1970$ (Table 1). This amount is independent of the reason why the eradication of *H. pylori* may represent the inappropriate treatment strategy for a particular ulcer type. In other words, the mistake would cost the same amount of money in patients with Zollinger–Ellison syndrome, NSAID-induced ulcer, or ulcers secondary to other causes. The threshold probability is influenced solely by the difference between the two treatment options, that is maintenance versus antibiotic therapy. As the difference between the two treatment options increases, the threshold probability decreases. If maintenance therapy becomes more expensive, the threshold for first trying to cure the ulcer by antibiotics becomes smaller. For instance, maintenance therapies using prostaglandin analogues, omeprazole, or twice the regular H_2RA dose would all result in higher drug expenses than the regular low-dose H_2RA maintenance prophylaxis considered in the present model.

COMMENTS

The outcome of the present analysis indicates that the clinical threshold for instituting antibiotic therapy should be set at a very low level in all patients with gastroduodenal ulceration. As a physician, one would need to be quite certain about another aetiology rather than infection with *H. pylori*, before forgoing the rather simple and cheap option to treat with antibiotics. Since management with antibiotics is so inexpensive in comparison with all other forms of long-term management, it pays to use antibiotics, for instance, also in peptic ulcer patients on NSAIDs who test positive for *H. pylori*. In general, the financial benefit of the antibiotic treatment approach outweighs by far the additional costs arising from what in retrospect may prove to be an inappropriate antibiotic treatment of an ulcer unrelated to *H. pylori*.

Usually, a medical decision analysis is based on a particular case with a set of detailed assumptions about the clinical circumstances. In the present model it was assumed that the patient had already been diagnosed with a peptic ulcer and that the patient's status with respect to *H. pylori* was known at the onset of decision-making. In comparison with the cost of establishing an ulcer diagnosis, testing for *H. pylori* adds little to the overall costs; that is, less than $100. The efficacy and low cost of ulcer management with antibiotics should provide a strong incentive to test for *H. pylori* in all patients with peptic lesions of doubtful aetiology. In the majority of the available tests for *H. pylori* the negative predictive value ranges between 85% and 100%. This value means that 85% or more of all negative tests truly indicate the absence of infection with *H. pylori*[22,23]. Such 85% certainty regarding causes other than *H. pylori* would be sufficiently convincing for the physician to search for other potential causes of gastric or duodenal ulceration[24].

The present analysis compared the expected costs of different strategies to manage an ulcer over a time period of 15 years. In contradistinction with the initial costs, the expected costs include the future costs of treatment failures. In the case of antibiotics, for instance, treatment of the *acute ulcer* costs only $160, while management of the *disease* and its potential complications ranges between $660 and $995, depending on whether direct or total costs are considered. The difference between initial and expected costs becomes even more striking in treatments involving H_2RA. The expected costs were accumulated based on a detailed model of duodenal ulcer disease[3]. Since no similar calculations for gastric ulcer exist, duodenal ulcer was taken as a proxy for both ulcer types. In the past, gastric ulcer affected older patients than did duodenal ulcer. Gastric ulcer has been associated with higher complication and mortality rates, resulting in higher medical expenditures than pertain to duodenal ulcer[25]. The costs for long-term management of peptic ulcer, therefore, represent conservative estimates of the true cost. This type of bias affects long-term management with H_2RA more than antibiotics. A larger cost difference in these competing treatment strategies would lower the threshold probability even further.

The risk of serious side-effects with antibiotic therapy for peptic ulcer is low, and multiple clinical trials have proven antibiotics highly efficacious in curing ulcer disease[26]. Compared with all other treatment strategies, antibiotics are associated with the least direct costs, as well as indirect costs[3-5]. These obvious benefits result in a low threshold for treating ulcer patients with antibiotics, even before other potential aetiologies have been ruled out with certainty.

References

1. Graham DY, Go MF. *Helicobacter pylori*: current status. Gastroenterology. 1993;105:279–82.
2. Fennerty MB. *Helicobacter pylori*. Arch Intern Med. 1994;154:721–7.
3. Sonnenberg A, Townsend WF. Costs of duodenal ulcer therapy with antibiotics. Arch Intern Med. 1995;155:922–8.
4. Imperiale TF, Speroff T, Cebul RD, McCullough AJ. A cost analysis of alternative treatments for duodenal ulcer. Ann Intern Med. 1995;123:665–72.
5. Vakil N, Fennerty MB. Cost-effectiveness of treatment regimens for the eradication of *Helicobacter pylori* in duodenal ulcer. Am J Gastroenterol. 1996;91:239–45.
6. Griffin MR, Piper JM, Daugherty JR, Snowden M, Ray W. Nonsteroidal anti-inflammatory drug use and increased risk for peptic ulcer disease in elderly persons. Ann Intern Med. 1991;114:257–63.
7. Gabriel SE, Jaakkimainen L, Bombardier C. Risk for serious gastrointestinal complications related to use of nonsteroidal anti-inflammatory drugs. Ann Intern Med. 1991;115:787–96.
8. Allison MC, Howatson AG, Torrance CJ, Lee FD, Russell RI. Gastrointestinal damage associated with the use of nonsteroidal antiinflammatory drugs. N Engl J Med. 1992;327:749–54.
9. McCarthy DM. *Helicobacter pylori* infection and gastroduodenal injury by non-steroidal anti-inflammatory drugs. Scand J Gastroenterol. 1991;26(Suppl. 187):9–7.
10. Graham DY, Lidsky MD, Cox AM *et al*. Long-term nonsteroidal antiinflammatory drug use and *Helicobacter pylori* infection. Gastroenterology. 1991;100:1653–7.
11. Loeb DS, Talley NJ, Ahlquist DA, Carpenter HA, Zinsmeister AR. Long-term nonsteroidal anti-inflammatory drug use and gastroduodenal injury: the role of *Helicobacter pylori*. Gastroenterology. 1992;102:1899–905.
12. Heresbach D, Raoul JL, Bretagne JF *et al*. *Helicobacter pylori*: a risk and severity factor of nonsteroidal anti-inflammatory drug induced gastropathy. Gut. 1992;33:1608–11.
13. Schubert TT, Bologna SD, Nensey Y, Schubert AB, Mascha EJ, Ma CK. Ulcer risk factors: interactions between *Helicobacter pylori* infection, nonsteroidal use, and age. Am J Med. 1993; 94:413–18.
14. Taha AS, Russell RI. *Helicobacter pylori* and non-steroidal anti-inflammatory drugs: uncomfortable partners in peptic ulcer disease. Gut. 1993;34:580–3.
15. Kim JG, Graham DY, the Misoprostol Study Group. *Helicobacter pylori* infection and development of gastric or duodenal ulcer in arthritic patients receiving chronic NSAID therapy. Am J Gastroenterol. 1994;89:203–7.
16. Reinbach DH, Cruickshank G, McColl KEL. Acute perforated duodenal ulcer is not associated with *Helicobacter* infection. Gut. 1993;34:1344–7.
17. Cryer B, Feldman M. Effects of nonsteroidal anti-inflammatory drugs on endogenous gastrointestinal prostaglandins and therapeutic strategies for prevention and treatment of nonsteroidal anti-inflammatory drug-induced damage. Arch Intern Med. 1992;152:1145–55.
18. Graham DY, White RH, Moreland LW *et al*. and the Misoprostol Study Group. Duodenal and gastric ulcer prevention with misoprostol in arthritis patients taking NSAIDs. Ann Intern Med. 1993;119:257–62.
19. Pauker SG, Kassirer JP. The threshold approach to clinical decision making. N Engl J Med. 1980;302:1109–17.
20. First DataBank Division. Price alert. The official guide to average wholesale pricing. November 1993.
21. US Department of Commerce. Survey of current business. September 1993, p. 74.
22. Veldhuyzen van Zanten SJO, Tytgat KMAJ, deGara CJ *et al*. A prospective comparison of symptoms and five diagnostic tests in patients with *Helicobacter pylori* positive and negative dyspepsia. Eur J Gastroenterol Hepatol. 1991;3:463–8.
23. Cutler AF, Havstad S, Ma CK, Blaser MJ, Perez-Perez GI, Schubert TT. Accuracy of invasive and noninvasive tests to diagnose *Helicobacter pylori* infection. Gastroenterology. 1995;109:136–41.
24. Sonnenberg A, Townsend WF. Testing for *Helicobacter pylori* in the diagnosis of Zollinger–Ellison syndrome. Am J Gastroenterol. 1991;86:606–8.
25. Sonnenberg A. Peptic ulcer. In: Everhart JE, editor. Digestive diseases in the United States: epidemiology and impact. US Department of Health and Human Services. Washington, DC: US Government Printing Office, 1994; NIH publication no. 94-1447:357–408.
26. Chiba N, Rao BV, Rademaker JW, Hunt RH. Meta-analysis of the efficacy of antibiotic therapy in eradicating *Helicobacter pylori*. Am J Gastroenterol. 1992;87:1716–27.

P1
Population structure of *Helicobacter pylori* based on the *flaA* gene

M. U. GÖTTKE[1], C. A. FALLONE[2], V. LOO[2], A. N. BARKUN[3] and R. N. BEECH[1]

[1]*Institute of Parasitology,* [2]*Royal Victoria Hospital and* [3]*Montreal General Hospital, McGill University, Montreal, QC, Canada*

This study was aimed at a better understanding of the molecular mechanisms determining *Helicobacter pylori* genetic variability and overall adaptation to hostile host environments. The *flaA* gene chosen for analysis encodes a structural protein and is assumed to be under conservative evolutionary constraint. *flaA* DNA sequence diversity was determined in 37 clinical isolates from Montreal area hospitals using the standard molecular techniques of amplifying and cloning a gene fragment (508 bp) followed by dideoxy chain termination sequencing. DNA and protein diversity of *flaA* was 0.039 and 0.013 respectively. Diversity was well within the range of genes described for other enterobacteria and not higher, as has been deduced from several RFLP studies. Permutation tail probability analysis indicated significant population structure information present in the dataset. The minimum number of mutations required by maximum parsimony was 87 as compared to 93 mutations at the 95% confidence limit. However, phylogenetic reconstruction by the neighbour-joining method did not yield a clonal population structure, since in 1000 bootstrap replications none of the branches on either the DNA or amino acid level was statistically significant. A high degree of recombination was demonstrated by Sawyer analysis indicating panmyxis and explaining our findings. The consequences of a population utilizing frequent recombination as a means of guaranteeing viability in and adaptability to a hostile environment are far-reaching. Questions of development and spread of antibiotic resistance and the finding of reliable genetic markers and stable epitopes that could serve as vaccine candidates are affected.

P2
Human serum antibody response against iron-repressible outer membrane proteins of *Helicobacter pylori*

D. J. WORST, M. SPARRIUS, E. J. KUIPERS, J. G. KUSTERS and J. DE GRAAFF

Department of Medical Microbiology, Vrije Universiteit, and Department of Gastroenterology, Vrije Universiteit Hospital, Amsterdam, The Netherlands

Iron-restrictive culture conditions induce the expression of several iron-repressible outer membrane proteins (IROMP) in *Helicobacter pylori*. To determine whether these IROMP are expressed *in vivo*, we tested if sera of patients with and without *H. pylori* infection contained antibodies against IROMP. Serum samples from 20 patients positive for *H. pylori* infection, as determined by standard culture and histology, all showed an immune response against the 77 kDa IROMP of *H. pylori* in an immunoblot assay. Antibody responses against the other IROMP were also found, but these occurred at lower frequencies. Serum samples from 18 patients negative for *H. pylori* infection did not show any immunoreactivity with IROMP. These results indicate that the IROMP of *H. pylori* are immunogenic and expressed *in vivo*. In a previous study we have shown that the 77, 50 and 48 kDa IROMP of *H. pylori* are capable of binding haem. We suggested the existence of a specific haem – iron uptake system in *H. pylori*. The present study shows that the 77 kDa haem-binding IROMP must contain some well-conserved antigenic epitope(s). This conservation may be the result of the function of this protein, that involves an essential interaction with haem compounds from the host. Because this protein is always expressed *in vivo*, haem binding could be essential for the pathogenesis of *H. pylori* infections. We conclude that the 77 kDa haem-binding IROMP of *H. pylori* could be an interesting vaccine candidate. Also, the protein may be of diagnostic value by using it in a serological detection assay for *H. pylori* infection.

P3
Variable structures and interactions of lipopolysaccharides from *Helicobacter pylori*

G. O. ASPINALL, C. M. LYNCH, A. S. MAINKAR and M. A. MONTEIRO

Department of Chemistry, York University, North York, Toronto, ON, Canada

Reports of antigenic variations between strains of *Helicobacter pylori* and of different roles played by lipopolysaccharides (LPS) in the disruption of the integrity of the gastric mucosa, and in the stimulation of pepsinogen leading to penetration of the gastric epithelium, prompted a detailed chemical examination of LPS from different strains.

LPS samples from phenol–water extraction of bacterial cells from individual strains were fractionated, and treated under the mildest possible conditions to liberate the polysaccharide components, and these in turn were submitted to controlled chemical or enzymic degradation.

The various products, LPS, polysaccharides, and derived oligosaccharides, were examined by chemical analyses in conjunction with mass spectrometry, and by NMR spectroscopy.

These studies established detailed structures for LPS from three strains[1,2] and structural analyses of LPS from five further strains are nearing completion. The most striking feature of all lipopolysaccharides is the presence of Lewis blood group antigens [Le^x, Le^y, and probably H-2] at the termini of the O antigen chains in mimicry of human cell surface antigens.

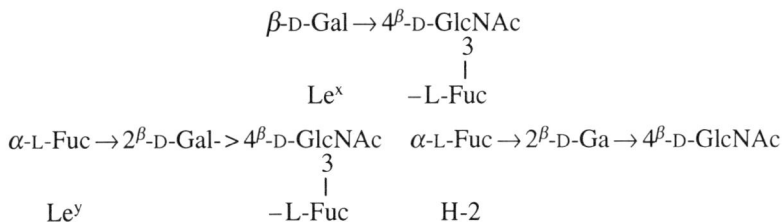

$$\beta\text{-}D\text{-}Gal \rightarrow 4^\beta\text{-}D\text{-}GlcNAc$$
$$3$$
$$|$$
$$Le^x \qquad -L\text{-}Fuc$$

$$\alpha\text{-}L\text{-}Fuc \rightarrow 2^\beta\text{-}D\text{-}Gal\text{-}>4^\beta\text{-}D\text{-}GlcNAc \qquad \alpha\text{-}L\text{-}Fuc \rightarrow 2^\beta\text{-}D\text{-}Ga \rightarrow 4^\beta\text{-}D\text{-}GlcNAc$$
$$3$$
$$|$$
$$Le^y \qquad\qquad -L\text{-}Fuc \qquad\qquad H\text{-}2$$

These epitopes terminate longer chains in which there are further variations in structure reflecting strain-to-strain diversity. In the type strain the Le^x epitope terminates in a repetitive sequence of Le^x units and extends the degree of mimicry. Other strains show considerable variations in the internal regions of the O antigen chains with partial or complete replacement of the Le^x structures with those *H. pylori* strains which induce the expression of anti-Lewis autoantibodies, and thus may have a pathogenic role in gastric atrophy, gastric cancer and MALT lymphoma.

1. Aspinall GO, Monteiro MA. Lipopolysaccharides of *Helicobacter pylori* strains P466 and MO19: structures of the O antigen and core oligosaccharide regions. Biochemistry. 1996;35:2498–504.
2. Aspinall GO, Monteiro MA, Pang H, Walsh EJ, Moran AP. Lipopolysaccharide of the *Helicobacter pylori* type strain NCTC 11637 (ATCC 43504): structure of the O antigen chain and core oligosaccharide regions. Biochemistry. 1996;35:2489–97.

Index